Neurotransmitter Interaction and Compartmentation

NATO ADVANCED STUDY INSTITUTES SERIES

A series of edited volumes comprising multifaceted studies of contemporary scientific issues by some of the best scientific minds in the world, assembled in cooperation with NATO Scientific Affairs Division.

Series A: Life Sciences

Recent Volumes in this Series

This series is published by an international board of publishers in conjunction with NATO Scientific Affairs Division

A	Life Sciences	Plenum Publishing Corporation
B	Physics	London and New York
C	Mathematical and Physical Sciences	D. Reidel Publishing Company Dordrecht, The Netherlands and Hingham, Massachusetts, USA
D	Behavioral and Social Sciences	Martinus Nijhoff Publishers The Hague, The Netherlands
E	Applied Sciences	

Neurotransmitter Interaction and Compartmentation

Edited by
H. F. Bradford
Imperial College of Science and Technology
London, United Kingdom

PLENUM PRESS • NEW YORK AND LONDON
Published in cooperation with NATO Scientific Affairs Division

Library of Congress Cataloging in Publication Data

NATO Advanced Study Institute on Compartmentation and Neurotransmitter Interaction (1981: Powys, Wales)
Neurotransmitter interaction and compartmentation.

(NATO advanced study institutes series. Series A, Life sciences; v. 48)
"Proceedings of a NATO Advanced Study Institute on Compartmentation and Neurotransmitter Interaction, held July 26–August 4, 1981, in Powys, Wales" — Verso t.p.
Bibliography: p.
Includes index.
1. Neurotransmitters — Congresses. 2. Compartmental analysis (Biology) — Congresses.
I. Bradford, H. F. (Henry F.) II. North Atlantic Treaty Organization. III. Title. IV. Series.
QP364.7.N38 1981   599.01'88   82-5311
ISBN 0-306-41015-X   AACR2

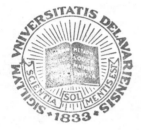

Proceedings of a NATO Advanced Study Institute on Compartmentation and Neurotransmitter Interaction, held July 26–August 4, 1981, in Powys, Wales

© 1982 Plenum Press, New York
A Division of Plenum Publishing Corporation
233 Spring Street, New York, N.Y. 10013

Printed in the United States of America

PREFACE

The NATO Advanced Study Institute held in the Hotel Metropole Llandrindod Wells, Powys, Wales from July 26th to August 4th 1981 provided an excellent platform for presentation and appraisal of our current knowledge of neurotransmitter systems. The proceedings comprise the present volume and these were arranged to allow study of the pathways and the interactions of specific transmitter systems, one with another, in the various sub-regions of the central nervous system. In addition several of the key factors involved in neurotransmitter release were highlighted. These include the structural and molecular organisation of the nerve terminal, its organelles (such as vesicles, neurotubules and synaptic densities) and the mechanisms involved in neurotransmitter release including the participation of calcium. The organisation of transmitter synthesis, storage and transport were discussed together with their linkage to other streams of metabolism, and the cellular compartmentation of these processes. In addition to the principal lectures given at the Institute, many participants presented short reports for discussion and these are all included in this volume.

The success of the Study Institute was due to the careful planning of the scientific programme to allow a smooth flow and integration of the topics included and this is reflected in the organisation of this book. The programme committee members were, R.Balázs (London), H.F.Bradford (London, Director), J.B.Clark (London), J.E. Cremer (MRC, Carshalton), J.S.Kelly (London), L.Lim (London), M.J. Neal (London) and P.J.Roberts (Southampton).

The major part of the funds were obtained from NATO, Scientific Affairs Division but additional financial support was generously provided by Beechams Pharmaceuticals Ltd., Imperial Chemical Industries Ltd. (Pharmaceuticals) Division, Glaxo Laboratories Ltd., and The Boots Pure Drug Co.Ltd.

I should also like to thank my secretary Mrs. Barbara Cowen for her energetic and thoughtful assistance in both the preparations for the Study Institute, and the preparation of these proceedings for publication which has greatly eased my task as Scientific Director of the ASI and editor of this book.

H.F.Bradford

London, October 1981.

CONTENTS

                    PART III: NEUROTRANSMITTERS AND
                             THEIR INTERACTIONS AT
                             THE CELLULAR LEVEL

PART IV: TRANSMITTER
METABOLISM

PART VII: NEUROTRANSMITTERS
IN THE RETINA

NERVE-TERMINAL ULTRASTRUCTURE: A ROLE FOR NEUROTUBULES?

E. George Gray, Phillip R. Gordon-Weeks and
Robert D. Burgoyne

National Institute for Medical Research
The Ridgeway, Mill Hill
London NW7 1AA

INTRODUCTION

The absence of microtubules (mt) from the presynaptic terminal
has long been regarded as dogma ever since the first EM studies of
synapses in the early fifties. They can be seen in the preterminal
axon (Fig. 1A) but they peter out as the axon expands into the bag.
Strangely enough the functional significance of "vanishing microtubules" has gone largely unheeded. Smith et al. (1970) and Smith
(1971), using conventional techniques, showed regular arrays of
synaptic vesicles (the ones away from the active zones) associated
with mt's in axons of the lamprey spinal cord and they postulated
a translocation mechanism. However the vesicle-clothed mt's were
never seen to run into the active zones of the synapse where the
vesicles form aggregates and so this last critical part of the
synaptic vesicle translocation remained unexplained. Also the
vesicle/mt association was only demonstrated in the lamprey, and
not in other groups of animals, another curious enigma.

Synapses teased in albumin

Some years later I was studying the effects of protein solutions
on synapse fixation (Gray, 1975). I teased frog brain in 10-20%
albumin for about 3 min. and then fixed with 4% unbuffered osmium
followed by aqueous uranyl staining. I was astonished to see,
emerging from the preterminal axon, mt's, clothed in synaptic
vesicles and running up to and in apparent contact with the dense
projections of the active zone (Fig. 1B, Figs. 2 and 3). Various
amphibian and mammalian synapses showed similar phenomena (Gray,
1975, 1976a,b, 1977, 1978a,b, Gray & Westrum, 1976a,b, 1977, Bird,
1976) and these papers should be consulted for details. In most

1

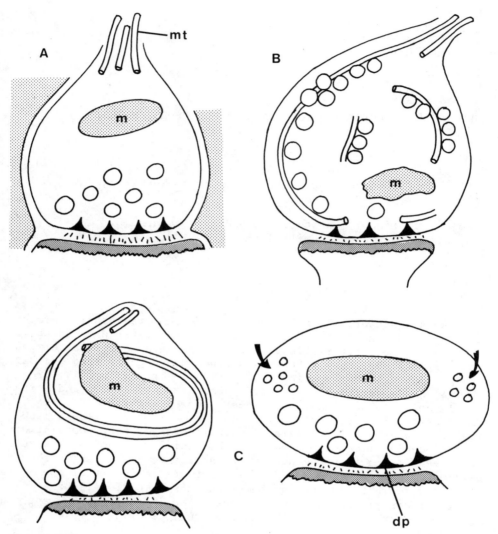

Fig. 1A. Synapse seen in section of whole brain using conventional
         fixation. Mt's do not enter the terminal.

    1B. Hypotonic albumin-treated synapse. Vesicle-clad mt's run
        down to the dense projections (dp).

    1C. Krebs-incubated synaptosome with coil or annulus of mt's
        (left). (Right) Two groups of mt profiles seen where the
        coil has been cut across (arrows).
        m, mitochondrion

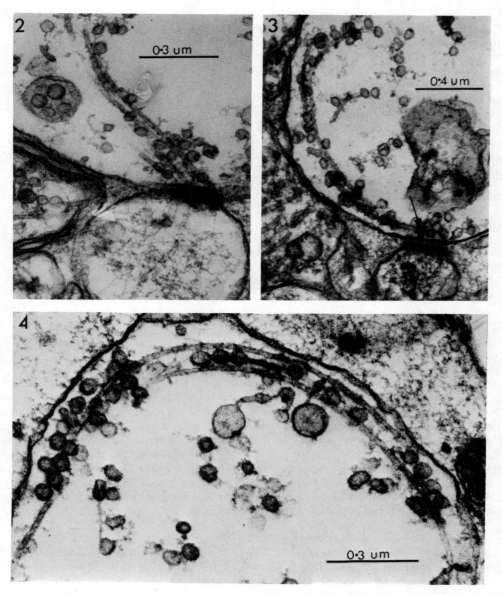

Fig. 2. Albumin-treated synapse, showing vesicle-clothed mt's focussed on the active zone.

Fig. 3. Mt apparently anchored to dense projection (arrow) (albumin).

Fig. 4. Circular bundles of mt's in albumin-treated synapse.

cases the initial immersing solution was hypotonic.

The implications of these observations are obvious. The dense projections could now be explained as the attachment points of the mt's along which the vesicles were translocated to discharge at the active zone. The mt's within the bag were assumed to be highly labile (see Discussion), hence their apparent termination at the end of the preterminal axon in conventionally fixed material.

These observations with their far-reaching implications have not yet been accepted in the literature. Some points to note are that in a teased albuminised brain fragment only about 1% of the endings show the mt/synaptic vesicle system. They are located in a zone about 20 µm into the fragment. It could be argued that only here are the diffusion gradients right to preserve the labile mt system. This could mean that most if not all synaptic bags in vivo possess the mt/synaptic vesicle system. Since the albumin used is hypotonic, the endings affected and showing the mt system, appear swollen 2-3 times of normal size (Figs. 1, 2 and 3). Also the vesicle-clad mt's often appear in section as arcs or semicircles (Fig. 4). Further observations relevant to this section are considered below.

Synaptosome mt's

This topic has been dealt with in detail by Gordon-Weeks et al. (1981). Briefly, Chan and Bunt (1978) and Hajós et al. (1979) showed annular bundles of mt's in incubated synaptosomes prepared from mammalian brain. The bundle lies parallel with the active zone and separated from it by clusters of synaptic vesicles (Fig. 1C). The mt bundle usually embraces a horse-shoe shaped mitochondrion and the mt's can often be shown to be continuous with those of the preterminal axon (just as are those in the albumin preparations - suggesting that they are the same things as the synaptosome ones under present consideration). Counts suggest that the mt bundle may in fact be one wound microtubule, in which case the term mt 'coil' is more appropriate and has been used below. EM's of mt coil-containing synaptosomes are shown cut in the different planes in Figs. 5 and 7.

Fractions of synaptosomes in Krebs show that up to 80% contain mt coils. The mt's of the coil are sensitive to cold, the numbers being reduced in 20 min. at 1°C to 17% without further reduction in numbers. Numbers recover to control values in 40 min. at 37°C. Colchicine disassembled these synaptosome mt's in a concentration-dependent manner. The IC_{50} of colchicine for disassembly was found to be 3 x 10^{-4}M. A small proportion (10%) of mt's were insensitive to colchicine. Reassembly was not attempted in the colchicine experiment for various reasons. Thus the synaptosome coil mt's respond to cold and colchicine in a manner typical of mt's in general. It is of special interest that the mt coil can reassemble (just as in

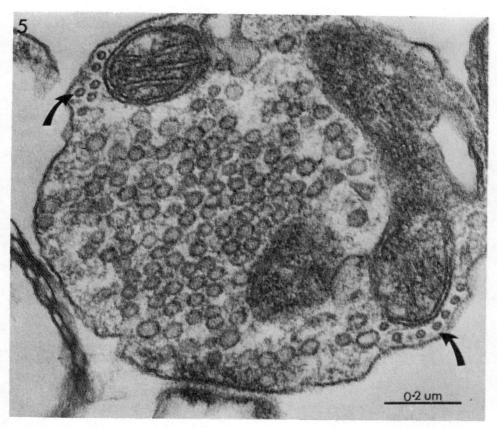

Fig. 5.   Krebs-incubated synaptosome – circular bundle of mt's cut
in t.s. (arrows).

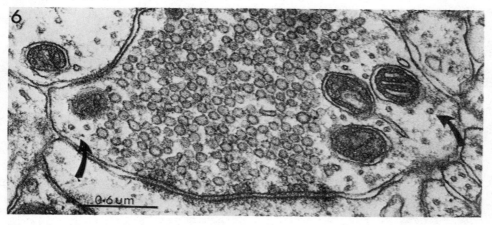

Fig. 6.   Synapse in brain perfused with EGTA in fixative.   Mt's in
in section (arrows).

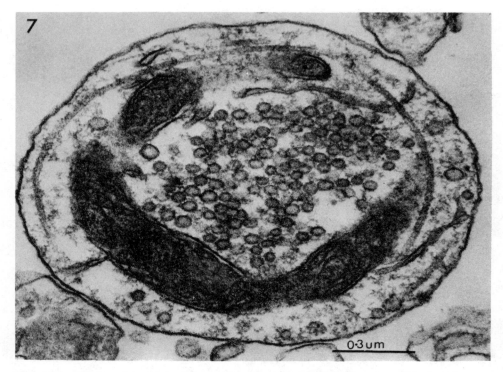

Fig. 7.   Krebs-incubated synaptosome showing the mt coil in the
plane of section.

platelets – Dustin, 1978) and one wonders whether there is a special
template present or whether the mt coil is indeed just one elongated
tubule, the coil shape simply imposed by the geometry of the globular
synaptosome. Homogenates of synaptosomes often show mt's (or one mt)
profiles apparently disorientated, whereas subsequent incubation
shows coils in the synaptosomes. The ability to form coils in this
way seems truly remarkable. There is evidence that mt coils are
already present in vivo in the intact brain (Fig. 6) but that the
high concentrations of extracellular Ca²⁺ makes them difficult to
fix (see below).

     Finally, a very interesting similarity can be seen between the
mt coil of the synaptosomes and that of the vertebrate platelet (and
nucleated red blood cell) (Dustin, 1978).   In the platelet the mt
coil embraces the one or more horse-shoe shaped mitochondria just as
is often seen in the synaptosome. In the platelet the mt coil plays
a role perhaps in both forming and maintaining its shape. Certainly
the synaptosome does not lose its shape when the mt coil is depolymerised with colchicine or cold (see above). The consideration of

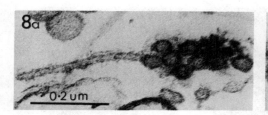
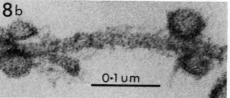

Fig. 8. Synaptic vesicle/mt complexes in the supernatant shown at
different magnifications (a and b).

the function of mt coils in synapses in vivo must await further
investigations.

The binding of synaptic vesicles to microtubules

     Smith et al. (1970) were the first to show, using conventional
fixation, the binding of synaptic vesicles to mt's away from but not
in the region of the active zone in lamprey spinal cord synapses.
Subsequently, Gray (1975, 1976b, 1978a) using 10-20% albumin and
various other hypotonic media (in some cases hypertonic media) showed
vesicle-clothed mt's. Bird (1976) was able to show a similar effect
in tissue culture synapses (but only after section of the preterminal
axons). The all-important question, of course, is whether or not the
synaptic vesicles are bound to the mt's in vivo indicating a translocation mechanism. Briefly, we (Gray & D.H. Jones, in preparation)
prepared separate fractions of mt's and synaptic vesicles, mixed them
together in vitro and fixed the fraction by suspension fixation. In
spite of numerous attempts, we were unable to show positive binding.
Best results were obtained when mt's were prepared by the Shelanski
et al. (1973) method. The synaptic vesicles and mt's remained
distinguishable in sections, and occasionally a few were seen bound
to an mt but usually the mt seemed absent or depolymerised where it
was in contact with the vesicle. It was as if some factor (Ca^{2+}?)
had leaked from the fixed vesicle and depolymerised the adjacent mt.
Albumin-treated synapses or motor end-plates (Gray, 1975, 1976b,
1978a) often showed a similar phenomenon, i.e. an mt passing into a
string of vesicles apparently disappearing and then reappearing at the
other end. This phenomenon was seen too often to be the result of the
mt passing out and back in the place of section. Also tilting and
cutting synaptic vesicle strings in cross section confirmed this view.

     A consistent observation was that the synaptic vesicle population
was heterogeneous, i.e. most vesicles in the fraction were 4-500 Å but
some were larger - 800-1000 Å or more. The size of the smaller ones
indicates that they are probably synaptic vesicles. Interestingly,
only these smaller ones were seen bound to mt's. Thus in future
experiments one can use the larger vesicles as controls: binding of

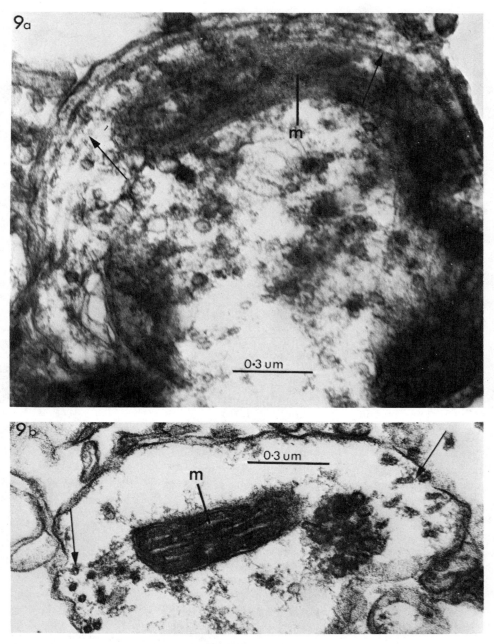

Fig. 9. <u>Xenopus</u> synaptosome. Arrows show the mt coils cut in both planes (a and b).   m, mitochondrion

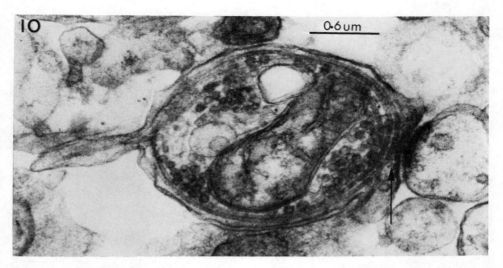

Fig. 10. Synaptosome (with spine attachment) showing mt coil passing through the active zone (arrow).

these would, of course, indicate a non-specific effect. Also in this experiment we used mt's artificially polymerised by the Shelanski et al.(1973) method. Such mt's lack certain proteins which could obscure the results of the experiment.

For this reason we used native brain mt's (Kirkpatrick et al., 1970) but such fractions were contaminated with coated vesicles and various tissue fragments and when added to the vesicle fraction the mt's disintegrated into debris. Thus mixing mt's with synaptic vesicles to study binding is far from straightforward both in method-ology and interpretation.

Our frustrations led us to retrace our path and we are studying brain homogenates with the EM using various media, to try and obtain an insight into the way the brain elements fragment under different conditions. Our main finding so far is that brain homogenised in RAB (with EGTA, etc.) (see Jones, Gray and Barron, 1980) and made hypertonic with hexalene glycol (500 mM) shows well-preserved mt's in the supernatant and more exciting they frequently have vesicles of the size of synaptic vesicles bound to them (Fig. 8). At this stage we cannot tell whether the vesicles have become specifically bound to the mt's when in the supernatant or whether the mt/synaptic vesicle complex (in vivo or in vitro) is already present in the synapse and comes out as a fragment when the presynaptic bag is ruptured during homogenisation. Of obvious importance is that we now know what is a suitable medium for the maintenance of an mt/synaptic vesicle complex for future experiments. If a similar solution is made hypotonic or

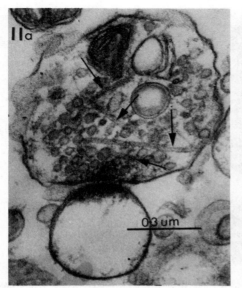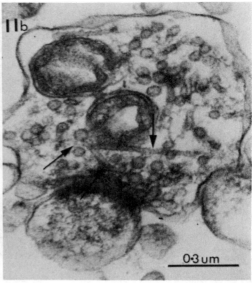

Fig. 11a and b. Synaptosomes prepared in hypertonic medium showing mt coils (arrows) extending down to the active zone.

if brain is homogenized in Krebs mt/synaptic vesicle complexes are not preserved in the supernatant and would therefore be unsuitable for fractionation studies (Gray and Jones, in preparation).

Amphibian synaptosome microtubules

The study of synaptosomes has, almost exclusively, been made on fractions prepared from the vertebrate brain, especially the rat (Gray and Whittaker, 1962). We used a very small hand homogenizer on an amphibian brain, Xenopus. The brain was removed and homogenized and incubated in Ringer at room temperature followed by aldehyde suspension fixation. EM revealed a small proportion of synaptosomes with the characteristic annular bundles of mt's (Fig. 9) usually with an associated horse-shoe mitochondrion. Of course, brains of other classes of vertebrates need examination, but this study suggests that the mt annulus is a universal feature of vertebrate brains, with all that this implies (see Discussion). We hope soon to investigate invertebrate synaptosomes.

Conclusions

In spite of thirty years intensive study of the synapse with the EM, we are still far from being able to deduce its in vivo structure (see Gordon-Weeks et al., 1981). In particular four main items need elucidating, the synaptic vesicles, mt's, dense projections and mitochondria.

How do the synaptic vesicles become clustered at the active zone? Obviously they would be strategically situated for transmitter release. We cannot be sure that the clustering is not a preparation artifact, however. Most methods show clustering, but some do not (KmnO₄ fixation - Gray, 1959, or freeze-substitution - Hirokawa and Kirino, 1980). Translocation along microtubules (Gray, 1975) seems a likely candidate, but mt/synaptic vesicle associations can (with the exception of Smith et al., 1970 - see above) only be demonstrated by using hypotonic albumin and certain other solutions (see above) or incubating brain slices in certain hypotonic media (Jones et al., 1980). In our coils of mt's (Gordon-Weeks et al., 1981) seen in synaptosomes, synaptic vesicles are virtually never found in contact with the mt of the coil.

Which brings us on to the nature of the dense projections. The mt's of the coil in the Krebs incubated synaptosomes never seem to run down to the dense projections. The plane of the coil nearly always lies parallel with the active zone, from which it is separated by the synaptic vesicles. Thus using this sort of preparation, two factors, namely lack of mt/synaptic vesicle association and absence of contact between mt and presynaptic membrane (to ensure completion of vesicle translocation) militate against an in vivo mt translocation system. On the other hand, using a high K medium (Jones et al., 1980) rings (possibly associated with synaptic vesicles) can be seen (Fig. 10) running through the active zone and in media made hypertonic with hexalene glycol (590 mM) mt rings can commonly be seen in synaptosomes with mt's running down the active zone (Fig. 11) although no synaptic vesicles contact these mt's - an essential feature of the mt translocation theory, of course.

The dense projections (Gray, 1963) are one of the most constant features to be seen in the synapse irrespective of the preparative technique used. In the albumin-type preparations the mt's are clearly in contact with the dense projections, which would appear ideal anchoring structures on the presynaptic membrane (especially if the synaptic vesicles are being translocated along the mt's). On the other hand the medium of albumin and related techniques is hypotonic and the presynaptic bag swells 2-3 times normal volume. Extensive arcs or circular profiles (vesicle-clad) mt's appear in the cytoplasm (Fig. 1B, 2-4). Probably they are derived from disrupted mt coils during the swelling. If the dense projections are very sticky the mt's could artifactually attach to them. If the dense projections are not in vivo attachment points of mt's, we are stuck with a raison d'etre for them.

The presynaptic mt coils and their disassembly and reassembly with temperature and colchicine have been described in detail elsewhere (Gordon-Weeks et al., 1981). There is no doubt of the high lability of presynaptic mt's. Attempts to demonstrate mt coils as a general presynaptic feature in whole brain have been made by Chan and

Bunt (1978) and Gordon-Weeks et al. (1981) using perfusion with
fixative plus EGTA (Fig. 6). The latter have pointed out the high
extracellular concentration of Ca^{2+} (3 orders of magnitude higher than
inside, Llinás and Heuser, 1977), to which, of course, mt's are highly
labile. Results look encouraging, perhaps all terminal synapses
contain an mt coil, remarkable in that they may have been overlooked
for 30 years!

Summary

Do microtubules bind synaptic vesicles as part of a mechanism
of vesicle translocation? Certainly under certain experimental
conditions of pretreatment before fixation they do. Whether binding
takes place as an in vivo phenomenon is still very much an open
question. Do mt's (probably attached to the dense projections)
in vivo reach the presynaptic membrane for vesicle translocation or
remain suspended as a coil above the synaptic vesicles? Thus the role
of presynaptic mt's remains an enigma. Probably the only safe state-
ment that can be made is that the presynaptic bag contains tubulin,
presumably at least in part, polymerised.

REFERENCES

Chan, K.Y., and Bunt, A.H., 1978, An association between mitochondria
        and microtubules in synaptosomes and axon terminals in cerebral
        cortex, J. Neurocytol. 7: 137.
Dustin, P., 1978, "Microtubules", Springer, Berlin.
Gordon-Weeks, P.R., Burgoyne, R.D., and Gray, E.G., 1981, Presynaptic
        microtubules: organisation and assembly/disassembly,
        Neuroscience (in press).
Gray, E.G., 1959, Axosomatic and axodendritic synapses of the cerebral
        cortex: an electron microscope study, J. Anat. Lond., 93: 420.
Gray, E.G., 1963, Electron microscopy of presynaptic organelles of the
        spinal cord. J. Anat. Lond., 97:101.
Gray, E.G., 1975, Presynaptic microtubules and their association with
        synaptic vesicles, Proc. Roy. Soc. B., 190:369.
Gray, E.G., 1976a, Microtubules in synapses of the retina,
        J. Neurocytol., 5: 361.
Gray, E.G., 1976b, Problems of understanding the substructure of
        synapses, Prog. Brain Res., 45: 207.
Gray, E.G., 1977, Presynaptic microtubules, agranular reticulum and
        synaptic vesicles, in: "Synapses," G.A. Cottrell and
        P.N.R. Usherwood, eds., Blackie, Glasgow.
Gray, E.G., 1978a, Synaptic vesicles and microtubules in frog motor
        end-plates, Proc. Roy. Soc. B., 203: 219.
Gray, E.G., 1978b, Synaptic ultrastructure, in: "Neurotransmitter
        systems and their disorders," N.J. Legg, ed., Academic Press,
        London.

Gray, E.G., Jones, D.H., and Barron, J., 1979, Aggregations of synaptic vesicles on the exposed inner membrane of presynaptic mitochondria in brain, J. Neurocytol., 8: 675.

Gray, E.G., Jones, D.H., and Barron, J., 1980, Cold stable microtubules in brain studied in fractions and slices, J. Neurocytol., 9: 493.

Gray, E.G., and Westrum, L.E., 1976a, Microtubules associated with nuclear pore complexes and coated pits in the CNS, Cell & Tissue Res., 168: 445.

Gray, E.G., and Westrum, L.E., 1976b, Microtubules and membrane specializations, Brain Res., 105: 547.

Gray, E.G., and Westrum, L.E., 1977, Microtubules associated with postsynaptic thickenings, J. Neurocytol., 6: 505.

Gray, E.G., and Whittaker, V.P., 1962, The isolation of nerve endings from brain: an electron microscope study of cell fragments derived by homogenization and centrifugation, J. Anat. Lond., 96: 79.

Hajós, F., Csillag, A., and Kálmán, M., 1979, The morphology of microtubules in incubated synaptosomes. Effect of low temperature and vinblastine, Exp. Brain Res., 35: 387.

Hirokawa, N., and Kirino, T., 1980, An ultrastructural study of nerve and glial cells by freeze-substitution, J. Neurocytol., 9: 243.

Jones, D.H., Gray, E.G., and Barron, J., 1980, Cold stable microtubules in brain studied in fractions and slices, J. Neurocytol., 9: 493.

Kirkpatrick, J.B., Hyams, L., Thomas, V.L., and Harley, P.M., 1970, Purification of intact microtubules from brain, J. Cell Biol., 47: 384.

Llinás, R.R., and Heuser, J.E., 1977, Depolarization-release coupling systems in neurons, Neurosci. Res. Prog., 15: 557.

Shelanski, M.L., Gaskin, F., and Cantor, C.R., 1973, Microtubule assembly in the absence of added nucleotides, Proc. Nat. Acad. Sci. (USA), 70: 765.

Smith, D.S., 1971, On the significance of cross-bridges between microtubules and synaptic vesicles, Phil. Trans. B., 261: 395.

Smith, D.S., Järlfors, U., and Beránek, R., 1970, The organisation of synaptic axoplasm in the lamprey (Petromyzon Marinus) central nervous system, J. Cell Biol., 46: 199.

PREPARATION OF SYNAPTIC JUNCTIONAL STRUCTURES BY PHASE PARTITIONING

IN THE PRESENCE OF n-OCTYL-GLUCOSIDE

James W. Gurd, Phillip R. Gordon-Weeks and
W. Howard Evans

National Institute for Medical Research
The Ridgeway, Mill Hill
London NW7 1AA

We have developed a simple and rapid method for the preparation
of post-synaptic densities (PSD's) and synaptic junctional complexes
from mammalian brain. By morphological criteria the PSD preparation
is pure, being essentially free of organised membrane and other
contaminants and the yield is high (70 μg protein/g wet weight
starting material). The method involves the use of the relatively
mild neutral detergent, n-octyl-glucoside (OG) in conjunction with
phase partitioning.

Synaptic plasma membranes were prepared according to Cotman and
Taylor (1972) and resuspended in water (8-12 mgm/ml). This suspension
(500 μl) was added to a mixture containing 500 μl of 0.5M $NaHCO_3$,
pH 9.6, 200 μl of OG (25% w/v), 1.25g of 20% w/v, polyethylene glycol
(PEG) and 1.45g of 20% (w/v) dextran T500 all at 4°C and made up to
5g by adding water. The mixture was then rapidly homogenised with
5 to 6 strokes of a tight fitting Dounce homogeniser and immediately
centrifuged at $2,250g_{av}$ for 7.5 min. to separate the PEG and dextran
phases. Material banding at the interface was removed for morphological and biochemical analysis.

The type of junctional preparation obtained and the extent of
contamination by extra-junctional membranes depended critically upon
the concentration of OG. When 0.5% OG was used, the interface
material was enriched in junctional structures relative to the parent
membrane fraction but contained large amounts of extra-junctional
membranes. With 0.75% OG, the amount of contamination was greatly
reduced and with 1% OG a morphologically pure PSD preparation was
obtained. Increasing the concentration of OG also produced a
progressive decrease in the presence of junctional membrane. With
0.5% OG, 85% of the junctional structures present had both pre- and

post-synaptic membranes (synaptic junctions), many (56.5%) with
intact pre-synaptic dense projections. With 0.75% OG, 42% of the
structures were synaptic junctions and 58% were PSD's, many of which
still retained post-synaptic membranes. With 1% OG a morphologically
pure PSD preparation was obtained.

Electrophoretic analysis of the isolated fractions demonstrated
that the enrichment of post-synaptic structures with increasing
detergent concentrations was associated with an increase in the
relative amount of the PSD-specific protein (M_r: 51K). All fractions,
however, showed a complex protein composition. Staining of gels with
[125]I-Concanavalin A revealed that the glycoprotein content of the
isolated PSD fraction was simple and consisted of 2 major components
of apparent M_r of 130K and 180K, corresponding to previously identified synapse-specific glycoproteins (Gurd, 1981).

REFERENCES

Cotman, C.W., and Taylor, D., 1972, Isolation and structural studies
        on synaptic complexes from rat brain, J. Cell Biol. 55: 696.
Gurd, J.W., 1981, Subcellular distribution and partial characteriza-
        tion of the three major classes of Concanavalin A receptors
        associated with rat brain synaptic junctions, Can. J. Biochem.
        58: 941.

MOLECULAR COMPOSITION OF SYNAPTIC JUNCTIONS AND POST-SYNAPTIC DENSITIES: A FUNCTIONAL PERSPECTIVE

C. W. Cotman, E. E. Mena and M. Nieto Sampedro

Department of Psychobiology
University of California, Irvine, California   92717

The development of subcellular methods to isolate central nervous system synapses and their subcomponents has made it possible to carry out detailed chemical analysis and to examine the capacities of the constituent molecules. The data gathered on the molecular structure and composition of synapses are making it possible to gain new insights into synapse development, maintenance and function. In this chapter we will first briefly review the molecular composition of isolated synaptic junctions and postsynaptic density fractions. We will then focus on the properties of synapse glycoproteins and receptor sites for excitatory neurotransmitters. Finally, in the last section we will describe the properties of a synapse-specific antibody which we have used as a probe for monitoring both the development of postsynaptic densities and their turnover following partial denervation. Several reviews on the general properties of synapse macromolecules have appeared (Cotman and Kelly, 1980; Mahler, 1977; Matus, 1981).

PREPARATION AND CHARACTERISTICS OF SYNAPTIC SUBFRACTIONS

When synaptic plasma membranes (SPMs) are treated with mild ionic or nonionic detergents, most extrajunctional membrane is solubilized so that synaptic junctions (SJs) or postsynaptic densities (PSDs) can be purified (Fig. 1). A number of procedures now exist for the isolation of SPM fractions. The main problem in preparing SPMs is their contamination by mitochondrial membranes of similar buoyant densities. These mitochondrial membranes will then contaminate SJ and PSD fractions if not removed prior to detergent treatment. Our procedure involves the incubation of crude synaptosomal-mitochondrial fractions with iodonitrotetra-

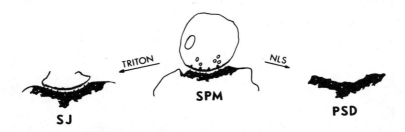

Figure 1. Preparation of synaptic junctions and postsynaptic densities. Treatment of synaptic plasma membranes with Triton X-100 solubilizes the extrajunctional membrane and leaves the synaptic junction. Treatment with the stronger detergent, N-lauroyl sarcosinate, leaves the postsynaptic density (from Kelly and Cotman, 1977).

zolium violet (INT) and succinate (Cotman and Taylor, 1972; Davis and Bloom, 1973). Mitochondrial succinate dehydrogenase creates a formazan deposit inside the mitochondria which increases mito-chondrial buoyant density. Thus, they can be separated from SPMs by density gradient centrifugation. In addition, INT treatment appears to stabilize the junction and preserve some of its consti-tuents.

SJ fractions are obtained by treatment of SPMs with Triton X-100 or a related detergent (Cotman and Taylor, 1972; Davis and Bloom, 1973; Cohen et al., 1976) or sodium deoxycholate (Matus and Walters, 1975), followed by centrifugation of the mixture of solubilized and particulate material on a density gradient. Our rat SJ fraction consists of 15-20% intact synaptic junctions which contain both pre- and postsynaptic membranes, and 55% postsynaptic specializations from which the presynaptic membrane has been lost. The remaining material consists of membrane fragments, micro-tubules and amorphous material (Churchill et al., 1976). Other procedures, even though varying in detail, also produce a fraction highly enriched in synaptic junctions. SJ fractions can be prepared from a variety of species with similar results (Rostas et al., 1979; Nieto Sampedro, M., Bussineau, C. M. and Cotman, C. W., submitted).

SPMs or SJs can be subfractionated to produce highly pure PSD fractions. Treatment of SPMs with sodium N-lauroyl sarco-sinate (NLS) solubilizes nearly all membranes while leaving PSD structures intact (Cotman et al., 1974). PSDs have a high bouyant density and can be isolated easily from other structures by centrifugation. The resulting fraction, as judged by quantitative electron microscopy, consists of about 80-85% PSDs. Isolated PSDs

retain many of the staining properties and certain of the
enzymatic properties characteristic of PSDs in intact tissue. The
yield is about 200 ug of PSDs/g brain wet weight. It would appear
that the PSD fraction represents about a 10^4-fold enrichment in
these structures from the total brain homogenate, assuming a nearly
quantitative recovery. Other methods now exist which produce somewhat similar fractions (Matus and Walters, 1977; Cohen et al.,
1977). Morphologically these two preparations look similar in the
electron microscope. However, the protein composition of PSD
prepared by using NLS is simpler. NLS is a stronger detergent and,
presumably, removes more PSD associated proteins than do milder
detergents, such as Triton X-100 or deoxycholate.

GENERAL COMPOSITION

    Isolated synaptic junctions consist primarily of protein and
a small amount of lipid and carbohydrate (Churchill et al., 1976).
The carbohydrate composition resembles that of the parent SPM
fraction, except that there is significantly less N-acetyl-
neuraminic acid and considerably more glucose. The overall amino
acid composition of protein in SPM, SJ and PSD fractions is
similar.

    As determined by polyacrylamide gel eletrophoresis, SJ and
PSD fractions contain polypeptides which range in apparent
molecular weight from 8,000 to 300,000 (Banker et al., 1974; Kelly
and Cotman, 1977). The overall protein pattern in SJs is somewhat
similar to that of SPMs, but the relative proportions of many
proteins are different in these two fractions.

    PSDs prepared by our procedure contain few major proteins.
The major component is a protein of 52,000 molecular weight that
represents more than 45% of the total Coomassie blue-staining
material in this fraction (Banker et al., 1974; Kelly and Cotman,
1977). There are also significant quantities of proteins in the
PSD fraction with molecular weights of 180,000, 86,000, 55,000,
45,000, 28,000 and 26,000, but most protein bands observed in SPMs
and SJs are absent from PSDs (Kelly and Cotman, 1977).

    In general, reports from different laboratories agree on the
major protein constituents of SJ and PSD fractions as resolved by
sodium dodecyl sulfate (SDS) polyacrylamide gel electrophoresis
(see Banker et al., 1974; Therien and Mushynski, 1976; Walters
and Matus, 1975; Cohen et al., 1976; Blomberg et al., 1977; Wang
and Mahler, 1976; Kelly and Cotman, 1977, 1978; Rostas et al.,
1979; Feit et al., 1977). Several of these proteins have now
been identified (Table 1).

    The major polypeptides of SJs and PSDs are not species
specific. They are present in similar fractions isolated from all

Table 1.   Identified proteins that are components of junctional fractions.

	MW x 10^{-3}	Reference
High mol. wt. microtubulin		
associated protein	300	Matus, 1981
Myosin	220	Beach et al., 1981
52K PSD protein	52	Kelly and Cotman, 1978
Actin	46	" "
		Bloomberg, et al., 1977
Tubulin	54	Kelly and Cotman, 1978
		Walters and Matus, 1975
		Westrum and Gray, 1977
Calmodulin	18	Grab et al., 1979
High affinity binding		
sites: GABA	unknown	Matus et al., 1980
Glutamate	unknown	Foster et al., 1981a
Aspartate	unknown	" "
Kainic acid	unknown	Foster et al., 1981b
Con A binding glyco-		
proteins: I	160	Rostas et al., 1979
II	123	" "
III	110	" "
IV	95	" "

vertebrate species examined from shark to man (Nieto Sampedro, M., Bussineau, C. M. and Cotman, C. W., submitted).   In addition, there is great similarity in the overall polypeptide composition of SJ fractions isolated from bovine brain regions which consist primarily of one class of postsynaptic neuron.   The CA1 field of the hippocampal formation, for example, consists of more than 90% pyramidal neurons and SJs isolated from this area have gel patterns nearly the same as those from other brain areas or whole brain. However, two-dimensional electrophoresis shows that minor proteins are enriched in some brain regions (Rostas et al., 1979). Interestingly, PSDs isolated from brainstem and cerebellum contained greatly diminished amounts of the major PSD polypeptide (Carlin et et al., 1980).

SYNAPSE GLYCOPROTEINS

As shown in Table 1, isolated synaptic junctions contain several glycoproteins.   The most studied are those characterized by their affinity for the lectin Concanavalin A.   These glyco-proteins, which have apparent molecular weights of 160,000, 123,000, 110,000 and 95,000 have been designated Con A-I, -II, -III, and -IV, respectively (Rostas et al., 1979).   Glycoproteins of identical size are present in SJs prepared from the brains of all vertebrates from bony fish to man, but not in shark (Rostas et al., 1979; Nieto Sampedro, M., Bussineau, C. M. and Cotman, C. W., submitted). Furthermore, little difference could be found in the relative amounts of these glycoproteins in SJs prepared from several different regions of the bovine brain (Rostas et al., 1979). Cytochemical studies with rat subcellular fractions have shown that these glycoproteins are localized within the synaptic cleft on the external surface of the postsynaptic plasma membrane (Kelly et al., 1976; Fig. 2). They are barely detectable in the synaptic plasma membranes from which the SJs originate (Rostas et al., 1979) and are found enriched only in those sub-cellular fractions that contain a high percentage of morphologically identifiable synaptic junctions (Mena et al., 1981). Thus, these glycoproteins appear to be synapse specific.

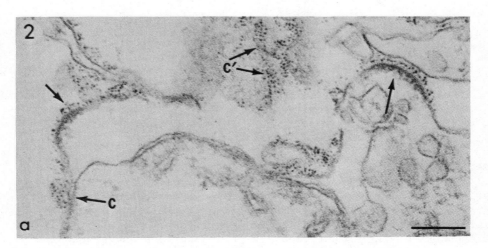

Figure 2. Ferritin-Con A conjugate binding to dendritic membranes. Junctional regions show numerous linear binding sites for Con A. Extrajunctional binding sites tend to be clustered (arrows C and C') probably due to the greater fluidity of extra-junctional Con A receptors (from Kelly and Cotman, 1976).

We have now isolated these Con A-positive glycoproteins from SJs by a modification of published procedures for affinity chromatography (March et al., 1974; Gurd, 1979) (Fig. 3). The total glycoprotein fraction isolated represents about 1.5-2% of the total 280 nm absorbing material applied to the column. Polyacrylamide gel electrophoresis in the presence of SDS showed that the major Con A-binding polypeptides had molecular weights of 160,000, 110,000 and 95,000 (Mena and Cotman, submitted). The rank order of Con A binding sites contained by these glycoproteins

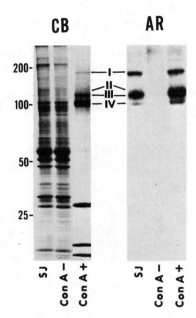

Figure 3. Purification of the Con A binding glycoproteins of the synaptic junction. The glycoproteins were isolated by affinity chromatography from solubilized synaptic junctions. Forty five micrograms of the solubilized synaptic junctions and Con A negative sample (Con A-), and 5 μg of the Con A positive material (Con A+) were subjected to polyacrylamide gel electrophoresis and stained with Coomassie blue (CB). The gels were incubated with ^{125}I-Con A and autoradiographed (AR) (from Mena, E. E. and Cotman, C. W., submitted).

is Con A-III>Con A-IV>Con A-I>Con A-II. This order is identical to that determined in SJs, indicating that the glycoprotein fraction isolated is representative of their distribution in the intact SJ (Rostas et al., 1979; Mena et al., 1981).

The three major Coomassie blue-staining glycoproteins and the area of the gel that corresponds to Con A-II were removed and ^{125}I tryptic peptide maps were prepared according to Elder et al., (1977). Con A-I, -II and -III contained a large percentage of identical patterns of radioactive peptides (Fig. 4). Approximately 50% of the peptides were common to all three glycoproteins as shown by comigration of peptides in a mixture of equivalent amounts of radioactivity of Con A-I and Con A-III (Fig. 4). Each of these glycoproteins also contained several unique radioactive peptides and, in addition, some of the peptides were common to only two of the three glycoproteins (Fig. 4). The peptide map of Con A-IV contained no pattern of peptides in common with Con A-I, -II and -III.

Thus, a large percentage of the primary structure of Con A-I, -II and -III must be identical, whereas Con A-IV is unrelated to the other three glycoproteins. The heterogenity in both apparent molecular weight and Con A binding capacity could be due to differences in length of the polypeptide chain or differences in additional moieties covalently attached to the protein, such as carbohydrate groups. Many examples of homologous proteins arising through gene duplication have been reported (Doolittle, 1981; Raftery et al., 1980). Usually these newly created proteins retain many of the functional features of the original protein. Since these glycoproteins are located in the same morphological structure, the SJ, they may have a role in some synaptic function that is fine-tuned by the unique portions of these molecules. Alternatively, these glycoproteins may differ only in carbo-hydrate sequence, composition, or the points of attachment of the carbohydrate to the protein. In this case, the specificity of each glycoprotein would be determined only by the carbohydrate structure. If these glycoproteins were recognition sites for lectin-like adhesive interactions at synapses, their carbohydrate diversity would allow a large variety of recognition sites without alteration of the polypeptide sequence. This possibility is supported by the finding that the carbohydrate moieties are not identical since these glycoproteins are retained to different degrees on Con A-Sepharose and fucose binding protein-Sepharose columns (Gurd, 1979).

RECEPTORS FOR PUTATIVE EXCITATORY TRANSMITTERS

If isolated synapses are to be useful for the study of synaptic function, they should contain receptors for major trans-mitters. The acidic amino acids, glutamate and aspartate, are at present the leading transmitter candidates at excitatory synapses in the CNS. In the mammalian CNS, previous studies with tritiated glutamate and aspartate have revealed a population of high affinity membrane binding sites which have characteristics similar to those of the physiological receptors for these amino acids

Figure 4. ^{125}I tryptic peptide maps of the Con A-binding glycoproteins of the synaptic junction. The bands on the gel that
corresponded to the Con A-positive glycoproteins were removed and
the peptide maps prepared. The radioactive peptides were
separated by electrophoresis in the X-axis and chromatographed in
the Y-axis. 1, Con A-I; 2, Con A-II; 3, Con A-III; 4, Con A-IV;
5, a mixture of Con A-I and -III; 6, peptides that Con A-I, -II,
and -III have in common (from Mena and Cotman, submitted).

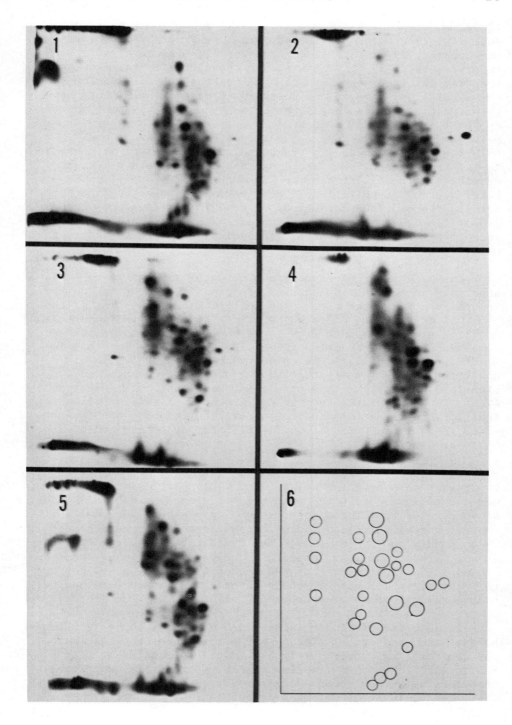

(Roberts, 1974; Michaelis et al., 1974; Fiszer de Plazas and De Robertis, 1976; De Robertis and Fiszer de Plazas, 1976; Foster and Roberts, 1978; Baudry and Lynch, 1979; Biziere et al., 1980; Roberts et al., 1980). However, in these studies the membrane preparations used were heterogenous and the subcellular locus of the binding was unknown. Electrophysiological experiments have shown that glutamate and aspartate receptors are present on many types of neurons, but such studies are unable to distinguish between junctional and extrajunctional receptors. In the invertebrate neuromuscular junction, where glutamate is known to be the transmitter, the junctional membrane possesses a high density of glutamate receptors (Takeuchi and Takeuchi, 1964; Usherwood and Machili, 1968), although extra-junctional receptors are also found (Takeuchi and Onedera, 1975; Onedera and Takeuchi, 1980). In order to study the characteristics of acidic amino acid receptors relevant to synaptic transmission, it is necessary to identify the characteristics of junctional receptors.

The values for the specific binding of glutamate and aspartate in several subcellular fractions are shown in Table 2. In all fractions, the mean values of glutamate were greater than those of aspartate. There was a trend towards an increase in the specific binding of both ligands as the purity of synaptic components in each fraction increased (i.e., whole particulate> P_2>SPM). Purified SJs were found to possess high levels of specific binding for aspartate and glutamate, approximately nine-fold greater than the values in whole particulate membranes (Table 2). Calculation of the total number of binding sites for individual preparations indicated that the recovery of binding sites in SJs from SPMs was $84.5 \pm 9.3\%$ for aspartate and $83.2 \pm 5.3\%$ for glutamate.

The nine-fold enrichment of both glutamate and aspartate binding in this fraction relative to whole particulate membranes, was due to an increase in the number of binding sites, since the K_D values for the binding of the two ligands were the same as those reported for crude synaptic membranes (Foster and Roberts, 1978; Baudry and Lynch, 1979; Sharif and Roberts, 1980; Roberts et al., 1980), and in P_2 and SPM fractions (unpublished observations). This indicates that the increase in binding was not due to a change in affinity of the binding site, caused for example, by the removal of an endogenous inhibitor.

The majority of binding sites in SPMs appear to be junctional, because the recovery of binding sites in SJs for both glutamate and aspartate is approximately 80%. This is consistent with findings in locust and crayfish muscle, where extra-junctional receptors have been found to exist only in low concentrations (Cull-Candy, 1978; Onedera and Takeuchi, 1980). Specific glutamate and aspartate binding sites were found in microsomal and

Table 2. Distribution of L-glutamate and L-aspartate binding
sites in various subcellular fractions. The fractions were
prepared and assayed as described by Foster et al., 1981a. The
binding in each fraction relative to whole particulate material
is also presented (from Foster et al., 1981a).

	Aspartate		Glutamate	
	Specific Binding pmol/mg protein	Relative to WP	Specific Binding pmol/mg protein	Relative to WP
WP	0.648 ± 0.197	1	1.202 ± 0.358	1
P_2	0.765 ± 0.175	1.18	1.539 ± 0.424	1.28
P_3	1.080 ± 0.520	1.67	1.808 ± 0.758	1.50
SPM	0.954 ± 0.120	1.74	2.860 ± 0.468	2.34
SJ	5.834 ± 1.685	9.00	11.638 ± 1.652	9.68

"light" SPM fractions, which may indicate the presence of extra-
junctional receptors. However, SJ-like membranes can be isolated
from these fractions and their polypeptide composition is
indistinguishable from that of SJs, indicating that some of the
glutamate and aspartate binding in microsomes and "light" SPMs may
be junctionally related (Mena, et al., 1981). Thus, it is not
possible in these experiments to accurately assess the numbers of
extra-junctional receptors. Despite the high levels of specific
binding for glutamate and aspartate observed in SJs, it is clear
that binding sites are also present on other subcellular particles
from the small enrichment of L-glutamate and L-aspartate binding
obtained in P_2 and SPM fractions (compared to whole particulate
membranes). This suggests that in order to study binding sites
for glutamate and asparate that are relevant to synaptic
processes, it is necessary to use a purified synaptic membrane
fraction.

     At least some of the glutamate receptors appear physiologically
relevant. Kinetic analyses of the inhibition of L-glutamate binding
by the α-amino-ω-phosphonic acid derivatives of propionic (APP),
butyric (APB) and valeric (APV) acids demonstrated that these homologues competed with different affinities for the same L-glutamate
binding site, which represented about 80% of the total L-glutamate
bound. The K_I values calculated for inhibition of L-glutamate
binding at this site were 18 μM (APB), 39 μM (APV) and 1 mM (APP);
the L-isomer of APB was 15-fold more potent than the D-form (K_I
values 5 μM and 75 μM, respectively)(Fagg, G. E., Foster, A. C., Mena,
E. E. and Cotman, C. W., submitted). These K_I values were in close
agreement with those determined electrophysiologically for the
antagonism of perforant path-evoked field potentials in the outer
molecular layer of the rat dentate gyrus in vitro (Koerner and
Cotman, 1981).

We have also examined the subcellular distribution of kainic acid binding sites. Lesions caused by injections of kainic acid (KA) into the rat striatum and hippocampus cause patterns of damage similar to those seen in Huntington's disease and status epilepticus, respectively (Coyle et al., 1978; Nadler et al., 1978, 1980). Although KA was originally thought to be a glutamate agonist (Johnston et al., 1974), it is now clear that it does not act on the majority of the receptors for glutamate (Hall et al., 1978; London and Coyle, 1979), and in fact, it appears to act on a class of receptors which are distinct from those which mediate responses to other excitatory amino acids (McLennan and Lodge, 1979). The potent and selective neurotoxic effects of this compound may be mediated by these same receptors. Some evidence favors a nonsynaptic (extrajunctional) localization, other evidence favors a synaptic one. Table 3 shows the relative values for specific binding (the [^{3}H]-KA binding which can be displaced by 100 µM unlabeled KA) in isolated fractions. Membranes from crude mitochondrial pellet (P$_2$) were not enriched in KA binding sites compared to the whole particulate fraction. However, upon subfractionation of P$_2$ the highest specific binding values were found in the SPM and SJ fractions.

Table 3. Distribution of kainic acid binding sites in isolated brain subcellular fractions (whole particulate material = 1). Specific binding to whole particulate material was 81.31 fmoles per mg protein (from Foster et al., 1981b).

Fraction	Specific ^{3}H-KA binding relative to whole particulate material (WP; =1)
WP	1
P$_2$	0.73 + 0.34
P$_3$	0.56, 0.25
Crude Myelin	0.05, 0.13
SPM	2.08 + 0.41
Mitochondria	0.95 + 0.21
SJ	22.37 + 5.79

Specific KA binding sites in SJs were enriched 22 times over those measured in the whole brain particulate fraction, and 10 times over those in SPMs. This enrichment in SJ fractions was greater than that shown previously for any other receptor or receptor related function. It was found that the majority of specific KA binding sites in the SPMs could be recovered in SJs (73 + 14% of binding sites; 9.4 + 0.6% protein; n = 4).

If KA binding sites are predominantly synaptic, they might be localized to discrete terminal fields. KA binding sites can be viewed directly in rat brain slices by using an _in vitro_ auto- radiographic technique (Young and Kuhar, 1979). Using this method KA binding sites were seen to be particularly enriched in discrete parts of the hippocampus, pyriform cortex, cerebellum and striatum. In the hippocampus a small band of silver grains was associated with the inner part of the molecular layer of the dentate gyrus, corresponding to the terminal field of the commissural/ associational fibers. However, the greatest density of grains was seen over stratum incidium in the CA3 region corresponding to the terminal zone of the mossy fiber input to the CA3 pyramidal cells (Fig. 5). Other brain areas also showed KA sites but in general these were of lower concentration than the CA3 field (Monaghan, D. T. and Cotman, C. W., in preparation).

Specific and localized synaptic receptors imply that the appropriate natural ligands exist. Our data, together with evidence that KA does not act on glutamate sites and that KA receptors are a discrete population (Davies et al., 1980; McLennan and Lodge, 1979), suggests that endogenous ligands for KA receptors exist. Such a compound would be a mediator or modulator of synaptic transmission, at sites where KA receptors are present.

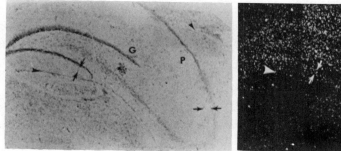 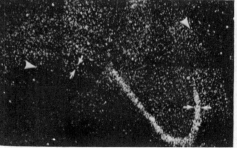

Figure 5. Distribution of kainic acid binding sites in the rat hippocampus. Left: cresyl violet stained tissue section, small arrows indicate identical area in dark field (from Foster et al., 1981b). Right: dark field illumination; small arrows indicate area of high silver grain density.

SYNAPSE SPECIFIC ANTISERA

As individual synapse molecules are identified and characterized, probes are needed which can be used to follow the appearance of these molecules during development and to further elucidate their function. Some of the most successful probes are

antibodies (see Matus, this volume). Accordingly, we have sought
to prepare synapse specific antibodies. At present we have not
developed antibodies to synapse specific glycoproteins or
receptors, although we are working in that direction. Our efforts
have been directed toward preparing an antibody specific for PSDs.

The appearance of the PSD seems to mark the commitment of two
neurons to engage in synaptic contact (Cotman, 1978; Rees et al.,
1976) both in the course of development (Jacobson, 1978; Lund,
1978) and following damage of the nervous system (Cotman et al.,
1981). The precise functional role of these specializations and
the mechanisms that control their biosynthesis and turnover are
not known. Antibodies directed against molecules that are
specific to the PSD would be extremely valuable tools with which
to approach these problems and would also provide much needed
information and potential markers to help in ascertaining the
unique composition of the PSD. Therefore, we prepared PSDs on a
comparatively large scale and immunized rabbits with high levels
of PSD protein over extended periods of time.

The sera from six immunized animals (R1 to R6) tested
positive to PSDs and could be separated into three groups,
according to their titer and antigenic specificity. The titer,
determined by testing the binding of sequential dilutions of the
sera to bovine PSD increased steadily in three animals (R4, R5 and
R6) after the second injection of immunogen. After the eighth
immunization the sera of these rabbits had titers that ranged from
1/2,000 to 1/5,000. The sera of the remaining three animals (R1,
R2 and R3) had a maximum titer of 1/300 after the fourth
immunization, decreasing thereafter. Serum R6 had the highest
titer and was characterized in detail (Nieto Sampedro et al.,
1981a).

The major antigens of bovine PSD preparations were three
polypeptides of molecular weight 95,000 (PSD-95), 82,000 (PSD-82)
and 72,000 (PSD-72), respectively (Fig. 6). Antigen PSD-95 was
present in mouse and rat PSDs and virtually absent in cytoplasm,
myelin, mitochondria, and microsomes from rodent or bovine brain.
Antigens PSD-82 and PSD-72 were present in all subcellular fractions from bovine brain, especially in mitochondria, but were almost absent from rodent brain. The antiserum also contained low
affinity antibodies directed against tubulin.

Immunohistochemical studies were performed in mouse and rat
brain, where antigen PSD-95 accounted for 90% of the antiserum
binding after absorption with purified brain tubulin. At the
light microscope level, antibody binding was observed in those
regions of the brain sections where synapses are known to be
present. No reaction was observed in myelinated tracts, inside

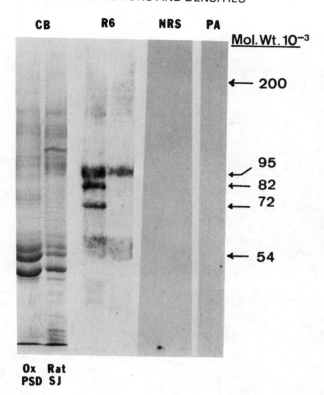

Figure 6. Antigenic specificity of rabbit anti-PSD antiserum R6.
Bovine postsynaptic densities and rat synaptic junctions were
subjected to electrophoresis in the presence of sodium dodecyl
sulfate on 8% polyacrylamide gel slabs. From left to right,
Coomassie blue-staining pattern (CB) and autoradiograms of ox and
rat PSD, respectively after sequential treatment of the gels with
antiserum (R6) and ^{125}I-labelled protein A. Non-immune rabbit
serum (NRS), anti-PSD sera exhaustively absorbed with bovine PSD
and ^{125}I-protein A alone (PA) did not bind to any junctional
component (from Nieto Sampedro et al., 1981a).

neuronal cell bodies or on non-neuronal cells. Strong reactivity
was observed in the molecular layer of the dentate gyrus, stratum
radiatum of the hippocampus, and the molecular layer of the
cerebellum. At the electron microscopic level, immunoreactivity
occurred exclusively at PSDs (Nieto Sampedro et al., 1981a).

Taken together, the reported observations indicate that
antigen PSD-95, in common with the major PSD-52 polypeptide (Kelly
et al., 1976), is highly enriched in PSDs. Therefore, PSD-95 can

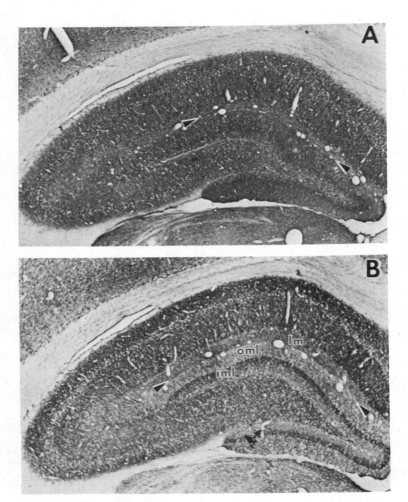

Figure 7. Immunohistochemical staining with anti-PSD antiserum of
the hippocampal formation of the A) normal rat, B) 3 days after
the ipsilateral entorhinal cortex of the animal was ablated.
Sections of brain tissue (25 μm thick) were stained using antiserum
R6 (1/500 dilution) exhaustively absorbed with tubulin. Arrowheads
point to the hippocampal fissure that separates hippocampus from
dentate gyrus. In the latter, inner third of the molecular layer
(iml); outer two-thirds of molecular layer (oml). The oml of the
dentate gyrus and stratum lacunosum moleculare (lm) of the hippocampus are deafferented by entorhinal ablation.
Magnification: x30 (from Nieto Sampedro et al., 1981b).

be proposed as a marker for SJs and PSDs during the purification of these structures by subcellular fractionation, as well as in the study of their biosynthesis. Other potential uses of antibodies against PSD-95 include the chemical determination of changes in synapse density following various experimental manipulations. The reaction of the antibody with slices of brain tissue, followed by treatment with radioactive protein A allows us to make this a quantitative estimate. We have tested the use of anti-PSD-95 in this capacity in the hippocampal formation and lateral septal nucleus of the rat.

Previous electron microscopic studies have demonstrated that following partial denervation of the hippocampus by an entorhinal lesion, 46% of the PSDs are rapidly lost and then eventually restored as part of the denervation-reinnervation cycle in the outer two-thirds of the molecular layer of the dentate gyrus ipsilateral to the lesion (Cotman, 1978).

Immunohistochemical staining with R6 serum also detected these selective changes in number of PSDs in discrete regions of the brain following experimental lesions. Unilateral ablation of the rat entorhinal cortex caused a localized decrease ($38 \pm 10\%$) in immunostaining in the outer two-thirds of the dentate molecular layer with respect to the side contralateral to the lesion or to unoperated animals (Fig. 7). Elimination of commissural/associational fibers by means of intraventricular injection of the neurotoxin kainic acid denervates the inner one-third of the molecular layer of the dentate gyrus (Nadler, et al., 1978; Nafstad, 1967). This event also correlated with a loss of specific immunohistochemical staining in the same area, the zone of termination of commissural/associational fibers (Nieto Sampedro et al., 1981b).

Thus, in the dentate gyrus PSDs appear to turnover following partial denervation. The agreement between electron microscopic and immunocytochemical data indicates that the antigens are lost from the outer two-thirds of the molecular layer, not simply rendered undetectable by electron microscopy. In contrast to results in the dentate gyrus, Raisman and Field (1973) reported electron microscopic evidence that PSD persist in the septum after partial denervation. Binding of anti-PSD antibody after unilateral fimbria transection also failed to show loss of PSDs, again in agreement with the electron microscopic evidence (Nieto Sampedro et al., 1981b).

ACKNOWLEDGEMENTS

We would like to thank Susanne Bathgate for assistance with the manuscript. This work was supported by grant numbers NS08957 and MH19691.

REFERENCES

Banker, G., Churchill, L., and Cotman, C. W., 1974, Proteins of
    the post-synaptic density, J. Cell Biol. 63:456-465.
Baudry, M., and Lynch, G., 1979, Two glutamate binding sites in
    rat hippocampal membranes, Eur. J. Pharmacol. 57:283-285.
Beach, R. L., Kelly, P. T., Babitch, J. A., and Cotman, C. W.,
    1981, Identification of myosin in isolated synaptic junctions,
    Brain Res. 225, 75-93.
Biziere, K., Thompson, H., and Coyle, J. T., 1980, Characterization
    of specific, high-affinity binding sites for L-[^{3}H]-glutamic
    acid in rat brain membranes, Brain Res. 183:421-423.
Blomberg, F., Cohen, R. S., and Siekevitz, P., 1977, The structure
    of post-synaptic densities isolated from dog cerebral cortex.
    II. Characterization and arrangement of some of the major
    proteins within the structure, J. Cell Biol. 74:204-225.
Carlin, R. K., Grab, D. J., Cohen, R. S., and Siekevitz, P., 1980,
    Isolation and characterization of postsynaptic densities from
    various brain regions. Enrichment of different types of post-
    synaptic densities, J. Cell Biol. 86:831-843.
Churchill, L., Cotman, C., Banker, G., Kelly, P., and Shannon, L.,
    1976, Carbohydrate composition of central nervous system
    synapses: analysis of isolated synaptic junctional complexes
    and post-synaptic densities, Biochim. Biophys. Acta 448:57-92.
Cohen, R. S., Blomberg, F., and Siekevitz, P., 1976, Studies of
    post-synaptic densities isolated from dog cerebral cortex, J.
    Cell Biol. 70:93a.
Cohen, R., Blomberg, F., Berzius, K., and Siekevitz, P., 1977, The
    structure of postsynaptic densities isolated from dog cerebral
    cortex, J. Cell. Biol. 74:181-203.
Cotman, C. W. and Kelly, P. T., 1980, Macromolecular architecture
    of CNS synapses, Cell Surface Rev. 6:505-533.
Cotman, C. W., Nieto Sampedro, M., and Harris, E. W., 1981, Synapse
    replacement in the nervous system of adult vertebrates,
    Physiol. Rev. 61:684-784.
Cotman, C. W., and Taylor, D., 1972, Isolation and structural
    studies on synaptic complexes from rat brain, J. Cell Biol.
    55:696-711.
Cotman, C. W., Banker, G., Churchill, L., and Taylor, D., 1974,
    Isolation of postsynaptic dendrites from rat brain, J. Cell
    Biol. 63:441-455.
Coyle, J.T., McGeer, E.G., McGeer, P.L., and Schwarcz, R., 1978,
    Neostriatal injections: a model for Huntingtons's chorea,
    in Kainic acid as a tool in neurobiology, McGeer, E. G.,
    Olney, J. W., and McGeer, P. L., Raven Press, New York, pp.
    139-160.
Cull-Candy, S. G., 1978, Glutamate sensitivity and distribution of
    receptors along normal and denervated locust muscle fibres,
    J. Physiol. (Lond.) 276:165-181.

Davis, G. A., and Bloom, F. E., 1973, Isolation of synaptic junctional complexes from rat brain, Brain Res., 62:135-153.

De Robertis, E., and S. Fiszer de Plazas, 1976, Isolation of hydrophobic proteins binding amino acids. Stereoselectivity of the binding of L-[^{14}C]-glutamate in cerebral cortex, J. Neurochem. 26:1237-1243.

Doolittle, R. F., 1981, Similar amino acid sequences: chance or common ancestry?, Science 214:149-159.

Elder, J. H., Pickett, R. A., Hampton, J. and Lerner, R. A., 1977, Radioiodinations of proteins in single polyacrylamide gel slices, J. Biol. Chem, 252, 6510-6515.

Feit, H. P., Kelly, P., and Cotman, C. W., 1977, The identification of a protein related to tubulin in the postsynaptic density, Proc. Natl. Acad. Sci. USA 74:1047-1051.

Fiszer de Plazas, S., and De Robertis, E., 1976, Isolation of hydrophobic proteins binding amino acids. L-Aspartic acid binding protein from rat cerebral cortex, J. Neurochem. 27: 889-894.

Foster, A. C., Mena, E. E., Fagg, G. E., and Cotman, C. W., 1981a, Glutamate and aspartate binding sites are enriched in synaptic junctions isolated from rat brain, J. Neurosci. 1: 620-625.

Foster, A. C., Mena, E. E., Monaghan, D. T., and Cotman, C. W., 1981b, Synaptic localization of kainic acid binding sites, Nature 281:73-75.

Foster, A. C., and Roberts, P. J., 1978, High affinity L-[^{3}H]-glutamate binding to postsynaptic receptor sites on rat cerebellar membranes, J. Neurochem. 31:1467-1477.

Grab, D. J., Berzins, K., Cohen, R. S., and Siekevitz, P., 1979, Presence of calmodulin in postsynaptic densities isolated from canine cerebral cortex, J. Biol. Chem. 254:8690-8696.

Gurd, J. W., 1979, Molecular and biosynthetic heterogeneity of fucosyl glycoproteins associated with rat brain synaptic junctions, Biochim. Biophys. Acta. 555:221-229.

Hall, J.G., Hicks, T.P., and McLennan, H., 1978, Kainic acid and the glutamate receptor, Neurosci. Letters 8:171-175.

Jacobson, M., 1978, Developmental Neurobiology, Plenum Press, New York.

Johnston, G.A.R., Curtis, D.R., Davies, J., and McCulloch, R.M., 1974, Spinal interneurone excitation by conformationally restricted analogues of L-glutamic acid, Nature 248:804-805.

Kelly, P. T., and Cotman, C. W., 1977, Identification of proteins and glycoproteins at synapses in the central nervous system, J. Biol. Chem. 252:786-793.

Kelly, P. T., and Cotman, C. W., 1978, Synaptic proteins: characterization of tubulin and actin and identification of a distinct postsynaptic density, J. Cell Biol. 79:173-183.

Kelly, P. T., Cotman, C. W., Gentry, C., and Nicolson, G. L., 1976, Distribution and mobility of lectin receptors on synaptic membranes of identified neurons in the central nervous system, J. Cell Biol. 71:487-496.

Koerner, J. F., and Cotman, C. W., 1981, Micromolar L-2-amino-4-
    phosphonobutyric acid selectively inhibits perforant path
    synapses from lateral entorhinal cortex, Brain Res. 216:192-
    198.
London, E. D., and Coyle, J. T., 1979, Cooperative interactions at
    [³H] kainic acid binding sites in rat and human cerebellum,
    Eur. J. Pharmac. 56:287290.
Lund, R. D., 1978, Development and plasticity of the brain, Oxford
    University Press, New York.
Mahler, H. R., 1977, Proteins of the synaptic membrane, Neurochem.
    Res. 2:119-147.
March, S. C., Parikh, I., and Cuatrecasas, P., 1974, A simplified
    method for cyanogen bromide activation of agarose for affinity
    chromatography, Anal. Biochem. 60:149-162.
Matus, A., 1981, The postsynaptic density, Trends in Neuroscience
    4:51-53.
Matus, A. I., Pehling, G and Wilkinson, D. A., 1980, γ-Aminobutyric
    acid receptors in brain postsynaptic densities, J. Neurobiol.
    12:67-73.
Matus, A. I., and Walters, B. B., 1975, Ultrastucture of the
    synaptic junctional lattice isolated from mammalian brain, J.
    Neurocytol. 4:357-367.
McLennan, H., and Lodge, D., 1979, The antagonism of amino acid-
    induced excitation of spinal neurons in the cat, Brain Res.
    169:83-90.
Mena, E. E., Foster, A. C., Fagg, G. E., and Cotman, C. W., 1981,
    Identification of synapse specific components, synaptic glyco-
    proteins, proteins and transmitter binding sites, J. Neuro-
    chem., in press.
Michaelis, E. K., Michaelis, M. L., and Boyarsky, L. L., 1974,
    High-affinity glutamate binding to brain synaptic membranes,
    Biochim. Biophys. Acta. 367:338-348.
Nadler, J. V., Perry, B. W., and Cotman, C. W, 1978, Preferential
    vulnerability of hippocampus to intraventricular kainic acid,
    in Kainic acid as a tool in neurobiology, McGeer, E. G.,
    Olney, J. W., and McGeer, P. L., eds., Raven Press, New York,
    pp. 219-237.
Nadler, J. V., Perry, B. W., and Cotman, C. W., 1980, Loss and
    reacquisition of hippocampal synapses after selective
    destruction of CA3-CA4 afferents with kainic acid, Brain Res.
    191:397-403.
Nafstad, P. H. J., 1967, An electron microscope study on the
    termination of the perforant path fibres in the hippocampus
    and the fascia dentata, Zeitsch. Zellforsch. 76:532-542.
Nieto Sampedro, M., Bussineau, C., and Cotman, C.W., 1981a, Post-
    synaptic density antigens: preparation and characterization
    of an antiserum against postsynaptic densities, J. Cell Biol.
    90:675-686.

Nieto Sampedro, M., Bussineau, C., and Cotman, C. W., 1981b, Selective changes in brain synapse number estimated with antibodies to a postsynaptic density component, Neuroscience Abst. 7:5.

Onedera, K., and Takeuchi, A., 1980, Distribution and pharmacological properties of synaptic and extra-synaptic glutamate receptors on crayfish muscle, J. Physiol. (Lond.) 306:233-250.

Olney, J. W., Fuller, T., and DeGubareff, T., 1979, Acute dendrotoxic changes in the hippocampus of kainic treated rats, Brain Res. 176:91-100.

Raftery, M. A., Hunkapiller, M. W., Strader, C. O., and Hood, L. E., 1980, Acetylcholine receptor complex of homologous subunits, Science 208:1454-1456.

Raisman, G., Cowan, W. M., and Powell, T. P. S., 1965, The extrinsic afferent, commissural and association fibres of the hippocampus, Brain 88:963-996.

Rees, R. P., Bunge, M. B., and Bunge, R. P., 1976, Morphological changes in the neuritic growth cone and target neuron during synaptic junction development in culture, J. Cell Biol. 68:240-263.

Roberts, P. J., 1974, Glutamate receptors in the rat CNS, Nature 252:399-401.

Roberts, P. J., Sharif, N. A., and Swait, J. C., 1980, Characteristics of L-[^{3}H]-aspartate binding to cerebellar synaptic membranes, Br. J. Pharmacol. 70:146P.

Rostas, J. A. P, Kelley, P. T., Pesin, R. H., and Cotman, C. W., 1979, Protein and glycoprotein composition of synaptic junctions prepared from discrete synaptic regions and different species, Brain Res. 168:151-167.

Sharif, N. A., and Roberts, P. J., 1980, Problems associated with the binding of L-glutamic acid to cerebellar synaptic membranes: Methodological aspects, J. Neurochem. 34:779-784.

Takeuchi, A., and Onedera, K., 1975, Effects of kainic acid on the glutamate receptors of crayfish muscle, Neuropharmacology 14:619-625.

Takeuchi, A., and Takeuchi, N., 1964, The effect on crayfish muscle of iontophoretically-applied glutamate, J. Physiol. (Lond.) 170:296-317.

Therien, H. M., and Mushynski, W. E., 1976, Isolation of synaptic junctional complexes of high structural integrity from rat brain, J. Cell Biol. 1:807-822.

Usherwood, P. N. R., and Machili, P., 1968, Pharmacological properties of excitatory neuromuscular synapses in the locust, J. Exp. Biol. 49:349-361.

Walters, B. B., and Matus, A. I., 1975, Tubulin in postsynaptic junctional lattice, Nature 257:496-498.

Wang, Y.-J., and Mahler, H. R., 1976, Topography of the synaptosomal membrane, J. Cell Biol. 71:639-658.

Westrum, L. E., and Gray, E. G., 1977, Microtubules associated
    with postsynaptic thickenings, J. Neurocytology, 6, 505-518.
Young, W. S., and Kuhar, M.J., 1979, A new method for receptor
    autoradiography: [^{3}H]-opiod receptors in rat brain, Brain
    Res. 179:255-270.

USING ANTIBODIES TO PROBE BRAIN DEVELOPMENT

Richard Hawkes, Evelyn Niday and Andrew Matus

Friedrich Miescher Institut, P. O. Box 273
4002 Basel, Switzerland

INTRODUCTION

When neuroblasts in the developing brain stop dividing, they enter a terminal differentiation sequence during which they extend axons and dendrites and make synapses with one another. Several fundamental features of this process are as yet poorly understood. For example, what controls the size and degree of branching of axonal and dendritic arborizations and what determines the numbers of synapses which two neurons make with each other? Historically, these questions have been investigated by microscopy, but microscopy alone cannot reveal the molecular mechanisms inside the neuron which drive the morphological events of differentiation. For this reason we are using antibodies as specific reagents to identify molecules which are associated with each morphological compartment of the differentiating neuron. Once identified, these "markers" can be used to quantitate changes in the extent of the neuronal structure they represent. For example, a protein associated exclusively with dendrites could be used as the basis of an immunochemical assay to quantitate dendrite growth.

It makes good sense to select as markers molecules which are already implicated in the establishment of specific parts of neurons. We use the term neuronal microstructures to designate distinctive subdivisions of nerve cell structure such as dendrites or synapses. Thus neurofilament proteins provide a useful marker for axons where they are very abundant compared to dendrites (1). As another example, the 50,000 molecular weight protein of postsynaptic densities (PSD-50) appears to be a good candidate as a marker for postsynaptic junctional structures, to which it seems

39

to be unique (2,3,4) and with whose development its appearance
correlates (5).

Antibodies are already widely accepted as reagents of choice
for studying developmental marker proteins by immunocytochemistry
(6,7). Now, with the advent of protein blotting technology (8)
they can be used both to precisely identify neural polypeptides
(9) and as highly sensitive immunoassay reagents (Hawkes,R., Niday,
E. and Gordon,J.; MS submitted). Below we give examples from
our recent work which illustrate this approach and the methods
we employ.

MATERIALS AND METHODS

The methods for subcellular fractionation, gel electrophoresis, the production of polyclonal rabbit antisera and immunochemical staining of gel blots have all been described in detail
before (9,13).

Monoclonal Antibody Production

Our method for the production of lymphocyte hybridomas is
essentially that of Galfré et al. (14). In the experiments described in detail below, a panel of BALB/c mice were immunized
three times intraperitoneally with 3-5 mg of rat cerebellar SPM
(synaptosomal plasma membrane) proteins. We have found that these
high doses are very effective with SPM antigens. Three days after
the third immunization, the two mice with the highest anti-SPM
serum titers (determined by a dot immunobinding assay - see below)
were chosen for hybridoma production. 10^8 spleen cells were fused
by polyethylene glycol 1500 with 10^7 cells of the 8-azaguanine-
resistant (HGPRT-deficient) myeloma line X63Ag8.6.5.3 and cultured
in selective medium (15) in 500 x 1.0 ml culture wells over a
feeder layer of 10^6 spleen cells per well. The cultures were
maintained at 37°C in a 95% air/5% CO_2 incubator with the medium
replaced every three days. Hybridoma colonies appeared in about
2/3 of the wells and the culture supernatants were tested for
anti-SPM antibody after 2-3 weeks.

Dot Immunobinding Assay

Approximately 0.5 µl of a 1.0 mg/ml suspension of SPM in
saline is "dotted" onto a nitrocellulose filter and allowed to
dry, thereby becoming tightly bound. To test for anti-SPM antibodies,
the filter is first incubated for 30 minutes in 10% normal horse
serum in TBS (50 mM tris buffer pH 7.4, 200 mM NaCl) to block
the remaining non-specific protein binding sites on the filter

and then incubated in the putative anti-SPM antibody solution.
In the case of polyclonal antisera, dilutions of between 1/10,000
and 1/100,000 are usually appropriate, monoclonal antibodies in
culture medium are usually tested undiluted. The incubation period
needed varies from 2 hours to overnight. Once the incubation
is complete, the filter is washed for 30 minutes in several changes
of TBS and then incubated for 2-3 hours in a solution of horseradish
peroxidase-conjugated antibody directed against the test antibody.
(Thus, for mouse anti-SPM we use HRP-rabbit anti-mouse Ig). The
filter is again washed and then antibody binding is detected by
incubation of the filter in a solution of 0.06% 4-chloro-1-naphthol
(from a 0.3% w/v methanol stock solution) and 0.01% hydrogen peroxide
in TBS. Positive results appear after 5-10 minutes as blue dots
against the white filter background. We use the dot immunobinding
assay to titer the sera of hyperimmunized mice, to test culture
media for anti-SPM antibodies and, by dotting a range of tissue
homogenates, to determine the tissue distribution of specific
determinants (Hawkes,R., Niday,E. & Gordon,J.; MS submitted).

POLYCLONAL ANTIBODIES

     For several years we have been investigating synaptic surface
proteins biochemically and immunocytologically (3,9,10). Recently
we have combined these two approaches. Working with three rabbit
antisera raised against subcellular fractions enriched in synaptosomal
plasma membranes, we have characterized a series of synapse-related
protein antigens. Our initial evidence that these antisera react
selectively with synaptic antigens came from immunofluorescence
staining of brain sections. This gave a dot-like pattern of fluorescent labelling whose distribution was strikingly similar to that
given by conventional silver "bouton" stains (10). Other laboratories have obtained essentially identical results using other
anti-SPM antisera (11,12).

     More recently we have identified the polypeptides with which
these antisera react by immunoperoxidase staining cellulose nitrate
blots made from sodium dodecyl sulphate-polyacrylamide gels (Matus,
A., Pehling,G., Ackermann,M. & Hauser,K.; in preparation). Some
of the results obtained with one of these antisera are shown in
Figure 1. This particular antiserum was raised against SPM from
rat cerebral cortex. Immunohistochemistry shows that the antigens
which it recognizes are associated exclusively with synapses.
The antigens were identified by staining immunoblots of SPM polypeptides with anti-SPM (Figure 1A). Among the reactive bands
are several which are detected by all three of the anti-SPM sera
we have used and which therefore appear to be particularly prominent
synaptic antigens. To characterize these antigens further we
tested the antiserum against subcellular fractions containing
PSDs (Figure 1B). This revealed that among the antibodies in

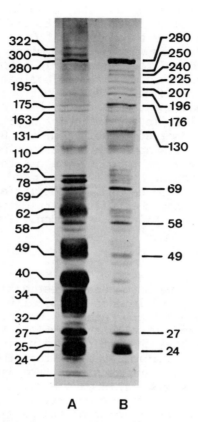

Figure 1:   An SDS-immunoblot to identify polypeptides reacting
with a polyclonal rabbit antiserum against synaptic plasma membranes
from rat cerebral cortex.   In Channel A the antiserum was tested
against SPM proteins and in Channel B against the separated proteins
of postsynaptic densities.   The molecular weights of prominent
bands in kDaltons appear to either side.

this polyclonal antiserum there is a subset which reacts with
what are apparently PSD-specific polypeptides. These PSD antigens
are all of very high molecular weight (above 200 kDalton) compared
to the major antigens seen in the unfractionated SPM (compare
Figures 1A and B).   Once again this result was replicated with
all three of our anti-SPM sera; they all stain a set of very high

molecular weight bands in PSD. These polyclonal antisera have
proven very useful for surveying synaptic antigens. With them
we have been able to identify a large number of antigenic synaptic
polypeptides in each SDS-gel immunoblot. However, ultimately
we want to refine our techniques to deal with single proteins
and individual cellular components. For this purpose monoclonal
antibodies are proving more appropriate.

MONOCLONAL ANTIBODIES

     The pre-eminent virtue of monoclonal antibodies is that each
lymphocyte hybridoma clone produces a unique antibody whose antigenic
specificity can be unequivocally defined. This overcomes one
of the major limitations upon the interpretation of results obtained
with conventional polyclonal sera where it is impossible to be
certain that the immunocytological and immunochemical results
reflect the behaviour of the self-same antibody. With monoclonal
antibodies this problem is removed because culture media from
clonal hybridoma lines contain antibody of only one specificity;
it and it alone must be responsible for all antibody-mediated
effects. In short, we have an homogeneous and specific reagent
for studying individual components of neural tissue.

     There is another advantage of monoclonal antibodies which
is of even greater immediate value. The cloning procedures allow
single antibody specificities to be recovered from an animal immunized
with a complex mixture of antigens. Because of this we are able
to immunize a mouse with a crude subcellular fraction containing
components from numerous cellular sources and realistically hope
to recover antibodies specifically directed against individual
brain regions, cell types or subcellular components. As we will
demonstrate, this ability to clone out complex antigenic mixtures
is the decisive advantage which monoclonal antibodies have to
offer.

     We are using our monoclonal antibodies to study cell differ-
entiation in the rat cerebellar cortex. With them we can identify
antigens whose spatial or temporal patterns of expression are
related to the molecular events of development. Similar studies
with monoclonal antibodies are beginning to emerge from other
laboratories (16-22). We use the cerebellum for the same reasons
that attracted other workers interested in brain development in
the past; simple cytoarchitecture, readily distinguishable cell
types and, in the rat, mainly postnatal histogenesis.

     So far we have raised monoclonal antibodies in two separate
fusion experiments. The second of these produced 176 independent
cultures of anti-SPM-secreting hybridomas as detected by the dot
immunobinding assay to isolated SPM. We have screened the antibodies

produced in two ways, by immunoblotting of SDS gels to identify
polypeptide antigens (8,9) and immunocytochemically to study the
distribution of antibody binding within the cerebellum (13). The
majority of clones were positive in all three assays, but there
were also examples of antibodies which (i) recognized polypeptide
bands on immunoblots but were negative by immunocytochemistry,
(ii) were negative on immunoblots but positive cytochemically
and (iii) were negative in both tests while remaining positive
in the original dot immunobinding assay. This emphasizes that
if the full range of antibody variability is to be detected then
several independent assay procedures must be employed.

The range of polypeptide specificities can be appreciated
by consideration of Figure 2 in which immunoblots from a selection
of independent cultures are compared. Several general points
can be made. Firstly, it is evident that any assumption that
a monoclonal antibody is specific for a particular molecule as
opposed to a specific epitope must be discounted; while several
antibodies do indeed recognize a single band (e.g. 20A3, 11C5),
others recognize either a small number of bands (e.g. 7D5, 20D6)
and some very many bands (e.g. 21A5, 7A2). In some cases numerous
stained bands may reflect a family of breakdown products from
a high molecular weight precursor in vivo, but it is clear in
general that many strongly antigenic determinants in brain are
shared by more than one polypeptide. Secondly, there is great
variability in the intensity with which different bands are stained.
Some (e.g. 12D5) are reproducibly very weak, others (e.g. 7D5)
are consistently strong. There are three obvious explanations
for this: that the antibody titer or affinity is low, that the
determinant conformation is only poorly preserved through immunoblotting or that the determinant is rare. In the example of 12D5,
the staining intensity on the immunoblot is always weak
(Figure 4A) and is unaffected by a tenfold antibody dilution.
On the other hand, staining of cerebellar tissue sections is strong
(Figure 4B). We suspect therefore that we lose most of the antigenic
activity during the isolation and immunoblotting of SPM.

The range of antigen diversity revealed by immunoblotting
is also reflected in the range of immunocytochemical results of
which we present three examples below.

MIT-23: A neuron-specific polypeptide whose expression
correlates with terminal differentiation.

The characteristics of MIT-23 are illustrated in Figure 3.
Immunoblotting shows that the monoclonal antibody recognizes a
single polypeptide band of 23 kDalton (Figure 3A). Immunoperoxidase

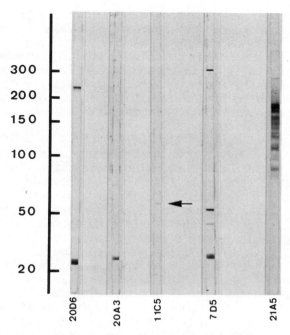

Figure 2: SDS–gel immunoblots identifying SPM polypeptide antigens
recognized by monoclonal antibodies. The identification codes
of the clones appear below each channel. The molecular weight
scale to the left is in kDalton. The weakly reactive band in
11C5 is arrowed. Compare the single SPM bands stained by 20A3
and 11C5 with the complex pattern given by the polyclonal antiserum
in Figure 1.

staining of adult rat cerebellum gives strong labelling of the
cell body, dendrites and axon hillock of Purkinje cells which
is deposited at discrete granular sites rather than continuously
distributed. The rest of the cerebellar cortex is less strongly
stained and the white matter is not stained at all. Staining
in the granular layer is associated with both granule and Golgi
II cells. In the molecular layer we also find stained basket
and stellate cells amongst the strongly–stained Purkinje cell
dendrites. A similar pattern of punctate staining also occurs
in the hippocampus as well as in cultured neuroblastoma
(Figure 3C).

When viewed in the electron microscope, the anti–MIT-23 staining appears to be associated with neuronal mitochondria (not shown), hence the name MIT(ochondria)-23(kdalton). We are well aware that apparent mitochondrial peroxidase staining can occur artifactually but it is unlikely in this case because (i) areas of Purkinje cell bodies where there are no mitochondria, are not stained at all and (ii) tests on brain subcellular fractions show that MIT-23 is enriched along with mitochondria (Hawkes,R., Niday,E. & Matus,A.; MS submitted).

Although MIT-23 is a prominent feature of most (probably all) neurons of the adult cerebellar cortex, its distribution in the neonate is strikingly restricted. From birth to 10 days postnatal, MIT-23 is confined exclusively to the growing Purkinje cells (Figure 3D). This may be significant as, unlike other neurons of the cerebellar cortex, the Purkinje cells have already entered terminal differentiation by birth (23). In older animals the expression of MIT-23 correlates with the terminal differentiation of the various classes of neurons and the adult staining pattern is qualitatively established by day 20. It is noteworthy that the external granular layer, which contains dividing neuroblasts, remains completely unstained by anti–MIT-23 throughout cerebellar histogenesis. This suggests that MIT-23 is a neuron-specific mitochondrial polypeptide which is only expressed after terminal cell division. On this basis it appears to be a good marker for the entry of neurons into terminal differentiation.

12D5: A monoclonal antibody which specifically recognizes components of the granular layer.

MIT-23 is an example of an antigen which is probably associated with all neurons. The antigen recognized by 12D5 is an example of a further level of restriction, a determinant specific to the granular layer. In SDS–gel immunoblotting, 12D5 reacts with a single polypeptide band of apparent molecular weight 270 kDalton (Figure 4A). In sections of cerebellar cortex immunoperoxidase–

Figure 3: Characteristics of monoclonal antibody MIT-23.   (A) It reacts with a single polypeptide, molecular weight 23 kDalton; (B) gives granular staining of Purkinje cell bodies, dendrites and axon hillock (arrow); (C) induces granular immunofluorescence in cell bodies of neuroblastoma NB_2A; and (D) stains only the developing Purkinje cells in 5–day old rat cerebellar cortex (ex.g. = external granular layer; in.g. = inner granular layer; dotted line indicates the division between adjacent cerebellar folia). Marker bars: B = 10 μm; C = 10 μm; D = 100 μm.

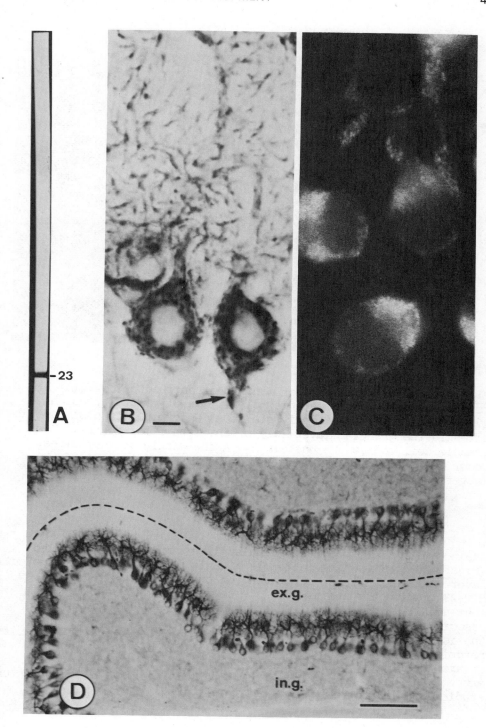

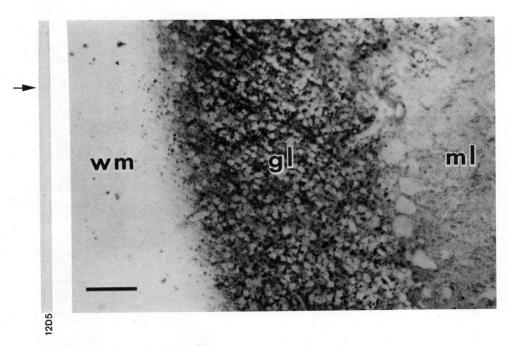

12D5

Figure 4: Characteristics of monoclonal antibody 12D5. (A) It reacts (faintly) with a single polypeptide of molecular weight 270 kDalton. (B) It strongly stains a dense population of punctate sites in the granular layer (gl) of the cerebellar cortex. The granule cell bodies are unstained. A few weakly stained sites occur in the molecular layer (ml). There is no staining of white matter (wm). Marker = 50 μm.

stained with 12D5, only the granular layer is strongly labelled (Figure 4B). The white matter is totally unreactive and the molecular layer contains a sparse scattering of punctate deposits. Whereas MIT-23 prominently stains Purkinje cells, 12D5 does not label them at all. The strong 12D5 staining in the granular layer is associated with the synaptic glomeruli which occur in between the islands of granule cell bodies. This is suggestive of a specific reaction with a neuronal element, such as granule cell dendrites or axon terminals, but we cannot exclude the possibility of some extreme, hitherto unconsidered, glial specialization. Ultrastructural studies are in progress to settle this point.

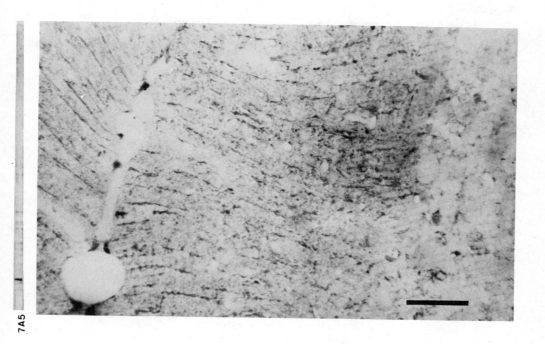

7A5

Figure 5: Characteristics of monoclonal antibody 7A5. (A) It reacts with widely varying intensities with many polypeptides. (B) It stains the cerebellar cortex with a characteristic glial pattern of radiating Bergmann glia fibers. There is no neuronal staining.Marker = 50 μm.

7A5: A monoclonal antibody which recognizes a glial-specific determinant associated with many polypeptide chains.

Three of the independent cell lines isolated from the S2 fusion (7A5, 18B1 and 12D2) give antibodies which share the same very striking characteristics. SDS-gel blots show that the determinant they recognize is present on numerous different polypeptides (at least 30), ranging in apparent molecular weights from 10 to more than 300 kDalton (Figure 5A). This, by itself, is unsuprising; the antibody might be directed against a "trivial" determinant such as a short amino acid sequence occurring randomly in numerous proteins, or alternatively it could be of low specificity and cross-react with a variety of antigens. However these explanations cannot be correct because when the cerebellar cortex is immunoperoxidase-stained using 7A5, the labelling is confined exclusively

to glial cells (Figure 5B). There is strong staining of both
cell bodies and radial fibres of Bergmann glia, and at the periphery
of blood vessels where the endfeet of astroglial cells are concentrated. There is no detectable reaction with any neuronal component.

It is possible, in principle, that 7A5 recognizes a family
of proteins but we find this implausible because of the diversity
and number of stained bands. We suspect instead that 7A5 may
be recognizing a specific label of some kind, such as a signal
peptide sequence or specific glycosylation, which is found in
glia but not neurons and is associated with a large number of
different polypeptide chains.

ACKNOWLEGEMENTS

We thank M. Ackermann and G. Pehling for technical assistance
and D. Monard for helpful discussions.

REFERENCES

1. Peters,A., Palay,S.L. & Webster,H. de F. (1976) "The Fine
   Structure of the Nervous System". Saunders, Philadelphia.
2. Cohen,R.S., Blomberg,F., Berzins,K. & Siekevitz,P. (1977)
   The structure of postsynaptic densities isolated from dog
   cerebral cortex. I. Overall morphology and protein composition.
   J. Cell Biol. 74, 181-203.
3. Matus,A.I. & Taff-Jones,D.H. (1978) Morphology and molecular
   composition of isolated postsynaptic junctional structures.
   Proc. Roy. Soc. Lond.(B) 203, 135-151.
4. Kelly,P.T. & Cotman,C.W. (1978) Synaptic proteins. Characterization of tubulin and actin and identification of a distinct
   postsynaptic density polypeptide. J. Cell Biol. 79, 173-183.
5. Kelly,P.T. & Cotman,C.W. (1981) Developmental changes in morphology and molecular composition of isolated synaptic junctional
   structures. Brain Res. 206, 251-271.
6. Raff,M.C., Fields,K.L., Hakamori,S., Mirsky,R., Pruss,R.M.
   & Winter,J. (1979) Cell-type-specific markers for distinguishing
   and studying neurons and the major classes of glial cells
   in culture. Brain Res. 174, 283-308.
7. Schachner,M. (1979) Cell surface antigens of the nervous system.
   Curr. Topics in Dev. Biol. 13, 259-279.
8. Towbin,H., Staehelin,T. & Gordon,J. (1979) A procedure for
   the electrophoretic transfer of proteins from polyacrylamide
   gels to nitrocellulose sheets and some applications. Proc.
   Natl. Acad. Sci. (U.S.A.) 76,4350-4354.
9. Matus,A., Pehling,G., Ackermann,M. & Maeder,J. (1980) Brain
   postsynaptic densities: their relationship to glial and neuronal

10. Matus,A.I., Jones,D.H. & Mughal,S. (1976) Restricted distribution of synaptic antigens in the neuronal membrane. Brain Res. 103, 171–175.
11. Rostas,J.A. & Jeffrey,P.L. (1975) Restricted mobility of neuronal membrane antigens. Neuroscience Lett. 1, 47–53.
12. Howe,P.R.C., Fenwick,E.M., Rostas,J.A.P. & Livett,B.G. (1977) Immunochemical comparison of synaptic plasma membrane and synaptic vesicle membrane antigens. J. Neurocytol. 6, 339 352.
13. Matus,A.I., Ng,M.L. & Jones,D.H. (1979) Immunohistochemical localization of neurofilament antigen in rat cerebellum. J. Neurocytol. 8, 513–525.
14. Galfré,G., Howe,S., Milstein,C., Butcher,G.W. & Howard,J.C. (1977) Antibodies to major histocompatibility antigens produced by hybrid cell lines. Nature(Lond.) 266, 550–552.
15. Littlefield,J.W. (1964) Selection of hybrids from matings of fibroblasts in vitro and their presumed recombinants. Science 145, 709.
16. Lagenauer,C., Sommer,I. & Schachner,M. (1980) Subclass of astroglia in mouse cerebellum recognized by monoclonal antibody. Dev. Biol. 79, 367–378.
17. Barnstable,C.J. (1980) Monoclonal antibodies which recognize different cell types in the rat retina. Nature (Lond.) 286, 231–235.
18. Bartlett,P.F., Noble,M.D., Pruss,R.M., Raff,M.C., Rattray,S. & Williams,C.A. (1981) Rat neural antigen-2 (RAN-2): a cell surface antigen on astrocytes, ependymal cells, Müller cells and lepto-meninges defined by a monoclonal antibody. Brain Res. 204, 339–351.
19. Vulliamy,T., Rattray,S. & Mirsky,R. (1981) Cell surface antigen distinguishes sensory and autonomic peripheral neurones from central neurones. Nature (Lond.) 291, 418–420.
20. Cohen,J. & Selvendran,Y. (1981) A neuronal cell-surface antigen is found in the CNS but not in peripheral neurones. Nature (Lond.) 291, 421–423.
21. Trisler,G.D., Schneider,M.D. & Nirenberg,M. (1981) A topographic gradient of molecules in retina can be used to identify neuron position. Proc. Natl. Acad. Sci. (U.S.A.) 78, 2145–2149.
22. Zipser,B. & McKay,R. (1981) Monoclonal antibodies distinguish identifiable neurones in the leech. Nature (Lond.) 289, 549 554.
23. Ramon y Cahal, S. (1911) "Histologie du Système Nerveux de l'Homme et des Vertébrés". Maloine, Paris.

GLUTAMATE DEPOLARIZATION-INDUCED RELEASE IN THE CEREBELLUM

AND ITS REGULATION BY GABA

Giulio Levi and Vittorio Gallo

Istituto di Biologia Cellulare, CNR, Via Romagnosi 18/A
00196 Roma, Italy

INTRODUCTION

The cerebellum is an area of the CNS particularly suitable for
biochemical studies on neurotransmission for a number of reasons.
In fact, its structure is very well characterized, and so are the
connections among its neurons (Palay and Chan-Palay, 1974). Techniques have been developed for the selective destruction of specific
systems of neurons (Mc Bride et al., 1976b; Perry et al., 1976;
Mc Bride et al., 1978; Tran and Snyder, 1979; Rohde et al., 1979).
Methods are available, not only for the preparation of slices and
synaptosomes, but also for a satisfactory bulk purification of different cell types (Purkinje cells, granule cells and astrocytes) (Wilkin
et al., 1976) and for the in vitro culture of some of them (namely,
granule cells and astrocytes) (Cohen et al., 1979; Balàzs et al., 1980;
Woodhams et al., 1981). Mutants carrying specific lesions of cerebellar neuronal systems provide an additional tool for functional
and biochemical studies (Sidman et al., 1965; Mc Bride et al., 1976a;
Roffler-Tarlov and Sidman, 1978).
    The studies conducted in the last years have shown that neuro-
transmission mediated by amino acids plays a particularly important
role in the cerebellum, as compared to other areas of the CNS. GABA
is known to be the inhibitory neurotransmitter of Purkinje cells, and
probably of most inhibitory interneurons (like Golgi , stellate and
basket cells) (Curtis and Johnston, 1974; Mc Laughlin et al., 1976;
Storm-Mathisen, 1976). It has been proposed that glycine may be the

53

transmitter of some Golgi cells (Wilson et al., 1975), and taurine
has been suggested as a possible transmitter of stellate cells (Mc
Bride and Frederickson, 1980), and is probably present in high concentration in the climbing fiber terminals (Descline and Escubi, 1974;
Rea et al., 1980).

The cerebellum receives two excitatory inputs, represented by
the mossy fibers and the climbing fibers. The transmitter of the
mossy fibers is largely unknown, but it is known that the excitation
of these fibers is conveyed to the Purkinje cells through the mediation of the granule cells, which give origin to the parallel fibers
in the molecular layer. A fairly large amount of evidence, mainly
biochemical, suggests that glutamate is the excitatory transmitter
released from parallel fiber terminals (Young et al., 1974; Mc Bride
et al., 1976b; Roffler-Tarlov and Sidman, 1978; Sandoval and Cotman,
1978; Rohde et al., 1979). As to the transmitter of the climbing
fibers, which originate from the inferior olives, glutamate or aspartate have been proposed as candidates (Guidotti et al., 1975; Rea
et al., 1980).

In the present report we shall treat some biochemical aspects
of the excitatory neurotransmission presumably mediated by glutamate.
In the first part, biochemical evidence in favour of a neurotransmitter
role of glutamate, and data on the localization and on the origin of
the glutamate released will be presented. The second part will concern
a GABAergic presynaptic mechanism which appears to control glutamate
release in the cerebellum.

AUTORADIOGRAPHIC LOCALIZATION OF ^{3}H-D-ASPARTATE IN CEREBELLAR SLICES
AND CULTURED CELLS

In general, the neurons and nerve endings utilizing a given
substance as a transmitter can be identified autoradiographically,
since they selectively take up that particular substance from the
extracellular space. With the aim of identifying the neurons presumably utilizing glutamate as a transmitter, the autoradiographic
localization of ^{3}H-D-aspartate in prelabelled cerebellar slices was
analyzed by light and electron microscopy (Wilkin et al., 1982; Levi
et al., 1982). D-Aspartate is a non metabolized glutamate analogue
which is transported by the L-glutamate carrier (Balcar and Johnston,
1972), and is frequently used to label the glutamate "reuptake pool".

In the granule cell layer, very few silver grains were present
over the neurons, while astrocytes often showed a heavy labelling.

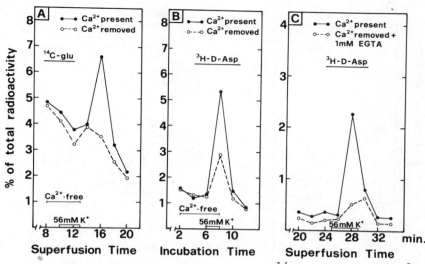

Fig. 1. Depolarization-induced release of ^{14}C-glutamate and ^{3}H-D-aspartate from rat cerebellar slices. Panel A: chopped "mini-slices" prelabelled with 10 μM ^{14}C-glutamate for 5 min were superfused (Raiteri et al., 1974) first with standard medium, then with a depolarizing medium as indicated in the figure. Panel B: chopped sagittal slices prelabelled for 10 min with 15 nM ^{3}H-D-aspartate were incubated at 37°C in a medium which was renewed every 2 min, in order to minimize reuptake. Panel C: had-cut surface slices prelabelled for 30 min with 0.5 μM ^{3}H-D-aspartate were superfused at 37°C in 0.1 ml chambers and depolarized as indicated. In all cases, the radioactivity released in each 2 min fraction is given as a percentage of the radioactivity recovered in all fractions plus that remaining in the slices at the end of the experimental period (Data from Levi et al., 1982).

In the molecular and Purkinje cell layer, the processes and perikarya of the Bergmann glia exhibited the greatest accumulation of radioactivity, but a substantial number of nerve endings were also labelled, almost half of which could be identified as granule cell terminals (Wilkin et al., 1982). Autoradiographic studies performed on cultured cerebellar cells confirmed the preferential accumulation of ^{3}H-D-aspartate in glial cells, as compared to granule cells.

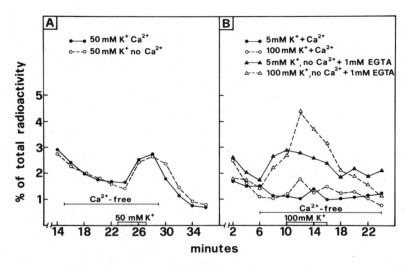

Fig. 2. Effect of high KCl concentrations on the release of
[3]H-D-aspartate from glia. Panel A: glia-enriched cell suspensions from 8-day rat cerebella (Cohen et al., 1979) were
prelabelled with 0.5 μM ^{3}H-D-aspartate and then superfused
(Raiteri et al., 1974) as indicated in the figure. Panel B:
cerebellar glial confluent cultures (Cohen et al., 1979)
prelabelled with 1.0 μM ^{3}H-D-aspartate were incubated at 37°C
in media which were renewed every 2 min. The results are
expressed as in Fig. 1 (Data from Levi et al., 1982).

DEPOLARIZATION-INDUCED RELEASE OF ACIDIC AMINO ACIDS FROM CEREBELLAR PREPARATIONS "IN VITRO"

In view of the preferential localization of ^{3}H-D-aspartate in
glia, mentioned in the previous paragraph, it seemed interesting to
study the characteristics of glutamate (or ^{3}H-D-aspartate) release
from cerebellar slices during depolarization. In fact, it is known
that putative neurotransmitters are released from nerve endings by
depolarizing stimuli in a Ca^{2+}-dependent way (Blaustein, 1975; Redburn et al., 1978; Sandoval and Cotman, 1978), while release from
glia is not believed to be triggered by Ca^{2+} (Blaustein, 1975; Sellström and Hamberger, 1977; Bowery et al., 1979). The depolarization-
-induced release of radioactive acidic amino acids was studied in
superfusion and incubation conditions, using different types of

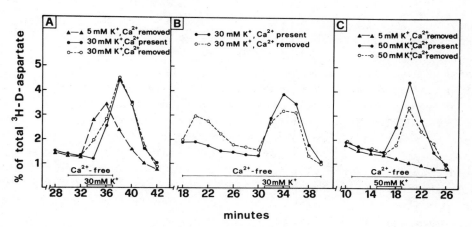

Fig. 3. Depolarization-induced release of ^{3}H-D-aspartate from rat
cerebellar synaptosomal fractions. Crude synaptosomal fractions (P_2) were prelabelled with ^{3}H-D-aspartate (<0.1 μM))
and then superfused (Raiteri et al., 1974). Panel A: the
synaptosomes were labelled during the first part of superfusion with 12 μM ^{14}C-glutamine, and then superfused with
standard medium, followed by media whose composition was
altered as indicated. The figure reports the data on the
release of ^{3}H-D-aspartate, while the release of endogenous
glutamate and of ^{14}C-glutamate derived from ^{14}C-glutamine
are reported in Fig. 4. For other experimental details, see
Levi and Gallo, 1981 and Levi et al., 1982. Panel B: the
time of superfusion with Ca^{2+}-free medium was increased, as
compared to the experiments of panel A, to allow the baseline efflux to resume normal values, before depolarization.
Panel C: the superfusion was performed with media in which
all the NaCl was replaced by Na^+-isethionate, which did not
alter the spontaneous efflux of ^{3}H-D-aspartate, but prevented
the releasing effect of Ca^{2+}-free media. Other changes in the
media are indicated in the figure. The results are expressed
as in Fig. 1 (Data from Levi et al., 1982).

cerebellar slices, showing a different degree of structural integrity,
and, in particular, of glial preservation (Garthwaite et al., 1979).
Minislices (1 x 0.3 x 0.3 mm) (Fig. 1A) prepared by a mechanical
chopper, show a good preservation only of nerve endings, while the
other structures, including glial cells, are badly damaged. Hand-cut

surface slices (0.4 mm thick) (Fig. 1C) exhibit an excellent preservation of all structures (Garthwaite et al., 1979), and chopped
sagittal slices (0.42 mm) (Fig. 1B) are expected to have features in
between these two extremes. In all cases, the release of exogenous
glutamate or D-aspartate induced by high K^+ showed a large Ca^{2+}-de-
pendent component. ^{3}H-D-Aspartate release from hand-cut slices could
be induced also by depolarizing the tissue with veratrine, and this
release could be prevented by tetrodotoxin (Levi et al., 1982). In
conclusion, in spite of the predominant localization of exogenous
acidic amino acids in glia, the release of ^{3}H-D-aspartate from cerebellar slices has features that are characteristic of neurotranmitter
release from neuronal structures, rather than from glia. Studies
performed with freshly isolated glia-enriched fractions and with
glial cultures (Cohen et al., 1979) are consistent with this view
(Fig. 2). With freshly isolated cells, depolarization with high K^+
elicited a non Ca^{2+}-dependent efflux of preaccumulated ^{3}H-D-aspartate,
while with cultured glial cells the depolarizing stimulus did not
evoke ^{3}H-D-aspartate release in the presence of Ca^{2+}, and the removal
of Ca^{2+} from the medium had, by itself, a substantial releasing
effect.

     In order to obtain further information on the characteristics
and on the origin of the glutamate released by depolarization, we
studied the release of exogenous ^{3}H-D-aspartate and of endogenous
and neosynthesized glutamate from cerebellar synaptosomal preparations. These experiments are summarized in Figs. 3 and 4. Crude
synaptosomal fractions were preincubated in the presence of ^{3}H-D-
-aspartate (to label the "reuptake pool") and then superfused with
a medium containing a low concentration of ^{14}C-glutamine, as glutamate precursor (to label the "new synthesis pool"). It has been previously shown that, when glutamine is used as a precursor, the glutamate deriving from glutamine is preferentially released from nerve
endings (Bradford et al., 1978; Hamberger et al., 1979). The labelling
with ^{14}C-glutamine was performed in superfusion conditions (Raiteri
et al., 1974; Raiteri and Levi, 1978), to avoid that the neosynthesized glutamate progressively released is recaptured by the nerve
endings. The depolarization-induced release of ^{3}H-D-aspartate does
not appear to be Ca^{2+}-dependent (Fig. 3A), in contrast with what
was observed with cerebellar slices (see Fig. 1). It will be noted,
however, that Ca^{2+} removal had, by itself, a substantial releasing
effect, which complicates the interpretation of this experiment.
Interestingly, when it was attempted to minimize the releasing effect
of the Ca^{2+}-free medium (either by exposing the synaptosomes to a

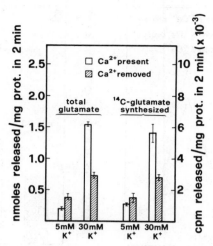

Fig. 4. Ca^{2+}-dependence of the depolarization-induced release of endogenous and newly synthesized glutamate from cerebellar
synaptosomal fractions. Total glutamate and ^{14}C-glutamate previously formed from ^{14}C-glutamine were measured (Levi and Gallo, 1981) in samples from the experiments reported in Fig. 3A.
The spontaneous release was measured in aliquots of the fractions collected at min 32–34, the stimulated release was measured at min 38 (see Fig. 3A) (from Levi and Gallo, 1981).

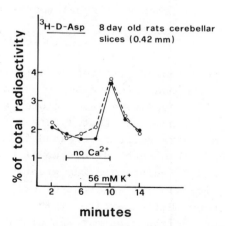

Fig. 5. High K^+-induced release of ^3H-D-aspartate from 8-day rat cerebellar slices. For experimental details, see legend for
Fig. 1B (from Levi et al., 1982).

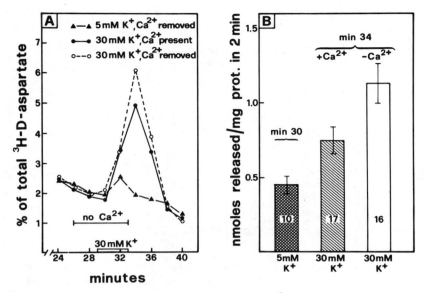

Fig. 6. Depolarization-induced release of ^{3}H-D-aspartate and of endogenous glutamate from 8-day old rat cerebellar synaptosomal
fractions. Crude synaptosomal fractions prelabelled with 90
nM ^{3}H-D-aspartate were superfused for 26 min with standard
medium, and then as indicated in panel A. The release of
^{3}H-D-aspartate is reported in panel A, while panel B shows
the release of endogenous glutamate, as measured during
spontaneous release (min 30) and at the peak of the depolarization-evoked release (min 34) (Data from Levi et al, 1982).

Ca^{2+}-free medium for a longer time before stimulation, or by replac-
ing NaCl with Na$^+$-isethionate in the superfusion medium) a modest
Ca^{2+}-dependence of ^{3}H-D-aspartate release became apparent (Figs. 3B
and 3C). It is evident, however, that a larger Ca^{2+}-dependence would
be expected for a neurotransmitter released from nerve endings. On
the other hand, the high K$^+$-evoked release of endogenous glutamate
and of neosynthesized ^{14}C-glutamate was greatly potentiated by the
presence of Ca^{2+} (Fig. 4). The apparent discrepancy between the
behaviour of exogenous ^{3}H-D-aspartate or ^{14}C-glutamate, and that of
endogenous or neosynthesized glutamate is probably due to the fact
that the exogenous amino acid is accumulated not only in nerve endings, but also in glial fragments (gliosomes) contaminating the preparation. According to the data presented in Fig. 2, the ^{3}H-D-asp-

artate accumulated by glia is not released in a Ca^{2+}-dependent way, and may be released by Ca^{2+}-free media, even in the absence of depolarization.

The Ca^{2+}-dependence of acidic amino acid release observed with cerebellar slices and synaptosomes from adult animals was not present in the same preparations obtained from 8-day old rats (Figs. 5 and 6). At this age, the granule cells are still replicating, and the parallel fibers are very poorly developed (Altman, 1972), while the climbing fibers are in a more advanced stage of development and have synaptic connections with the Purkinje cell perikarya (Balàzs, 1979). Although the lack of Ca^{2+}-dependent release of acidic amino acids at this stage of maturation suggests that, in the adult, the parallel fiber terminals are the main site of origin of the glutamate released, further evidence is necessary to substantiate this conclusion. In fact, even the climbing fibers will undergo a large rearrangement at later stages, and will establish definitive synaptic contacts with the Purkinje cell dendrites (Balàzs, 1979).

In view of the data presented so far, we can attempt the following conclusions:

1. Acidic amino acids appear to be avidly taken up by cerebellar glial cells, in slices and cultures, and by glial fragments present in homogenates. The ability of glia to take up glutamate or aspartate may be greater in the cerebellum than in other CNS areas, and it is possible that glia has, in the cerebellum, a particularly important role in the inactivation of synaptically released glutamate.

2. The behaviour of glia seems to differ in the various in vitro preparations used. The ^{3}H-D-aspartate accumulated by glial cells in slices does not appear to be easily released by depolarization and is not released by Ca^{2+} removal. On the other hand, glial cultures and "gliosomes" do not retain the preaccumulated ^{3}H-D-aspartate when exposed to a Ca^{2+}-free medium.

3. The exogenous ^{3}H-D-aspartate or ^{14}C-glutamate released from slices by depolarizing stimuli is likely to have a neuronal origin, since the release is Ca^{2+}-dependent, and the veratrine-induced release is prevented by tetrodotoxin.

4. The evoked release of endogenous and neosynthesized glutamate from synaptosomal preparations is Ca^{2+}-dependent. The amino acid released probably originates from nerve endings.

5. The absence of a Ca^{2+}-dependent release of glutamate at a developmental stage at which the parallel fibers have not yet developed may suggest that glutamate is released from the terminals of these fibers.

6. Alltogether, the data are consistent with a neurotransmitter role of glutamate in the cerebellum.

PRESYNAPTIC REGULATION OF GLUTAMATE DEPOLARIZATION-INDUCED RELEASE BY GABA

The putative glutamate-releasing terminals of the cerebellar cortex are localized in a "milieu" very rich in cells and terminals utilizing GABA as a neurotransmitter (Curtis and Johnston, 1974; Mc Laughlin et al., 1976; Storm-Mathisen, 1976). For this reason we

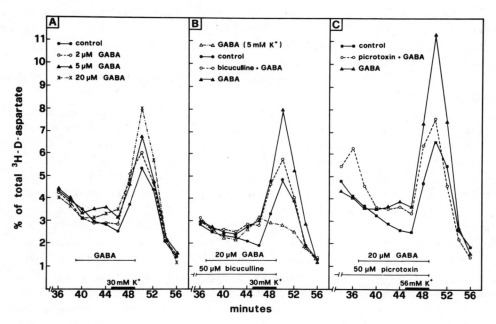

Fig. 7. Effect of GABA on the depolarization-induced release of ^{3}H-D-aspartate from rat cerebellar synaptosomal fractions. Crude synaptosomal fractions were superfused (Raiteri et al., 1974) for 15 min with a Krebs-Ringer medium containing 6 nM ^{3}H-D-aspartate (in some experiments the medium contained 90 nM ^{3}H-D-aspartate and 12 μM ^{14}C-glutamine; see Fig. 9 for results). After washing, the superfusion was continued as indicated in the various panels. Picrotoxin and bicuculline, when present, were added at min 32. The results are expressed as in Fig. 1 (From Levi and Gallo, 1981).

started an investigation aimed at analyzing whether the release of glutamate could be influenced by GABA or GABA agonists.

Figure 7 shows, on the left panel, that low concentrations of GABA (2-20 µM) are capable of potentiating the release of ^{3}H-D-aspartate from synaptosomal preparations depolarized with 30 mM KCl. The effect of GABA was concentration-dependent, and reached its maximum at a concentration of 20 µM. The two GABA antagonists bicuculline and picrotoxin, which, by themselves, did not influence ^{3}H-D-aspartate release, were both able to antagonize the potentiating effect of GABA on the depolarization-induced release of ^{3}H-D-aspartate (Fig. 7, panels B and C), even when the effect of GABA was increased by depolarizing the synaptosomes with a higher KCl concentration (Fig. 7C). Neither one of the two antagonists prevented the small releasing effect of GABA observed in the absence of depolarization (Fig. 7, panels B and C). Therefore, the effect of GABA on the spontaneous release was probably aspecific; as a matter of fact, it was not shared by muscimol (Fig. 8) which, otherwise, behaved very similarly to GABA, both in terms of magnitude of the effect, and of sensitivity to antagonists.

Experiments not presented showed that the release of preaccumulated radioactive glutamate was influenced by GABA and muscimol similarly to that of ^{3}H-D-aspartate. However, in view of the previously mentioned possibility that "gliosomes" present in the preparation accumulate exogenous acidic amino acids, it seemed important to determine whether the effect of GABA or muscimol could be detected also on pools of glutamate different from the "reuptake pool". Therefore, we studied the effect of GABA on the depolarization-evoked release of endogenous glutamate, and of ^{14}C-glutamate previously synthesized from ^{14}C-glutamine. As already mentioned, the latter pool (neosynthesized ^{14}C-glutamate) should be the most representative of the releasable glutamate pool present in nerve endings (Bradford et al., 1978; Hamberger et al., 1979). The results of these experiments, reported in Fig. 9, indicate that GABA potentiated the K^+-induced release of newly synthesized ^{14}C-glutamate, in a picrotoxin-sensitive way, but did not appear to affect the overall release of endogenous glutamate. Thus, it appears that GABA exerts its effect only on certain pools of glutamate, the "reuptake" and the "new synthesis" pool, and not on all the glutamate releasable by depolarization. It has to be noted that, in the experimental conditions used (tracer amounts of exogenous radioactive D-aspartate or glutamine), the "reuptake" and the "new synthesis" pools represent only a minimal fraction of the overall pool of glutamate. Altogether, the data

G. LEVI AND V. GALLO

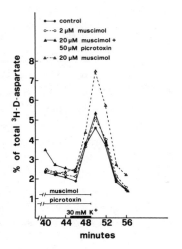

Fig. 8. Effect of muscimol on the depolarization-induced release of
^{3}H-D-aspartate from rat cerebellar synaptosomal fractions. Experimental details as in Fig. 7 (From Levi and Gallo, 1981).

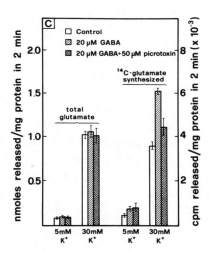

Fig. 9. Effect of GABA on the high K$^+$-induced release of endogenous
and neosynthesized glutamate from cerebellar synaptosomal
fractions. The release of endogenous 'glutamate and of ^{14}C-
glutamate formed from ^{14}C-glutamine was measured before depolarization (min 46) and at the peak of the K$^+$-evoked release
(min 50), in aliquots of effluent fractions of the experiment
reported in Fig. 7B (From Gallo et al., 1981).

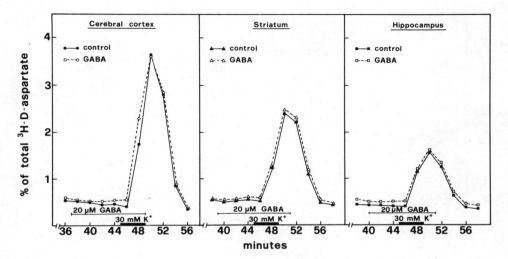

Fig. 10. Absence of GABA effect on ^{3}H-D-aspartate release from cor-
          tical, striatal and hippocampal synaptosomal preparations.
          Experimental details as in the legend for Fig. 7 (From Levi
          and Gallo, 1981).

presented in Figs. 7, 8 and 9 suggest that GABA and muscimol poten-
tiate the depolarization-evoked release of glutamate after interacting with a picrotoxin- and bicuculline-sensitive GABA receptor,
presumably localized on the membrane of glutamate-releasing terminals.

     A study on the regional specificity of the presynaptic GABA
effect is shown in Fig. 10. GABA, at a concentration giving a maximal stimulation of ^{3}H-D-aspartate release in the cerebellum, had
no detectable effect in the cerebral cortex, corpus striatum and
hippocampus.

     The effect of GABA and muscimol on ^{3}H-D-aspartate release was
not present at a developmental stage (8 days post-natal) at which
the parallel fibers have not yet developed (Altman, 1972) (Fig. 11)
and at which glutamate depolarization-induced release is not Ca^{2+}-
-dependent (see Figs. 5 and 6). This observation may suggest that
the GABA receptors responsible for the enhancement of glutamate release are located on the terminals of the parallel fibers. In this
respect, however, see the discussion of the results of Figs. 5 and
6. The right panel of Fig. 11 shows that, in 20-day old cerebella,
the effect of GABA was already similar to that observed in adults.

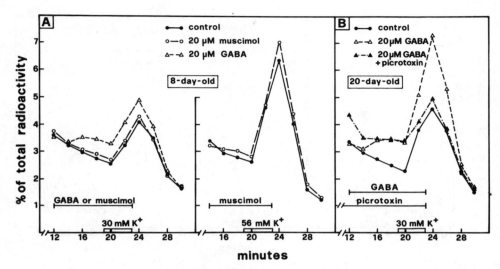

Fig. 11. Effect of GABA and muscimol on the depolarization-induced release of ^{3}H-D-aspartate in 8-day and 20-day rat cerebellar synaptosomal fractions. Experimental details as in Fig. 7.

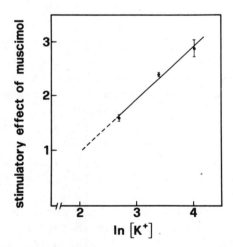

Fig. 12. Relationship between the stimulatory effect of muscimol on ^{3}H-D-aspartate release and the KCl concentration in the depolarizing medium. The stimulatory effect was calculated as ratio between maximal KCl-evoked ^{3}H-D-aspartate release in the presence and in the absence of muscimol. Muscimol concentration: 20 μM. For experimental details, see Fig. 7 (From Levi and Gallo, 1981).

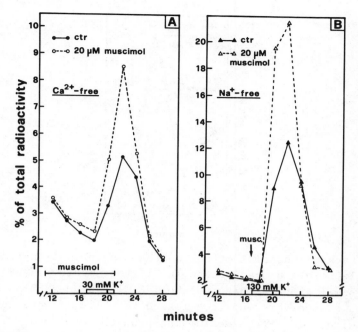

Fig. 13. Effect of muscimol on the depolarization-induced release of
^{3}H-D-aspartate from cerebellar synaptosomal preparations in
the absence of Ca^{2+} (panel A) or Na^+ (panel B). Experimental
conditions as described in the legend for Fig. 7, except
that Ca^{2+} was removed from the superfusion medium starting
from min 5 (panel A), and NaCl was completely replaced by
KCl in the stimulation phase (panel B).

Figure 12 presents a group of experiments performed to study
the relationship between the effect of muscimol on the release of
^{3}H-D-aspartate and the K^+ concentration in the depolarizing medium.
Within the range of K^+ concentrations tested (15-56 mM) the data
point to the existence of a linear relationship between muscimol
effect and logarithm of K^+ concentration. The extrapolation of the
straight line to a value of 1 on the ordinate (that is, to absence
of muscimol effect) corresponds to a K^+ concentration of 7.8 mM,
which is close to the concentration of 5 mM present in our standard
media, and probably too low to cause a significant depolarization of
synaptosomes. The data of this figure are compatible with at least
two models. Depolarization of the membrane may be necessary for the
binding of the ligand to the receptor. In this case, larger depola-

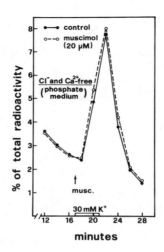

Fig. 14. Lack of muscimol effect on the depolarization-induced release of ^{3}H-D-aspartate in Cl$^-$-free medium. Crude synaptosomal preparations prelabelled with 6 nM ^{3}H-D-aspartate in
a standard medium (see legend for Fig. 7) were superfused
with a Ca^{2+}-free medium in which the NaCl and KCl were replaced by appropriate concentrations of Na$^+$- and K$^+$-phos-
phates. From min 17 to 21, the K$^+$ concentration was increased from 5 to 30 mM, by increasing the concentration of
K$^+$-phosphate.

rizations would allow greater binding. Alternatively, if binding
occurred even in the absence of depolarization, depolarization of the
membrane would be necessary to trigger the so far unknown event
leading to an enhancement of glutamate release. Yet another possibility is not excluded by the data of Fig. 12, namely that the K$^+$ ion
as such is necessary, either for the binding of the ligand, or for
triggering the biological effect.

    In order to understand more thouroughly the mechanism by which
GABA and muscimol exert their effect, we performed a systematic analysis of the ionic requirements of the effect of muscimol on ^{3}H-D-
-aspartate release.

    Figure 13 shows, in the left panel, that the muscimol effect is
not Ca^{2+}-dependent. In fact, the stimulation of ^{3}H-D-aspartate release by muscimol was similar in the absence and in the presence of
the divalent cation. It seemed important to determine whether the
effect of muscimol on the release of newly synthesized ^{14}C-glutamate

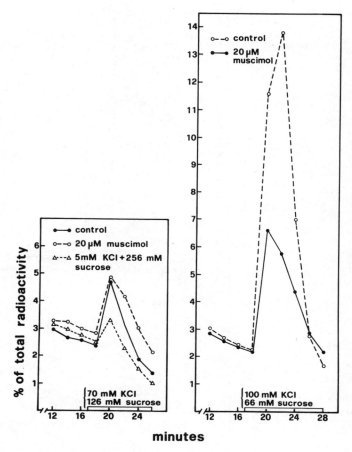

Fig. 15. Chloride-dependence of the effect of muscimol on the depolarization-induced release of ^{3}H-D-aspartate from cerebellar
synaptosomal preparations. Experimental details as in the
legend for Fig. 7, except that, in the depolarization phase,
the NaCl was replaced by KCl and sucrose, at the concentrations indicated in the two panels.

(see Fig. 9) was maintained also in the absence of Ca^{2+}. In a set
of preliminary experiments, we observed that, in spite of the low
depolarization-induced increase of ^{14}C-glutamate release present with
Ca^{2+}-free media (see Fig. 4), muscimol potentiated the evoked release
in a way which was similar, in relative terms, to that observed in

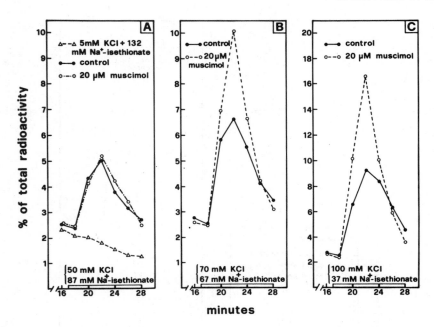

Fig. 16. Chloride-dependence of the effect of muscimol on the depolarization-induced release of ^{3}H-D-aspartate from cerebellar
synaptosomal preparations. Prelabelled (see Fig. 7) crude
synaptosomal fractions were superfused with a Ca^{2+}-free
medium in which the NaCl was replaced by Na^+-isethionate,
or, during the depolarization phase, by KCl and Na^+-ise-
thionate at the concentrations shown in the three panels.

the presence of the cation: in Ca^{2+}-free conditions, the ratio between the evoked release in the presence of muscimol and that in its
absence was 2.0, after subtracting the baseline efflux. In the
experiments with Ca^{2+} (see Fig. 9), in which GABA was used as an
agonist, the ratio was 1.8. It can be deduced that the efficiency
of the presynaptic mechanism regulating glutamate release is not
altered by the absence of Ca^{2+}.

Panel B of Fig. 13 demonstrates that Na^+ is not required for
muscimol to exert its effect. In this experiment, all the NaCl was
replaced by KCl, during the depolarization phase. Another experiment,
not presented here, showed that the effect of muscimol was maintained
unchanged in the absence of Mg^{2+}.

The following group of experiments was performed to assess the

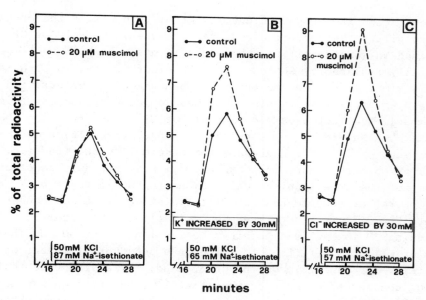

Fig. 17. Reappearance of the muscimol effect upon increasing the K⁺
        or the Cl⁻ concentration. The experiments of panel A are
        the same as those reported in panel A of Fig. 16. In panel
        B, the concentration of K⁺ was brought from 50 to 80 mM by
        adding K⁺-phosphate buffer and the concentration of Cl⁻ was
        kept at 50 mM. In panel C, the concentration of Cl⁻ was
        brought from 50 to 80 mM by adding NaCl, and the concentra-
        tion of K⁺ was kept at 50 mM. In both cases, care was taken
        to maintain constant the osmolarity of the medium.

role of Cl⁻. Since the postsynaptic effects of GABA are mediated by
changes in the Cl⁻ permeability, which lead, in general, to a hyperpolarization of the membrane, it seemed particularly interesting to
examine whether Cl⁻ had a role also in the presynaptic effect of
GABA described in this report. Figure 14 shows an experiment in which
KCl and NaCl were replaced by appropriate concentrations of K⁺- and
Na⁺-phosphates; Cl⁻ was therefore totally removed from the medium.
In these conditions, a depolarization obtained by increasing the concentration of K⁺-phosphate (to give a K⁺ concentration of 30 mM) did
elicit ³H-D-aspartate release, but muscimol was devoid of effect.
This experiment tells us not only that the effect of muscimol can
not manifest itself in the absence of Cl⁻, but also that a high K⁺

concentration is not sufficient, by itself, to elicit the effect,
a possibility that had remained, so far, open. The role of Cl^- was
examined in more detail in other experiments, in which NaCl was
partially replaced by sucrose or by Na^+-isethionate. In both cases,
the muscimol effect became apparent when the Cl^- concentration was
above a critical level. When NaCl was replaced by sucrose (Fig. 15)
the muscimol effect became detectable at Cl^- concentrations above
70 mM. When Na^+-isethionate substituted NaCl (Fig. 16) a concentration
of Cl^- above 50 mM was necessary for muscimol to be effective. It
could be objected that, in these experiments, the appearance of the
effect of the GABA agonist could be due to the increase of K^+ concentration rather than to that of Cl^-. Therefore, in a subsequent experiment (Fig. 17) we brought the concentration of Cl^- from 50 to 80 mM
by adding 30 mM NaCl and leaving the level of K^+ at 50 mM. The addition of Cl^- was sufficient to evidence a substantial effect of muscimol (Fig. 17, panel C). On the other hand, it is also true that muscimol became effective even when the Cl^- concentration was maintained at 50 mM and that of K^+ was increased by adding K^+-phosphate
(Fig. 17, panel B). So, a Cl^- concentration at the borderline of
effectiveness, became effective when the magnitude of the depolarizing stimulus was increased.

        The above reported data on the ionic requirements of the musci-
mol effect on the depolarization-induced release of ^{3}H-D-aspartate
can be summarized as follows:

        1. Muscimol is effective only in the presence of depolarizing
concentrations of K^+. Potassium is not required as such (that is,
as ionic species), but as a depolarizing agent.

        2. Calcium, sodium and magnesium are not required.

        3. A depolarizing concentration of K^+ is a necessary, but not
sufficient condition to observe the effect. In the absence of Cl^-
no effect is present, and a minimum concentration of the anion is
required for muscimol to exert its effect. Depending on the composition of the medium, a Cl^- concentration higher than 50-70 mM is
necessary.

        4. The minimal effective Cl^- concentration becomes lower when
the magnitude of the depolarization is increased.

CONCLUDING REMARKS

        The problem of the molecular mechanism at the basis of the
activation of glutamate release elicited by GABA agonists is not

completely solved by the studies reported in the previous section. In particular, what is the role of depolarization and what is the role of Cl^-? Judging from the published data on GABA or muscimol binding to synaptic membrane preparations, neither K^+ nor Cl^- seem to be important for the binding of the ligand to its receptor (Möhler and Okada, 1978; Placheta and Karobath, 1980; Fujimoto and Okabayashi, 1981). Among the various models that can be proposed, we would like to suggest the following working hypothesis. The depolarization may expose the GABA binding sites on the membrane (or increase their affinity for GABA). The activation of the receptors following the binding of the agonist could produce a picrotoxin-sensitive entry of Cl^- into the presynaptic terminals. The entry of Cl^- would trigger some unknown event, leading to an increased release of glutamate. It may be worth stressing that, according to this hypothesis, the role of Cl^- would be completely different from the role that this anion has at the postsynaptic level. It is clear that the effect of GABA agonists on glutamate release, which is present only during depolarization, could not be explained by the hyperpolarizing action of Cl^- entry.

    As to the possible functional significance of our findings, it may appear paradoxical that an inhibitory neurotransmitter like GABA can promote an increase in the release of an excitatory transmitter like glutamate. However, the paradox may be resolved by considering the architecture of the cerebellar cortex (Palay and Chan-Palay, 1974). The only output of the cerebellar cortex is represented by the Purkinje cells, which are inhibitory in nature. On the other hand, the Purkinje cells represent the main target of cerebellar excitatory fibers, namely the parallel fibers and the climbing fibers. As previously mentioned, acidic amino acids are the likely transmitters of these fibers, and, in particular, glutamate is the putative transmitter of the parallel fibers. It is therefore clear that the ultimate result of the enhancement of glutamate depolarization-induced release elicited by GABA should be an increase in the inhibitory output of the cerebellum, mediated by the Purkinje cells. The cerebellum would thus be endowed with an auxiliary mechanism to increase its inhibitory output. This mechanism would become active only when the glutamate releasing terminals are excited, and would determine a potentiation in the excitation of the efferent inhibitory neurons.

    The origin of the GABA reaching the presynaptic GABAergic receptors located on the glutamate-releasing terminals remains to be established. Besides the possibility that GABA is synaptically released on the excitatory terminals from inhibitory neurons (for example, stellate or basket cells), it could be also conceived that GABA is released as a neuromodulator from Purkinje cell or Golgi cell dendrites onto the contiguous parallel fiber terminals.

Acknowledgements. We thank Mrs. M.T. Ciotti and Mr. A. Coletti for excellent assistance. Part of this work was done in collaboration with Dr. R. Balàzs and his group (MRC Developmental Neurobiology Unit, London, U.K.). The investigation was partly supported by NATO Research Grant n.58.80/DI and by a Grant of the Italian National Research Council (CNR) in the framework of the Italy–U.K. bilateral projects.

REFERENCES

Altman, J., 1972, Postnatal development of the cerebellar cortex in the rat. I. The external granule layer and the transictional molecular layer, J. Comp. Neurol., 1: 353.
Balàzs, R., 1979, Cerebellum: certain features of its development and biochemistry, in: "Development and Chemical Specificity of Neurons", M. Cuénod, G.W. Kreutzberg and F.E. Bloom, eds., Progr. Brain Res., 51: 357.
Balàzs, R., Reagan, C., Meier, E., Woodhams, P.L., Wilkin, G.P., Patel, A.J. and Gordon, R.D., 1980, Biochemical properties of neural cell types from rat cerebellum, in: "Tissue Culture in Neurobiology", E. Giacobini, A. Vernadakis and A. Shahar, eds., p. 155, Raven Press, New York.
Balcar, V.J. and Johnston, G.A.R., 1972, The structural specificity of the high affinity uptake of L-glutamate and L-aspartate by rat brain slices, J. Neurochem., 19: 2657.
Blaustein, M.P., 1975, Effects of potassium, veratridine and scorpion venom on calcium accumulation and transmitter release by nerve terminals in vitro, J. Physiol. (London), 247: 617.
Bowery, N.G., Brown, D.A. and Marsh, S., 1979, α-Aminobutyric acid efflux from sympathetic glial cells: effect of "depolarizing" agents, J. Physiol. (London), 293: 75.
Bradford, H.F., Ward, H.K. and Thomas, A.J., 1978, Glutamine – A major substrate for nerve endings, J. Neurochem., 30: 1453.
Cohen, J., Woodhams, P.L. and Balàzs, R., 1979, Preparation of viable astrocytes from the developing cerebellum, Brain Res., 161: 503.
Curtis, D.R. and Johnston, G.A.R., 1974, Amino acid transmitters in the mammalian central nervous system, Ergebn. Physiol., 69: 97.

Descline, J.C. and Escubi, J., 1974, Effects of 3-acetylpyridine on the central nervous system of the rat, as demonstrated by silver methods, Brain Res., 77: 349.

Fujimoto, M. and Okabayashi, T., 1981, Effect of picrotoxin on benzodiazepine receptors and GABA receptors with reference to the effect of Cl^- ion, Life Sci., 28: 895.

Gallo, V., Levi, G., Raiteri, M. and Coletti, A., 1981, Enhancement by GABA of glutamate depolarization-induced release from cerebellar nerve endings, Brain Res., 205: 431.

Garthwaite, J., Woodhams, P.L., Collins, M.J. and Balàzs, R., 1979, On the preparation of brain slices: morphology and cyclic nucleotides, Brain Res., 173: 373.

Guidotti, A, Biggio, G. and Costa, E., 1975, 3-Acetylpyridine: a tool to inhibit the tremor and the increase in cyclic GMP content in cerebellar cortex elicited by harmaline, Brain Res., 96: 201.

Hamberger, A.C., Chiang, G.M., Nylén, E.S., Scheff, S.W. and Cotman, C.W., 1979, Glutamate as a CNS transmitter. I. Evaluation of glucose and glutamine as precursors for the synthesis of preferentially released glutamate, Brain Res., 168: 513.

Levi, G. and Gallo, V., 1981, Glutamate as a putative transmitter in the cerebellum: stimulation by GABA of glutamic acid release from specific pools, J. Neurochem., 37: 22.

Levi, G., Gordon, R.D., Gallo, V., Wilkin, G.P. and Balàzs, R., 1982, Putative acidic amino acid transmitters in the cerebellum: I. Depolarization-induced release, Brain Res., submitted.

Mc Bride, W.J. and Frederickson, R.C.A., 1980, Taurine as a possible inhibitory transmitter in the cerebellum, Fed. Proc., 39: 2701.

Mc Bride, W.J., Aprison, M.H. and Kusano, K., 1976a, Contents of several amino acids in the cerebellum, brain stem and cerebrum of "staggerer", "weaver" and "nervous" mutant mice, J. Neurochem., 26: 867.

Mc Bride, W.J., Nadi, N.S., Altman, J. and Aprison, M.H., 1976b, Effects of selective doses of X-irradiation on the levels of several amino acids in the cerebellum of the rat, Neurochem. Res., 1: 141.

Mc Bride, W.J., Rea, M.A. and Nadi, N.S., 1978, Effects of 3-acetylpyridine on the levels of several amino acids in different CNS regions of the rat, Neurochem. Res., 3: 793.

Mc Laughlin, B.J., Wood, J.G., Saite, K., Barber, R., Vaughen, J.E., Roberts, E. and Wu, J.Y.,1976, The fine structural localization of glutamate decarboxylase in synaptic terminals of rodent cerebellum, Brain Res., 76: 377.

Möhler, M. and Okada, T., 1978, Properties of α-aminobutyric acid
    receptor binding with (+)-[³H] bicuculline methiodide in rat
    cerebellum, 1978, Molec. Pharmacol., 14: 256.

Palay, S.L. and Chan-Palay, V., 1974, "Cerebellar Cortex - Cytology
    and Organization", Springer-Verlag, Berlin.

Perry, T.L., Mac Lean, J., Perry, T.L.Jr. and Hensen, S., 1976,
    Effects of 3-acetylpyridine on putative neurotransmitter amino
    acids in rat cerebellum, Brain Res., 109: 632.

Placheta, P. and Karobath, M., 1980, In vitro modulation by SQ 20009
    and SQ 65396 of GABA receptor binding in rat CNS membranes,
    Eur. J. Pharmacol., 62: 225.

Raiteri, M. and Levi, G., 1978, Release mechanisms for catecholamines
    and serotonin in synaptosomes, in: "Reviews of Neuroscience",
    vol. 3, S. Ehrenpreis and I. Kopin eds., p. 77, Raven Press,
    New York.

Raiteri, M., Angelini, F. and Levi, G., 1974, A simple apparatus for
    studying the release of neurotransmitters from synaptosomes,
    Eur. J. Pharmacol., 25: 411.

Rea, M.A., Mc Bride, W.J. and Rohde, B.M., 1980, Regional and synapto-
    somal levels of amino acid neurotransmitters in the 3-acetyl-
    pyridine deafferentated rat cerebellum, J. Neurochem., 34: 1106.

Redburn, D.A., Broome, D., Ferkany, J. and Enna, S.J., 1978, Develop-
    ment of rat brain uptake and calcium dependent release of GABA,
    Brain Res., 152: 511.

Roffler-Tarlov, S. and Sidman, R.L., 1978, Concentrations of glutamic
    acid in cerebellar cortex and deep nuclei of normal mice and
    weaver, staggerer and nervous mutants, Brain Res., 142: 269.

Rohde, B.H., Rea, M.A., Simon, J.R. and Mc Bride, W.J., 1979, Effects
    of X-irradiation induced loss of cerebellar granule cells on
    the synaptosomal levels and high affinity uptake of amino acids,
    J. Neurochem., 32: 1431.

Sandoval, M.E. and Cotman, C.W., 1978, Evaluation of glutamate as
    a neurotransmitter of cerebellar parallel fibers, Neuroscience,
    3: 199.

Sellström, A. and Hamberger, A., 1977, Potassium-stimulated α-amino-
    butyric acid release from neurons and glia, Brain Res., 119: 189.

Sidman, R.L., Green, M.C. and Appel, S.H., 1965, "Catalog of the
    Neurological Mutants of the Mouse", Harvard University Press,
    Cambridge.

Storm-Mathisen, J., 1976, Distribution of the components of the GABA
    system in neuronal tissue: cerebellum and hippocampus - effects
    of axotomy, in: "GABA in Nervous System Function", E. Roberts,

T.N. Chase and D.B. Tower eds., p. 149, Raven Press, New York.

Tran, V.T. and Snyder, S.H., 1979, Amino acid neurotransmitter candidates in rat cerebellum: selective effects of kainic acid lesions, Brain Res., 167: 345.

Wilkin, G.P., Balàzs, R., Wilson, J.E., Cohen, J. and Dutton, G.R., 1976, Preparation of cell bodies from the developing cerebellum: structural and metabolic integrity of the isolated "cells", Brain Res., 115: 181.

Wilkin, G.P., Garthwaite, J. and Balàzs, R., 1982, Putative acidic amino acid transmitters in the cerebellum. II. Electron microscopic localization of transport sites, Brain Res., submitted.

Wilson, J.E., Wilkin, G.P. and Balàzs, R., 1975, Biochemical dissection of the cerebellum. Functional properties of the "glomerulus particles", in: "Metabolic Compartmentation and Neurotransmission", S. Berl, D.D. Clarke and D. Schneider eds., p. 427, Plenum Press, New York.

Woodhams, P.L., Wilkin, G.P. and Balàzs, R., 1981, Rat cerebellar cells in tissue culture. II. Immunocytochemical identification of replicating cells in astrocyte-enriched cultures, Dev. Neurobiol., in press.

Young, A.B., Oster-Granite, M.L., Herndon, R.M. and Snyder, S.H., 1974, Glutamic acid: selective depletion by viral-induced granule cell loss in hamster cerebellum, Brain Res., 73: 1.

DEVELOPMENTAL ANALYSIS OF NEUROTRANSMITTER SYSTEMS IN RABBIT RETINA

D.A. Redburn, C.K. Mitchell and C.K. Hampton

Department of Neurobiology and Anatomy
University of Texas Medical School, Houston, TX 77025

The efficacy of chemical transmission is dependent upon a number of transmitter-specific processes associated with both pre and post-synaptic compartments of the synapse. Neurotransmitters are synthesized in the presynaptic compartment of the neuron and maintained in a metabolically protected storage site which can subsequently be made available for release in response to incoming stimuli. Appropriate postsynaptic receptors for each specific transmitter are synthesized by the postsynaptic neuron and maintained in high density at synapses according to the nature of transmitter used at that particular synapse. Degradative enzymes and uptake systems are present in cellular elements surrounding the synapse in order to clear the synaptic cleft of released transmitter, and to replenish pre-synaptic transmitter pools. How this complex set of transmitter-specific processes is established during development is a basic and intriguing question.

The retina offers a highly suitable model system for approaching this question. It is easily accessible, the general structural and functional maturation of its synaptic layers has been characterized (McArdle, et al., 1977; Masland, 1977), and the neurotransmitters utilized by some retinal neurons have been reasonably well-established. (For a review, see Rodieck, 1973). In addition, the five major neuronal cell types of the retinal can be readily identified, even at the light microscopic level, because of the discrete laminar arrangement of cell bodies and synapse with the tissue. (see Fig. 1).

Information flow through the retina is essentially undirectional through three of the cell types. The visual signals generated in the photoreceptor cells are passed through bipolar cells to ganglion cells whose axons form the optic

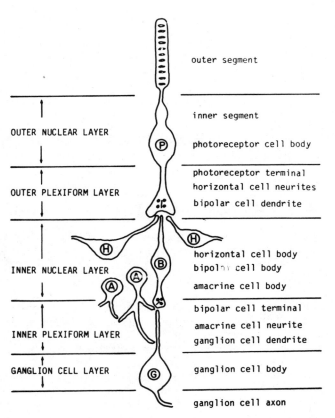

OUTER NUCLEAR LAYER

OUTER PLEXIFORM LAYER

INNER NUCLEAR LAYER

INNER PLEXIFORM LAYER

GANGLION CELL LAYER

outer segment

inner segment

photoreceptor cell body

photoreceptor terminal
horizontal cell neurites
bipolar cell dendrite

horizontal cell body
bipolar cell body

amacrine cell body

bipolar cell terminal

amacrine cell neurite

ganglion cell dendrite

ganglion cell body

ganglion cell axon

Figure 1.   Schematic Representation of the Neurons in the
Vertebrate retina.   On the left are listed the major laminar
divisions of the retina.   On the right are listed the major
cellular elements in each layer. The term "neurite" is used to
designate processes which may be both pre and post-synaptic.

nerve.   Synapses between these cells are restricted to two
well-defined plexiform layers.   Photoreceptor terminals contact
bipolar cell dendrites in the outer plexiform layer; bipolar
terminals synapse with ganglion cell dendrites in the inner
plexiform layer.   Lateral integration occurs within both layers
and is mediated to a large degree by two types of retinal
interneurons: horizontal cells associated with the outer
plexiform layer and amacrine cells associated with the inner
plexiform layer.   There is considerable evidence that amacrine
cells can be divided into a variety of distinct subclasses of
cells   based   upon   differencs   in   electrophysiological,
morphological and neurochemical properties.   We have previously
described a variety of different neurotransmitter systems in
retina, all of which appear to be associated with different

subclasses of amacrine cells (Redburn, 1979). We are now utilizing this well-defined system to follow the developmental pattern of both pre and post-synaptic compartments of the specific neurotransmitter systems present in identified amacrine cell types in the rabbit retina. We report here the general characteristics of the dopamine and GABA systems in adult rabbit retina and the temporal sequence which defines the maturation of these systems during postnatal development.

Two experimental approaches have been utilized in our studies of the dopamine system in rabbit retina. The first is a morphological approach in which ^{3}H-dopamine accumulating neurons were identified by light autoradiography and dopamine containing neurons were identified by glyoxylic acid-induced histofluorescence. (see Fig. 2). As previously reported (Dowling and Ehinger, 1978; Haggendahl and Malmfors, 1973), the population of presumptive dopaminergic cells observed by these methods are localized in the amacrine cell layer in the rabbit retina. There are relatively few dopaminergic cell bodies compared with either cholinergic, glycinergic or GABAergic cell bodies which are also located in the amacrine cell layer. The three distinct bands of dopamine terminals are present within the inner plexiform layer. They are non-uniform in apparent density with the outermost band being the most prominent. It is not clear whether each dopaminergic cell is multistratified or whether each cell terminates in a single layer. However, because of the relatively low number of cell bodies, it is clear that the aborization of each cell whether horizontal and/or vertical, is very extensive.

It is interesting to note that dopaminergic terminals are present in both the outermost portion (sublamina a) as well as the innermost portion (sublamina b) of the inner plexiform layer. Based on the current hypothesis concerning functional organization of the inner plexiform layer, dopamine transmission may play a complex or multifunctional role in processing visual information. Hartline (1938) first observed that the vertebrate retina segregates information processing into two separate channels. The ON channel generates excitatory input at the onset of a focal light stimulus through distinct bipolar, amacrine, and ganglion cell pathways. The OFF channel generates excitatory input at the termination of the stimulus through separate pathways. Elements of the ON pathway are restricted to the innermost portion (sublamina b) of the inner plexiform layer and elements of the OFF pathway are restricted to the outermost portion (sublamina a) (Famiglietti and Kolb, 1976). Cells with more complex responses (on-off type cells) have dendrites in both sublaminae. Since dopaminergic amacrine cell terminals occur in both sublaminae, dopamine function is probably not limited to ON or OFF channels but rather serves a more complex function.

In addition to morphological analyses, we have examined biochemical properties associated with dopamine transmitter function using in vitro assays for uptake, release, receptor binding and dopamine stimulation of adenylate cyclase. These assays allow a more quantitative assessment of the dopamine system compared to the morphological studies and, in addition, a more complete pharmacological analysis including dose response studies are more feasible under in vitro conditions.

A variety of fractionation procedures were analyzed to determine which fraction would be most suitable for these studies. The procedure selected was based on the procedures developed for brain synaptosomal fractions (Redburn, 1977). The highly membranous portions of the retina, the photoreceptor outer segments, were first removed by gentle agitation and rinsing. Homogenization by hand was required to maintain synaptic integrity especially in the large (3μ diameter) terminals from photoreceptors. The homogenate was centrifuged at 150xg for 10 min to remove cell debris and many nuclei. Centrifugation of the resulting supernatant produced a fraction (P_1) containing many large photoreceptor terminals plus significant contamination from inner segments, nuclei and large Muller cell (glial) fragments. A P_2 fraction was obtained after centrifugation at 25,000xg for 12 min. The general composition of this fraction was similar to a synaptosomal fraction from brain and was highly enriched in conventional sized synaptosomes. It is reasonable to assume that most of these terminals are of amacrine cell, inner plexiform layer origin since the amacrine cell terminals constitute the vast majority of conventional sized terminals in retina. The P_2 or inner plexiform layer fraction, as expected, provided an excellent substrate for all of the dopamine functions we have examined. The P_1 or other plexiform layer fraction provided an excellent control fraction for comparison since it clearly contained synaptosomes of photoreceptor cell origin but displayed few of the characteristics associated with dopamine transmitter function.

The uptake of ^{3}H–dopamine by retinal tissue demonstrated the characteristics described for a variety of neurotransmitters in brain: saturation kinetics with increasing time and with increasing ligand concentration; and dependency upon external sodium ions and temperature (Thomas, et al. 1978). The rate of maximum ^{3}H–dopamine uptake/mg protein was approximately 3 to 4 fold higher in the P_2 fraction than in the P_1 fraction or the homogenate. Values for K_m (μM) and V_{max} (pmole/mg protein) were calculated from double reciprocal plots and are as follows: homogenate K_m=0.206, V_{max}=3.497; P_1 K_m=0.181, V_{max}=5.780; P_2 K_m=0.246, V_{max}=14.417.

In order to determine the amount of ^{3}H–dopamine released by potassium–induced depolarization, samples of P_1 and P_2 fractions were incubated in ^{3}H–dopamine, entrapped on a filter and superfused. The small amount of ^{3}H–dopamine taken up by the P_1 fraction was readily lost due to high rates of spontaneous release during perfusion with standard buffer. This may indicate the lack of long-term dopamine storage sites (synaptic vesicles) within the elements of the P_1 fractions. In spite of the high spontaneous release rates, no potassium-evoked release was observed in P_1 fractions either in the presence or absence of calcium. Thus the small amount of ^{3}H-dopamine taken up in the P_1 fraction appears to enter a pool which is not released in a Ca^{++}-dependent manner. In contrast, the P_2 fraction showed a relatively low rate of spontaneous release and a marked increase in release rates in the presence of depolarizing levels of K^+ and 3mM Ca^{++}.

The dopamine system was further characterized by analysis of dopamine receptors in rabbit retina synaptosomes using a ^{3}H-spiperone binding assay (Redburn and Kyles, 1980). Spiperone, formerly known as spiroperidol, is a butyrophenone neuroleptic whose affinity for dopamine receptors in brain tissue is greater than that of any other known drug (Burt, Creese and Snyder, 1977). In addition, ^{3}H-spiperone has been found to label dopamine receptors in vivo and in vitro (Creese, Schneider and Snyder, 1977).

The binding characteristics of rabbit retina appear to be similar to those previously reported for brain (Creese and co-workers, 1977; Fields and colleagues, 1977). The binding of ^{3}H-spiperone was saturable at nmolar concentrations. Scatchard analysis revealed only a single dissociation constant of approximately 0.3 nM which compares to 0.25 nM reported for the highly dopaminergic brain region, the striatum. Receptor density was calculated by Scatchard analysis and equalled approximately 190 pmol/mg protein. Reported values for human, bovine and rat caudate range from approximately 300-500 pmol/mg protein; whole rat brain receptor density is roughly 150 pmol/mg protein (Fields and others, 1977).

The ability of a variety of receptor antagonists to inhibit ^{3}H-spiperone binding indicated a high degree of pharmacological specificity associated with the receptor. Potent antipsychotic drugs such as fluphenazine and haloperidol which are also potent dopamine antagonists, were able to displace receptor binding at nmolar concentrations. Agonists such as dopamine and the inactive (-) stereoisomer of the antagonist (+) butaclamol were less potent displacers.

Although butyrophenones such as spiperone and (+) butaclamol have a very high affinity for the dopamine receptor, there are reports that at higher concentrations they also bind to serotonin receptors (Leysen and others, 1978). In the experiments reported here, low concentrations were used for both the ligand, ^{3}H-spiperone, and the displacer, (+) butaclamol, which should assure that most of the displaceable binding measured was associated with the dopamine receptor. As a further test, an additional compound 2 amino-6,7-dihydroxy-1,2,3,4 tetrahydronaphthalene (ADTN), which binds only to dopamine receptors, was used as displacer in the retina. The amount of

^{3}H-spiperone displaced by 10 μM ADTN and 0.1 μM (+) butaclamol were similar. These data suggest that most of the displaceable [^{3}H]-spiperone binding measured under our conditions was associated with the dopamine receptor.

In the brain, there is considerable evidence that some postsynaptic actions which are stimulated by dopamine-receptor interaction are in fact mediated via the activation of adenylate cyclase (Kebabian and co-workers, 1972). It has been suggested that dopamine receptors can be divided into two classes, one which is associated with adenylate cyclase (D_1); the other which is not (D_2) (Kebabian, 1978). In attempt to further characterize the dopamine receptor, retinal adenylate cyclase activity was analyzed in the presence and absence of dopamine.

In the rabbit retina, dopamine produced a dose dependent increase in cyclic AMP formation. A fifty percent increase in enzyme activity was observed with 100 μM dopamine which is very similar to that seen in brain (Thomas and co-workers, 1978; Clement-Cormier and Redburn, 1978). The highest specific activity of adenylate cyclase was found in the P_2 fraction. Adenylate cyclase activity was also observed in the P_1; however, adenylate cyclase sensitivity to dopamine was not associated with this fraction.

A high degree of pharmacological specificity was demonstrated for the receptor-cyclase complex. Dopamine agonists, apomorphine, N-methyldopamine (epinine) and ADTN mimicked the action of dopamine on adenylate cyclase activity in retinal homogenates and subcellular fraction P_2. Chlorpromazine, a dopamine antagonist, competitively inhibited the activity of the enzyme in the P_2 fraction with a calculated inhibition constant of 5×10^{-8}M. A study of the relative effects of the cis-trans isometric forms of fluphenthixol (a thioxanthene), showed that the (α) isomer of fluphenthixol was a more potent antagonist of adenylate cyclase activity in the retina than the ( ) isomer. In addition, the (+) isomer of butaclamol was more potent than the (−) isomer in blocking the stimulation of adenylate cyclase by dopamine. The inhibition constant for (+) butaclamol was calculated to be 4.5×10^{-8}M.

Characterization of GABA Systems in Adult Retina

Autoradiographic analysis of ^{3}H-GABA accumulating neurons in mammalian retina is complicated by the fact that Muller cell uptake of ^{3}H-GABA is much more pronounced than neuronal uptake (Ehinger, 1977). General methods have been devised to obviate this problem. Yazulla and Brecha (1980) have recently demonstrated that ^{3}H-muscimol competes for the neuronal GABA transport site but not the glia uptake site. The affinity of muscimol for the site is relatively low compared to its affinity for the receptor site, however, it is metabolized slowly and therefore significant amounts can be accumulated and visualized autoradiographically in the absence of appreciable glial labeling.

We have utilized a method for specific labeling of neurons based on the relatively high rates of ^{3}H-GABA metabolism in glial compartments as compared to neuronal compartments (Redburn, 1981). Autoradiograms of adult rabbit retina after 15 min incubation in 2 μM ^{3}H-GABA show heavy accumulation in Muller cells, cells of the amacrine cell layer, and elements of the inner plexiform layer. Postincubation in label-free medium causes a loss of Muller cell labeling, while neuronal cell labeling is enhanced. Three faint bands of label can be discerned in the inner plexiform layer after postincubation. (See Fig. 3).

Inclusion of aminoxyacetic acid, a GABA-transaminase inhibitor, in the incubation medium blocks the loss of Muller cell labeling normally seen after postincubation. Thus, it is suggested that GABA is metabolized by Muller cells while neuronal stores are relatively protected from metabolism.

It is interesting to note that kainic acid, under certain conditions, has a potentiating effect on ^{3}H-GABA uptake into neurons. A variety of laboratories have demonstrated that kainic acid has potent effects on the rabbit retina causing massive depolarization of many neurons, release of some neurotransmitters such as acetylcholine(Massey, S. personal communication) and morphological damage to certain neuronal cell types (Hampton et al, 1981). When kainic acid (10^{-4}M) is included during a 15 min in vivo incubation of rabbit retina in buffer containing 2μM ^{3}H-GABA, neuronal accumulation is virtually eliminated, while Muller cell accumulation is only slightly decreased. However, after a subsequent 30 min postincubation of the tissue in the absence of kainic acid, a dramatic enhancement of neuronal labeling is observed. Our suggestion is that kainic acid causes tonic release of ^{3}H-GABA by depolarization, thus decreasing net accumulation. After removal of kainic acid, the increased accumulation of ^{3}H-GABA may result from a compensatory replenishment of these GABA-depeted neurons.

^{3}H-GABA and ^{3}H muscimol accumulating neuronal cell bodies are relatively numerous compared to ^{3}H-dopamine accumulating somas. Labeled cell bodies are observed both in the amacrine cell layer and in the ganglion cell layer. Labeled cell bodies in the ganglion cell layer may represent displaced amacrine cells rather than ganglion cells since no labeling has been observed in ganglion cell axons. The multistratified distribution of GABA terminals in both sublamina a and b of the innerplexiform layer suggests that GABA, like dopamine, may be functionally involved in both ON and OFF pathways.

We have also characterized the uptake, release and receptor binding properties of the GABA transmitter system in homogenates and subcellular fractions from adult rabbit retinal. ^{14}C-GABA was taken up by homogenates, P_1 and P_2 fractions; however, the greatest binding activity was measured in the P_2 fraction

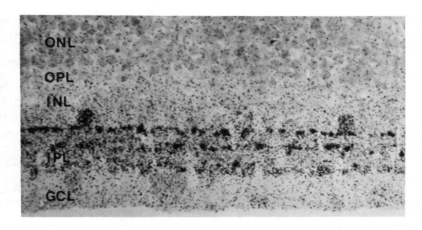

Figure 2. Autoradiography of ^{3}H–dopamine Uptake in Rabbit Retina. Tissue was incubated in vitro for 15 min in buffer containing ^{3}H–dopamine. Label is present in amacrine cell bodies in the inner nuclear layer and in their processes which form 3 distinct bands in the inner plexiform layer. X 600. ONL, outer nuclear layer; OPL, outer plexiform layer; INL, inner nuclear layer; IPL, inner plexiform layer; GCL, ganglion cell layer.

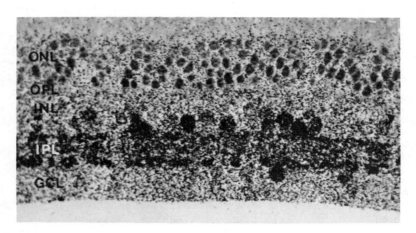

Figure 3. Autoradiography of ^{3}H–GABA Uptake in Rabbit Retina. Tissue was incubated in vitro for 15 min in buffer containing ^{3}H GABA, then post-incubated for 30 min in buffer alone. Amacrine cell bodies in the INL and displaced amacrine cells in the GCL are heavily labeled. The autoradiograph has been overexposed to enhance the labelled bands present in the IPL which represent ^{3}H–GABA uptake into amacrine cell processes. X 520. Designation of layers is the same as in Fig. 2.

which represented less than 5 percent of the total protein in the homogenate (Redburn, 1977). The P_2 fraction sequestered about three times the amount bound by other fractions, when compared on a per milligram protein basis.

The uptake of ^{14}C-GABA was temperature and sodium dependent. The ^{14}C GABA uptake was inhibited in P_1 (75 percent $\pm$ 5 percent, n=3) and in P_2 (74.0 percent $\pm$ 2.1 percent, n=3) by lowering the incubation temperature from 37° to 4^oC. Replacement of sodium chloride with choline chloride in the incubation medium, also reduced uptake: 74.3 $\pm$ 2 percent (n=3) for P_1 fractions and 78.3 $\pm$ 8 percent (n=3) for P_2 fractions. The demonstration of sodium and temperature dependent characteristics illustrate the similarity of the uptake system in retina to the high affinity, GABA uptake system previously described in brain.

Efflux rates of previously accumulated ^{14}C-GABA from retinal fractions were also determined. Addition of depolarizing levels of potassium to samples of a P_2 fraction caused a significant increase in the amount of ^{14}C-GABA released. Subsequent addition of 6 mM calcium caused an additional increase in the release of ^{14}C-GABA from the P_2 fraction of about 3 to 5 percent of the available ^{14}C-GABA pool per minute. A small Ca^{++}-dependent increase in release was observed in homogenates but the increase was not statistically significant. Ca^{++}-dependent release was not observed in P_1 fractions. Addition of 10 mM $MnCl_2$ to the perfusing medium blocked the calcium response in the P_2 fraction.

In order to determine the specificity of the uptake and release mechanisms for ^{14}C-GABA within these retinal fractions, ^{3}H-leucine was substituted for ^{14}C-GABA during incubations. Under these conditions a significantly different release profile was observed. ^{3}H-leucine was accumulated by retinal fractions, however, much less was taken up/mg protein as compared to ^{14}C-GABA. In addition, the efflux of ^{3}H-leucine from the retinal fraction was insensitive to potassium, calcium and manganese.

GABA receptors in rabbit retina homogenates and subcellular fractions were analyzed using an in vitro binding assay with ^{3}H-muscimol as a ligand (Redburn and Mitchell, 1981). ^{3}H-muscimol is a potent GABA receptor agonist that is widely used to tag the GABA receptor because of its high affinity for the site. Yazulla and Brecha (1980) demonstrated that muscimol does bind to the GABA transport site in intact retina; however, in membrane preparations, the amount of binding to the transport site is negligible compared to the binding at the receptor site.

Rabbit retinal synaptosomal fractions bind ^{3}H-muscimol with high affinity and limited capacity. Scatchard analysis revealed two sites with K_D's of 17 and 91 nM. Potent GABA agonists and antagonists were effective displacers of ^{3}H-muscimol binding. Agonists were, in general, better displacers than antagonists with muscimol itself being the most potent displacer tested. GABA and 3-amino-propane-sulfonic acid were equipotent and THIP was the least potent of the agonists tested.

^{3}H-GABA was also used as a ligand in in vitro binding assays of rabbit retinal homogenates (Madtes and Redburn, 1981). Binding characteristics were essentially identical to those of ^{3}H-muscimol binding except that the affinity of ^{3}H-GABA for the receptor was lower than ^{3}H-muscimol and ranged from 40nM for the high affinity site to 400nM for the low affinity site.

Based on these studies, as well as the work from a variety of other laboratories(Dowling and Ehinger, 1978; Brandon et al., 1979), both GABA and dopamine appear to be functional neurotrannsmitters for separate subclasses of amacrine cells. General transmitter properties of both pre and post-synpatic components of these two systems are similar to those described in brain. However, in comparison to brain, these systems in retina represent more well-defined, discretely localized systems which are more amenable for both morphological and biochemical analyses. We have therefore utilized this preparation in order to study characteristics of the postnatal development of neurotransmitter systems. It was of interest to determine not only the temporal sequence of overall transmitter maturation but more specifically, the individual developmental patterns for each component of the two transmitter systems.

Post-natal Development of Dopamine and GABA Transmitter Systems

We have analyzed the development of both pre and post-synaptic components of the dopamine systems in rabbit retinas from 1 day to 20 days postnatal (Redburn et al., 1981). Receptor binding activity was determined first in an in vitro binding assay using ^{3}H-spiperone as a ligand and ADTN as a displacer. Secondly, dopamine stimulation of cAMP formation was assayed. Presynaptic stores of dopamine were visualized by histofluorescence using the glyoxylic acid method. Increases in localized fluorescence after incubation in micromolar concentrations of dopamine were used as an indication of the activity of the high affinity uptake system for dopamine.

Our results showed that at birth, endogenous levels of dopamine were not detectable by histofluorescence. Likewise, no dopamine fluorescence was observed in retinas after a 15 min incubation in 50 μM dopamine in the presence of ascorbate and pargyline. At day 5 endogenous levels were still undetectable; however, in two of the three retinas examined, dopamine fluorescence was observed after incubation with dopamine. A faint band of fluorescence was observed in the outermost portion (sublamina a), of the inner plexiform layer. At day 9, endogenous fluorescence of dopamine first appeared in a band in sublamina a. (See. Fig. 4). Between days 9 and 12, gradual increases were observed in the amounts of endogenous dopamine and

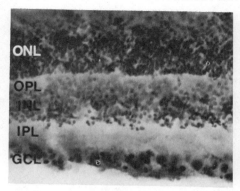 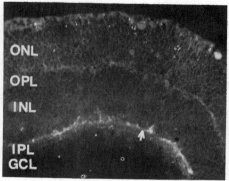

Figure 4-A. Five Day Old Rabbit Retina. Left, a 20 micron frozen section stained with hematoxylin and eosin demonstrates the morphology of the retina at 5 days. X 690. Right, glyoxylic acid-stained 5 day old retina after incubation in 50 µM dopamine. Histofluorescence of dopamine is observed in the outermost band of the IPL (arrow). No endogenous dopamine was observed in this tissue, indicating that although endogenous levels of dopamine are below the limit of detectability using histofluorescence, dopaminergic uptake systems are already present and can accumulate sufficient amounts of dopamine for histofluorescence detection. X 688. Designation of layers is the same as in Fig. 2.

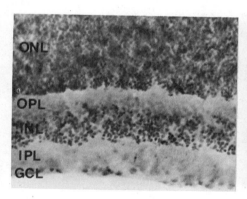 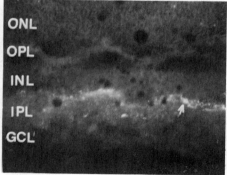

Figure 4-B. Nine Day Old Rabbit Retina. Left, a 20 micron frozen section demonstrates the morphology of the retina at this age (hematoxylin and eosin). X 690. Right, endogenous levels of dopamine are sufficient to be detected by histofluorescence in the 9 day old retina. Dopamine histofluorescence is primarily observed in the outermost band of the IPL (arrow). X 688. Designation of layers is the same as in Fig. 2.

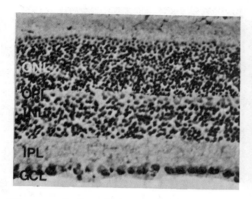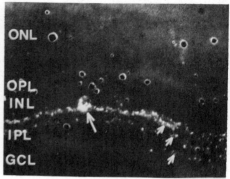

Figure 4-C. Sixteen Day Old Rabbit Retina. Left, a 20 micron frozen section demonstrates the morphology of the retina at this age which is comparable to adult retina (hematoxylin and eosin). X 690. Right, dopamine histofluorescence in 16 day old retina has attained its adult pattern. Fluorescent amacrine cell bodies are present in the INL (large arrow) and three fluorescent bands are visible in the IPL (small arrows). X 688. Designation of layers is the same as in Fig. 2.

in the amount of dopamine taken up by amacrine cells in the inner plexiform layer. Adult patterns of these pre-synaptic markers were observed by day 12.

^{3}H-spiperone binding to the dopamine receptor and dopamine stimulated adenylate cyclase activity displayed similar developmental profiles. At birth no appreciable amount of specific ^{3}H-spiperone binding was observed, and dopamine had no effect on cAMP production. Dramatic increases in these two functions were noted between postnatal days 5 and 9. We observed a significant overshoot in receptor binding and dopamine stimulated adenylate cyclase activity on days 7-9, followed by a decrease to adult levels by day 11.

In a subsequent series of experiments, we have also examined the development of GABA receptor binding using both ^{3}H-muscimol and ^{3}H-GABA as ligands (Redburn and Mitchell, 1981). The binding of ^{3}H-muscimol to GABA receptors in retinal homogenates not treated with Triton X-100 showed a distinct developmental profile. At day 1 through day 5, binding remained at approximately 15 percent of adult levels. A precipitous increase was observed between days 7 and 12, at which time adult levels were reached. Virtually identical results were obtained using ^{3}H-GABA as a ligand and pretreating the tissue with Triton X-100 (Madtes and Redburn, 1981).

We have observed a significant amount of specific binding of ^{3}H-GABA in rabbit retinal homogenates not treated with Triton X-100, which is stimulated by sodium ions and inhibited by low concentrations of nipecotic acid (Redburn, Mitchell, unpublished data). The apparent affinity of this site is approximately 4μM. Binding under these conditions is not significantly inhibited by GABA receptor blockers such as bicuculline or muscimol. These characteristics suggest that the binding observed may be associated with the neuronal GABA transport site. Using 1 mM unlabeled GABA as a displacer and 3 μM ^{3}H–GABA as the ligand in the presence of sodium perchlorate, we observed significant amounts of binding in retinas from one day old rabbits. The concentration of presumptive transport sites doubled by day 3 and remained stable with a slight decrease between 9 and 11 days postnatal.

In contrast, when unlabeled nipecotic acid, a potent uptake blocker was used as a displacer; a significantly different developmental profile was observed. A significant amount of nipecotic acid–sensitive binding was observed at birth and remained virtually unchanged until day 9 postnatal. However, a dramatic two and one–half fold increase in the amount of binding was observed at day 11 with a continued upward trend on day 13. These data suggest that the GABA transport site may be present at birth, but that final maturation may not be reached until after 13 days postnatal.

Conclusions

The biochemical and morphological analyses of dopaminergic and GABAergic systems in rabbit retina provided a highly suitable preparation for investigations of transmitter maturation in a well–defined system. Our results demonstrate that the emergence of endogenous pools of dopamine and a high affinity dopamine uptake system closely coincide with the appearance of dopamine receptor binding sites as well as those systems which couple the receptor to regulators of adenylate cyclase.

The dopamine histofluorescent pattern appears to be an appropriate marker for the presynaptic compartment of neurons which are destined to become the dopaminergic amacrine cells of the adult retina. Dopamine histofluorescence observed throughout development is restricted to cell bodies in the amacrine cell layer and a trilaminar arrangement of terminals in the inner plexiform layer. The most prominent lamina is located directly adjacent to the inner nuclear layer. The other two minor bands are located in the middle and innermost aspect of the inner plexiform layer. Autoradiographic, histochemical and histofluorescent studies have clearly shown that dopaminergic amacrine cells of the adult rabbit retina display precisely the same morphological characteristics (Dowling and Ehinger, 1978). Thus, it appears that the adult pattern of morphological relationships among dopaminergic cell bodies, their processes and other retinal neurons is established at the onset of dopaminergic differentiation and remains, for the most part, unchanged during development. One minor change was observed in that the more prominent lamina of dopamine terminals was frequently observed at earlier stages of maturation than the two minor bands. This observation may suggest that growing neurites of developing amacrine cells reach their most distant synaptic targets in the more proximal retina at a later stage in development. Alternatively, the level of dopamine present in the relatively less dense bands at early stages of development, may be below the sensitivity of the assay.

The absolute sensitivity of the histofluorescent technique is difficult to ascertain. In a recent study, dopamine levels in retinal homogenates from different aged rabbits were determined by radioenzymatic assay (Lam et al., 1981). Dopamine concentration was reported to be approximately 0.25 μM through day 7 with an abrupt increase to 0.6μM on day 9 and 1μM by day 12 postnatal. Our histofluorescent studies are in agreement with these findings in that distinct endogenous pools are first visualized on day 9.

In the adult retina, the endogenous fluorescence of dopaminergic cells was significantly enhanced when the tissue is pre-incubated in μmolar concentrations of dopamine. The increase in fluorescence is thought to be an indication of the activity of the specific uptake system for dopamine. In retinas from newborn rabbits, we were unable to demonstrate any fluorescence, either endogenous or taken up. At day 5 postnatal, fluorescence was observed only after incubation. By day 9, endogenous fluorescence was observed and the fluorescence was enhanced after incubation with dopamine. The data suggest that the uptake system for dopamine can function to accumulate detectable stores of dopamine at a time during early development (at about 5 days postnatal) when synthetic enzymes have not yet produced detectable stores of endogenous dopamine.

Autoradiographic studies also suggest that dopamine uptake systems are functional very early in development. However, autoradiographic localization of dopamine was observed at birth (Lam et al., 1981) which preceded our observation by about 5 days. Our failure to observe dopamine accumulation by histofluorescence at birth may simply reflect the greater sensitivity of the autoradiographic technique for these measurements.

Several interesting points were noted in the postnatal development of dopamine receptors. The binding site and its ability to stimulate adenylate cyclase displayed identical developmental profiles. At no time in development did the amount of receptor binding increase without a similar increase in the activity of dopamine stimulated adenylate cyclase. Thus it appears that the coupling of the receptor to the cyclase enzyme is established at the time of emergence of the receptor system.

The increase in dopamine receptors from non-detectable levels to twice adult levels within a 2-3 day span, was striking. Such a precipitous rise in receptors is in conspicuous contrast to developmental patterns of many other transmitter functions. It is tempting to speculate that the increase in receptor function may be specifically triggered or induced and may in fact involve unmasking or activation of sites rather than de novo synthesis.

There is an obvious overshoot in dopamine receptor function at days 7-9, followed by a decrease to adult levels by day 11. The total number of retinal neurons decrease significantly from birth to adult stages (McArdle et al., 1977). Thus the loss of dopamine receptor function may reflect the loss of cells which are dopamine-receptive. Alternatively, the decrease may be due to a specific down-regulation of dopaminergic input. It is interesting to note that the decrease in dopamine receptor function coincides with the time at which eyes open and mature receptive field responses can be recorded in ganglion cells (Masland, 1977).

Our studies of GABAergic development in rabbit retina have primarily focused on receptor binding with some preliminary data on binding which may be associated with the GABA uptake site. Similar data was obtained using ^{3}H-muscimol as a receptor ligand without Triton X-100 pretreatment and using ^{3}H-GABA as a ligand after Triton X-100 treatment. Our data suggest that GABA receptors appear at a later stage in development than dopamine receptors. In addition, there is no apparent overshoot in the developmental profile of the GABA receptor but rather a simple increase to adult levels which occurs between day 7-8 to day 14. The period of rapid increase in GABA receptor binding coincides with the period of maximum increase in retinal synaptic density. Also, receptor binding reaches 80 percent of adult levels at approximately the time of the appearance of mature receptive field responses in some ganglion cells (Masland, 1977).

Binding to the presumptive GABA transport site suggests that the uptake system may be present very early during development. These results are consistent with autoradiographic studies which demonstrate neuronal localization of ^{3}H-GABA at birth (Lam et al., 1980). In our studies, significant levels of binding were observed at birth; adult levels were reached by day 3 postnatal. However, sensitivity of the site to nipecotic acid changed significantly at day 9. The amount of nipecotic acid displaceable binding had not fully reached adult levels by day 13. These data suggest that GABA uptake sites may be present in an immature form at birth and that some developmental change occurs at about day 9 which establishes the pharmacological sensitivity of the system seen in the adult.

The change in pharmacological sensitivity may be also related to functional maturity of the system. As shown by Lam et al. (1980) Ca^{++}-dependent, K^+-stimulated release of ^{3}H-GABA was not demonstrable in rabbit retinas until day 5. Thus the GABA sequestered by retinas prior to that time does not reside in a releaseable pool. We have previously shown that synaptosomes isolated from developing rat brain demonstrate active uptake of

Table I. Developmental analysis of dopaminergic and GABAergic components in rabbit retina. Quantitative determinations are listed at each postnatal day as an approximate percentage of the values observed at 13 days postnatal. Qualitative observations of relative levels of histofluorescence are noted by the relative number of arrows. Nondetectable levels are noted by a dash.

Dopamine

days postnatal	endogenous fluorescence	accumulated fluorescence	receptor binding	dopamine stimulated adenylate cyclase
1.	–	–	–	–
3.	–	–	–	–
5.	–	↑	100	100
9.	↑	↑↑	200	180
11.	↑↑	↑↑↑	200	190
13.	↑↑↑	↑↑↑	100	100

GABA

days postnatal	transport binding displaced by GABA	transport binding displaced by nipecotic acid	receptor binding
1.	50	50	20
3.	100	50	20
5.	100	50	20
9.	100	80	50
11.	100	90	80
13.	100	100	100

^{3}H—GABA long before Ca^{++}—dependent K$^+$ —stimulated release can be demonstrated (Redburn et al., 1978). Thus a similar phenomenon is present in brain.

The composite of developmental patterns shown in Table I takes into account most of the data described above. Significant differences are noted in the profiles of specific components of the GABAergic and dopaminergic systems. However, it is clear that both systems begin to emerge before the retina is exposed to partially focused light at the time of eye opening. In fact, the developmental changes appear to be orchestrated so as to provide near—maximal function in each component on the day the eyes are opened. Most components of the neurotransmitter systems develop postnatally with the possible exception of uptake systems which may develop prenatally and, in the case of GABA, undergo further maturational changes after birth. The rabbit retina has provided a highly suitable substrate for developmental analysis of emerging transmitter systems and will be analyzed in even greater detail in our future studies.

REFERENCES

Brandon, C., Lam, D.M.K. and Wu, J.-Y, 1979. The GABA system in the rabbit retina: localization by immunocytochemistry and autoradiography. Proc. Nat. Acad. Sci. USA 76:3557–3561.

Burt, D.R., Creese, I. and Snyder, S.H., 1977. Properties of ^{3}H—haloperidol and ^{3}H—dopamine binding associated with dopamine receptors in calf brain membranes. Molec. Pharmacol. 12:800–812.

Clement-Cormier, Y. and Redburn, D.A., 1978. Dopamine sensitive adenylate cyclase in retina: subcellular distribution. Biochem. Pharmacol. 27:2281–2282.

Creese, I., Schnieder, R. and Snyder, S.H., 1977. ^{3}H—spiroperidol labels dopamine receptors in pituitary and brain. Eur. J. Pharm. 46:377–81.

Dowling, J. and Ehinger, B., 1978. Synaptic organization of the dopaminergic neurons in the rabbit retina. J. Comp. Neurol. 180:203–220.

Ehinger, B., 1977. Glial and neuronal uptake of GABA, glutamic acid, glutamine and glutathione in the rabbit retina. Exp. Eye Res. 25:221–234.

Famiglietti, E.V. and Kolb, H., 1976. Structural basis for ON and OFF—center responses in retinal ganglion cells. Science 194:193–195.

Fields, J.Z., Reisine, T.D. and Yamamura, H.I., 1977. Biochemical demonstration of dopaminergic receptors in rat and human brain using ^{3}H-spiroperidol. Brain Res. 136:578-584.

Haggendahl, J. and Malmfors, T., 1973. Evidence of dopamine-containing neurons in the retina of rabbits. Acta Physiol. Scand. 62:295-296.

Hampton, C.K., Garcia, C. and Redburn, D.A., 1981. Localization of kainic acid-sensitive cells in mammalian retina. J. Neurosci. Res. 6:99-111.

Hartline, H.K., 1938. The response of single optic nerve fibers of the vertebrate eye to illumination of the retina. Am. J. Physiol. 121:400-415.

Kebabian, J.W., Petzald, G.L. and Greengard, P., 1972. Dopamine sensitive adenylate cyclase in caudate nucleus of rat brain and its similarity to the dopamine receptor. Proc. Nat. Acad. Sci. U.S.A 69:2145.

Kebabian, J.W., 1978. Multiple classes of dopamine receptors in mammalian central nervous system: the involvement of dopamine-sensitive adenylate cyclase. Life Sci. 23:479-484.

Lam, D.M.K., Fung, S.C. and Long, Y.C., 1980. Postnatal development of GABAergic neurons in the rabbit retina. J. Comp. Neurol. 193:89-102.

Lam, D.M.K., Fung, S.C. and Kong, Y.C., 1981. Post-natal development of dopaminergic neurons in rabbit retina. J. Neurosci. In press.

Leysen, J.E., Niemegeers, C.J.E., Tollenaere, J.O. and Laudron, P.M., 1978. Serotonergic components of neuroleptic receptors. Nature 272:168-171.

McArdle, C.B., Dowling, J.E. and Masland, R.H., 1977. Development of outersegments and synapses in the rabbit retina. J. Comp. Neurol. 175:253-264.

Madtes, P. and Redburn, D.A., 1981. GABA binding in developing rabbit retina. Submitted for publication.

Masland, R.H., 1977. Maturation of function in the developing rabbit retina. J. Comp. Neurol. 175:275-286.

Redburn, D.A. 1977. Uptake and release of ^{14}C-GABA from rabbit retina synaptosomes. Exp. Eye Res. 25:265-275.

Redburn, D.A., Broome, D.S. and Enna, S., 1978. Developmental analysis of synaptosomal uptake and release of ^{14}C-GABA. <u>Brain Res.</u> 152:511-519.

Redburn, D.A., 1979. A review of neurotransmitters in retina. <u>Tex. Soc. Electron Microscopy</u> 10:12-19.

Redburn, D.A. and Kyles, C.B., 1980. Localization and characterization of dopamine receptors within two synaptosome fractions of rabbit and bovine retina. <u>Exp. Eye Res.</u> 30:699-708.

Redburn, D.A., 1981. GABA and glutamate as neurotransmitters in rabbit retina in "Glutamate as a Neurotransmitter" (G. DiChiaramel G.L. Gessa eds.) pp. 79-89, Raven Press, New York.

Redburn, D.A. and Mitchell, C.K., 1981. ^{3}H-muscimol binding in synaptosomal fractions from bovine and developing rabbit retinas. <u>J. Neurosci. Res.</u> In press.

Redburn, D.A., Mitchell, C.K., Hampton, C.K. and Clement-Cormier, Y., 1981. Developmental analysis of dopamine histofluorescence, receptor binding and adenylate cyclase activity in rabbit retina. Submitted for publication.

Rodieck, R.W., 1973. "The Vertebrate Retina" W.H. Freeman and Co., San Francisco.

Thomas, T.N., Clement-Cormier, Y. and Redburn, D.A., 1978. Dopamine uptake and dopamine sensitive adenylate cyclase activity of retinal synaptosomal fractions. <u>Brain Res.</u> 155:394-396.

Yazulla, S. and Brecha, N., 1980. Binding and uptake of the GABA analogue, ^{3}H-muscimol, in the retinas of goldfish and chicken. <u>Invest. Ophthalmol. Vis. Sci.</u> 19:1415-1426.

GRANULAR VESICLES OF THE POSTERIOR PITUITARY : A MODEL FOR PEPTIDE

SYNTHESIS AND TRANSPORT

B.T. Pickering

Department of Anatomy, University of Bristol
The Medical School, Bristol BS8 1TD, England

The hormones of the posterior pituitary, oxytocin and vasopressin, are secreted by neurones which have their perikarya in the supraoptic and paraventricular nuclei of the hypothalamus, and their axon terminals in the posterior pituitary or neuro-hypophysis. Since polypeptide synthesis occurs in the perikaryon and release is from the axon terminals, there is an anatomical distribution of the various phases of the secretory process and the hypothalamo-neurohypophysial neurone is therefore an excellent model for the study of polypeptide secretion (Pickering, 1978).

Along with the hormones the neurones secrete a family of 90-95 residue polypeptides, the neurophysins. Each hormone is biosynthetically related to its own neurophysin through the sharing of a common precursor polypeptide - propressophysin giving rise to vasopressin and vasopressin-neurophysin, and pro-oxyphysin yielding oxytocin and oxytocin-neurophysin (Russell et al, 1980). Since the neurophysins as well as the hormones are rich in cystine residues, their biosynthesis and passage through the cell can be followed using $[^{35}S]$cysteine as a tracer. In this way it has been shown that the precursor can be synthesised, packaged into granules and transported to axon terminals within 1-1½h. Thus secretory granules are transported at a velocity of about 75 mm/day and processing of the precursor occurs within the granule during transport (Pickering et al, 1975; Brownstein et al, 1980).

Granule transport can be inhibited with colchicine. The arrested granules build up in the perikaryon but processing continues normally so that fully-formed products also build up

99

(Parish et al, 1981). The inhibitor of glycosylation, tunicamycin,
also leads to a build-up of secretory product in the perikaryon, but
in this case packaging is inhibited and the product accumulates
within the cisternae and dilatations of the rough endoplasmic
reticulum (González et al, 1981). Thus glycosylation of product
or a membrane component is essential for the normal formation of
secretory granules. Preliminary experiments suggest that
processing is incomplete in the tunicamycin-treated cell so
that packaging into granules is necessary to complete the synthetic
pathway as well as to convey the secretory product from site of
synthesis to release site.

References

Brownstein, M.J., Russell, J.T. and Gainer, H., 1980, Synthesis,
    transport and release of posterior pituitary hormones,
    Science NY, 207:373-378.
González, C.B., Swann, R.W. and Pickering, B.T., 1981, Effects of
    tunicamycin on the hypothalamo-neurohypophysial system of the
    rat, Cell Tissue Res., 217:199-210.
Parish, D.C., Rodríguez, E.M., Birkett, S.D. and Pickering, B.T.,
    1981, Effects of small doses of colchicine on the components
    of the hypothalamo-neurohypophysial system of the rat, Cell
    Tissue Res., (in press).
Pickering, B.T., 1978, The neurohypophysial neurone : a model for
    the study of secretion, Essays in Biochemistry, 14:45-81.
Pickering, B.T., Jones, C.W., Burford, G.D., McPherson, M., Swann,
    R.W., Heap, P.F. and Morris, J.F., 1975, The rôle of
    neurophysin proteins : suggestions from the study of their
    transport and turnover, Ann. NY Acad. Sci., 248:15-35.
Russell, J.T., Brownstein, M.J. and Gainer, H., 1980, Biosynthesis
    of vasopressin, oxytocin and neurophysins : isolation and
    characterization of two common precursors (propressophysin
    and pro-oxyphysin), Endocrinology, 107:1880-1891.

CALMODULIN MODULATION OF THE

CALCIUM SIGNAL IN SYNAPTIC TRANSMISSION

Robert John DeLorenzo

Department of Neurology
Yale Medical School, 333 Cedar Street
New Haven, CT 06510

INTRODUCTION

Ca^{2+} plays a major role in the function of nervous tissue[1,2]. One of the most widely recognized roles of Ca^{2+} in synaptic function is its action in neurotransmission. Early studies showed that the release of neurotransmitter substances by vertebrate neuromuscular junctions was dependent upon the Ca^{2+} ion concentration in the media[1-3]. Elegant studies at the synaptic level most convincingly demonstrated that the effects of Ca^{2+} on neurotransmission were not secondary to effects of Ca^{2+} on the presynaptic action potential, but were directly dependent upon the entry of Ca^{2+} into the nerve terminal[4-7]. The role of Ca^{2+} in stimulus-secretion coupling has also been demonstrated in a variety of secretory processes in several tissues[8]. Thus, the role of Ca^{2+} in synaptic function is well established. One of the major questions in neuroscience research at the present time is what is the molecular mechanism mediating the effects of Ca^{2+} on synaptic activity.

Research in my laboratory over the last ten years has been directed at providing a molecular approach to studying the biochemistry of the Ca^{2+}-signal in neurotransmitter release and synaptic modulation. In vitro and in vivo preparations were developed and employed to study the effects of Ca^{2+} on neurotransmitter release[9,11], synaptic protein phosphorylation[11-18], and synaptic vesicle and synaptic membrane interactions[9,19-21]. These studies provided an experimental framework to demonstrate that calmodulin, a major Ca^{2+}-receptor protein in brain[22], modulates many of the biochemical effects of Ca^{2+} on synaptic preparations. From this evidence the calmodulin hypothesis of neuronal transmission was developed[9,11,19,21]. This hypothesis states that as Ca^{2+} enters the presynaptic nerve terminal,

101

it binds to calmodulin and activates several Ca^{2+}-calmodulin regulated processes that modulate synaptic activity. In this paper the
evidence from my laboratory for the role of calmodulin in synaptic
activity will be presented.

SYNAPTIC CALMODULIN

Calmodulin is a heat stable, Ca^{2+}-binding protein that is
structurally very similar to troponin C from skeletal muscle[22].
Calmodulin is present in many tissues and animal and plant species[22].
The importance of this Ca^{2+} receptor protein in mediating the actions
of Ca^{2+} in cellular functions has been emphasized. As recently
reviewed[22,23], it is now becoming accepted that calmodulin may be a
universal receptor, mediating the many diverse effects of Ca^{2+} on
cellular functions. Calmodulin is found in high concentrations in
brain[22,23]. However, to implicate this Ca^{2+} regulator protein in
synaptic function, it is necessary to demonstrate that calmoduin is
present at the synapse.

A vesicle-bound heat stable protein was isolated from highly
enriched preparations of synaptic vesicles from rat cortex that had
the same molecular weight as calmodulin[11]. This vesicle bound
protein could be removed from the vesicles in the presence of EGTA
and was found to bind Ca^{2+} at micromolar concentrations[9,19]. When
compared to calmodulin isolated from whole rat brain, the vesicle-
Ca^{2+} binding protein was found to be identical to calmodulin in
molecular weight (Figure 1), amino acid composition, isoelectric
point, and in its ability to stimulate vesicle protein kinase, adenylate cyclase and phosphodiesterase activity[9,19]. Vesicle calmodulin
represented 0.92% of the total protein in synaptic vesicle fractions[9].

A heat stable, Ca^{2+} binding protein,was also isolated from
nerve terminal synaptoplasm prepared by standard procedures[9,19].
Approximately 80-90% of the protein in this synaptoplasmic preparation
has been shown to originate in the presynaptic terminal[24]. This
synaptic protein (Figure 1) was found to be identical to whole brain
calmodulin in molecular weight, isoelectric point, amino acid composition, and ability to stimulate protein kinase and phosphodiesterase activity[9,19]. Synaptic calmodulin comprised 0.71% of the total
protein in the synaptoplasm preparation[9]. Since the concentration
of calmodulin in whole brain fractions is approximately 1% of the
total brain protein, the high percentage of calmodulin in synaptoplasm and synaptic vesicle fractions strongly indicate the presence
of this Ca^{2+} receptor protein in the presynaptic nerve terminal.

Calmodulin has been shown to be present in postsynaptic density
regions of cerebral cortex by immunological procedures[25]. In
addition, calmodulin has been isolated from postsynaptic density
preparations[25-27].

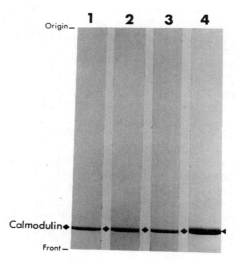

Figure 1. Electrophoretic protein patterns on SDS-polyacrylamide gel of calmodulin isolated from whole rat brain cytosol, synaptosome cytosol, and synaptic vesicles, and a mixture of all three calmodulin preparations as shown in channels 1-4, respectively. Whole brain cytosol[30], synaptosome cytosol[9], and synaptic vesicle[11] preparations were prepared by standard procedures. Each fraction was then subjected to heat treatment, column chromatography, and preparative gel electrophoresis to obtain a highly enriched preparation of calmodulin as described by Lin et al[30]. Calmodulin isolated from synaptosome cytosol and synatpic vesicles behaved identically during the isolation procedure to calmodulin isolated from whole brain. Calmodulin represented approximately 0.96%, 0.71%, and 0.92% of the total protein in brain cytosol, synaptosome cytosol, and synaptic vesicle preparation, respectively (reproduced from Reference 9).

These results strongly indicate that calmodulin is present in both presynaptic and postsynaptic regions of the synapse. Thus, calmodulin is present at the synapse and capable of mediating the effects of Ca^{2+} on synaptic function.

CALMODULIN-DEPENDENT NEUROTRANSMITTER RELEASE

Since the evidence strongly indicates that calmodulin is present at the synapse, this Ca^{2+}-receptor protein is an attractive pre-synaptic protein for modulating the effects of Ca^{2+} on neurotransmitter release. As Ca^{2+} enters the presynaptic ending, it can bind to this high affinity receptor and initiate several biochemical processes involved in synaptic function[9,19]. The first evidence that Ca^{2+}-stimulated neurotransmitter release may be calmodulin dependent was obtained from studies on isolated synaptic vesicles[10,11].

A more physiological procedure for isolating synaptic vesicles was developed[10,11] and vesicles from this isolation procedure were shown to be much more responsive to Ca^{2+} than vesicles prepared under the standard hypotonic isolation methods[28,29]. Ca^{2+} in the presence of ATP and Mg^{2+} simultaneously initiated the release of vesicle neurotransmitter substances[9-12], vesicle protein phosphorylation[10-14], and vesicle and membrane interactions[9,19-21]. The Ca^{2+} responsive synaptic vesicle preparation was then studied to determine if cal-modulin mediated the effects of Ca^{2+} on vesicle neurotransmitter release.

The vesicles prepared under more physiological procedures that simulated the intracellular environment[10] also contained calmodulin[9]. The calmodulin in the vesicle preparation was tightly bound to the vesicle surface and could be selectively removed by washing the vesi-cles with the Ca^{2+} chelating agent, EGTA[9-12]. Thus, it was possible to obtain preparations of calmodulin containing (plain vesicles) and calmodulin depleted (treated vesicles) vesicles. These vesicle fractions were then studied for neurotransmitter release (Table 1).

Ca^{2+} in the presence of calmodulin stimulated the release of norepinephrine[9,11], acetylcholine[9,19], and dopamine[9,11], from calmodu-lin depleted vesicles (Table 1). Ca^{2+} or calmodulin alone, however, had no significant effect on neurotransmitter release (Table 1). Trifluoperazine, a phenothiazine that inactivates calmodulin[23,31], also inhibited Ca^{2+}-calmodulin stimulated vesicle neurotransmitter release[19,21] (Table 1). The calmodulin kinase inhibitors, pheny-toin[12,16,17] and diazepam[32-34], were also found to inhibit Ca^{2+}-calmodulin stimulated vesicle neurotransmitter release (Table 1). The Ca^{2+}-calmodulin stimulation of release was also shown to be dependent on Mg^{2+} and ATP[9-11] and vesicles prepared under hypotonic conditions[28,29] didn't show significant Ca^{2+}-calmodulin stimulated re-lease of neurotransmitter substances. These results demonstrate

Table 1. Effects of Calmodulin and Ca^{2+}-Calmodulin Kinase Inhibitors on Ca^{2+}-Calmodulin Stimulated Protein Phosphorylation and Neuro-transmitter Release in Isolated Synaptic Vesicles

Condition	Neurotransmitter Release (%)		Protein DPH-M Phosphorylation (%)
	Acetylcholine	Norepinephrine	
Control	34	38	21
Ca^{2+}	41	44	25
Calmodulin	36	39	22
Ca^{2+} + Calmodulin	100	100	100
Ca^{2+} + Calmodulin			
+ Trifluoperazine	62	68	55
+ Phenytoin	69	72	49
+ Diazepam	61	63	47

Calmodulin depleted synaptic vesicles were isolated and studied for neurotransmitter release and protein DPH-M phosphorylation as described previously.[9],[11] The data give the means of 10 determinations and are expressed as percent of the maximally stimulated condition (100%). The largest ± S.E.M. was 5.6. The effects of trifluoperazine (15 μM), phenytoin (80 μM), and diazepam (15 μM) were found to be statistically significant in comparison to maximally stimulated values. P < 0.001 (reproduced from Reference 19).

Table 2. Effects of Calmodulin and Ca^{2+}-Calmodulin Kinase Inhibitors on Neurotransmitter Release and Protein Phosphorylation in Intact Nerve Terminal Preparations

Condition	Neurotransmitter Release(%)		Protein Phosphorylation(%)	
	Acetylcholine	Norepinephrine	Whole Synaptosome	Synaptic Vesicles
Control	45	52	58	39
Ca^{2+}	51	56	61	44
Ca^{2+}, K	100	100	100	100
+ Trifluoperazine	63	68	69	61
+ Phenytoin	68	70	68	67
+ Diazepam	64	59	72	67
Ca^{2+}, A 23187	94	98	91	96
+ Trifluoperazine	69	73	72	76
+ Phenytoin	74	76	73	70
+ Diazepam	78	75	75	72

Intact synaptosomes were incubated under various conditions after preincubation with ^{32}P followed by quantitation of neurotransmitter release and protein DPH-M phosphorylation as described.[11] Concentrations of trifluoperazine, phenytoin, and diazepam were 15 µM, 80 µM, and 20 µM, respectively. The data give the means of eight determinations and are expressed as percent of the maximally stimulated condition (100%). The largest ± S.E.M. was ± 6.3. The effects of changes produced by all three drugs in comparison to the maximally stimulated condition was statistically significant. $P < 0.001$. (reproduced from Reference 19).

that the effects of Ca^{2+} on vesicle neurotransmitter release were mediated by calmodulin and required an intact biological system that was dependent on Mg^{2+} and ATP and was sensitive to methods of vesicle isolation.

Although vesicle preparations offer several advantages for studying the effects of Ca^{2+} on neurotransmitter release, it is important to correlate the results from the isolated vesicle fractions with data obtained from neurotransmitter release studies on intact nerve terminal preparations. Isolated intact nerve terminals (synaptosomes) have been shown to be an excellent preparation for studying the effects of Ca^{2+} and membrane depolarization on neurotransmitter release[35].

Studies in this laboratory have employed the intact synaptosome system[9,11,12,19] to study the role of calmodulin in neurotransmitter release as summarized in Table 2. The disadvantage of the synaptosome system for studying the effects of calmodulin on release is that it is not yet possible to remove calmodulin from the synaptosome without destroying the viability of the preparation. However, various inhibitors of calmodulin (trifluoperazine) and Ca^{2+}-calmodulin protein kinase activity (phenytoin and diazepam) that were shown to inhibit Ca^{2+}-calmodulin release in vesicle preparations were used to probe the possible involvement of calmodulin in neurotransmitter release from intact nerve terminals[19,21].

The effects of trifluoperazine on depolarization dependent neurotransmitter release are shown in Table 2. Conditions that induce Ca^{2+} entry by the depolarization of the synaptosome membrane (high K+ or veratridine[35]) or by producing Ca^{2+} channels (Ca^{2+} ionophore A 23187) caused significant synaptosomal release of norepinephrine and acetylcholine. This increased release of neurotransmitter substances produced by both elevated K+ and A 23187 was significantly inhibited by trifluoperazine (Table 2) in micromolar concentrations. These results suggest that inhibition of calmodulin by trifluoperazine blocks the release process. However, it is not possible from these experiments to determine if trifluoperazine is inhibiting release by blocking Ca^{2+}-uptake or by inhibiting a specific Ca^{2+}-regulated process within the nerve terminal.

To test these possibilities, the effects of trifluoperazine on Ca^{2+}-uptake was investigated. It was shown that trifluoperazine inhibits the depolarization dependent-uptake of Ca^{2+} into intact synaptosomes induced by both elevated K+ and veratridine[19,21]. However, the Ca^{2+} uptake produced by A 23187 was not inhibited by trifluoperazine[19,21]. Thus, trifluoperazine inhibits release in two ways: 1) by inhibiting depolarizion-dependent Ca^{2+} uptake, and 2) by blocking a Ca^{2+} regulated process that modulates release even when Ca^{2+} is entering the nerve terminal in the presence of A 23187.

The anticonvulsant, phenytoin, and the benzodiazepine, diazepam, also blocked norepinephrine and acetylcholine release from intact synaptosomes produced by elevated K+ and A 23187[9],[21] (Table 2). These inhibitors of calmodulin kinase activity also blocked the Ca^{2+} calmodulin-dependent release of neurotransmitter substances from isolated vesicles, further suggesting that calmodulin is involved in neurotransmission. Thus, studies from both isolated vesicles and intact synaptosome preparations indicate that calmodulin may act as the Ca^{2+} receptor mediating the effects of Ca^{2+} on neurotransmission.

Ca^{2+}-CALMODULIN STIMULATED SYNAPTIC PROTEIN PHOSPHORYLATION AND NEUROTRANSMISSION

The evidence presented above suggests that Ca^{2+}-calmodulin regulated synaptic biochemical processes may regulate the effect of Ca^{2+} on synaptic activity. Thus, it would be important to determine which calmodulin regulated enzyme systems are involved in specific aspects of synaptic function. Ca^{2+}-stimulated endogenous protein phosphorylation was initially described in whole rat and human brain homogenates and synaptosome preparations[13-17],[36] and it was suggested that the effects of Ca^{2+} on protein kinase activation might mediate the effects of Ca^{2+} on neurotransmitter release and synaptic function[14],[36]. Calmodulin has been shown to mediate the activation of specific kinase systems in non-neuronal tissues,[37],[38]   crude brain membrane[39] and highly enriched synaptic preparations, including synaptic vesicle,[11],[12] synaptic membrane,[9],[19] synaptic junction[9], and postsynaptic density fractions[9],[19],[26]. Thus, Ca^{2+}-regulated protein kinase activity is a major enzyme system that may mediate the effects of calmodulin on synaptic function.

Experiments in this laboratory[10-12] demonstrated that the Ca^{2+}-calmodulin dependent release of neurotransmitter substances from synaptic vesicles was also dependent on Mg^{2+} and ATP[10-12], suggesting that utilization of ATP by synaptic protein kinases may be involved in the release process. Experiments that simultaneously studied Ca^{2+}-calmodulin stimulated neurotransmitter release and protein phosphorylation in isolated vesicles and intact synaptosomes led to the hypothesis that Ca^{2+}-calmodulin regulated synaptic protein phosphorylation, a distinct phosphorylation system from the cyclic AMP protein kinases[9],[18],[19], may mediate the effects of Ca^{2+} on neurotransmission[10-12],[36]. The evidence supporting this hypothesis is summarized below.

Studies on calmodulin depleted synaptic vesicles showed that protein phosphorylation (Figure 2) and neurotransmitter release (Table 1) were both simultaneously stimulated by Ca^{2+} and calmodulin[9-12]. In addition it was shown that vesicle protein phosphorylation and neurotransmitter release had the same requirements for Mg^{2+}, ATP, Ca^{2+}, and calmodulin[9],[10]. Various incubation conditions

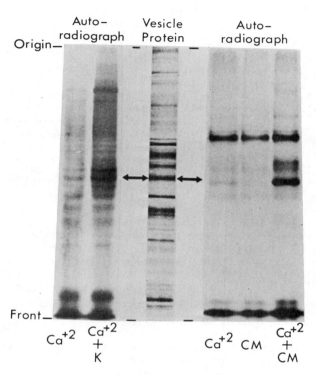

Figure 2. Phosphorylation of vesicle protein. Effects of calmodulin (CM) and Ca²⁺ on protein phosphorylation in isolated calmodulin-depleted synaptic vesicles (right)[10],[11] and of depolarization dependent Ca²⁺ uptake on protein phosphorylation of synaptic vesicles isolated from ³²P-labeled intact synaptosomes (left)[9],[10]. For experiments with isolated vesicles, γ-³²P-ATP was added to the reaction mixture and incubated for one minute in the presence and/or absence of Ca²⁺ (free [Ca²⁺] 10 μM) and CM (5 μg). For experiments with intact synaptosomes, synaptosomes were preincubated with ³²P and then incubated with Ca²⁺ (1 mM) or Ca²⁺ (1 mM) plus K⁺ (65 mM). Following incubation, synaptic vesicles were rapidly isolated from each incubated synaptosome reaction and analyzed for vesicle protein phosphorylation (from Reference 9). Protein DPH-M is designated by arrows.

such as pH and buffer solutions that produced maximal Ca^{2+} stimulated release, also gave maximal levels of phosphorylation[9,18-20]. Phenytoin[12] and diazepam[32,33] which specifically inhibit the vesicle Ca^{2+}-calmodulin kinase system were also shown to signficantly inhibit neurotransmitter release (Table 1). Trifluoperazine also simultaneously inhibited vesicle protein phosphorylation and neurotransmitter release[19,20] (Table 1). Vesicles prepared under conditions that inactivated the labile Ca^{2+}-calmodulin kinase system, also showed no significant Ca^{2+}-calmodulin stimulated release[19,20]. Thus, in the isolated vesicle preparation, there is convincing evidence that protein phosphorylation and neurotransmitter release are simultaneously activated by Ca^{2+} and calmodulin and that the release of neurotransmitter substances is directly dependent on the stimulation of vesicle protein phosphorylation. Several proteins are phosphorylated in the vesicle system, but proteins DPH-M and DPH-L (Figure 2) were the most consistently observed phosphoproteins that showed the greatest Ca^{2+}-calmodulin stimulated incorporation of ^{32}P-phosphate and the most significant inhibition by phenytoin[12,19].

In intact synaptosome preparations, depolarization of the synaptosome membrane in the presence of Ca^{2+} stimulated the phosphorylation of an 80,000 dalton protein, designated protein I[40]. Depolarization-dependent Ca^{2+}-uptake was also shown to stimulate the phosphorylation of proteins DPH-L and DPH-M in intact synaptosomes[9,11]. Since synaptosome preparations are not pure, it was important to demonstrate that the depolarization-dependent increase in protein phosphorylation was actually occurring within the synaptosomes. Experiments were conducted to isolate synaptic vesicle, synaptic membrane, synaptic junction, and postsynaptic density fractions from ^{32}P labeled synaptosomes incubated under various conditions[9]. These experiments demonstrated that depolarization stimulated phosphorylation of proteins DPH-L and DPH-M was occurring in specific synaptosome fractions[9] (Figure 2).

It was subsequently shown that depolarization-dependent Ca^{2+} uptake simultaneously stimulated protein phosphorylation and neurotransmitter release in intact synaptosome preparations[9,19-21] (Table 2). The phosphorylation of proteins DPH-L, DPH-M, and several other proteins correlated with release in these studies. Furthermore, the level of phosphorylation of protein DPH-M in synaptic vesicle, synaptic junction, and postsynaptic density fractions from intact synaptosomes was shown to also correlate with neurotransmitter release[9]. Since the Ca^{2+}-stimulated levels of phosphorylation of proteins DPH-L and DPH-M and several other proteins were shown to be dependent on calmodulin in vesicle[11,12], membrane[9,19], and synaptic junction preparations[9,19,26], it is reasonable to conclude that depolarization dependent Ca^{2+}-uptake simultaneously stimulates Ca^{2+}-calmodulin dependent protein phosphorylation and neurotransmitter release in intact synaptosome preparations.

Although it has been shown that Ca^{2+} entry into the nerve terminal simultaneously stimulates neurotransmitter release and protein phosphorylation[9,18,20], a more definitive correlation is needed to clearly implicate Ca^{2+}-calmodulin kinase activity in the process of neurotransmission. Studies in this laboratory employing trifluoperazine, diazepam, and phenytoin demonstrated a more direct relationship between phosphorylation and release (Table 2).

Trifluoperazine inhibited both synaptic protein phosphorylation and neurotransmitter release in intact synaptosome preparations[18-20]. The effect of trifluoperazine on protein phosphorylation was exactly the same as its effect on neurotransmitter release (described above). Trifluoperazine inhibited phosphorylation by both inhibiting depolarization-dependent Ca^{2+} uptake induced by high K+, and by directly inactivating the calmodulin-kinase system, as seen in the presence of A 23187. Phenytoin and diazepam also inhibited the activation of calmodulin kinase activity in intact synaptosomes while simultaneously inhibiting neurotransmitter release[18,20] (Table 2). Thus, direct inactivation of calmodulin and the calmodulin kinase system inhibited the Ca^{2+}-dependent release process in intact synaptosomes. Combining the direct studies on the isolated vesicle system with the pharmacologic data obtained in the intact synaptosome preparation, it is reasonable to suggest that synaptic Ca^{2+}-calmodulin kinase activity may play an important role in modulating the effects of Ca^{2+} on synaptic transmission[9-17,18-21].

Ca^{2+}-CALMODULIN SYNAPTIC VESICLE AND SYNAPTIC MEMBRANE INTERACTIONS

Evidence has been accumulating to suggest that vesicle and membrane interactions during exocytosis may be the fundamental step in neurotransmission[41,42]. It would be important to study the possible role of calmodulin in mediating Ca^{2+}-stimulated membrane interactions. The following studies indicate that calmodulin is involved in modulating vesicle-membrane interactions at the synapse[9,18-21].

Under conditions that stimulate vesicle and membrane protein phosphorylation and neurotransmitter release, it has been shown that vesicles become attached to and possibly interact with synaptic membrane[9,18-21]. These results are presented in Table 3. Ca^{2+} plus calmodulin caused a statistically significant increase in vesicle membrane interactions. Ca^{2+} or calmodulin alone did not significantly affect membrane interactions (Table 3). Vesicle-membrane interactions were also found to be dependent on Mg^{2+} and ATP[9,19,21]. Trifluoperazine in micromolar concentrations inhibited the Ca^{2+}-calmodulin stimulated membrane interactions (Table 3)[9,19-21]. In addition, vesicle membrane interactions were also inhibited by phenytoin and diazepam[9,19,20].

Table 1. Effects of Calmodulin and Ca^{2+} on Synaptic Vesicle and
          Synaptic Membrane Interactions

Condition	Synaptic Vesicle and Synaptic Membrane Interactions (Number Vesicles/μ Membrane)
Control	2.58 $\pm$ 0.21
Ca^{2+}	5.33* $\pm$ 0.36
Calmodulin	2.66 $\pm$ 0.19
Ca^{2+} + Calmodulin	12.36*† $\pm$ 0.91
+ Trifluoperazine	6.33* $\pm$ 0.55

Calmodulin-depleted synaptic vesicles were incubated
under various conditions with synaptic membrane, prepared
for electronmicroscopy, and quantitated for vesicle-
membrane interactions as described previously[9],[19-21].
The data give the mean values of 500 determinations.
*P < 0.001 in comparison to control condition. †P <
0.001 in comparison to Ca^{2+} condition (from Reference 21).

        These results demonstrate that like neurotransmitter release
and synaptic protein phosphorylation, vesicle-membrane interactions
may be mediated by calmodulin. The requirements of ATP and the
inhibition by Ca^{2+} calmodulin kinase inhibitors(phenytoin and diazepam)
suggest that Ca^{2+}-calmodulin stimulated phosphorylation of synaptic
proteins may trigger physical changes in the surface properties of
the synaptic vesicle   and membrane, initiating interaction between
these membrane structures.

Ca^{2+}-CALMODULIN TUBULIN KINASE ACTIVITY IN NEUROTRANSMISSION

        To investigate the role of Ca^{2+}-calmodulin stimulated protein
phosphorylation in mediating vesicle-membrane interactions, studies
were initiated to determine the identity and possible function of
two of the major synaptic phosphoproteins, proteins DPH-L and DPH-M.
Since the levels of phosphorylation of these two proteins have been
shown to correlate with neurotransmitter release and vesicle membrane
interactions,[9-12],[19-21] it was important to elucidate the specific
function of these phosphoproteins at the synapse.

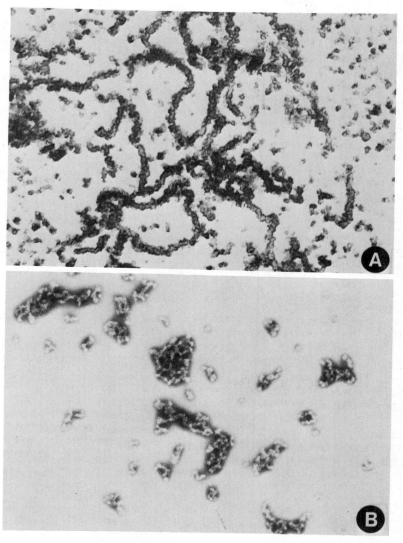

Figure 3. Effects of Ca²⁺ and calmodulin-stimulated phosphorylation on the morphology of tubulin. Following phosphorylation by the Ca²⁺-calmodulin tubulin kinase, tubulin became insoluble as determined by turbidity measurements and centrifugation. A. Glutaraldehyde - osmium fixed pellet of the phosphorylated tubulin following dehydration, epon embedding, and thin sectioning (x 200,000). The fibril-like structures were uniformly seen in the pellet. B. Negatively stained phosphorylated tubulin showing the same fibril-like structure seen in A. (x 100,000) (from Reference 19).

Protein bands DPH-L and DPH-M were observed to have similar molecular weights as α and β tubulin, respectively[18]. It was then shown that a major proportion of protein bands DPH-L and DPH-M were composed of α and β tubulin[18]. Tubulin was found to be a major substrate for a Ca^{2+}-calmodulin protein kinase system in brain cytosol and synaptosome preparations[18,19,21]. This Ca^{2+}-calmodulin tubulin kinase was demonstrated to be a distinct kinase from the previously described Mg^{2+}-cyclic AMP kinase system[18]. These results demonstrated a direct biochemical effect of Ca^{2+} on tubulin and suggested that the Ca^{2+}-stimulated phosphorylation of synaptic tubulin may play a role in neurotransmission.

Tubulin is a major cytoskeletal protein in the nervous system[43] that is present at the synapse and has been previously implicated in vesicle function and neurotransmitter release[44]. It was observed that phosphorylation of tubulin by the Ca^{2+}-calmdoulin tubulin kinase system, results in marked alterations in the physiochemical properties of tubulin[18,21]. Tubulin is transformed into nonrandom, insoluble, "filamentous-like" structures that were clearly distinct form microtubules by electronmicroscopic examination[18,21]. The insoluble structures formed by phosphorylated tubulin are shown in Figure 3.

Phosphorylation of several proteins has been shown to allosterically regulate their function and structure[45]. The rapid and dramatic change of tubulin from a soluble to an insoluble aggregated phase that is induced by phosphorylation by a Ca^{2+}-calmodulin regulated kinase represents a biochemical mechanism for converting the Ca^{2+} signal at the synapse into a structural change. The aggregation of tubulin following its phosphorylation by the calmodulin kinase may provide the mechanism for explaining the possible role of synaptic protein phosphorylation in mediating vesicle membrane interactions. This major synaptic cytoskeletal protein may be involved in Ca^{2+}-regulated vesicle movement or membrane fluidity changes at the synapse. The role of tubulin phosphorylation in modulating the effects of Ca^{2+} and calmodulin at the synapse are being actively investigated.

A MOLECULAR APPROACH TO NEUROTRANSMISSION

Developing a molecular approach to neurotransmission is an especially complex task, since it requires the functional integration of biochemical, physiological, and morphological parameters to explain

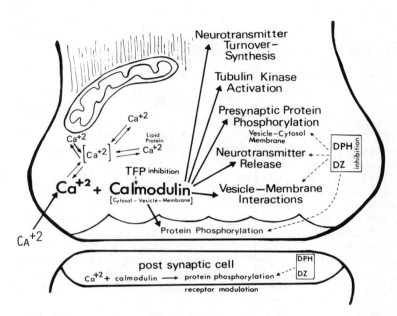

Figure 4. Schematic model representing a summary of existing evidence
supporting a role for calmodulin in modulating some of the effects
of Ca^{2+} at the synapse. Presynaptic and postsynaptic calmodulin
serves as a Ca^{2+} receptor activating several enzyme processes and
synaptic events. The inhibition of calmodulin by trifluoperazine
(TFP) is shown and the model indicates that this drug would be
expected to affect all calmodulin dependent processes. The Ca^{2+}-
kinase inhibitors (phenytoin, DPH; Diazepam, DZ) have been shown to
inhibit not only kinase activity but vesicle-membrane interactions
and neurotransmitter release, suggesting that synaptic protein
phosphorylation may play a role in modulating these processes
(from Reference 19).

the dynamic process of synaptic transmission. The schematic model
shown in Figure 4 summarizes the evidence that has led to the calmodulin hypothesis of neurotransmission[9],[18-20]. This model illustrates that synaptic calmodulin serves as a synaptic Ca^{2+} receptor
protein that regulates several biochemical processes at the synapse.
It is not unreasonable to assume that other Ca^{2+} receptor proteins
may exist at the synapse, but at the present time calmodulin appears
to be the major synaptic Ca^{2+} receptor.

Calmodulin has been shown to regulate synaptic protein phosphorylation, neurotransmitter release, vesicle-membrane interactions,
and tubulin phosphorylation in both isolated and intact synaptic
preparations. It has also been recently demonstrated that calmodulin
mediates the effects of Ca^{2+} on neurotransmitter turnover[46] and
synaptic adenylate cyclase and phosphodiesterase activity[22],[23].
These effects of calmodulin on synaptic events are shown in Figure 4
and suggest that many of the effects of Ca^{2+} at the synapse may be
mediated via calmodulin.

In an attempt to provide a dynamic role for calmodulin at the
synapse, I have attempted to correlate the effects of Ca^{2+} and calmodulin on protein phosphorylation, vesicle-membrane interactions
and neurotransmitter release. These results represent an initial
insight into a biochemical mechanism mediating the effects of Ca^{2+}
on synaptic transmission. As Ca^{2+} enters the nerve terminal during
depolarization, it is immediately bound by synaptic vesicle or synaptic membrane associated calmodulin that is localized within 100 Å
units of the synaptic cleft[9],[12]. Although synaptic calmodulin
may regulate many synaptic processes, my laboratory has been investigating its effects on the synaptic vesicle and membrane Ca^{2+}-kinase
systems, especially the Ca^{2+}-calmodulin tubulin kinase.

Activation of membrane and vesicle associated tubulin kinase
systems by the binding of Ca^{2+} to calmodulin in close proximity to
the synaptic junction results in the phosphorylation of synaptic
vesicle and synaptic membrane tubulin. Phosphorylation of tubulin
by the calmodulin kinase would then produce a rapid allosteric change
in the physiochemical properties of the tubulin molecule resulting in
vesicle-membrane interactions, changes in membrane permeability, or
possibility altered expression of membrane receptors. This conceptual
model based on the experimental evidence summarized in this paper
provides a molecular approach to converting the Ca^{2+} signal into a
dynamic force at the synapse.

Whether the effects of Ca^{2+} and calmodulin on synaptic protein
phosphorylation can mediate some of the dynamic effects of Ca^{2+} at
the synapse must still be more clearly established. However, the
growing evidence from this laboratory and others for the numerous
effects of Ca^{2+} on synaptic processes, strongly suggests that calmodulin is a major receptor protein for Ca^{2+} at the synapse, medi-

ating many of the presynaptic and postsynaptic effects of
Ca^{2+}[9],[19-21]. The experimental systems developed in this investigation
provide new insights into the release process and will hopefully provide an impetus for obtaining a molecular understanding of neurotransmission.

ACKNOWLEDGMENTS

        This research was supported by Research Career Development
Award NSI-EA-1-K04-NS245 and U.S. Public Health Service Grant NS 1352.

REFERENCES

1. R.P. Rubin, The role of calcium in the release of neurotrans-
    mitter substances and hormones, Pharm. Rev. 22: 389-428 (1972).

2. H. Rasmussen and D.B.P. Goodman, Relationships between calcium
    and cyclic nucleotides in cell activation, Physiol. Rev. 57:
    421-509 (1977).

3. J. Del Castillo and L. Stark, The effects of calcium ions on the
    motor end-plate potentials, J. Physiol. 124: 553-559 (1952).

4. B. Katz and R. Miledi, Spontaneous and evoked activity of motor
    nerve endings in calcium Ringer, J. Physiol. 203: 689-706 (1969).

5. B. Katz and Miledi, Further study of the role of calcium in
    synaptic transmission, J. Physiol. 207: 789-801 (1970).

6. R. Miledi and C.R. Slater, The action of calcium on neuronal
    synapses in the squid, J. Physiol. 184: 473-478 (1966).

7. R. Miledi, Transmitter release induced by injection of calcium
    ions into nerve terminals, Proc. Roy. Soc., Lond. 183: 421-425
    (1973).

8. W.W. Douglas, Stimulus-secretion coupling: The concept and
    clues from chromaffin and other cells, Brit. Pharmacol. 34:
    451-474 (1968).

9. R.J. DeLorenzo, Role of calmodulin in neurotransmitter release
    and synaptic function, Ann. N.Y. Acad. Sci. 356: 93-109 (1980).

10. R.J. DeLorenzo and S.D. Freedman, Calcium-dependent neurotrans-
    mitter release and protein phosphorylation in synaptic vesicles,
    Biochem. Biophys. Res. Commun. 80: 183-192 (1978).

11. R.J. DeLorenzo, S.D. Freedman, W.B. Yohe, and S.C. Maurer,
     Stimulation of Ca^{2+}-dependent neurotransmitter release and
     presynaptic nerve terminal protein phosphorylation by calmodulin
     and a calmodulin-like protein isolated from synaptic vesicles,
     Proc. Natl. Acad. Sci. U.S.A. 76: 1838-1842 (1979).

12. R.J. DeLorenzo, Phenytoin: Calcium and calmodulin-dependent
     protein phosphorylation and neurotransmitter release, in
     "Antiepileptic Drugs: Mechanisms of Action", G.H. Glaser,
     D. Woodbury, and K. Penry eds. pp. 399-414, Raven Press, New York
     (1980).

13. R.J. DeLorenzo, Calcium-dependent phosphorylation of specific
     synaptosomal fraction proteins: Possible role of phosphorylation
     in mediating neurotransmitter release, Biochem. Biophys. Res.
     Commun. 71: 590-597 (1976).

14. R.J. DeLorenzo, Antagonistic action of diphenylhydantoin and
     calcium on the level of phosphorylation of particular rat and
     human brain proteins, Brain Res. 134: 125-138 (1977).

15. R.J. DeLorenzo and S.D. Freedman, Possible role of calcium-
     dependent protein phosphorylation in mediating neurotransmitter
     release and anticonvulsant action, Epilepsia 18: 357-365 (1977).

16. R.J. DeLorenzo, G.P. Emple, and G.H. Glaser, Regulation of the
     level of endogenous phosphorylation of specific brain proteins
     by diphenylhydantoin, J. Neurochem. 28: 21-30 (1977).

17. R.J. DeLorenzo and G.H. Glaser, Effect of diphenylhydantoin on
     the endogenous phosphorylation of brain protein, Brain Res. 105:
     381-386 (1976).

18. B. Burke and R.J. DeLorenzo, Calcium and calmodulin dependent
     phosphorylation of neurotubulin, Proc. Natl. Acad. Sci. U.S.A.
     78: 991-995 (1981).

19. R.J. DeLorenzo, Calmodulin in neurotransmitter release and
     synaptic function, Fed. Proc., in press.

20. R.J. DeLorenzo, Calcium, calmodulin, and synaptic function,
     in "Regulatory Mechanisms of Synaptic Transmission", R. Tapia
     ed., in press, Plenum Press, New York.

21. R.J. DeLorenzo, The calmodulin hypothesis of neurotransmission,
     Cell Calcium, in press.

22. W.Y. Cheung, Calmodulin plays a pivotal role in cellular regu-
     lation, Sci. 207: 19-27 (1980).

23. C.B. Klee, T.H. Crouch, and P.G. Richman, Calmodulin, Ann. Rev. Biochem. 49: 489-515 (1980).

24. S.H. Barondes, Synaptic macromolecules: Identification and metabolism, Ann. Rev. Biochem. 43: 147-194 (1974).

25. J.G. Wood, R.W. Wallace, J.N. Whitaker, and W.Y. Cheung, Immuno-cytochemical localization of calmodulin in regions of rodent brain, Ann. N.Y. Acad. Sci. 356: 75-82 (1980).

26. D.J. Grab, R.K. Carlin, and P. Siekevitz, The presence and functions of calmodulin in the postsynaptic density, Ann. N.Y. Acad. Sci. 356: 55-72 (1980)

27. D.J. Grab, K. Berzins, R.S. Cohen, and P. Siekevitz, Presence of calmodulin in postsynaptic densities isolated from canine cerebral cortex, J. Biol. Chem. 254: 8690-8696 (1979).

28. U.P. Whittaker, I.A. Michaelson, and R.J.A. Kirkland, The separation of synaptic vesicles from nerve ending particles (Synaptosomes), Biochem. J. 90: 293-305 (1964).

29. K. Kodota and T. Kodota, Isolation of coated vesicles, plain synaptic vesicles, and floculent material from a crude synapto-some fraction of guinea pig whole brain, J. Cell Biol. 58: 135-151 (1973).

30. Y.M. Lin, Y.P. Lin, and W.Y. Cheung, Cyclic 3':5'-nucleotide phosphodiesterase: Purification, characterization and active forms of the protein activator from bovine, J. Biol. Chem. 249: 4943-4954 (1974).

31. B. Weiss, W. Proxialeck, M. Cimino, M.S. Barnette, and T.L. Wallace, Pharmacological regulation of calmodulin, Ann. N.Y. Acad. Sci. 356: 319-345 (1980).

32. S. Burdette and R.J. DeLorenzo, Benzodiazepine inhibition of calcium-dependent protein phosphorylation in synaptosome and synaptic vesicle preparations, Neurol. 30: 449 (1980).

33. R.J. DeLorenzo, S. Burdette, and J. Holderness, Benzodiazepine inhibition of the calcium-calmodulin protein kinase systems in brain membrane, Sci. 212: 1157-1159 (1981).

34. R.J. DeLorenzo, Calcium-calmodulin protein phosphorylation in neuronal transmission, in "Status Epilepticus", C. Waserlain and A.V. Delgado-Escueta eds., Raven Press, New York, in press.

35. M.P. Blaustein, E.M. Johnson, and P. Needleman, Calcium-dependent norepinephrine release from presynaptic nerve endings in vitro, Proc. Natl. Acad. Sci. U.S.A. 69: 2237-2240 (1972).

36. R.J. DeLorenzo and S.D. Freedman, Calcium-dependent phosphorylation of synaptic vesicle proteins and its possible role in mediating neurotransmitter release and vesicle function, Biochem. Biophys. Res. Commun. 77: 1036-1043 (1977).

37. R.S. Adelstein, M.A. Conti, and M.O. Pato, Regulation of myosin light chain kinase by reversible phosphorylation and calcium-calmodulin, Ann. N.Y. Acad. Sci. 356: 142-150 (1980).

38. P. Cohen, C.B. Klee, C. Picton, and S. Shenolikar, Calcium control of muscle phosphorylase kinase through the combined action of calmodulin and troponin, Ann. N.Y. Acad. Sci. 356: 151-161 (1980).

39. H. Shulman and P. Greengard, Stimulation of brain membrane protein phosphorylation by calcium and an endogenous heat-stable protein, Nature 271: 478-479 (1978).

40. B. Krueger, J. Forn, and P. Greengard, Depolarization-induced phosphorylation of specific proteins mediated by calcium influx in rat brain synaptosomes, J. Biol. Chem. 252: 2764-2773 (1977).

41. J.E. Heuser, T.S. Reese, M.J. Dennis, Y. Jan, and L. Evan, Syanptic vesicle exocytosis captured by quick freezing and correlated with quantal transmitter release, J. Cell Biol. 81: 275-300 (1979).

42. J.E. Heuser and T.S. Reese, Structural changes after transmitter release at frog neuromuscular junction, J. Cell Biol. 83: 564-580 (1981).

43. H. Feit, G.R. Dutton, S.H. Barondes, and M.L. Shelanski, Microtubule protein: Identification in and transport to nerve endings, J. Cell Biol. 51: 138-146 (1971).

44. N. Zisapel, M. Levi, and D. Gozes, Tubulin: An integral protein of mammalian synaptic vesicle membranes, Neurochem. 34: 26-32 (1980).

45. Y. Gazitt, I. Ohen, A. Loyter, Phosphorylation and diphosphorylation of membrane proteins as a possible mechanism for structural rearrangement of membrane components, Biochem. Biophys. Acta 436: 1-14 (1976).

46. M. Kuhn, and W.M. Lovenberg, Calmodulin: Neurotransmitter synthesis (tryptophane hydorxylase), Fed. Proc., in press.

THE STUDY OF RECEPTORS AND Ca MOVEMENTS IN SMOOTH MUSCLE AS A MODEL FOR PRESYNAPTIC EVENTS

Theophile Godfraind and Robert C. Miller

Lab. Pharmacodyn. Gen. and Pharmacol
Universitié Catholique de Louvain
73 Ave. E. Mounier B-1200 Bruxelles, Belgium

Transmitter release from central and peripheral nervous tissue evoked by membrane depolarization is a calcium dependent process although the precise relationship between calcium influx and exocytosis is not known (Rahamimoff, 1970; Blaustein et al., 1978). This release of transmitter can be modulated by transmitters and autocoids interacting with specific receptors on the nerve cell membrane (see reviews by Starke, 1977; Langer et al., 1981). In particular modulation of noradrenaline release from sympathetic nerve terminals by stimulation of presynaptic α-adrenoceptors has been extensively investigated. It has been found that a reduction of the external calcium concentration increases the ability of presynaptic α-adrenoceptor agonists to inhibit transmission at low frequencies of stimulation (Langer et al., 1975; Marshall et al., 1977) while Kalsner(1981) found that noradrenaline depressed ^{3}H-noradrenaline release from guinea-pig atria in low calcium (0.26 mM) solution to a constant level regardless of stimulation frequency. All workers have found a reduction in the pre-junctional effects of α-adrenoceptor agonists when peripheral neurones are exposed to increased calcium concentrations and similar effects have been noted in brain tissue (Dismukes et al., 1977).

These results indicate that the ability of prejunctional α-adrenoceptor stimulation to regulate transmitter release can be overcome at higher calcium concentrations, which correlates with the known fall in efficacy of prejunctional regulation of transmitter release at higher frequencies of stimulation (Starke, 1977), when it might be expected that intracellular calcium concentrations were higher than normal.

In view of evidence in favour of a distinction between these prejunctional α-adrenoceptors modulating noradrenaline release and postsynaptic α-adrenoceptors in smooth muscle, Langer (1974) proposed that the classical post-junctional receptors be designated α_1 and prejunctional receptors α_2.It has been emphasized that this should not be regarded as an anatomical division but rather as a pharmacological one along the lines of the division of β-adrenoceptors into subgroups depending on their affinities for various agonists and antagonists (Starke and Langer, 1979). In fact, evidence has been presented for the presence of both α_1 and α_2-adrenoceptor subtypes in the plasma membrane of vascular smooth muscle, stimulation of both receptor types by noradrenaline mediating vasoconstriction.(Docherty et al., 1979; Drew and Whiting, 1979; Timmermans et al., 1979; Constantine et al., 1980; De Mey and Vanhoutte, 1980; Drew, 1980, Yamaguchi and Kopin, 1980) and both types of receptor may also be present presynaptically (Kobinger and Pichler, 1980).

A further suggestion has been made that vascular postjunctional α_1 and α_2 receptors might be further differentiated in their degree of innervation. Yamaguchi and Kopin (1980) have examined the relative effects of α-adrenergic antagonists on increases in plasma noradrenaline levels and increases in blood pressure produced by sympathetic stimulation in the pithed rat and compared them to the effects of exogenous noradrenaline. They have concluded that the pressor effects of exogenous noradrenaline are mediated by α_2-adrenoceptors and that the pressor response to stimulation of sympathetic outflow appears to be mediated by α_1 receptors. That is α_1-adrenoceptors are innervated and α_2-adrenoceptors are not. A similar conclusion has been reached by others (Langer et al., 1981). However Hirst and Neild (1980), examining the effects of iontophoretic application of noradrenaline to arterioles concluded that classical α-adrenoceptors (α_1) which are sensitive to phentolamine are extrajunctional and effectively uninnervated. A second type of α-receptor, not sensitive to phentolamine corresponded to the α-receptors stimulated by noradrenaline released from sympathetic nerve terminals. This contradiction might be a result of species differences or of type of vascular bed studied.

SMOOTH MUSCLE AS A MODEL FOR MEMBRANE RECEPTOR MEDIATED EFFECTS

It is obvious that calcium is involved in transmitter release and since it is experimentally difficult to obtain a homogenous nerve ending preparation in which calcium exchange and biological responses dependent on receptor activation can be easily studied, it seems reasonable to use postjunctional membranes as a model.

Vascular smooth muscle is a convenient, relatively homogenous tissue in which to study receptor mediated effects since it responds to many types of stimulation with an easily quantified contraction and enough tissue is available to faciliate measurements of ion fluxes across the cell membrane. It has been suggested that the proportions of α_1 and α_2 receptors differ in various vascular tissues (De Mey and Vanhoutte, 1980) and the α-adrenoceptors of the rat aorta, which is not functionally innervated (Patil et al., 1972) have been classified as α_2 on the basis of their comparative sensitivity to clonidine and yohimbine (Ruffolo et al., 1980; 1981).

However Godfraind and Dieu (1981) obtained slightly different results when comparing the α-adrenoceptors of the rat mesenteric artery and aorta. They found no difference between these tissues in their sensitivity to yohimbine, phentolamine or prazosin using noradrenaline as agonist. It is probable therefore that both types of receptor are present postsynaptically in these tissues but perhaps to varying extents, α_2-receptors being more numerous in the aorta.

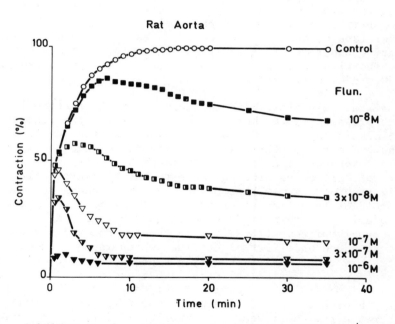

Fig. 1. Inhibition of maximal depolarization (100 mM K^+) induced contractions of rat aorta by various concentrations of flunarizine. Tissues were incubated with the calcium entry blocker for 90 min before contractions were induced. Contractions in the absence and presence of the blockers were then followed for 35 min. Each point represents the mean of at least 6 determinations.

We have compared the effects of the contractile agents noradrenaline and PGF$_2\alpha$ in these two tissues. Both of these agonists stimulate specific prejunctional receptors to produce an inhibition of transmitter release and it might be expected that stimulation of the same type of receptors situated postjunctionally would mediate similar membranal effects.

CALCIUM ENTRY BLOCKERS

Effects on contraction

An analysis of calcium movements in smooth muscle is facilitated by the use of calcium blocking agents, which were originally defined as compounds which inhibit contractions produced by the addition of calcium to a calcium free depolarized preparation. Figure 1 shows the effect of various concentrations of the calcium entry blocker, flunarizine on maximal contractions of rat aorta induced by depolarization in a medium containing 100 mM K$^+$ and 1.25 mM Ca^{++}. Similar effects are produced by cinnarizine, nifedipine and D600. All these calcium entry blockers produce a dose related reversible depression of contraction and there is an increase in the degree of inhibition of contraction with time, or a use-dependent effect, which is most marked with flunarizine and least with nifedipine.
The faster rate of onset of action of nifedipine can be demonstrated by comparing the rates of relaxation of depolarization constricted aortae. The time to peak effect is about 20 min with nifedipine and about 150 min with flunarizine.

Qualitatively similar inhibitions of depolarization induced contractions are seen in rat mesenteric arteries. Large concentrations of the blockers (about 10^{-5}M) produce complete blockade of these contractions. The reason for this use-dependent effect is unknown, but perhaps the opening of calcium channels by depolarization presents more, or more effective binding sites to the blockers. Alternatively, depolarization of the membrane might produce a sudden release of calcium bound closely to the exterior of the cell membrane (perhaps in the glycocalix) and this might produce a high local calcium concentration capable of competing with the calcium entry blockers for binding sites. Such an effect of calcium, which is however not truely competitive in the classical sense, has been described for verapamil and cinnarizine (Godfraind and Kaba, 1969; Haeusler, 1972; Godfraind et al., 1973; Godfraind and Morel, 1978; Godfraind, 1978). These calcium entry blockers can also inhibit agonist induced contractions in both the rat aorta and mesenteric arteries (Godfraind and Dieu, 1981; Godfraind and Miller, 1981).

No use-dependent effect of calcium entry blockers is seen when maximal contractions of aorta and mesenteric arteries are elicited by noradrenaline (Godfraind and Dieu, 1981) or PGF$_2\alpha$ (Godfraind and Miller, submitted for publication) and this might be taken as an indication that these agonists produce contractions without an associated membrane depolarization, as has been reported in various vascular smooth muscles (Su et al., 1964; Mekata and Niu, 1972; Haeusler,1978; Casteels, 1980; Holman and Surprenant, 1980).

Noradrenaline stimulated contractions of the rat aorta and mesenteric arteries are not however completely inhibited by calcium entry blockers, (Godfraind and Dieu, 1981) the maximal inhibition of contraction in these tissues produced by flunarizine is about 50 % in the aorta and about 90 % in the mesenteric arteries. Similar maximal inhibitory effects are produced by nifedipine, lidoflazine,D600 and cinnarizine (unpublished observations). When these arteries are washed in a Ca^{++} free solution for 10 min they are then incapable of contracting in response to depolarization but contract to noradrenaline, the extent of the contraction in aorta being about 44 % of that in normal physiological solution and in mesenteric arteries about 10-15 %. This residual contraction in calcium free solution and the degree of inhibition of contraction by the calcium entry blockers is an indication that noradrenaline can also stimulate the release of some intracellular store of calcium, not sensitive to membrane polarity (Hinke et al., 1964; Hiraoka et al., 1968; Godfraind and Kaba, 1969; Keatinge, 1972; Bohr, 1973; Godfraind et al., 1973; Karaki et al., 1974; Bülbring, 1979; van Breemen and Siegel, 1980, van Breemen et al., 1980) and evidently the extent of this intracellular store of noradrenaline-releasible calcium varies in different vessels.

<u>Effect on calcium movements</u>

That contractions of vascular smooth muscle sensitive to these antagonists are indeed due to an influx of calcium has been shown by direct measurement of agonist stimulated cellular ^{45}Ca influx and efflux using the lanthanum method of Godfraind (1976). Lanthanum does not penetrate cell membranes unless they are damaged (dos Remedios, 1981) and displaces extracellular calcium from its binding sites with little or no effect on intracellular calcium (Mayer et al., 1972; van Breemen et al., 1973; Godfraind, 1974, 1976). While the non-stimulated influx of ^{45}Ca into the La^{++}-resistant calcium fraction is not much altered by the calcium entry blocking drugs (Godfraind and Dieu, 1981; Godfraind and Miller, submitted for publication), Table 1 shows the concentration related inhibition by cinnarizine of ^{45}Ca uptake and contraction produced by depolarization in rat aorta and also shows the close correlation between depression of contraction and inhibition of ^{45}Ca influx.

It is notable that depolarization, which is dependent on extracellular calcium to produce a contraction, also produces an immediate efflux of ^{45}Ca which diminishes in parallel with the depression of ^{45}Ca influx and contraction.

Both the entry blockers cinnarizine and flunarizine produce a similar concentration related inhibition of ^{45}Ca influx and contraction produced by $PGF_{2\alpha}$ in the mesenteric artery (Godfraind and Miller

Table 1. Action of cinnarizine on depolarization (100
mM K^+) dependent contraction (measured after
2 min) and ^{45}Ca influx and efflux measured
as the difference between changes in ^{45}Ca content of the La^{+++} resistant Ca fraction of
control rat aorta and of aorta stimulated in
depolarizing solution for 2 min. Aortae were preincubated for 90 min in the presence of
cinnarizine. Each value is the mean $\pm$ SE of
at least 6 observations).

	C I N N A R I Z I N E (M)		
	0	10^{-7}	10^{-6}
% maximal contraction	100	67.5 $\pm$ 2.2	6.6 $\pm$ 1.8
Ca influx $\mu mol.kg^{-1}$	107.2 $\pm$ 9.1	68.9 $\pm$ 11.0	10.9 $\pm$ 8.7
Ca efflux $\mu mol.kg^{-1}$	58.7 $\pm$ 6.3	37.0 $\pm$ 9.5	6.2 $\pm$ 10.1

1981) and by noradrenaline in both the mesenteric artery and aorta
(Godfraind and Dieu, 1981). Table 2 illustrates the concentration
dependent inhibition by flunarizine of ^{45}Ca influx into the rat superior mesenteric artery stimulated by noradrenaline and also illustrates the specific effect of flunarizine on ^{45}Ca influx, noradrenaline stimulated ^{45}Ca efflux being little affected even at the highest
concentrations of antagonists (Godfraind and Dieu, 1981). This comparative lack of effect on ^{45}Ca efflux, seen with all the calcium entry blockers even though ^{45}Ca influx is almost completely abolished
also implies a noradrenaline stimulated release of intracellular calcium. However the ability to release this intracellular calcium store is not a universal property of agonist-receptor interactions.
For example in rat mesenteric arteries where noradrenaline and $PGF_{2\alpha}$
produce similar maximal contractions,the turnover of ^{45}Ca (i.e. influx plus efflux) produced by noradrenaline is much greater than that
produced by $PGF_{2\alpha}$ (measured over the first 2 min of agonist contact),
largly because the ^{45}Ca efflux stimulated by noradrenaline is about
twice that due to $PGF_{2\alpha}$ (Godfraind and Miller,submitted for publication). $PGF_{2\alpha}$ induced contractions also exhibit a much slower initial
rate of increase in tension and could be completely inhibited   by
higher concentrations of flunarizine or prior exposure to a calcium
free medium (Godfraind and Miller, 1981).

These observations indicate that $PGF_{2\alpha}$ induced contractions
in this artery are totally dependent on extracellular calcium. Also
serotonin induced contractions of rat aorta can be inhibited by a

Table 2. Action of flunarizine on noradrenaline depedent ^{45}Ca influx and efflux in rat aorta. Aortae were preincubated for 90 min in the presence of flunarizine. Each value is the difference $\pm$ SE between changes in ^{45}Ca content of La^{+++} resistant Ca fraction of control rat aorta and of aorta stimulated with 10^{-5}M noradrenaline. Numbers in parenthesis are number of pairs   (Godfraind and Dieu, 1981).

	FLUNARIZINE (M)				
	0	10^{-7}	3×10^{-7}	10^{-6}	10^{-5}
Ca influx	20 ± 0.9	17 ± 2	12 ± 2	9 ± 1	2 ± 1
$\mu mol/kg^{-1}.min^{-1}$	(80)	(6)	(6)	(12)	(12)
Ca efflux	29 ± 1	25 ± 4			23 ± 5
$\mu mol/kg^{-1}.min^{-1}$	(60)	(9)			(9)

variety of calcium entry blockers to a much greater extent (about 97 % inhibition, unpublished observations) than can noradrenaline induced contractions, indicating that serotonin is not able to release as much, if any of the internal calcium accessible to noradrenaline.

MEMBRANE CALCIUM CHANNELS

     It is evident that both depolarization, and agonists interacting with specific membrane receptors can increase smooth muscle membrane permeability to calcium and produce a contraction. It has been assumed that under these different circumstances separate mechanisms or channels for the admission of calcium are activated(see Bolton, 1979). That this is actually the case for smooth muscle has been demonstrated in several ways; firstly such calcium entry blocking drugs as D600, caroverine fumerate, verapamil and flunarizine have been shown to inhibit depolarization induced contractions at lower concentrations than those necessary to inhibit noradrenaline induced contractions in the same tissue (Peiper et al., 1971; Ishida et al., 1980; van Breemen et al., 1980; Godfraind and Dieu, 1981). The reverse situation occurs with amrinone, which is more potent as an antagonist of noradrenaline stimulated ^{45}Ca influx than of ^{45}Ca influx induced by depolarization (van Breemen et al., 1980) but unfortunately it also has other effects on the excitation-contraction process (Meisheri et al., 1980). Secondly, van Breemen et al. (1980), have shown that the initial rates of ^{45}Ca influx into rabbit aorta due to depolarization and noradrenaline are additive, that is when all the potential sensitive channels are open noradrenaline will still produce a further influx of ^{45}Ca.

The concentrations of nifedipine producing 50% of the maximal reduction of the contractile response (IC_{50} values) are not different in the aorta and mesenteric arteries (Table 3). This indicates that the interaction of nifedipine with the membrane potential sensitive calcium channels could occur at a common membrane site related to these channels in the two tissues although this is not the case for flunarizine which is 10 fold more potent in the mesenteric artery (IC_{50} 2.0 x $10^{-9}M$) than in the aorta (IC_{50} 1.9 x $10^{-8}M$). It has been suggested that calcium channels sensitive to membrane potential have different properties in different tissues (see review by Hagiwara and Byerly, 1981) and in particular electrically stimulated release of noradrenaline from cardiac sympathetic nerves is unaffected by concentrations of verapamil which completely inhibit myocardial contractions (Haeusler, 1972; Göthert et al., 1979a). However any effect that membrane depolarization might exert on the relative ability of verapamil to block the potential sensitive calcium channels in each membrane, as described for other calcium entry blockers is unknown, and verapamil itself is able to increase smooth muscle membrane permeability to calcium in some circumstances (Bohr and Webb, 1981).

The next question is that of the receptor operated channels, do all receptors activate the same calcium channels or do different receptors activate their own separate channels having differing characteristics ?
To investigate this we have compared the sensitivities of the agonists noradrenaline and $PGF_{2\alpha}$ to the calcium entry blockers flunarizine, cinnarizine and nifedipine in rat aorta and mesenteric arteries. Although both agonists produce contractions in both tissues, they exhibit different sensitivities to the calcium entry blockers, both between tissues and in the same tissue, as can be seen in table 3 which compares the IC_{50} concentrations of cinnarizine, flunarizine and nifedipine.

In aorta, $PGF_{2\alpha}$ induced contractions and ^{45}Ca influx are insensitive to both cinnarizine and flunarizine but are inhibited by nifedipine, while noradrenaline induced contractions and ^{45}Ca influx are inhibited by all three compounds but are 10 fold more sensitive to nifedipine than to cinnarizine and flunarizine. In the mesenteric artery $PGF_{2\alpha}$ induced contractions and ^{45}Ca influx are much more sensitive (about 20-30 fold) to flunarizine and nifedipine than to cinnarizine while noradrenaline induced contractions are approximately equally sensitive to all the antagonists. These results indicate a likely difference between the calcium channels activated by these two agonists both in each tissue and between tissues.

Table 3. Concentrations of cinnarizine, flunarizine and nifedipine (M) producing 50 % of the maximal reduction of the contractile response (IC_{50}) induced by depolarization (100 mM K^+), noradrenaline (10 µM) and $PGF_{2\alpha}$ (33.3 µM) in rat aorta and mesenteric arteries.

	Cinnarizine	Flunarizine	Nifedipine
Rat aorta			
Depolarization	2.7×10^{-8}	1.9×10^{-8}	2.5×10^{-9}
Noradrenaline	1.7×10^{-7}	2.0×10^{-7}	2.0×10^{-8}
$PGF_{2\alpha}$	resistant	resistant	1.0×10^{-7}
Rat mesenteric artery			
Depolarization	9.1×10^{-8}	2.0×10^{-9}	3.8×10^{-9}
Noradrenaline	6.0×10^{-8}	2.4×10^{-8}	1.3×10^{-8}
$PGF_{2\alpha}$	3.3×10^{-6}	1.4×10^{-7}	1.0×10^{-7}

In the case of the α-adrenoceptor operated calcium channels an interesting possibility is that receptor subtypes are associated with their own particular type of calcium channel and that some of these compounds exhibit a selectivity for a particular channel associated with a particular receptor, these apparent differences then might be due to the presence of varying proportions of α-adrenoceptor subtypes in the tissues. Cinnarizine does not antagonize α receptor mediated constriction of the rabbit aorta (Godfraind et al., 1968) a tissue which is though to contain mostly α_1 receptors (Wikberg, 1978), and is also inactive against single bolus injections of noradrenaline in the perfused rat mesenteric bed, but does inhibit vasoconstriction produced by a continuous noradrenaline perfusion (Godfraind and Dieu, unpublished observations). Possibly single bolus injections of noradrenaline are most effective at stimulating a single receptor subtype, most likely the adrenoceptor not associated with nerve terminals, which in this vascular bed could also be the α_1-adrenoceptor (Hirst and Nield, 1980). Perfused noradrenaline presumeably reaches equilibrium throughout the tissue and stimulates all types of α receptors. Flunarizine, on the other hand inhibits both the bolus injections and the continuous infusion of noradrenaline. Thus a possible explanation for these differences might be that cinnarizine exhibits selectivity for the calcium channel associated with α_2-adrenoceptors. Such an interpretation raises the possibility that $PGF_{2\alpha}$ is also acting on more than one type of receptor.

On the basis of these experiments with calcium entry blockers it can be concluded that there are at least 3 separate types of calcium channel in vascular smooth muscle membranes. Firstly, there is the calcium entry channel into unstimulated smooth muscle which is insensitive to any of the blocking agents so far investigated (the leak channel). Secondly, there are membrane potential sensitive calcium channels which have slightly differing characteristics in various vascular smooth muscles but much greater variations might exist between the channels in different types of tissues. Activation of these channels does not release intracellularly bound calcium. Thirdly there are receptor operated channels, it being likely that in any one tissue each type of receptor is coupled to a separate distinct type of calcium channel. However the calcium channel associated with a particular receptor is either not necessarily identical in each tissue, as exemplified by $PGF_{2\alpha}$ responses which are completely resistant to the calcium entry blockers cinnarizine and flunarizine in the aorta, but not in the mesenteric arteries, or each tissue contains differing proportions of receptor subtypes, each subtype being associated with a unique calcium channel. It seems that stimulation of both α_1 and α_2 adrenoceptors produces an influx of calcium into the cell but the importance of the release of intracellularly stored calcium varies in different tissues. Stimulation of other receptor types does not necessarily release intracellularly bound calcium. The calcium entry blockers cinnarizine and flunarizine display a degree of selectivity for the α-receptor operated channels of the mesenteric artery but nifedipine is nonselective.

DISCUSSION

Excitation-contraction and excitation-secretion coupling share many features in common. Excitation-secretion coupling is calcium dependent, activation of α receptors producing a rise in intracellular free calcium levels by either increasing membrane permeability to Ca^{++} or by releasing intracellularly bound calcium or both, and this rise in free calcium levels leads to a characteristic increase in membrane permeability to potassium (see review by Putney, 1979) and perhaps other ions. Noradrenaline also produces a K^+ efflux from rat aorta in a concentration dependent manner (Jones, 1973; Jones et al., 1977; 1981) and increased intracellular Ca^{++} levels produce an increase in K^+ permeability in nervous tissue of various origins (Meech, 1976; Ascher et al., 1978; Gorman and Thomas, 1980). Thus it seems that the common primary event of α receptor stimulation is an increase in intracellular free calcium, which in turn mediates an increase in membrane permeability to K^+. The end result of these changes in permeability will probably depend on the strengh of the initial stimulus, on the number and type of receptors present and on the characteristics of the calcium channel to which they are coupled.

        In this regard it is of interest that sympathomimetic amines
produce hyperpolarization of secretory and liver cells (see review
by Putney, 1979) and of nervous tissue by stimulating α-receptors
(Lundberg, 1952; De Groat and Volle, 1966; Dun and Nishi, 1974) and
these have been classified as α_2-adrenoceptors (Cederbaum and Agha-
janican, 1977; Brown and Caufield, 1979; Cole and Shinnick-Gallagher,
1981). However, a large increase in intracellular free calcium might
be sufficient to reduce any hyperpolarization and even inhibit Na^+,
K^+-ATPase (Schwartz et al., 1975) which would tend to further depolarization of the membrane.

        On the basis of the experimental evidence several hypothesis
have been proposed to explain the action of α receptor stimulation in
reducing transmitter release. Firstly, a direct link between α-adre-
noceptors and potential sensitive channels, receptor stimulation producing an inhibition of potential sensitive calcium channel opening,
and it has been observed that the release of noradrenaline from sympathetic neurones stimulated by calcium when the membrane has been
firstly depolarized in a calcium free medium is inhibited by noradrenaline and enhanced by phentolamine (Göthert, 1977; Göthert et al.,
1979b). However in some neurones a large elevation in intracellular
free calcium concentration, such as might be produced under these conditions when both α-adrenoceptor and potential activated calcium channels are open, itself depresses membrane calcium permeability (Hagiwara & Byerely, 1981) and a similar phenomenon exists in smooth muscle
(Bohr, 1963; Bohr and Webb, 1981).
Secondly, since it has been observed that the Na^+, K^+-ATPase of nerve
is stimulated by catecholamines (Schaefer et al., 1972; Godfraind et
al., 1974; Gilbert et al., 1980; Cohen et al., 1980) and an increased
transmitter release has been demonstrated when the enzyme activity is
likely to be reduced (Kirpekar and Wakade, 1968; Blaszkowski and Bogdanski, 1971; Garcia and Kirpekar, 1973; Bonaccorsi et al., 1977; Lorenz et al., 1980) it has been suggested (Vizi, 1977) that stimulation of the Na^+, K^+-ATPase of neuronal cell membranes plays a role in
the regulation of transmitter release by α-adrenoceptor stimulation.
Inhibition of Na^+, K^+-ATPase enhancing, and stimulation reducing neurotransmitter release. However evidence for a direct effect of sym-
pathomimetics on the enzyme is inconclusive (see review by Powis,1981)
and these effects may be secondary to other cellular changes, such as
alterations in membrane permeability.
Thirdly, a relatively small increase in the free intracellular calcium concentration, particularly close to the membrane, which in turn
produces an increase in membrane permeability to potassium would tend
to hyperpolarize the cell membrane and reduce the effectiveness of
the next action potential (Stjarne, 1978). Any stimulation of Na^+,
K^+-ATPase would also tend to hyperpolarize the cell membrane, particularly if the Na^+, K^+-ATPase in electrogenic (see review by Fleming,
1980).
In view of the effects of α-adrenoceptor stimulation on membranal
calcium and potassium permeabilities this third possibility seems
to be the most likely at the present time.

REFERENCES

Ascher, P., Marty, A., and Neild, T.O., 1978, Life time and elemen-
    tary conductance of the channels mediating the excitatory ef-
    fects of acetylcholine in Aplysia neurones, J. Physiol. (Lond.),
    278:177.
Blaszkowski, T.P., and Bogdanski, D.F., 1971, Possible role of so-
    dium and calcium ions in retention and physiological release of
    norepinephrine by adrenergic nerve endings, Biochem. Pharmacol.,
    20:3281.
Blaustein, M.P., Ratzlaff, R.W., and Kendrick, N.K., 1978, The regu-
    lation of intracellular calcium in presynaptic nerve terminals,
    Ann. N.Y. Acad. Sci., 307:195.
Bohr, D.F., 1963, Vascular smooth muscle : duel effect of calcium,
    Science, 139:597.
Bohr, D.F., 1973, Vascular smooth muscle updated, Circulation Res.,
    32:665.
Bohr, D.F., and Webb, R.C., 1981, Membrane excitation in vascular
    smooth muscle, changes in hypertension, in : "Cell Membrane in
    Function and Dysfunction of Vascular Tissue", Godfraind, T.,
    and Meyer, P., eds, Elsevier/North Holland Biomedical Press,
    Amsterdam, New York, Oxford.
Bolton, T.B., 1979, Mechanisms of action of transmitters and other
    substances on smooth muscle, Physiol. Rev., 59:606.
Bonaccorsi, A., Hermsmeyer, K., Smith, C.B., and Bohr, D.F., 1977,
    Norepinephrine release in isolated arteries induced by K-free
    solution, Am. J. Physiol., 232:H140.
Brown, D.A., and Caufield, M.P., 1979, Hyperpolarizing "α_2"-adreno-
    ceptors in rat sympathetic ganglia, Br. J. Pharmacol., 65:435.
Bülbring, E., 1979, Postjunctional adrenergic mechanisms, Br. Med.
    Bull., 35:285.
Casteels, R., 1980, Electro-and pharmacomechanical coupling in vas-
    cular smooth muscle, Chest, 79:150 (supplement).
Cederbaum, J.M., and Aghajanian, G.K., 1977, Catecholamine receptors
    on locus coeruleus neurones : pharmacological characterization,
    Eur. J. Pharmacol., 44:375.
Cohen, J., Eckstein, L., and Gutman, Y., 1980, The mechanism of α-
    adrenergic inhibition of catecholamine release, Br. J. Pharma-
    col., 71:135.
Cole, A.E., and Shinnick-Gallagher, P., 1981, Comparison of the re-
    ceptors mediating the catecholamine hyperpolarization and slow
    inhibitory postsynaptic potential in sympathetic ganglia, J.
    Pharmacol. Exp. Ther., 217:440.
Constantine, J.W., Gunnell, D., and Weeks, R.A., 1980, α_1 and α_2
    vascular adrenoceptors in the dog, Eur. J. Pharmacol., 66:281.
De Groat, W.C., and Volle, R.L., 1966, The actions of the catecho-
    lamines on transmission in the superior cervical ganglion of
    the cat, J. Pharmacol. Exp. Ther., 154:1.

De Mey, J.G., and Vanhoutte, P.M., 1980, Differences in pharmacological properties of postjunctional α-adrenergic receptors among arteries and veins, Arch. Int. Pharmacodyn., 244:328.

Dismukes, K., De Boer, A.A., and Mulder, A.H., 1977, On the mechanism of α-receptor mediated modulation of ³H-noradrenaline release from slices of rat brain neocortex, Naunyn-Schmiedeberg's Arch. Pharmacol., 299:115.

Docherty, J.R., Mac Donald, A., and Mc Grath, J.C., 1979, Further sub-classification of α-adrenoceptors in the cardiovascular system, vas deferens and anococcygeus of the rat, Br. J. Pharmacol., 67:421P.

dos Remedios, C.G., 1981, Lanthanide ion probes of calcium-binding sites on cellular membranes, Cell Calcium, 2:29.

Drew, G.M., 1980, Postsynaptic α₂-adrenoceptors mediate pressor responses to 2-N, N-dimethylamine-5, 6-dihydroxy-1,2,3,4-tetrahydrophthalene (M-7), Eur. J. Pharmacol., 65:85.

Drew, G.M., and Whiting, S.B., 1979, Evidence for two distinct types of postsynaptic α-adrenoceptor in vascular smooth muscle in vivo, Br. J. Pharmacol., 67:207.

Dun, N., and Nishi, S., 1974, Effects of dopamine on the rabbit superior cervical ganglion, J. Physiol. (Lond.),239:155.

Fleming, W.W., 1980, The electrogenic Na⁺, K⁺-pump in smooth muscle : physiologic and pharmacologic significance, Ann. Rev. Pharmacol. Toxicol., 20:129.

Garcia, A.G., and Kirpekar, S.M., 1973, Release of noradrenaline from the cat spleen by sodium deprivation, Br. J. Pharmacol., 47:729.

Gilbert, J.C., Sawas, A.H., and Wyllie, M.G., 1980, Stimulation and inhibition of synaptosome ATPase by noradrenaline. The involvement of cytoplasmic factor, Arch. int. Pharmacodyn. Ther., 245:42.

Godfraind, T., 1974, The action of cinnarizine and of phentolamine on the noradrenaline-dependent calcium influx in vascular smooth muscle, Br. J. Pharmacol., 52:120P.

Godfraind, T., 1976, Calcium exchange in vascular smooth muscle, action of noradrenaline and lanthanum, J. Physiol. (Lond.), 260:21.

Godfraind, T., 1978, Cellular metabolism of calcium and control of smooth muscle function, in : "Progress in Pharmacology", vol. 2, van Zwieten, P.A., and Schönbaum, E., eds., Gustav Fischer Verlag, Stuttgart, New York.

Godfraind, T., and Dieu, D., 1981, The inhibition of flunarizine of the norepinephrine-evoked contraction and calcium influx in rat aorta and mesenteric arteries, J. Pharmacol. Exp. Ther., 217-510.

Godfraind, T., and Kaba, A., 1969, Blockade or reversal of the contraction induced by calcium and adrenaline in depolarized atrial smooth muscle, Br. J. Pharmacol., 36:549.

Godfraind,T., Kaba,A., and Polster,P.,1968, Differences in sensitivity of arterial smooth muscles to inhibition of their contractile response to depolarization by potassium,Arch.int.Pharmacodyn.

Ther., 172:235.

Godfraind, T., Kaba, A., and Rojas, R., 1973, Inhibition by cinnarizine of calcium channels opening in depolarized smooth muscle, Br. J. Pharmacol., 49:164P

Godfraind, T., Koch, M.-C., and Verbeke, N., 1974, The action of EGTA on the catecholamine stimulation of rat brain Na-K-ATPase, Biochem. Pharmacol., 23:3505.

Godfraind, T., and Miller, R.C., 1981, Prostaglandin $F_{2\alpha}$ mediated contraction and ^{45}Ca influx into rat mesenteric arteries. Inhibition by flunarizine a calcium entry blocker, Br. J. Pharmacol., 73:252P.

Godfraind, T., and Morel, N., 1978, Inhibitors of calcium influx, in : "Mechanisms of Vasodilatation", Vanhoutte, P.M., and Leusen, I., eds., S. Karger, Basel.

Gorman, A.L.F., and Thomas, M.V., 1980, Potassium conductance and internal calcium accumulation in a mollescan neurone, J. Physiol. (Lond.), 308:287.

Göthert, M., 1977, Effects of presynaptic modulators on Ca^{++}-induced noradrenaline release from cardiac sympathetic nerves, Naunyn-Schmiedeberg's Arch. Pharmacol., 300:267.

Göthert, M., Nawroth, P., and Neumeyer, H., 1979a, Inhibitory effects of verapamil, prenylamine and D600 on Ca^{++}-dependent noradrenaline release from the sympathetic nerves of isolated rabbit hearts, Naunyn-Schmiedeberg's Arch. Pharmacol., 310:11.

Göthert, M., Pohl, I.M., and Wehking, E., 1979b, Effects of presynaptic modulators on Ca^{++}-induced noradrenaline release from central noradrenergic neurones : noradrenaline and enkephalin inhibit release by decreasing depolarization induced Ca^{++} influx, Naunyn-Schmiedeberg's Arch. Pharmacol., 307:21.

Haeusler, G., 1972 : Differential effect of verapamil on excitation-contraction coupling in smooth muscle and on excitation-secretion coupling in adrenergic nerve-terminals, J. Pharmacol. Exp. Ther., 180:672.

Haeusler, G., 1978, Relationship between noradrenaline-induced depolarization and contraction in vascular smooth muscle, Blood Vessels, 15:46.

Hagiwara, S., and Byerly, L., 1981, Calcium channel, Ann. Rev. Neusci., 4:69.

Hinke, J.A.M., Wilson, M.C., and Burnham, S.C., 1964, Calcium and the contractility of arterial smooth muscle, Am. J. Physiol., 206:211.

Hiraoka, M., Yamagishi, S., and Sano, T., 1968 : Role of calcium ions in the contraction of vascular smooth muscle, Am. J. Physiol., 214:1084.

Hirst, G.D.S., and Neild, T.O., 1980, Evidence for two populations of excitatory receptors for noradrenaline on arteriolar smooth muscle, Nature, 283:767.

Holman, M.E., and Suprenant, A., 1980, An electrophysiological analysis of the effects of noradrenaline and α-receptor antagonists on neuromuscular transmission in mammalian muscular arteries, Br. J. Pharmacol., 71:651.

Ishida, Y., Ozaka, H., and Shibata, S., 1980, Vasorelaxant action
of caroverine fumarate (a quinoxaline derivative) a calcium
blocking agent, Br. J. Pharmacol., 71:343.

Jones, A.W., 1973, Altered ion transport in vascular smooth muscle
from spontaneously hypertensive rats and influences of aldo-
sterone, norepinephrine and angiotensin, Circ. Res., 33:563.

Jones, A.W., Sandler, P.D., and Kampschmidt, D.L., 1977, The effect
of norepinephrine on aortic ^{42}K turnover during deoxycortico-
sterone acetate-hypertension and antihypertensive therapy in
the rat, Cir. Res., 41:256.

Jones, A.W., Dutta, P., Garwitz, E.T., Heidlage, J.F., and Warden,
D.H., 1981, Altered active and passive transport in vascular
smooth muscle during experimental hypertension, in :"Cell Mem-
brane in Function and Dysfunction of Vascular Tissue",Godfraind,
T., and Meyer, P., eds., Elsevier/North-Holland Biomedical Press
Amsterdam, New York, Oxford.

Kalsner, S., 1981, The role of calcium in the effects of noradrenaline and phenoxybenzamine on adrenergic transmitter release from
atria : no support for negative feedback of release, Br. J.
Pharmacol., 73:363.

Karaki, H., Kubota, H., and Urakawa, N., 1979, Mobilization of stored
calcium for phasic contraction induced by norepinephrine in rabbit aorta, Eur. J. Pharmacol., 56:237.

Keatinge, W.R., 1972, Mechanical response with reversed electrical
response to noradrenaline by Ca-deprived arterial smooth muscle,
J. Physiol. (Lond.), 224:21.

Kirpekar, S.M., and Wakade, A.R., 1968, Release of noradrenaline from
the cat spleen by potassium, J. Physiol. (Lond.), 194:595.

Kobinger, W., and Pichler, L., 1980, Investigation into different types of post and presynaptic α-adrenoceptors at cardiovascular
sites in rats, Eur. J. Pharmacol., 65:393.

Langer, S.Z., 1974, Presynaptic regulation of catecholamine release,
Biochem. Pharmacol., 23:1793.

Langer, S.Z., Dubocovich, M.L., and Celuch, S.M., 1975, Prejunctional regulatory mechanisms for noradrenaline release elicited
by nerve stimulation, in : "Chemical Tools in Catecholamine
Research", vol.II, Almgren, O., Carlson, A., and Engel, J.,
eds., North Holland Publishing Co., Amsterdam.

Langer, S.Z., Shepperson, N.B., and Massingham, R., 1981, A critical evaluation of the evidence for regulation of noradrenergic
neurotransmission by presynaptic α-receptors, in : "Cell Membrane in Function and Dysfunction of Vascular Tissue",Godfraind,
T., and Meyer, P., eds., Elsevier/North Holland Biomedical Press
Amsterdam, New York, Oxford.

Lorenz, R.R., Powis, D.A., Vanhoutte, P.M., and Shepherd, J.T.,1980,
The effects of acetylstrophanthidin and ouabain on the sympathetic adrenergic neuroeffector junction in canine vascular
smooth muscle, Circ. Res., 47:845.

Lundberg, A., 1952, Adrenaline and transmission in the sympathetic ganglion of the cat, Acta Physiol. Scand., 26:252.

Marshall, I., Nasmyth, P.A., and Shepperson, N.B., 1977, The relationship between pre-synaptic α-adrenoceptors, stimulation frequency and calcium, Br. J. Pharmacol., 61:128P.

Mayer, C.J., van Breemen, C., and Casteels, R., 1972, The action of lanthanum and D600 on the calcium exchange in the smooth muscle cells of the guinea-pig taenia coli, Pflügers Arch., 337:333.

Meech, R.W., 1976, Intracellular calcium and the control of membrane permeability, in : "Calcium in Biological Systems", Duncan, C.J. ed., Cambridge University Press, Cambridge-London, New York, Melbourne.

Meisheri, K.D., Palmer, R.F., and van Breemen, C., 1980, The effects of amrinone on contractility, Ca^{++} uptake and cAMP in smooth muscle, Eur. J. Pharmacol., 61:159.

Mekata, F., and Niu, H., 1972, Biophysical effects of adrenaline on the smooth muscle of the rabbit common carotid artery, J. Gen. Physiol., 59:92.

Patil, P.N., Fudge, K., and Jacobowitz, D., 1972, Steric aspects of adrenergic drugs XVIII. α-Adrenergic receptors of mammalian aorta, Eur. J. Pharmacol., 19:79.

Peiper, U., Griebel, L., Wende, W., 1971, Activation of vascular smooth muscle of rat aorta by noradrenaline and depolarization: Two different mechanisms, Pflügers Arch., 330:74.

Powis, D.A., 1981, Does Na, K-ATPase play a role in the regulation of neurotransmitter release by prejunctional α-adrenoceptors, Biochem. Pharmacol., in press.

Putney, J.W., 1979, Stimulus-permeability coupling : role of calcium in the receptor regulation of membrane permeability, Pharmacol. Rev., 30:209.

Rahamimoff, R., 1970, Role of calcium ions in neuromuscular transmission, in : "Calcium and Cellular Function", Cuthbert, A.W., ed., Macmillan, London-Basingstoke.

Ruffolo, R.R., Waddel, J.E., and Yaden, E.L., 1981, Postsynaptic alpha adrenergic receptor subtypes differentiated by yohimbine in tissues from the rat. Existence of alpha-2 adrenergic receptors in rat aorta, J. Pharmacol. Exp. Ther., 217:235.

Ruffolo, R.R., Yaden, E.L., and Waddell, J.E., 1980, Receptor interactions of imidazolines, V. Clonidine differentiates postsynaptic alpha adrenergic receptor subtypes in tissues from the rat, J. Pharmacol. Exp. Ther., 213:557.

Schaefer, A., Unyi, G., and Pfeifer, A.K., 1972, The effect of a soluble factor and of catecholamines on the activity of adenosine triphosphatase in subcellular fractions of rat brain, Biochem. Pharmacol., 21:2289.

Schwartz, A., Lindenmayer, G.E., and Allen, J.C., 1975, The sodium-potassium adenosine triphosphatase : pharmacological, physiological and biochemical aspects, Pharmacol. Rev., 27:3.

Starke, K., 1977, Regulation of noradrenaline release by presynaptic receptor systems, Rev. Physiol. Biochem. Pharmacol., 77 : 1.

Starke, K., and Langer, S.Z., 1979, A note on terminology for presy-
    naptic receptors, in : "Presynaptic Receptors", Langer, S.Z.,
    Starke, K., and Dubocovich, M.L., eds., Pergamon Press, Oxford.
Stjärne, L., 1978, Facilitation and receptor-mediated regulation of
    noradrenaline secretion by control of recruitment of varicosi-
    ties as well as by control of electro-secretory coupling, Neuro-
    science, 3:1147.
Su, C., Bevan, J.A., and Ursillo, R.C., 1964, Electrical quiescence
    of pulmonary artery smooth muscle during sympathomimetic stimu-
    lation, Circ. Res., 15:20.
Timmermans, P.B.M.W.M., Kwa, H.Y., and van Zwieten, P.A., 1979, Pos-
    sible subdivision of postsynaptic α-adrenoceptors mediating
    pressor responses in the pithed rat, Naunyn-Schmiedeberg's Arch.
    Pharmacol., 310:189.
van Breemen, C., Aaronson, P., Loutzenhiser, R., and Meisheri, K.,
    1980, Ca^{++} movements in smooth muscle, Chest, 78:157 (suppl.).
van Breemen, C., Farinas, B.R., Casteels, R., Gerba, P., Wuytack, F.,
    and Deth, R., 1973, Factors controlling cytoplasmic Ca^{++} concen-
    trations, Phil. Trans. R. Soc. B., 265:57.
van Breemen, C., and Siegel, B., 1980, The mechanism of α-adrenergic
    activation of the dog coronary artery, Circulation Res., 46:426.
Vizi, E.S., 1977, Termination of transmitter release by stimulation
    of sodium-potassium activated ATPase, J. Physiol. (Lond.), 267:
    261.
Wikbirg, J., 1978, Differentiation between pre- and post-junctional
    α-receptors in guinea-pig ileum and rabbit aorta, Acta Physiol.
    Scand., 103:225.
Yamaguchi, I., and Kopin, I.J., 1980, Differential inhibition of α_1
    and α_2 adrenoceptor-mediated pressor responses in pithed rats,
    J. Pharmacol. Exp. Ther., 214:275.

ROLE FOR CONTRACTILE PROTEINS IN TRANSMITTER RELEASE?

S. Berl, R. Nunez and A.D. Colon

Dept. of Neurology, Mt. Sinai School of Medicine
New York, New York, 10029

D.D. Clarke

Dept. of Chemistry, Fordham University
New York, New York 10458

Actin, myosin and tropomyosin have been identified in synaptosomal preparations (Puszkin et al., 1972; Blitz and Fine, 1974). Furthermore, actin (Blomberg et al., 1977; Cohen et al., 1977; Kelly and Cotman, 1978; Wang and Mahler, 1976; Schwartz et al., 1977; Mahler, 1977), myosin (Beach and Cotman, 1979) and the calcium regulator protein calmodulin (Grab et al., 1979; Lin et al., 1980; Wood et al., 1980) have been shown to be present in synaptic membrane sites. The physiological activity of the contractile proteins in synaptic membranes has not been established. It has been suggested that the actomyosin system present in nerve terminals may function in the release of transmitter materials at synaptic junctions (Poisner, 1970; Berl et al., 1973). Little direct evidence in support of such a function has been reported (Babitch et al., 1979).

Several of the proteins associated with this system e.g., actin (Krans et al. 1965; Gaetjens and Barany, 1966, myosin (Offer, 1964), tropomyosin (Stone and Smillie, 1978; Mak et al., 1980), troponin C (Collins et al., 1977) and calmodulin (Watterson et al., 1980) have a property in common, namely, their N-terminal amino acid is blocked by the acetyl moiety covalently bound to the α amino group. The functional significance of this terminal group is not known.

A number of years ago we observed that radiolabeled acetate probably can be incorporated into brain proteins from which it can be readily released by acid hydrolysis and lost upon drying in vacuo. This

139

suggested to us that acetate may be rapidly turning over in proteins as the acetyl moiety and may perhaps serve as a marker for synaptosomal activity. Therefore a study was undertaken to determine whether or not labile acetate incorporation can be demonstrated in synaptosomes and whether or not such incorporation would be affected by conditions which cause stimulated release of neurotransmitters.

Materials and Methods. The synaptosomes were prepared from the cerebral hemispheres of Sprague-Dawley rats by the floatation procedure of Booth and Clark (1978). Critical examination of this preparation has shown its purity to be approximately 85% or more (Deutsch et al., 1981). The yield of washed protein was 2.5-3 mg/ml of synaptosomal suspension. The incubation medium in all these studies was Krebs-Ringer phosphate fortified with 5.5 mM glucose (KRP) and oxygenated with 95% O_2-5% CO_2 prior to use. The incubation temperature was 37°C.

The $[^3H]$-acetate (2 Ci/mmole) was obtained from New England Nuclear and the veratridine and tetrodotoxin (TTX) were obtained from Sigma Chemical Co. The concentration of added $[^3H]$-acetate was 0.05 mM (100 μCi/ml), of veratridine was 10-100 μM, and of TTX was 2 μM.

Effect of veratridine and TTX on labeling of proteins. In one set of experiments the veratridine, TTX or their combination was added to the synaptosomal suspension prior to the addition of the $[^3H]$-acetate, and samples taken at 1, 5, 10 and 15 minutes. The 1 ml samples were immediately placed in 0.1 ml of 4N perchloric acid and kept in ice until centrifuged. The precipitates were exhaustively washed 6 times with 4 ml of 0.4 N perchloric acid, and then with organic solvents. In early experiments the protein was repeatedly washed with organic solvents by the procedure of Siekevitz, (1952). In most of the experiments the protein was washed with acidified chloroform-methanol 3:2. In either case the last wash contained no radioactivity; the results were also not affected by either procedure. The protein was dissolved in 1 ml of 1 N NaOH at 60°C, its concentration determined (Lowry et al., 1951) and counted by liquid scintillation spectrometry in a Packard Tricarb Instrument. Internal standards of ^3H_2O were used for the conversion of cpm to dpm.

The labeling of the protein was rapid and non-linear beyond approximately 1.5 minutes (Fig. 1). At 1 minute the veratridine treated synaptosomal protein contained approximately 17% less radioactivity than did the control protein (Table 1) and this difference increased gradually with time largely due to further labeling of the control protein. Further labeling of the protein was inhibited by veratridine (Fig. 1). The presence of TTX completely blocked the effect of veratridine. As seen in Fig. 1 the major effect of the veratridine occurred in the first 1-2 minutes. This Figure is typical of the results obtained with 4 other synaptosomal preparations.

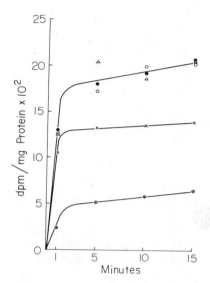

Fig. 1. Effect of veratridine on the labeling of synaptosomal protein with [³H]-acetate. Suspensions of synaptosomes in KRP were preincubated for 10 min at 37°C. At 1 minute intervals TTX, veratridine and [³H]-acetate (100 μCi/ml. 0.05 μmole) were added and 1 ml samples taken at the indicated times after addition of the [³H]-acetate.

●- control, no drug; o - TTX, 2 μM; Δ - TTX, 2 μM + veratridine, 75 μM. Line drawn through the averaged values; x - Veratridine, 75 μM; ⊖ - Difference between the averaged and the veratridine values.

TABLE I. EFFECT OF VERATRIDINE ON LABELING OF
SYNAPTOSOMAL PROTEINS WITH $[^3H]$-ACETATE

Minutes	1	5	10	15
		\% of Control		
		89.6	62.4	
	79.0	76.0	69.5	64
	91.5	81.7	76.1	61.5
	77.6	62.4	62.0	
	83.6	82.3	77.5	69.7
Ave.	82.9	78.4	69.5	65.1

Synaptosomes preincubated for 10 minutes at 37° in KRP, veratridine added (75 μM final conc.) and after 1 minute 100 μCi/ml (2 Ci/mmole) $[^3H]$-acetate was added. Samples taken at indicated time periods.

Effect of veratridine on distribution of labile radioactivity in the proteins. To determine how much of the radioactivity was incorporated in a hydrolyzable and acid volatile state, probably as acetate, and how much was incorporated into the protein, probably as amino acids, portions of the protein were heated at 100°C in 1N NaOH for 1-2 hours. Aliquots of hydrolyzed protein (0.4 ml) were acidified with 1 ml of 2N HCl and taken to dryness in vacuo at $60-65^\circ$C, the residue dissolved in 1 ml 2 N HCl and dried. Four ml of water were added and the protein dried again. The residue was dissolved in 1.1 ml of H_2O and 1 ml was counted (Fig. 2). Approximately 2/3 of the radioactivity was lost under these conditions and 1/3 was non-acid volatile. This latter fraction was apparently not affected by the presence of veratridine; it was the hydrolyzable and acid volatile radioactivity that was inhibited by the veratridine from incorporation into the protein as shown by the decreased amount in the protein.

Effect of veratridine on prelabeled proteins. In another set of experiments the synaptosomes were incubated with labeled $[^3H]$-acetate for 20 min prior to the addition of veratridine, TTX or their combination. The synaptosomal protein was labeled by the $[^3H]$-acetate but further labeling was again completely inhibited by the veratridine, while that in the control samples continued to rise at a slow rate (Fig. 3A). At 1 minute the veratridine treated synaptosomal protein contained approximately 15% less radioactivity as compared to the control preparation without veratridine (Table II). The decreased percentage of label in the veratridine treated samples is due to an absolute loss of radioactivity as well as an increased labeling of the

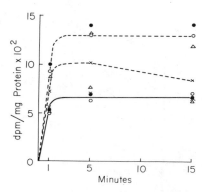

Fig. 2. Effect of veratridine on the distribution of labile radioactivity in synaptosomal protein. Experimental conditions and symbols are the same as in Fig. 1. Aliquots of the protein were base hydrolyzed, acidified and dried as described in the text.

—— Non-volatile radioactivity
— — — — Volatile radioactivity

control sample. It appears that in the presence of veratridine a portion of the radioactive acetate previously attached to protein is removed. The presence of TTX blocks the effect of the veratridine and the labeling of the protein is even greater than that in the control samples (Fig. 3A). In Fig. 3B, the radioactivity lost after base hydrolysis and drying under acidic conditions is described. The same general effects of veratridine and TTX were observed under these conditions as previously. The loss of radioactivity due to incubation with veratridine is in the volatile fraction following hydrolysis. It should be noted that the same difference curves between control and veratridine treated

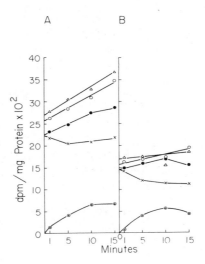

Fig. 3. Prelabeling of synaptosomal protein with $[^{3}H]$ -acetate and the effect of veratridine. Suspensions of synaptosomes in KRP were preincubated for 5 min at $37^{\circ}C$, $[^{3}H]$ -acetate (100 μCi/ml, 0.05 μmole) added and incubation continued for 20 minutes. At 1 minute intervals TTX and veratridine were added and 1 ml samples taken at indicated times after addition of the veratridine.

    A.   Total radioactivity in the protein.
    B.   Radioactivity removed from the protein by base hydrolysis and drying under acidic conditions. Symbol ●, o, Δ , x are the same as in Figure 1, ⊙ = control - veratridine.

TABLE II. EFFECT OF VERATRIDINE ON SYNAPTOSOMAL
PROTEIN LABELED WITH [^{3}H] -ACETATE

Minutes	1	5	10
		% of Control	
Veratridine			
10 µM		88.9	
10 µM		77.8	
100 µM	86.8	84.2	81.3
100 µM	85.1	75.1	78.3
100 µM	82.7	82.6	72.3
Ave.	84.9	81.7	77.3

Synaptosomes incubated for 20 minutes at 37° in KRP + 100 µCi/ml (2 Ci/mmole) [^{3}H] -acetate, veratridine added and samples taken at indicated time periods.

Control without veratridine = 100%.

samples is obtained before and after hydrolysis (compare Fig. 3A and 3B).   Extrapolation back to zero time (point of addition of veratridine) suggests that the effect of veratridine is extremely rapid with no time lag.

Since the inhibition and decreased labeling of the protein by veratridine occurs whether the protein is labeled by [^{3}H] -acetate prior to or after addition of the veratridine indicates that the effect of the veratridine is not due to altered uptake of the acetate.

Effect of Ca^{2+} and K$^+$.   The presence or absence of calcium did not affect this action of veratridine (Table III). High concentrations of K$^+$ (100 mM) did not inhibit the labeling of the synaptosomal protein by acetate (data not shown). Therefore the inhibition of incorporation of acetate does not appear to be related to depolarization of the membrane.

Discussion. It is well established that veratridine has a major effect on sodium channels causing them to open, thereby stimulating the entrance of Na$^+$ and Ca^{++} and the release of transmitter materials from presynaptic sites (Ulbricht, 1969; Marahashi, 1974; Blaustein et al., 1972; De Belleroche and Bradford, 1973; Abita et al., 1977). These effects are completely inhibited by TTX. It is clear that TTX acts externally on membranes and has only a single known pharmacological action, that is

TABLE III. EFFECT OF CA^{2+} ON SYNAPTOSOMAL PROTEIN
LABELED WITH [^{3}H]-ACETATE

	*Ca^{2+}	$\dfrac{dpm}{mg\ Pr}$	% decrease
Control	+	7768	
10 μM Veratridine	+	5960	23.3
Control	−	7478	
10 μM Veratridine	−	5893	22.2

Synaptosomes incubated for 20 minutes at 37° in KRP + 100 μCi/ml (2 Ci/mmole) [^{3}H]-acetate, veratridine added and samples taken at 5 minutes.

        * + Ca^{2+} - 1.7 mM
           - Ca^{2+} - 2 mM EGTA, no Ca^{2+} added to KRP

TABLE IV. EFFECT OF VERATRIDINE ON SYNAPTOSOMAL ACTIN
FRACTION LABELED WITH [^{3}H] ACETATE

	dpm/mg Protein		%
	Control	Veratridine	
Total Protein	1298	1003	77.3
Actin Fraction	1245	846	68.0
Supernatant	694	374	53.9

Synaptosomes preincubated for 10 min at 37° in KRP, veratridine was added (75 μM final concentration) and after 1 min 100 uCi/ml (2 Ci/mmole) [^{3}H] -acetate was added. Samples taken at 10 min. Actin fraction obtained from synaptosomal acetone powder extract by polymerization. Supernatant remained after centrifugation of polymerized actin.

the specific blocking of sodium channels (Ritchie and Rogart, 1977; Catterall, 1980).

The data presented here suggests that incorporation of acetate into protein probably as the acetyl group, is associated with the action of veratridine. It is not as yet proven, although logical to expect, that this incorporation is in the N-terminal amino acid since a number of proteins are known in which the N-terminal amino acid is blocked by the acetyl moiety.

It has been demonstrated that actin acetylation probably occurs as a post-translational process and that under certain conditions a small amount of non-acetylated actin may exist in brain preparations (Palmer and Saborio, 1978; Rubenstein and Deuchler, 1979; Garrels and Hunter, 1979; Palmer et al., 1980). In the present study, hydrolyzable, acid volatile radioactivity was found associated with crude synaptosomal actin. However, the radioactivity did not concentrate as the actin was carried through several steps of purification (Table IV). These findings suggest that actin may not be the major protein into which the acetate is incorporated.

The identification of the protein or proteins into which the acetate is incorporated is rendered difficult by the small amount of ^{3}H-acetate which is fixed into the protein. We estimate on the basis of the added acetate that 1-2 pmoles/mg protein is bound. If the synaptosomes contain acetate in concentrations usually found in tissue (Knowles et al., 1974; Tyce et al., 1981) then the amount fixed could be 3-6 pmoles/mg protein. This amount is in the same order of magnitude as that found for the binding of TTX to synaptosomal membranes (Abita et al., 1977) and of TTX or saxitoxin to other conducting membranes (Ritchie and Rogart, 1977). The binding of these toxins is related to the density of the Na^+ channels in the membranes.

Although cause and effect is not established, it does appear that acetate fixation into protein is associated with Na^+ channel dynamics. It is conceivable that deacetylation and acetylation of protein terminals can sufficiently change their conformation or polarity to permit movement of protein from less polar to more polar regions of the membrane and vice versa and thus affect opening and closing of ionic channels.

Dr. Eder at this meeting has presented evidence to the effect that stimulated release of acetylcholine from nerve-electroplaque junction of Torpedo is associated with release of acetate in excess of that which would be expected in acetylcholine as judged by the radioactivity in the labeled choline. This would be consistent with the major premise of this report, namely that acetate is released from acetylated protein during synaptic stimulation.

ACKNOWLEDGEMENT

This research was supported in part by NIH Grant NS 11824 and the Clinical Center for Research in Parkinson's and Allied Disorders. Grant NS 11631 from NINCDS.

REFERENCES

Abita, J.-P., Chickeportiche, R., Schweitz, H. & Lazdunski, M., 1977. Effects of neurotoxins (veratridine, sea anemone toxin, tetrodotoxin) on transmitter accumulation and release by nerve terminals in vitro. Biochem. 16: 1838-1844.

Babitch, J.A., Gage, F.H. & Valdes, J.J., 1979. Effects of phalloidin on K^+-dependent, Ca^{2+}-independent neurotransmitter efflux and K^+-facilitated, Ca^{2+}-dependent neurotransmitter release. Life Sci. 24: 117-124.

Beach, R.L. & Cotman, C.W., 1979. Myosin is a component of synaptic plasma membranes and synaptic junctions. J. Cell Biol. 83: 133a.

Berl, S., Puszkin, S. & Nicklas, W.J., 1973. Actomyosin-like protein in brain. Actomyosin-like protein may function in release of transmitter material at synaptic endings. Science 179: 441-446.

Blaustein, M.P., Johnson, Jr., E.M. & Needleman, P., 1972. Calcium-dependent norepinephrine release from presynaptic nerve endings in vitro. Proc. Natl. Acad. Sci., U.S.A. 69: 2237-2240.

Blitz, A.L. & Fine, R.E., 1974. Muscle-like contractile proteins and tublin in synaptosomes. Proc. Natl. Acad. Sci., U.S.A. 71: 4472-4476.

Blomberg, F., Cohen, R.S. & Siekevitz, P., 1977. The structure of post-synaptic densities isolated from dog cerebral cortex. II. Characterization and arrangement of some of the major proteins within the structure. J. Cell Biol. 74: 204-225.

Booth, R.F. & Clark, J.B., 1978. A rapid method for the preparation of relatively pure, metabolically competent synaptosomes from rat brain. Biochem. J. 176: 365-370.

Catterall, W.A., 1980. Neurotoxins that act on voltage-sensitive sodium channels in excitable membranes. Ann. Rev. Pharmacol. Toxicol. 20: 15-43.

Cohen, R.S., Blomberg, F., Berzins, K. & Siekevitz, P., 1977. The structure of postsynaptic densities isolated from dog cerebral cortex. I. Overall morphology and protein composition. J. Cell. Biol. 74: 181-203.

Collins, J.H., Greaser, M.L., Potter, J.D. & Horn, M.J., 1977. Determination of the amino acid sequence of troponin C form rabbit skeletal muscle. J. Biol. Chem. 252: 6356-6362.

De Belleroche, J.S. and Bradford, H.F., 1973. The synaptosome: An isolated, working neuronal compartment, in "Progress in Neurobiology"

(G. Kerkut, and J.W. Phyllis, eds.), Vol. I, pp. 277-298, Pergamon Press, Oxford.

Deutsch, C., Drown, C., Rafalowski, U. & Silver, I., 1981. Synaptosomes from rat brain: Morphology, compartmentation, and transmembrane pH and electrical gradients. J. Neurochem. 36: 2063-2072.

Gaetjens, E. & Barany, M., 1966. N-acetyl-aspartic acid in G-actin. Biochim. Biophys. Acta. 117: 176-183.

Garrels, J.I. & Hunter, T., 1979. Post-translational modification of actins synthesized in vitro. Biochim. Biophys. Acta. 564: 517-525.

Grab, D.J., Berzins, K., Cohen, R.S. & Seikevitz, P., 1979. Presence of calmodulin in postsynaptic densities isolated from canine cerebral cortex. J. Biol. Chem. 254: 8690-8696.

Kelly, P.T. & Cotman, C.W., 1978. Synaptic proteins: Characterization of tubulin and actin and identification of a distinct post-synaptic density protein. J. Cell Biol., 79: 173-183.

Knowles, S.E., Jarrett, I.G., Filsell, O.H. & Ballard, F.J., 1974. Production and utilization of acetate in mammals. Biochem. J. 142: 401-411.

Krans, H.M.J., Van Eijk, H.G. & Westenbrink, H.G.K., 1965. A study of G-actin. Biochim. Biophys. Acta. 100: 193-201.

Lin, C.T., Dedman, J.R., Brinkley, B.R. & Means, A.R., 1980. Localization of calmodulin in rat cerebellum by immunoelectron microscopy. J. Cell Biol. 85: 473-480.

Lowry, O.H., Rosebrough, M.J., Farr, A.L. & Randall, R.J., 1951. Protein measurements with the Folin phenol reagent. J. Biol. Chem. 193: 265-275.

Mahler, H.R., 1977. Proteins of the synaptic membrane. Neurochem. Res. 2: 119-147.

Mak, A.S., Smillie, L.B. & Stewart, G.R., 1980. A comparison of the amino acid sequences of rabbit skeletal muscle α- and β- tropomyosins. J. Biol. Chem., 255: 3647-3655.

Narahashi, T., 1974. Chemicals as tools in the study of excitable membranes. Physiol. Rev. 54: 813-889.

Offer, G.W., 1964. Myosin: An N-acetylated protein. Biochim. Biophys. Acta. 90: 193-195.

Palmer E. & Saborio, J.L., 1978. In vivo and in vitro synthesis of multiple forms of rat brain actin. J. Biol. Chem. 253: 7482-7489.

Palmer, E., de la Vega, H., Grana, D. & Saborio, J.L., 1980. Posttranslational processing of brain actin. J. Neurochem. 34: 911-915.

Poisner, A.M., 1970. Release of transmitters from storage: A contractile model. Adv. Biochim. Psychopharmacol. 2: 95-108.

Puszkin, S., Nicklas, W.J. & Berl, S., 1972. Actomyosin-like protein in brain; subcellular distribution. J. Neurochem. 19: 1319-1333.

Ritchie, J.M. & Rogart, R.B., 1977. The binding of saxitoxin and tetrodotoxin to excitable tissue. Rev. Physiol. Biochem. Pharmacol., 79: 1-43.

Rubenstein, P. & Deuchler, J., 1979. Acetylated and non-acetylated actins in Dictyostelium discoideum. J. Biol. Chem. 254: 11142-11147.

Schwartz, J., Berl, S., Nicklas, W.J., Mahendran, C. & Elizan, T., 1977. Further characterization of brain actin by electron microscopy. J. Neuropath. Exp. Neurol. 36: 398-410.

Siekevitz, P., 1952. Uptake of radioactive alanine in vitro into the proteins of rat liver fractions. J. Biol. Chem. 195: 549-565.

Stone D. & Smillie, L.B., 1978. The amino acid sequence of rabbit skeletal α-tropomyosin. J. Biol. Chem. 253: 1137-1148.

Tyce, G.M., Ogg, J. & Owens, Jr., C.A., 1981. Metabolism of acetate to amino acids in brains of rats after complete hepatectomy. J. Neurochem. 36: 640-650.

Ulbricht, W., 1969. The effect of veratridine on excitable membranes of nerve and muscle. Ergeb. Physiol. Biol. Chem. Exptl. Pharmakol. 61: 18-71.

Wang, Y. & Mahler, H.R., 1976. Topography of the synaptosomal membrane. J. Cell. Biol. 71: 639-658.

Watterson, D.M., Sharief, F. & Vanaman, T.C., 1980. The complete amino acid sequence of the Ca^{2+}-dependent modulator protein (calmodulin) of bovine brain. J. Biol. Chem. 255: 962-975.

Wood, J.G., Wallace, R.W., Whittaker, J.N. & Cheung, W.Y., 1980. Immunocytochemical localization of calmodulin and a heat-labile calmodulin-binding protein (CaM-BP$_{80}$) in basal ganglia of mouse brain. J. Cell. Biol. 84: 66-76.

NEW INSIGHTS INTO VESICLE RECYCLING IN A MODEL CHOLINERGIC SYSTEM

V.P. Whittaker and I.S. Roed

Abteilung Neurochemie
Max-Planck-Institut für Biophysikalische Chemie
D-3400 Göttingen

THE ELECTROMOTOR SYSTEM OF TORPEDO AS A MODEL CHOLINERGIC SYSTEM

There are many advantages, when studying the molecular basis
of transmitter function, to select a hypertrophied system which
utilizes a single transmitter. The use of adrenal medullary cells
as models for adrenergic nerve terminals is well known. For the
investigation of cholinergic function we have used the electromotor
neurones of *Torpedo marmorata* (Whittaker and Zimmermann, 1976;
Whittaker and Stadler, 1980). The cholinergic electrocytes of the
electric organ of this fish are derived embryologically from muscle
(Fox and Richardson, 1979). Each fish provides 0.4 - 0.5 kg of
electric tissue with a nerve-terminal content 500 - 1000 times
greater than that of muscle. Preparations of small (so-called
T-sacs; Dowdall and Zimmermann, 1977), large (Morel, Israël,
Manaranche and Mastour-Franchon, 1977) and improved (Richardson and
Whittaker, 1981) cholinergic synaptosomes, presynaptic plasma
membranes (Stadler and Tashiro, 1979) and synaptic vesicles
(Sheridan and Whittaker, 1964; Whittaker, Essman and Dowe, 1972;
Ohsawa, Dowe and Whittaker, 1979; Tashiro and Stadler, 1978) can
all be readily obtained.

ORGANIZATION OF THE CHOLINERGIC TERMINAL

The generally accepted organization of the cholinergic terminal
is summarized in Fig. 1. Choline, taken up by a high-affinity
saturable uptake mechanism (Dowdall and Simon, 1973; Yamamura and
Snyder, 1973; Kuhar, Sethy, Roth and Agajanian, 1973) is acetylated

151

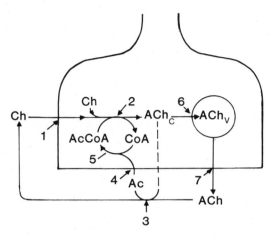

Fig. 1   Compartmentation of acetylcholine in cholinergic nerve terminals. Choline (Ch) is transferred via a high affinity permease (1) into the cytoplasm, where it mixes with endogenous Ch and is acetylated by the enzyme choline acetyltransferase (2), the other substrate of which is acetylcoenzyme A (AcCoA). The cytoplasmic acetylcholine so formed (ACh_c) leaks out in a non-quantized manner, is hydrolyzed by acetylcholinesterase (3) and the products are recycled. The concentration of ACh_c is determined by a balance of these processes. Internal recycling may also take place. Little is known about the uptake of acetate (Ac) (4) and its reconversion to AcCoA (5), except that there is an endogenous pool of AcCoA in the terminal and that acetate itself is a preferred source for the acetyl group of acetylcholine (ACh) in Torpedo *and lobster but not in mammals (Tuček, 1978).*

Uptake of ACh_c into vesicles (6) and the release of vesicular acetylcholine (ACh_v) via vesicular exocytosis (7) occurs only sporadically in resting tissue but is greatly increased by stimulation, providing the basis of quantized release. The high concentration of ACh_v when released temporarily inhibits esterase action (3) until it is dissipated by diffusion, when ACh_v is recycled in the same way as ACh_c.

by a soluble acetyltransferase which is fairly (but not completely) specific for its physiological substrates, choline and acetylco-enzyme A. The cytoplasmic acetylcholine pool so formed serves as the source of acetylcholine for vesicular uptake. The acetylcholine of fully charged vesicles does not appreciable exchange with the cytoplasmic pool (Marchbanks and Israël, 1971; Zimmermann and Denston, 1977b) but vesicular uptake is greatly stimulated by loss of stored vesicular acetylcholine following stimulus-induced trans-mitter release (Zimmermann and Denston, 1977b). By labelling vesicles with dextran, vesicles that have recycled can be readily distinguished from those of the reserve population (Zimmermann and Denston, 1977a). They can also be physically separated from them, at least in preparations derived from the electromotor nerve terminals of *Torpedo marmorata,* by utilizing their smaller size (Giompres, Zimmermann and Whittaker, 1981a) or lower density (Zimmermann and Denston, 1977b). As the recycled vesicles fill up their size and density return to that of the reserve population, due to inbibition of water from the cytoplasm (Giompres, Zimmermann and Whittaker, 1981b).

Specificity

The specificity of the high-affinity choline uptake system has been extensively studied (Dowdall, 1977); some recent results (Roed, 1980) for electromotor synaptosomes are given in Table 1. The insertion of additional carbon atoms into the choline molecule reduces both affinity for the carrier ('permease') and the maximum rate of uptake. The rates of acetylation of some of these homologues in the same system have been studied (Luqmani and Richardson, 1981) and are listed in Table 1.

Isolated vesicles show a saturable uptake of acetylcholine (Giompres and Luqmani, 1980); the affinity of the substrate for the putative permease is much lower than that of choline for the plasma membrane choline permease and this system is also not highly speci-fic (Table 1). Thus the specificities of the two permeases and the acetylation step are such that near homologues of choline and acetylcholine can gain excess, in varying degrees, to both the cytoplasmic and vesicular pools, but may distribute themselves differently from acetylcholine. Such compounds are released on stimulation (i.e. behave as false transmitters); they thus provide a means whereby the source of the transmitter released on stimu-lation can be identified (Luqmani, Sudlow and Whittaker, 1980; Whittaker and Luqmani, 1980; Schwarzenfeld, Sudlow and Whittaker, 1979). This turns out, as might be expected, to be the population of recycling vesicles (Luqmani et al., 1980).

TABLE 1 SPECIFICITY OF THE CHOLINE PERMEASE, CHOLINE ACETYLTRANSFERASE AND VESICULAR UPTAKE SYSTEM OF TORPEDO ELECTROMOTOR NERVE TERMINALS

Results are means ± SEM expressed as a percentage of choline or acetylcholine as indicated.

	Choline permease[1]		Choline acetyltransferase[2]		Vesicular uptake system[3]
	$1/K_T$	V_{max}	$1/K_m$	V_{max}	(vesicle/medium ratio)
Acetylcholine	-	-	-	-	(100)
Choline	(100)	(100)	(100)	(100)	(100)
MEC	27 ± 1 (3)	57 ± 1 (3)	90 ± 6	53 ± 6	84
DEC	17 ± 1 (7)	24 ± 2 (7)	57 ± 3	17 ± 1	65
TEC	6 ± 1 (4)	10 ± 1 (4)	8 ± 1	4 ± 1	-
Homocholine	comparable to choline[4]		1 ± 0	2 ± 0	74

1 Roed (1980), synaptosomes. Choline had $1/K_T$ 0.5 μM^{-1}, V_{max} 75 $\mu mol.min^{-1}$. (mg of protein)$^{-1}$.

2 Luqmani and Richardson (1981), washed synaptosome preparation. Choline had $1/K_m$ 2.3 mM^{-1}, V_{max} 10 $nmol.min^{-1}$. (mg of protein)$^{-1}$. Values are means of 3-11 experiments.

3 Luqmani and Giompres (1981). Conditions: substrate concentration, 30 μM, uptake ratio for acetylcholine 9.1, incubation at 26°C for 1 h

4 Data from Dowdall 1975; kinetic constants were not determined.

Size of the cytoplasmic pool

The size of the cytoplasmic pool has recently been determined for resting electromotor terminals by incubating slices of electric tissue at 20-22°C in *Torpedo* Ringer's solution containing 10 mM deuterated (d$_4$) choline (Weiler, Roed and Whittaker, 1981). The results are shown in Fig. 2. The isotopic ratio of the acetylcholine of the slices remained constant at only 22% of that of the tissue choline at all time-points studied from 1 to 24 h. On the two-compartment model (Fig. 1) this implies that the recycling, i.e. cytoplasmic pool of acetylcholine is 22% of the total and that nearly 80% of the acetylcholine is stored in vesicles.

VESICLE STRUCTURE AND METABOLIC HETEROGENEITY

Vesicle structure

Fig. 3 summarizes our recent work on the chemical structure of the *Torpedo* synaptic vesicle. Estimates of the amount of lipid and protein per vesicle (Ohsawa et al., 1979) and the discovery that there is no extractable core protein in vesicles purified to constant composition (Ohsawa et al., 1979; Stadler and Whittaker, 1978) reveals (Ohsawa et al., 1979) that there is just enough lipid and protein to form a lipid-rich lipoprotein membrane of the required surface area and density around a core of the observed diameter.

The water spaces of vesicles have been measured by a simple biophysical technique in which their density in an iso-osmotic density gradient in water is compared to that in a similar gradient to which a dense, penetrating solute has been added (Giompres, Morris and Whittaker, 1981). The water spaces measured vary according to the penetrating solute. Deuterium oxide gives the largest value (83%), glycerol the smallest (65%) and dimethylsulphoxide an intermediate value (72%). The observation that the glycerol and dimethylsulphoxide spaces become equal and amount to 75% of vesicle volume when vesicles are lysed to form 'ghosts' with loss of acetylcholine and ATP and that the glycerol space is zero in hyper-osmotically collapsed vesicles suggests that glycerol measures the osmotically active water but cannot replace the water bound to diffusible solutes. This water can apparently be replaced by dimethylsulphoxide (and by deuterium oxide) and occupies a volume of 7% (difference between dimethylsulphoxide and glycerol spaces). The acetylcholine and ATP in their non-solvated form occupy 3% (difference between dimethylsulphoxide spaces of ghosts and intact vesicles) and in their solvated form, 10% (difference between glycerol space of ghosts and intact vesicles) of vesicle volume. The further water space replaceable by deuterium oxide but inaccessible to dimethylsulphoxide is thought to be the water of hydration of the lipoprotein membrane of the vesicle.

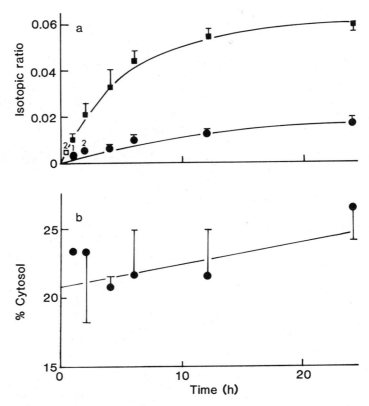

Fig. 2 (a)   Isotopic ratios for choline (squares) and acetyl-choline (circles) as a function of time of incubation. Unless indicated by small numbers near them the points are means of 3 values obtained from paired measurements of endogenous (d_o) and labelled (d_4) choline or acetylcholine. Bars indicate SEM or range (2 expts) when these are larger than the points. The curves through the points are exponential curves fitted by a linear transformation.

(b)   Isotopic ratio at different times of acetylcholine plotted as a percentage of that of choline. On the two-compartment model described in the text this is equal to the cytosolic compartment of acetylcholine expressed as a percentage of the total tissue pool. Points are means of 3 paired measurements or are single values or the means of 2 when indicated by the small figures near them, and the bars are SEM or range (2 expts). The straight line through the points is the straight line of nearest fit to all data; this has a slope of 0.2 and a y intercept of 20 at zero time. However the correlation coefficient is only 0.3, so that the slope does not significantly differ from zero. The mean of all points is 22 ± 3 (15)%.

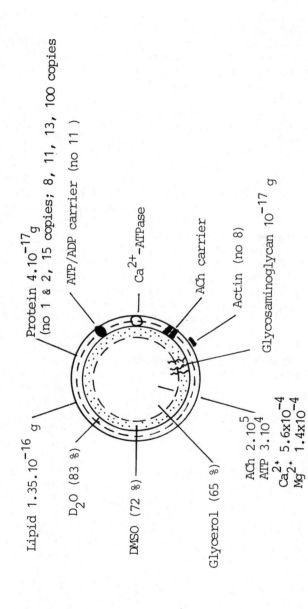

Fig. 3   Summary of synaptic vesicle structure. The 135 ag of lipid and 40 ag of protein are just sufficient to construct a membrane of the observed size and density. The protein consists of five main components, of which 1 and 2, present in 15 copies, probably constitute the Ca^{2+}-activated ATPase, 8 is actin (Zechel and Stadler, 1979), 11 and 13 are probably the ATP and acetylcholine (ACh) carriers, 8, 11 and 13 being present in about 100 copies each. The 2×10^5 molecules of ACh and 3×10^4 molecules of ATP constitute solutions, in the core water, of 0.9 and 0.1 M respectively.

A hydrated membrane volume of 25% is consistent with the observed vesicle diameter ($\sim$90 nm) and membrane thickness ($\sim$4.5 nm) and when combined with the observed density of the membrane (itself consistent with its observed lipid and protein composition) and of a liquid core containing acetylcholine and ATP of the requisite concentration, the density of the intact vesicle is precisely accounted for. The model also accounts for the density of the vesicle ghost in which the core contains only water. Thus a self-consistent vesicle structure emerges in which the biochemical, biophysical and morphological data are satisfactorily combined.

The concept of the vesicle as a highly hydrated osmometer in which acetylcholine and ATP are present in the core in essentially free solution is confirmed by recent ^{1}H- and ^{31}P-NMR results (Stadler and Füldner, 1980; Füldner and Stadler, 1981). In the case of acetylcholine there is little line broadening or reduction in peak height (Fig. 4 e,f) in spectra derived from vesicular acetylcholine relative to the free transmitter, such as would be expected if the acetylcholine were bound to a solid matrix, but there is a chemical shift, attributable to the shielding effect of the vesicle membrane, so that in isolated vesicle preparations intra-and extravesicular acetylcholine may be readily distinguished. In ^{31}P-NMR of whole electric organ, two sets of ATP resonances may be distinguished (Fig. 4b). One set corresponds to free ATP and must be generated by cytoplasmic ATP (not necessarily only confined to presynaptic nerve terminals), the other to the vesicular ATP of vesicles isolated in a K^+-glycine buffer. All peaks attributable to

Fig. 4 (a, b) ^{31}P-NMR spectrum of (a) a crude cholinergic synaptic vesicle preparation isolated from Torpedo *electric organ in a Na-containing buffer (0.4 M NaCl – 3.5 mM EGTA – 10 mM Tris-HCl, pH 7.2) compared to (b) that obtained from intact tissue suspended in* Torpedo *Ringer solution. Note that in (b) peaks attributable to the α, β and γ phosphate groups of ATP appear twice, one series (subscripted v) occurring in the positions characteristic of the vesicles, the other (subscripted c) attributable to free, presumambly cytoplasmic, ATP. The peak due to creatine phosphate (CP), present in high concentration in electric tissue, and an extravesicular contaminant in (a), serve to index the two spectra.*

(c, d) Spectra of vesicles prepared in (c) 0.1 M KCl – 0.6 M glycine – 3 mM MgCl$_2$ – 3.5 mM EGTA – 10 mM Tris-HCl, pH 7.2, (d) same NaCl medium as (a). The scale is expanded compared to (a) and (b) to show differences in peaks. Note that in K medium peaks due to γ- and β-P of ATP are broader and shifted upfield compared to Na medium, and the spectrum in K more closely resembles that of vesicles in situ (b). The peak broadening (attributable to restricted rotation) and upfield shift (possibly due to a ΔpH of 1.5 between vesicle core and medium) disappear rapidly on adding 4 mM nigericin (not shown) and (insert) slowly on aging.

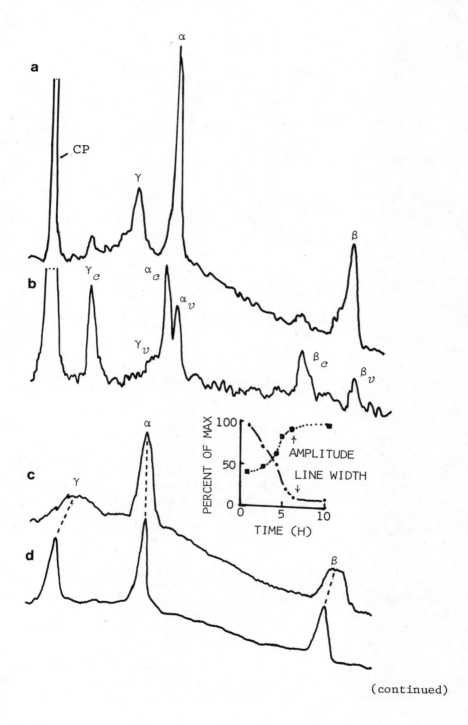

(continued)

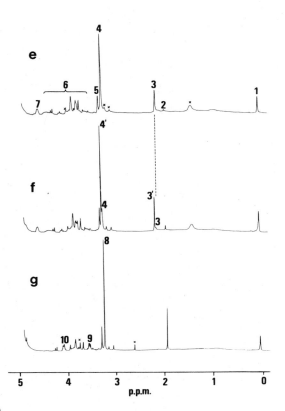

Fig. 4 (cont.)

(e) ^{1}H-NMR spectrum of isolated synaptic vesicles from Torpedo showing peaks attributed to (1) trimethylsilyl-d_2-d_2-propionic acid added as a calibrating compound, (2) free acetate, (3) acyl, (4) methyl, (7) methylene hydrogens of acetylcholine, (5) trimethylamine oxide (present in high concentrations in Torpedo tissues), (6) sucrose; (X) indicates peaks due to unidentified substances.

(f) Spectrum of vesicles lysed by repeated freezing and thawing in presence of an anticholinesterase showing (3', 4') peaks due to free acetylcholine. Note virtual lack of peak broadening indicating unrestricted rotation and upfield shift attributable to a shielding effect of the vesicle membrane in the acetylcholine peaks of (e) compared to (f).

(q) Lysis in the absence of an anticholinesterase causes hydrolysis of the released acetylcholine by traces of cholinesterase in the preparation and the appearance of peaks due to free acetate (2) and choline (8-10).

vesicular ATP show a chemical shift relative to free ATP and the β-
and γ-P resonances show significant line broadening. This is thought
to be due to exchange broadening since it can be duplicated in model
solutions of acetylcholine, Mg^{2+} (but not Ca^{2+}) and ATP at pH 5.8;
vesicles do contain significant amounts of Mg^{2+} (Schmidt,
Zimmermann and Whittaker, 1980) and if treated with nigericin, an
ionophore which exchanges K^+ for H^+ thus collapsing pH gradients
across membranes whose outer surface is bathed in K^+-containing
solutions, the line broadening disappears. Line broadening also disappears slowly on standing and is not seen in vesicles prepared in
NaCl. Acidification of the vesicle core may be brought about by the
Ca^{2+}-activated ATPase, tentatively identified with vesicle components
1 and 2, acting as a proton translocating system. Another type of
line broadening, paramagnetic line broadening, is shown by the β-
and γ-P groups of ATP in the presence of 10 μM Cu^{2+} but there is
no reason to suppose that this amount of Cu^{2+} is actually present
in vesicles (Schmidt et al., 1980).

Metabolic heterogeneity: its cause and significance

When innervated blocks of electric tissue corresponding to the
territory of an electromotor nerve and its accompanying blood
vessels are perfused and stimulated at 0.1 Hz, acetylcholine is
released, tissue levels of acetylcholine fall but vesicle numbers
are not significantly depleted (Zimmermann and Whittaker, 1977;
Zimmermann and Denston, 1977a). If dextran of molecular mass 10^4
to 4 x 10^4 is perfused a high proportion of the vesicles will
eventually contain dextran particles which are readily visible in
the electron microscope (Fig. 5). Dextran of this molecular mass
cannot cross membranes so that the presence of dextran in the
vesicles implies that it entered during exocytosis. The dextran-
containing vesicles have a mean diameter 20-25% less than that of
unlabelled vesicles.

When vesicles are prepared from such blocks and separated on
a density gradient in a zonal rotor (Zimmermann and Denston, 1977b)
the distribution of the remaining vesicular acetylcholine (and ATP)
is bimodal (Fig. 6, lower diagram), in contrast to the unimodal
distribution in preparations from unstimulated tissue (Fig. 6,
upper diagram). On examination in the electron microscope, the
peaks are found to contain numerous synaptic vesicles; those from
the less dense peak (labelled VP_1) are similar in size distribution
to those from unstimulated blocks (Fig. 6, upper diagram, VP) and
contain no dextran particles; those from the denser peak (labelled
VP_2) are about 20% smaller and up to 80% of the profiles may
contain dextran particles.

If a radioactive acetylcholine precursor (choline or acetate)
is perfused, radioactive acetylcholine is formed, but there is
relatively little labelling of the vesicular pool in unstimulated

blocks, a finding that is consistent with a previously published report from another group (Marchbanks and Isräel, 1971). By contrast, in stimulated blocks, there is considerable labelling of the vesicular pool, but this is largely confined to the small dense vesicles (Fig. 6, lower diagram, filled circles). Thus *newly synthesized transmitter is preferentially taken up by vesicles that have undergone one or more cycles of exo- and endocytosis as evinced by their content of small dextran particles and in so doing have besome smaller and denser.* For uptake of newly formed transmitter to take place it seems reasonable that a vesicle must first have to be emptied by exocytosis and reformed as an empty, but still functional vesicle. The observed changes in size and density may be a consequence of this recycling.

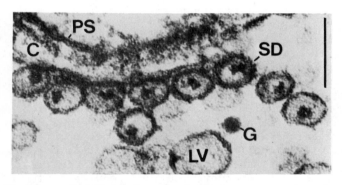

Fig. 5   Portion of a **Torpedo** *electromotor nerve terminal from an innervated tissue block that had been perfused with dextran (molecular mass 1 to 4 x 10^4) and stimulated. PS, post-synaptic membrane; C, synaptic cleft; LV, large light vesicle of reserve population; SD, small dense vesicles near the presynaptic plasma membrane that are actively undergoing recycling and have acquired dextran particles in their lumen. The dextran particles are smaller than and readily distinguished from the glycogen granules (G) visible in the cytoplasm. Vesicles similar to those marked SD, but without glycogen granules, are visible in stimulated blocks that were not perfused with dextran-containing solutions.*

We should predict that on restimulation at a rate and for a duration that did not seriously disturb the vesicle population the transmitter released should have the same specific radioactivity as that of the acetylcholine of the VP_2 fraction; on longer stimulation

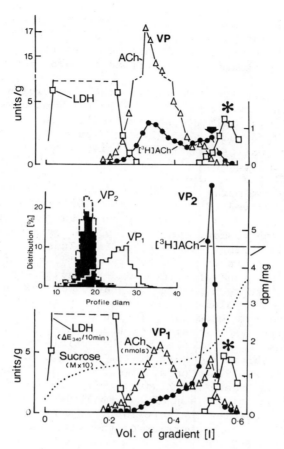

Fig. 6 Top and bottom: distribution of lactate dehydrogenase (LDH, squares), endogenous acetylcholine (ACh, triangles) and radioactive ACh (filled circles) in a zonal density gradient after centrifuging cytoplasmic extracts containing synaptic vesicles derived from (top) a control block, (bottom) a block that had been stimulated through the nerve at 0.1 Hz for 3 h. Control and stimulated blocks had been perfused with radioactive acetate and dextran. Note that whereas the control block gave one main vesicle peak (VP) the ACh of which is not much labelled, the stimulated block gave two vesicle peaks, VP₁ and VP₂. The lighter (VP₁) is identical in density and amount of label- led to VP; the denser (VP₂) is highly labelled. The insert diagram shows that the mean profile diameter of vesicles in VP₂ is about 30% less than that in VP₁, and that 80% of the vesicles in VP₂ but none in VP₁ had been labelled with dextran (black blocks)². The asterisks mark peaks (distinct from VP₂) containing synaptosomes and the arrow (upper diagram) marks a highly radioactive shoulder of VP which suggests that adventitious stimulation has generated a small VP₂ population even in the control block.

we should expect its specific radioactivity to fall below that of
the VP_2 vesicles due to recruitment of 'cold' (VP_1) vesicles into
the VP_2 pool. These expectations are fully realized (Suszkiw,
Zimmermann and Whittaker, 1978; Whittaker, 1978; Suszkiw, 1980).

The greater density and smaller size of vesicles undergoing
recycling are in no way dependent on the entry of dextran into them
and are most simply explained by osmotically induced changes in
water content. Measurements of glycerol space show that the recycled
vesicles have a smaller osmotically active water space than those
of the larger, lighter vesicles (45% compared to 63%) and it may
be calculated that a vesicle of this reduced core dimension but
with an unchanged membrane should have exactly the density and diameter thas is observed (Giompres et al., 1981b). The basis for this
change in water space is not exactly known but could result from
changes in internal osmotic pressure due to variations in small-
molecule content during vesicle recycling. Thus, on exocytosis,
a vesicle somewhat hyperosmotic to extracellular medium would
become iso-osmotic; on reformation and reloading, the core might
well eventually become hyperosmotic and would draw in water thus
increasing the core volume. Hyperosmotic conditions in the core of
an artificial vesicle undergoing fusion with a planar artificial
membrane stimulate the 'fission' of the apposed membranes (i. e.
assist the formation of a hole into the vesicle core from the side
of the planar membrane opposite to the vesicle)(Miller, Arvan,
Telford and Racker, 1976; Cohen, Zimmerberg and Finkelstein, 1980;
Pollard, Pazoles, Creutz and Zinder, 1979). The reconversion during recovery from stimulation of the small dense vesicles to the
larger, lighter vesicles characteristic of resting tissues has been
followed (Fig. 7). The properties of the small dense vesicles are
summarized in Table 2.

Fractions of small, dense vesicles, even when these are separated on high-resolution gradients in zonal rotors (Suszkiw et al.,
1978) do contain residual membrane contamination; this can be
successfully removed by filtration through columns of porous glass
beads (Giompres et al., 1981a) so that there is no doubt that the
radioactive acetylcholine is vesicular and not trapped in larger
membranous vesicles contaminating the fraction, as suggested by
Dunant and Israel (1979). Furthermore synaptosomes can be clearly
separated in the gradient from fraction VP_2 (Zimmermann and Denston,
1977b) so that the radioactive acetylcholine in fraction VP_2 is not
due to cytoplasmic acetylcholine entrapped in synaptosomes.

Attempts to discredit the vesicle model of transmitter storage
and release by insisting that there should at all times be a
correspondence between the specific radioactivity of the acetylcholine of the entire vesicle population and that of the released
transmitter are clearly simplistic since they fail to recognize the
structural restraints on vesicle recycling and the experimental

fact of vesicle heterogeneity. Moreover, further positive evidence
that the vesicles are the source of transmitter released on stimulation has come from the study of false transmitters (Luqmani et al.,
1980; Whittaker and Luqmani, 1980; Schwarzenfeld et al., 1979). In
a typical experiment of this kind (Fig. 8) a mixture of the
triethyl analogue of choline ('triethylcholine') radioactive
acetate and an anticholinesterase were perfused through a tissue
block during stimulation to provoke the turnover of transmitter
stores. After a period of rest during which unutilized radioactive
acetate was washed out the block was restimulated and released
transmitter was collected. At the end of the experiment vesicle
fractions were prepared from the restimulated block and from a
control block that had not been restimulated. The labelled esters
were separated from whole tissue, vesicles and fractions of perfusate by liquid ion-exchange extraction and chromatography and the
ratio of newly synthesized true to false transmitter determined.
The metabolically active vesicular fraction of transmitter was
labelled differently from the cytoplasmic as evinced by the marked
difference in the ratio for vesicles and whole tissue; however the
ratio for the transmitters released by stimulation agreed with that
of the vesicular fraction and not with the cytoplasmic or whole
tissue fractions.

TABLE 2   PROPERTIES OF SMALL DENSE VESICLES

1   *They are generated by stimulation.*

2   *If the tissue is perfused with dextran, they acquire dextran
    particles (which cannot cross membranes), indicating that their
    formation involves one or more cycles of exo- and endocytosis.*

3   *On isolation they may be separated from the main vesicle
    population by physical methods utilizing their greater density
    or smaller size.*

4   *These physical differences are due to their lower water content.*

5   *They acquire labelled acetylcholine if the tissue is perfused
    with radioactive precursor during their formation.*

6   *On further stimulation, the acetylcholine released has the same
    specific activity as their acetylcholine.*

7   *They acquire false transmitters if the tissue is perfused with
    these or their precursors during stimulation.*

8   *On further stimulation transmitters are released in the same
    ratio as they are found in these vesicles.*

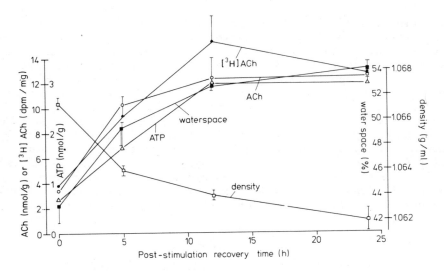

*Fig. 7   Changes in vesicular acetylcholine (ACh), ATP, [³H]ACh,
density and glycerol water space of innervated, perfused blocks
of electric tissue during post-stimulation (0.1 Hz for 5 h) recovery
Perfusate containing [³H]acetate was recycled until the 12 h time
point and then exchanged for a non-radioactive one. At 24 h the
water-space had recovered to 83% of control.*

Histochemical evidence for vesicle exocytosis

Fig. 9 shows the effect of stimulation on the accessibility of
a specific vesicle antigen, as revealed by indirect immunofluorescence histochemistry. The ventral, innervated surface of the
unstimulated electrocyte (Fig. 9a) fluoresces only weakly after
application of the vesicle antiserum and fluorescein-labelled IgG.
However, on stimulation (Fig. 9b), the vesicle antigen becomes
much more accessible and the innervated surface now fluoresces

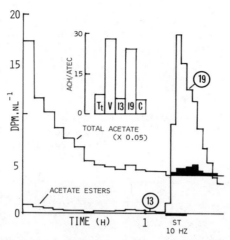

Fig. 8   Release of acetyltriethylcholine (ATEC) and acetylcholine (ACh) from an innervated, perfused block of electric tissue from Torpedo marmorata. *The tissue block corresponding to the territory of one electromotor nerve and its accompanying blood vessels was perfused with* Torpedo *Ringer solution containing triethylcholine (TEC) (250 μM), choline (25 μM) and [³H]acetate (16.7 μM, specific radioactivity 300 Ci/mol) for 3 h. Stimulation was then applied at 0.1 Hz for 1 h to promote incorporation of newly synthesized transmitter into tissue stores. After 2 h recovery in label and 70 min washout perfusion with radioactivity-free Ringer solution containing paraoxon (100 μM) to inhibit acetylcholinesterase the tissue was restimulated at 10 Hz for 10 min (release stimulus) while perfusion was continued. The continuous line shows the total concentration of [³H]acetate (free and esterified) in the perfusate, the broken line, the concentration of [³H]acetate (as esterified organic bases) passing into the organic phase when samples of perfusate were extracted with allylcyanide containing sodium tetraphenylboride (10 mg/ml). Note that the scale of extractable counts is 10 times greater than that of total counts and that as a result of stimulation the concentration of acetylated bases in the perfusate enormously increased from a very low baseline.*

The insert diagram shows the ratio of ACh to ATEC in total tissue (Tt), a crude vesicle pellet (V), in the perfusion fluid before (fraction no. 13) and during (no. 19) the release stimulus, and in the cytoplasmic fraction (C). The extracted acetyl esters were separated by paper chromatography.

Note the close agreement in the ratio of ACh to ATEC in the perfusate after the stimulated release of transmitter with that in vesicles, even though this ratio is almost 5 times higher than that found in the whole tissue.

brightly. We interpret these results to mean that stimulation has promoted exocytosis of vesicles and has exteriorized vesicle antigen whose determinant group is normally on the inside of the vesicle membrane and therefore, in the resting state is largely inaccessible.

CONCLUSIONS

The purpose of this article has been to show how a combination of morphological, physiological, biochemical and biophysical techniques, applied to a carefully selected model synapse, has led

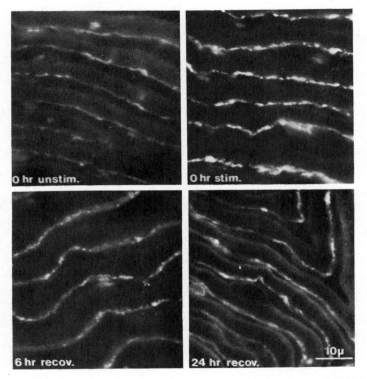

Fig. 9   Section of electric organ of Torpedo *after indirect immunofluorescence histochemical staining with an anti-serum directed to a specific synaptic vesicle antigen. (Top left) unstimulated tissue, (others) tissue stimulated through lobe (5 Hz, 17 min). Note increased fluorescence of innervated side of electrocyte after stimulation which decreases to control level on recovery (reinternalization of vesicle antigen). Unpublished results of R.T. Jones and J.H. Walker. Unlike the serum described by Hooper, Carlson and Kelly (1980) this serum is completely specific for cholinergic vesicles.*

to new insights into the mechanisms of transmitter storage and
release.

Much remains to be understood. We have little precise knowledge of, and are certainly some way yet from reproducing, in a
reconstituted system, the uptake mechanisms which enable a relatively simple structure, the synaptic vesicle to store acetylcholine
(and ATP) in such extremely high concentrations. Only the outline
of a solution, involving, possibly, the sequential uptake of ATP
and acetylcholine in response to the generation of a hydrogen-ion
gradient and membrane potential by a proton-translocating Ca^{2+}-
activated ATPase (Luqmani, 1981), is visible. On the other hand,
better knowledge of the physicochemical conditions prevailing in
vesicles *in situ* in resting and stimulated tissue are providing the
essential basis for successful uptake studies.

We are also basically ignorant of the mechanisms involved in
vesicle exocytosis and reformation as, indeed, we are of exo- and
endocytosis in any tissue. Here, the role of osmotic pressure in
generating the micellar rearrangement involved in membrane 'fission'
is becoming increasingly apparent and is supported by our studies
of the changes in water content of recycling vesicles.

Possibly the most important advance has been the recognition
of vesicle metabolic heterogeneity and the discovery that vesicles
in differing metabolic states can be separated due to these osmotically driven changes in water content. It can now be recognized
that the original mathematical description of the quantization of
transmitter release which assumed an equal probability that any
vesicle should undergo exocytosis and transmitter release (Katz,
1966) held by some assiduous reviewers (Marchbanks, 1975) to be of
the essence of the 'vesicle theory' is, in fact, only a convenient
mathematical oversimplification of a system in which there must
always be a much greater probability that vesicles near the region
of the presynaptic plasma membrane adjacent to the synaptic cleft
will recycle than those distant from it. Having recognized this, the
apparent paradox that in terminals in which the transmitter pool has
been labelled by a radioactive precursor, the transmitter released
on restimulation has a higher specific activity than the totality
of the vesicle population disappears since the relevant (and successful) comparison is with the actively recycling vesicle population.
This finding makes theories of release directly from the cytoplasm
superfluous. Transmitter storage and release is seen as a specialized,
modified and miniaturized version of a philogenetically old and
ubiquitous cellular mechanism: exo- and endocytosis of cellular
storage granules.

*Acknowledgements. We are grateful to various members of
our department for allowing us to mention their unpublished
results.*

REFERENCES

Cohen, F.S., Zimmerberg, J. and Finkelstein, A., 1980. Fusion of phospholipid vesicles with planar phospholipid bilayer membranes. II. Incorporation of a vesicular membrane marker into a planar membrane. J. gen. Physiol. 75: 251-270.

Dowdall, M.J., 1975. Nerve terminal sacs from Torpedo electric organ: a new preparation for the study of presynaptic cholinergic mechanisms at the molecular level, in 'Cholinergic Mechanisms and Psychopharmacology (D.J. Jenden ed.), pp 359-375. Plenum Press, New York.

Dowdall, M.J., 1977. The biochemistry of Torpedo cholinergic neurons, in 'Biochemistry of Characterised Neurons' (N.N. Osborne ed.), pp 171-216. Pergamon Press, Oxford.

Dowdall, M.J. and Simon, E.J., 1973. Comparative studies on synapto-somes: uptake of [N-Me-^{3}H]choline by synaptosomes from squid optic lobes. J. Neurochem. 21: 969-982.

Dowdall, M.J. and Zimmermann, H., 1977. The isolation of pure cholin-ergic nerve terminal sacs (T-sacs) from the electric organ of juve-nile Torpedo. Neuroscience 2: 405-421.

Dunant, Y. and Israël, M., 1979. When the vesicular hypothesis is no longer the vesicular hypothesis. Trends in Neurosciences 2: 130-132.

Fox, G.Q. and Richardson, G.P., 1979. The developmental morphology of Torpedo marmorata: electric organ-electrogenic phase. J. comp. Neurol. 185: 293-314.

Füldner, H.-H. and Stadler, H., 1981. The storage of acetylcholine and ATP in synaptic vesicles. Hoppe-Seyler's Z. Physiol. Chem. 362: 198.

Giompres, P.E. and Luqmani, Y.A., 1980. Cholinergic synaptic vesicles isolated from Torpedo marmorata: demonstration of acetylcholine and choline uptake in an in vitro system. Neuroscience 5: 1041-1052.

Giompres, P.E., Morris, S.J. and Whittaker, V.P., 1981. The water spaces in cholinergic synaptic vesicles from Torpedo measured by changes in density induced by permeating substances. Neuroscience 6: 757-763.

Giompres, P.E., Zimmermann, H. and Whittaker, V.P., 1981a. Puri-fication of small dense vesicles from stimulated Torpedo electric tissue by glass bead column chromatography. Neuroscience 6: 765-774.

Giompres, P.E., Zimmermann, H. and Whittaker, V.P., 1981b. Changes in the biochemical and biophysical parameters of cholinergic synaptic vesicles on transmitter release and during a subsequent period of rest. Neuroscience 6: 775-785.

Hooper, J.E., Carlson, S.S. and Kelly, R.B., 1980. Antibodies to synaptic vesicles purified from *Narcine* electric organ bind a subclass of mammalian nerve terminals. J. Cell Biol. 87: 104-113.

Katz, B., 1966. Nerve, Muscle and Synapse. McGraw-Hill, New York.

Kuhar, M.J., Sethy, V.H., Roth, R.H. and Agajanian, G.K., 1973. Choline: selective accumulation by central cholinergic neurones. J. Neurochem. 20: 581-593.

Luqmani, Y.A., 1981. Nucleotide uptake by isolated cholinergic vesicles: evidence for a carrier of adenosine 5-triphosphate. Neuroscience 6: 1011-1021.

Luqmani, Y.A. and Giompres, P.E., 1981. On the specificity of uptake by isolated *Torpedo* synaptic vesicles. Neurosci. Lett. 23: 81-85.

Luqmani, Y.A. and Richardson P.J., 1981. Homocholine and short-chain N-alkyl choline analogues as substrates for *Torpedo* choline acetyltransferase. Submitted for publication.

Luqmani, Y.A., Sudlow, G. and Whittaker, V.P., 1980. Homocholine and acetylhomocholine: false transmitters in the cholinergic electromotor system of *Torpedo*. Neuroscience 5: 153-160.

Marchbanks, R.M., 1975. The subcellular origin of the acetylcholine released at synapses. Int. J. Biochem. 6: 303-312.

Marchbanks, R.M. and Israël, M., 1971. Aspects of acetylcholine metabolism in the electric organ of *Torpedo marmorata*. J. Neurochem. 18: 439-448.

Miller, C., Arvan, P., Telford, J.N. and Racker, E., 1976. Ca^{2+}-induced fusion of proteoliposomes: dependence on transmembrane osmotic gradient. J. Membrane Biol. 30: 271-282.

Morel, N., Israël, M., Manaranche, R. and Mastour-Franchon, P., 1977. Isolation of pure cholinergic nerve endings from *Torpedo* electric organ. J. Cell Biol. 75: 43-55.

Ohsawa, K., Dowe, G.H.C., Morris, S.J. and Whittaker, V.P., 1979. The lipid and protein content of cholinergic synaptic vesicles from the electric organ of *Torpedo marmorata* purified to constant composition: implications for vesicle structure. Brain Res. 161: 447-451.

Pollard, H.B., Pazoles, C.J., Creutz, C.E. and Zinder, O., 1979. The chromaffin granule and possible mechanisms of exocytosis. Int. Rev. Cytol. 58: 159-197.

Richardson, P.J. and Whittaker, V.P., 1981. The Na^+ and K^+ content of isolated *Torpedo* synaptosomes and its effect on choline uptake. J. Neurochem. 36: 1536-1542.

Roed, I., 1980. Uptake of false transmitter precursors into synapto-somes derived from a purely cholinergic source. Hoppe-Seyler's Z. Physiol. Chem. 361: 1331.

Schmidt, R., Zimmermann, H. and Whittaker, V.P., 1980. Metal ion content of cholinergic synaptic vesicles isolated from the electric organ of *Torpedo*: effect of stimulus induced transmitter release. Neuroscience 5: 625-638.

Schwarzenfeld, I. von, Sudlow, G. and Whittaker, V.P., 1979. Vesicular storage and release of cholinergic false transmitters. Prog. Brain Res. 49: 163-174.

Sheridan, M.N. and Whittaker, V.P., 1964. Isolated synaptic vesicles: morphology and acetylcholine content. J. Physiol. (Lond.) 175: 25P-26P.

Stadler, H. and Füldner, H.-H., 1980. Proton NMR detection of acetyl-choline status in synaptic vesicles. Nature (Lond.) 286: 293-294.

Stadler, H. and Tashiro, T., 1979. Isolation of synaptosomal plasma membranes from cholinergic nerve terminals and a comparison of their proteins with those of synaptic vesicles. Eur. J. Biochem. 101: 171-178.

Stadler, H. and Whittaker, V.P., 1978. Identification of vesiculin as a glycosaminoglycan. Brain Res. 153: 408-413.

Suszkiw, J.B., 1980. Kinetics of acetylcholine recovery in *Torpedo* electromotor synapses depleted of synaptic vesicles. Neuroscience 5: 1341-1349.

Suszkiw, J.B., Zimmermann, H. and Whittaker, V.P., 1978. Vesicular storage and release of acetylcholine in *Torpedo* electroplaque synapses. J. Neurochem. 30: 1269-1280.

Tashiro, T. and Stadler, H., 1978. Chemical composition of cholin-ergic synaptic vesicles from *Torpedo marmorata* based on improved purification. Eur. J. Biochem. 90: 479-487.

Tuček, S., 1978. Acetylcholine synthesis in neurons. Chapman and Hall, London.

Weiler, M., Roed, I.S. and Whittaker, V.P., 1981. The kinetics of acetylcholine synthesis in resting cholinergic electromotor nerve terminals in *Torpedo marmorata*. Hoppe-Seyler's Z. Physiol. Chem. 362: 243.

Whittaker, V.P., 1978. The electromotor system of *Torpedo* as a model cholinergic system, in Cholinergic Mechanisms and Psychopharmacology' (D.J. Jenden, ed.), pp 323-345. Plenum Publishing Corp. New York.

Whittaker, V.P. and Luqmani, Y.A., 1980. False transmitters in the cholinergic system: implications for the vesicle theory of transmitter storage and release. Gen. Pharmacol. 11: 7-14.

Whittaker, V.P. and Stadler, H., 1980. The structure and function of cholinergic synaptic vesicles, in 'Proteins of the Nervous System' (R.A. Bradshaw and D.M. Schneider eds.), 2nd ed., pp 231-255. Raven Press, New York.

Whittaker, V.P. and Zimmermann, H., 1976. The innervation of the electric organ of *Torpedinidae*: a model cholinergic system, in 'Biochemical and Biophysical Perspectives in Marine Biology' (D.C. Malins and J.R. Sargent eds.), Vol 3, pp 67-116. Academic Press, London.

Whittaker, V.P., Essman, W.B. and Dowe, G.H.C., 1972. The isolation of pure cholinergic synaptic vesicles from the electric organs of elasmobranch fish of the family *Torpedinidae*. Biochem. J. 128: 833-846.

Yamamura, H.I. and Snyder, S.H., 1973. High affinity transport of choline into synaptosomes of rat brain. J. Neurochem. 21: 1355-1374.

Zechel, K. and Stadler, H., 1979. Identification of actin in purified synaptic vesicles of the electric organ of *Torpedo marmorata*. Hoppe-Seyler's Z. Physiol. Chem. 360: 409.

Zimmermann, H. and Denston, C.A., 1977a. Recycling of synaptic vesicles in the cholinergic synapses of the *Torpedo* electric organ during induced transmitter release. Neuroscience 2: 695-714.

Zimmermann, H. and Denston, C.R., 1977b. Separation of synaptic vesicles of different functional states from the cholinergic synapses of the *Torpedo* electric organ. Neuroscience 2: 715-730.

Zimmermann, H. and Whittaker, V.P., 1977. Morphological and biochemical heterogeneity of cholinergic synaptic vesicles. Nature (Lond.) 261: 633-635.

PHARMACOLOGY OF THE ACETYLCHOLINE RELEASE EVOKED BY ONE OR A FEW

NERVE IMPULSES AT THE NERVE-ELECTROPLAQUE JUNCTION OF TORPEDO

Lorenza Eder-Colli, Yves Dunant, Jacqueline Corthay
Anthony I. Walker* and Françoise Loctin

Département de Pharmacologie, Centre Médical Universitaire
1211 Geneva 4, Switzerland
*Present address: Emmanuel College, Cambridge, England

The release of acetylcholine(ACh) at synapses can be measured indirectly by recording the electrophysiological response generated by ACh at the postsynaptic membrane.However it is probable that the shape and the amplitude of the response are modified by postsynaptic changes affecting the availability of the receptor or the ionic gradient responsable for the discharge.On the other hand direct measurements of ACh release can be performed after repetitive stimulation provided that inhibitors of cholinesterases are present in the medium perfusing the tissue.However these drugs are expected to modify the metabolism of ACh since they inhibit the hydrolysis of the transmitter and therefore the subsequent recycling of the two precursors,acetate and choline.Thus a correlation between the electrophysiological and biochemical measurements has proved to be difficult.

In the present work a method will be first described which enabled us to directly measure the release of ACh in the absence of any inhibitor of cholinesterases (Dunant et al.,1980a).The amount of ACh released can then be compared to the electrophysiological response induced by different stimulation patterns.Secondly the results of a pharmacological analysis of the ACh release will be presented. Some of these results have been already presented as a short communication(Dunant and Walker,1981).These studies are performed with the electric organ of the fish Torpedo marmorata.This organ is composed of a large number of hexagonal prisms arranged side by side.Each prism consists of 400 to 500 superposed electroplaques which are embryologically derived from muscle cells.Each electroplaque receives on its ventral side a profuse innervation which is purely cholinergic. The electroplaque is totally devoid of any contractile material and is unable to generate and propagate action potentials.Thus the ele-

175

ctric discharge of Torpedo corresponds to the summation of the potentials generated by each electroplaque.The electroplaque potential
(epp) shares most of the properties which have been already described
for the endplate potential of the neuromuscular junction.

DIRECT MEASUREMENT OF ACh RELEASE

Israël and Tuček (1974) have demonstrated that the electric
organ of Torpedo incorporates preferentially acetate into ACh rather
than using glucose or pyruvate.Moreover external acetate and choline
are both used at the same rate for the synthesis of ACh.Because of
these properties it is possible to double label the ACh stores in
the electric organ by incubating small fragments(one or two prisms)
with acetate and choline used at the same molar concentrations
(8.4 uM) but radiolabelled with different isotopes.As shown in table
1. ,at the end of the incubation period (4 to 6 h at room temperature) the tissue retains equal amounts of total radioactive choline
and acetate.About 25 % of this total radioactivity is incorporated
into ACh and the ratio of the two precursors is not significantly
different from 1.Thus we conclude that the incorporation of choline
and acetate into ACh proceeds at the same rate.After a rather long
washing period (15 h at 7°C),the loss of total choline is greater
than the loss of total acetate.However the amount of ACh radiolabel
led from choline is not significantly changed during this period
although the amount of ACh radiolabelled from acetate decreases.This
suggests that a transfer of radiolabelled acetate occurs from ACh
to others constituents of the tissue.This is supported by the fact
that high voltage electrophoresis of tissue extracts shows that a
substantial incorporation of radiolabelled acetate into glutamine,
glutamate,aspartate and acetylcarnitine takes place.It must be
pointed out that only a small percentage of the total ACh of the tissue is radiolabelled.The total content of ACh measured by bioassay
remains stable troughout the experiment.

Table 1. Tissue ACh In A Double Label Experiment
(nmol/g wet tissue ±SE)

	Total ^{3}H-Choline	Total ^{14}C-Acetate	^{3}H-ACh	^{14}C-ACh	Total ACh
At the end of incubation	19.7+0.8	19.3+1.0	4.9+0.7	4.5+0.5	607+3
After washing	10.7+0.4	15.0+0.9	5.5+0.2	3.6+0.2	613+36

The double-labelled fragments are then mounted on small pieces
of nylon cloth between two stimulating electrodes which are situated
parallel to the prisms.The recording electrodes are inserted at the
dorsal and ventral ends of the prisms.The prisms are kept under profuse and continuous superfusion with the saline physiological medium.
A "field" stimulus(60 to 110 volts;0.5-0.8 ms) is applied to the tissue producing a well synchronized compound electroplaque potential
the amplitude of which varied between 0.2 to several volts according
to the size of the fragment.After an initial test of the response the
prisms are left at rest during 60 to 90 minutes.A drug to be tested
is added to the perfusion medium during this period.After stimulation
the compound epp is recorded and the radioactive choline and acetate
counted in the perfusion medium.The results of a typical experiment
are shown in figure 1.A surprising but constant finding is that the
resting release of acetate is significantly higher than the release
of choline whereas the ACh stores are more strongly labelled from
choline.This is independent of the isotope used.However the evoked
release of acetate and choline rises significantly over the resting
release in a ratio which reflects the ratio present in the ACh stores
and which is not different from 1.During the recovery period the
release of acetate returns to its background level more slowly than

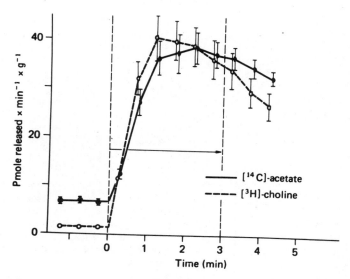

Fig.1. Release of radioactive ^{3}H-Choline and ^{14}C-Acetate in a double
labelling experiment.Fragments of tissue (1 or 2 prisms) are stimulated repetitively at 10 Hz during 3 minutes.The overflow of radioacti-
vities,expressed as absolute values of each precursor,is analysed be-
fore(1 minute),during(arrow) and after(1 minute) stimulation.During
stimulation the acetate and choline are released in a ratio not
significantly different from 1.(from Dunant et al.,1980a).

the release of choline.The higher resting release of acetate may be
explained by the release of some of the other compounds radiolabelled
from acetate and this release may be inhibited by the stimulation.

Using different stimulation patterns we have compared the amount
of radioactivity released to the electrophysiological response of
the tissue.In most of the experiments described here the results
with only one precursor of ACh will be presented.Figure 2. shows the
release of the radioactivity as a function of the number of stimuli
given in 1 second.Some fragments have been given a single impulse
while other received either 5,10 or 20 impulses in one second and
the radioactivity is counted in the medium during 4 minutes after
stimulation.In the short bursts the amplitude of the successive epps
decreases and the depression is more pronounced as the frequency of
stimulation is increased.In its physiological discharge the electric
organ of Torpedo produces short bursts of 5 to 10 impulses at approximately 100 Hz.Even in response to a single impulse the overflow of
radioactivity increases significantly over the background level.Larger
releases are obtained when more stimuli are delivered.However the relationship between the amount of radioactivity released and the number of impulses is not linear but hyperbolic this indicating that
the first impulse releases more radioactivity than the following ones
(Fig. 3).We have estimated that a saturation of the release occurs

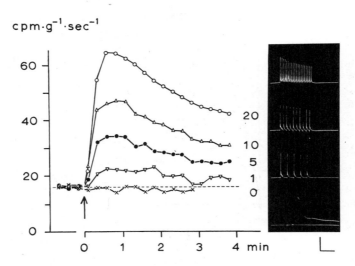

Fig.2 .Overflow of radioactivity and epps in function of the number
of impulses.Each curve is the mean of 2 different prisms which have
received : no stimulation(x),1 impulse(∇),5 impulses(•),10 impulses
(△) and 20 impulses(○) in 1 s.The arrow indicates the time of stimu-
lation.Label:3H-acetate.Bars:2V,4ms or 400ms(from Dunant et al.,1980a)

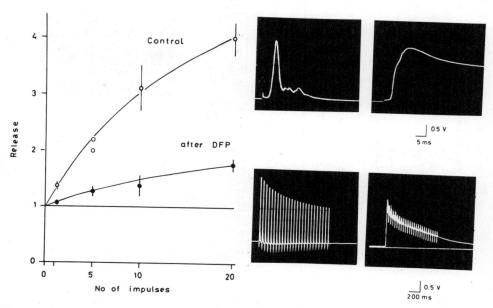

Fig. 3. Relationship between the evoked release of ACh and the number of stimuli.Labelling with 3H-acetate.The release measured in different experiments is expressed as the ratio of the peak of the
evoked release over the background level.Stimulation,as in Fig.2.,
consists of single impulse or short bursts of 5,10 or 20 stimuli in
1 s.The relationship between the number of stimuli and the release
is not linear but hyperbolic(o).Some fragments have been pretreated
with 1 µM DFP for 1 h before being mounted for stimulation.Before
stimulation the excess of the drug is washed out by perfusing the
fragments with the saline physiological medium during 90 minutes.
The spontaneous release is not modified by the drug.Means ± SE of
two to twenty values.The electrophysiological records show the
modification of the epp after pretreatment with DFP(right hand side
records). (from Dunant et al.,1980a)..

at approximately 100 impulses in one second.If this pattern of stimulation is repeated again after 30 to 60 minutes of rest,identical
results are obtained.It appears from this experiment that the depression of the electrophysiological response can be explained by a
decline in the amount of ACh released by the successive nerve impulses.

        This observation has been more properly analysed by measuring
the release due to paired stimuli separated by various time intervals
(Fig.4). In this experiment the amplitude of the second epp of the
pair is compared to the first one as a function of the time interval
separating them and is found to decrease as the interval decreases.

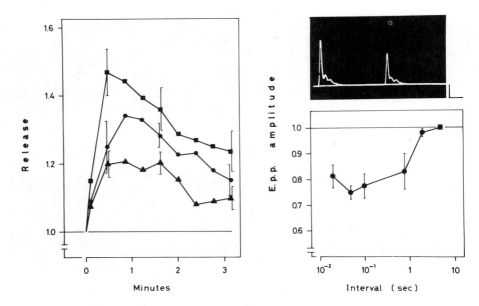

Fig.4. Release of ACh and depression of the synaptic transmission.
A single stimulus (▲) or paired stimuli separated by 50 ms (●) or
5 s(■) are applied to the tissue at the time t=o.The release of radioactivity is expressed as the ratio of the evoked release over the
resting release.Each curve is the mean + SE of 5 fragments stimulated for each condition.At 5 s interval the amplitude of the second
epp is identical to the first one ;the release is 2 times higher than
the release due to a single stimulus.Precursor as in Fig.2.The amplitude of the second epp in response to paired stimuli separated by
50 ms(see electrophysiological record) is depressed and the release
of radioactivity is significantly smaller than the one due to the
5 s paired stimuli.The right hand side graph shows the variation
of the ratio of the amplitudes of the second to the first epp as
a function of the time interval separating the two stimuli of the
pair.Calibration: 0.5 V and 10 ms.(from Dunant et al.,1980a).

A maximal depression occurs at 50 ms.The recovery from this depression
is very slow and is completed only after 5 s.The overflow of the radioactivity due to paired stimuli separated by 5 seconds appears to
be 2 times higher than the amount released by a single impulse.When
paired stimuli separated by 50 ms are delivered the release is significantly lower than after stimulation by paires pulses separated
by 5 seconds.Thus the depression of the amplitude of the second epp
of the pair is due to a decrease in the amount of ACh released by
the second stimulus of the pair.

        Finally the release of radioactivity has been tested as a func-
tion of the external concentrations of calcium and magnesium. As
shown in Figure 5 the release is strongly dependent on the calcium

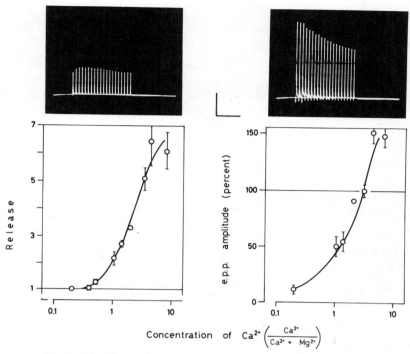

Fig.5. Effects of calcium and magnesium on the evoked release of ACh and on the epp.The release is expressed as in Fig.3.Means+SE of three to ten values.Labelling with 3H-Acetate.In the right⁻hand graph the epp amplitude is the percent of the epp amplitude measured in normal calcium and magesium concentrations(4.4 mM CaCl$_2$ and 1.3 mM MgCl$_2$).Electrophysiological records show the response to 20 impulses in one second;the one at the left :1.1 mM CaCl$_2$ ane no magnesium; the one at the right: 4.4 mM CaCl$_2$ and no magnesium.Calibration:1V and 400 ms .(from Dunant et al.,1980a).

concentration and is inhibited by magnesium.The slope of the concentration-release curve appears to be very steep and the Hill's coefficient measured in the absence of magnesium is 3.2.This confirms the results of many electrophysiological experiments which have shown that a co-operation of 3 to 4 calcium ions is required to trigger the ACh release.The calcium concentration corresponding to half of the maximal release is about 0.55 mM.The amplitude of the epps shows a parallel dependency on calcium concentration.The electrophysiological records in figure 4. show the response to 20 impulses in one second obtained either in low calcium and no magnesium or in normal calcium and no magnesium .In the first condition the amplitude of the first epp is depressed but the following epps remain rather constant and even show some degree of facilitation.In the second condition the amplitude of the first epp is increased but then the successive epps undergo a marked progressive depression.Therefore

the radioactivity measured in these experiments is faithfully related
to the ACh released by the nerve impulses and is not due to some nonspecific effect of the stimulating shocks.

In conclusion we can assume that the method described here
allows a direct measurement of the ACh release in the absence of
any anticholinesterases drug and provides a good correlation between
biochemical and electrophysiological measurements of the ACh released
even in response to a single nerve impulse.

PHARMACOLOGY OF THE ACh RELEASE

It has been suggested that neurotransmitters can inhibit their
own release by acting on presynaptic autoreceptors.In the nerve-
electroplaque junction of Torpedo the postsynaptic receptor is purely
nicotinic.Recently Kloog et al. (1978) have found muscarinic binding
sites in the electric organ of Torpedo whose localisation is probably
presynaptic.In order to characterize these presumed autoreceptors we
have tested the effects on the release of drugs known to interact
either with the nicotinic or with the muscarinic receptors.

Alpha-bungarotoxin binds irreversibly to the nicotinic receptor.
At 7 µm the toxin completely blocks the transmission in the electric
organ.However no modification at all was observed either of the spontaneous or of the evoked release of ACh. Curare ,a competitive inhibitor of the nicotinic receptor induces variable effects according
to the source from which it is provided.Indeed the drug from Vifor
Co(Geneva) produces only a very slight depression of the evoked release but the one from Sigma Co induces a marked depression.Neither
of them has an effect on the spontaneous release and both of them
at 0.1 mM completely inhibit the transmission.Carbachol a structural analogue of ACh is not hydrolysed by cholinesterases and is known
to stimulate both nicotinic and muscarinic receptors.In our preparations 1 mM carbachol depresses strongly the evoked release of ACh.

The effects of oxotremorine,a potent muscarinic agonist ,and
of atropine,an antagonist ,are shown in figure 6. The electrophysiological changes in response to 20 impulses in one second in the presence of 1 µm oxotremorine consist in a reduction of the amplitude
of the first epp of the train but the depression normally observed
does not occur.The depression of the transmission is followed by
spontaneous recovery after the drug is washed out.Atropine antagonizes completely oxotremorine when both drugs are used together.
The depression due to oxotremorine is very similar to the one obtained in low calcium concentration but oxotremorine has been shown not
to inhibit the intraterminal accumulation of calcium during repetitive stimulation.The drug at 1 and 10 µM reduces greatly the evoked
release of ACh in a concentration dependent manner.These effects
are totally inhibited by 1 µM atropine.Atropine itself (from 1 nM
to 10 µM) has no significant effect on ACh release and on the epp.

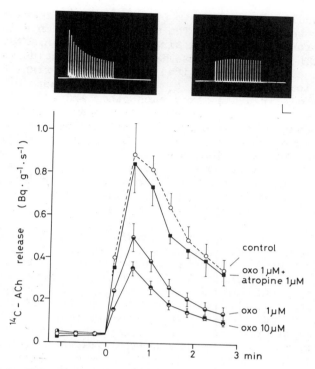

Fig. 6. Depression of the evoked release of ACh by oxotremorine and antagonistic effect of atropine.Stimulation : 20 impulses in one s. Electrophysiological records: control (left hand side record) and in the presence of 1 µM oxotremorine (right hand side record).Calibration: 0.5 V and 200 ms.The graphs show the release of 14C-ACh, labelled from 14 C-Choline,after the brief stimulation given at the time t=o.For each condition four prisms have been stimulated.(from Dunant and Walker, 1981).

Thus the effects of oxotremorine and atropine on the elctrophysiological response correlate well with a modification of the amount of ACh released by nerve impulses.Oxotremorine is found not to change the size of ACh stores in the tissue.Very surprisingly typical muscarinic agonists as muscarine,pilocarpine and betanechol do not impair at all the nerve electroplaque transmission and the ACh release.

There are good indications that ACh itself ,when it is not hydrolysed in the synaptic cleft inhibits its own release.Indeed we have found that anticholinesterases drugs produce a strong decrease in the evoked release of ACh.Similar effects have been obtained either in the presence of reversible inhibitors(physostigmine,neostigmine) or after pretreatment with irreversible inhibitor of cholinesterases

(DFP).The results obtained with DFP pretreated fragments of electric organ are shown in figure 3. The depression of ACh release appears to be more pronounced after a single impulse than after repetitive stimulation.The epp in response to a single stimulus is greatly prolonged(upper electrophysiological record at the right hand side). In response to 20 bursts in 1 s the individual epps of the train can no longer be distinguished from each other and a fused potential of long duration is produced(lower electrophysiological record at the right hand side).In the presence of anticholinesterases drugs the electric organ of Torpedo is unable to sustain repetitive stimulation (Feldberg and Fessard, 1942).When we depolarize the tissue by high potassium concentration no significant effect of the anticholinesterases drugs is noticed.The total amount of ACh in the tissue as well as the amount of radiolabelled transmitter are not altered after treatment with inhibitors of cholinesterases.

The addition of alpha-bungarotoxin or curare to preparations pretreated with DFP does not bring any further change of the release of ACh.However when atropine is added the depression is totally reversed and even some increase of the release can be detected (Fig.7). No additional change of the epp is noticed.This is expected since after inhibition of cholinesterases the epp is more strongly influenced by factors such as receptor desensitization and diffusion of ACh from the synaptic regions.After stimulation we can observe that the radioactivity released from DFP treated fragments returns only very slowly to its background level.This can be explained by the continuous diffusion of non-hydrolysed ACh from the more central regions of the prism into the perfusing medium,ACh being not taken up as easily as acetate and choline by the nerve endings.

Thus the non-hydrolysed ACh in the synaptic cleft seems to inhibit its own release.This has been more directly analysed by adding ACh to fragments pretreated with DFP (Fig. 8.).Indeed we obtain an additional decrease of the release and this effect seems to be concentration dependent.Oxotremorine at 10 μM mimics totally this effect of ACh.Both effects are competitively inhibited by 1 μM atropine.

All the drugs described so far have induced a depression of the evoked release of ACh.We have found only two drugs which are able to constantly increase the evoked release.These are oxythiamine and 4-aminopyridine (4 AP).Oxythiamine is a structural analogue of thiamine or vitamin B_1.Thiamine has been known for a long time to play a special but still not well-defined role in the function of the nervous tissues.We have measured very high amounts of this vitamin(120 nmol/g)in the electric organ of Torpedo(Eder et al.,1980a). Thiamine appears to be mainly localised in the nerves and the nerve endings of this tissue (Eder et al.,1978).Thiamine itself exerts a rather complex action on the evoked release of ACh,increasing it at concentrations lower than 1 mM but decreasing it at higher concentrations.However its analogue ,oxythiamine (from 0.01 to 1 mM)induces constantly a very significant increase of the evoked release(Fig.9.).

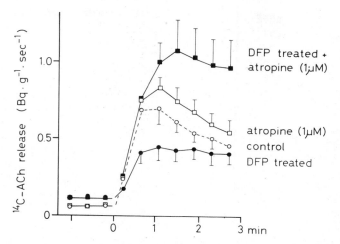

Fig. 7. Depression of the evoked release of ACh after pretreatment with DFP and reverse effect by atropine.Stimulation : 20 impulses in 1 s given at time t=o.Precursor: 14C-Choline.Half of the prisms have been pretreated with 1 mM DFP as described in Fig.3.The excess of DFP is washed out with saline physiological medium containing(■) or not (●) 1 μM atropine.Mean + SEM of 4 prisms for each condition. The significant decrease in ACh release due to DFP (p < 0.01) is largely reversed by atropine.Atropine alone (□) induces a nonsignificant increase in the ACh release.(from Dunant and Walker,1981).

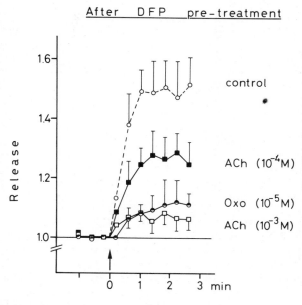

Fig. 8. Inhibition of the ACh release by ACh.In this experiment all the fragments have been pretreated with 1 mM DFP;therefore the release in controls(o) is reduced with respect to untreated tissue (see Fig.7) Addition of exogeneous ACh induces a further reduction in ACh release in a dose-dependent manner(p<0.001 for the two concentrations of ACh).Oxotremorine exerts same effect as ACh.For each condition four prisms have been given 20 bursts in one second.Precursor: 14C-Choline.(from Dunant and Walker,1981)*

*Fig. 6,7,8: paper in preparation for Eur.J.Pharmacol.

This effect is also significant in response to a single stimulus and is also expressed in the epp which shows a characteristic shoulder in its descending phase (Eder et al.,1980).

    The most dramatic increase of the evoked release of ACh is produced by 4 AP.As shown in figure 10 ,in response to a single nerve impulse a giant epp is formed which is followed constantly by a rebound which appears 250 to 300 ms after the stimulus artifact.Increasing concentrations of 4 AP enlarge mainly the duration rather than the amplitude of the epps.The overflow of radioactivity correlates well with the electrophysiological measurements ,that is the evoked release of ACh is enhanced in function of increasing concentrations of 4 AP.In the presence of 1 mM 4 AP a single impulse is able to release 68 times more ACh than in the absence of the drug.This potentiation concerns only isolated impulses and a second shock delivered 2 seconds later fails to produce an electrophysiological response. In the presence of the drug the resting content of ACh in the tissue is always reduced by about 50 %.This unexplained observation indicates that the effect of 4 AP cannot be explained simply by an increase in the available stores of ACh.

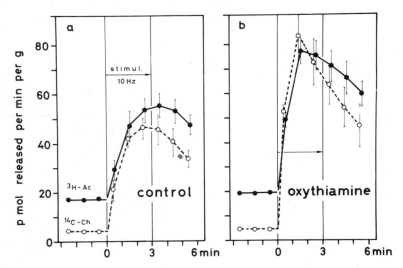

Fig.9.   Increase in the evoked release of ACh by oxythiamine. Precursors: 3H-Acetate and 14C-Choline.Experiment as in Fig.1.Five prisms have been treated with 0.1 mM oxythiamine and five others have been taken as controls.Oxythiamine,a structural analogue of thiamine(vitamin B$_1$) clearly potentiates the evoked release of ACh without changing the spontaneous release.Repetitive stimulation at 10 Hz during 3 minutes.(from Eder et al.,1980b).

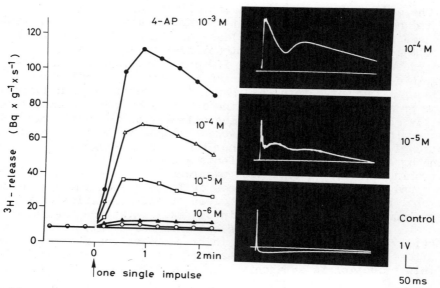

Fig.10. Potentiation of the evoked release of ACh and of the epp by 4 AP.Increasing concentrations of 4 AP induce a great prolongation of the epp which correlate well with the effect of the drug on the release.Stimulation (arrow) with a single impulse.The release from control fragments (o) increases significantly over the background level.For each condition four different fragments have been stimulated.Precursor: 3H-Acetate. (from Dunant et al.,1980b).

DISCUSSION

In the present work we have described a radiochemical assay for the release of ACh.This method is sensitive enough to detect the amount of neurotransmitter released even by a single nerve impulse. Moreover no addition of inhibitor of cholinesterase is required.This assay has been used in a number of different electrophysiological and pharmacological experiments.A very good correlation between the release of ACh and the electrophysiological events has been obtained.

Only two drugs have been found to increase significantly the evoked release of ACh.Oxythiamine is known to exert a metabolic anti-thiamine action when administred to animals.This structural analogue of thiamine has been shown by several other authors to be taken up actively by cells and to be phosphorylated intracellularly.It may be that this drug increases the release of ACh by acting inside the nerve terminals on the metabolism of the transmitter.A very strong potentiation of the electrophysiological response and of the evoked release has been observed with 4 AP.This drug is known to block the potassium efflux thus prolonging the axon terminal spike;this will increase the efficiency of the calcium uptake and consequently enhance the release

The major points of the results of the pharmacological analysis reported here are that the potent muscarinic agonist,oxotremorine, depresses strongly the evoked release of ACh and this effect is similar to the one observed with anticholinesterases drugs.In both cases the depression is antagonised by low concentrations of atropine,a muscarinic antagonist.The depression is more pronounced after a single or a few nerve impulses than after repetitive stimulation. In the presence of oxotremorine the decrease of the epp amplitude normally observed during repetitive stimulation does not occur. Moreover the depression of the evoked release by anticholinesterases is strongly reinforced by a further addition of exogeneous oxotremorine or ACh and again these effects are competitively antagonised by atropine.Similar results with oxotremorine and atropine have been also found in isolated synaptosomes of Torpedo when the ACh release is evoked by high potassium(Michaelson et al.,1979).Similarly in other tissues like mammalian brain or small intestine the release of ACh is reduced by oxotremorine but enhanced by atropine(Szerb and Somogyi,1973;Kilbinger ,1977).In these preparations cholinesterases inhibitors reduce the evoked release of ACh (Bourdois et al.,1974) and this reduction is antagonised by atropine(Szerb and Somogyi,1973).

At the neuromuscular junction discrepant results have been reported concerning the effects of oxotremorine on the evoked release(Ganguly and Das,1979;Gundersen and Jenden,1980).The inhibition of the ACh release by anticholinesterases seems to be reversed only by alpha-bungarotoxin or curare(Miledi et al.,1978).In the electric organ of Torpedo which is homologous to the neuromuscular junction we have been unable to elicit any change in the release by using inhibitors of the nicotinic receptor ;the depression due to anticholinesterases could not be reversed.Therefore the retrograde inhibition by ATP reported by Meunier et al.(1975) and by Israël et al.(1980) cannot account for these results.These authors have demonstrated that in the nerve-electroplaque junction of Torpedo,increasing concentrations of ACh in the synaptic cleft stimulate the nicotinic receptor thereby inducing a postsynaptic release of ATP;this ATP in turn will act presynaptically and inhibit further release of ACh.

The depression of the release of ACh produced by oxotremorine and the competitive action of atropine appear to be due to a direct effect on the nerve endings.However we cannot presently speak of a regulation of the release through a muscarinic receptor,localized presynaptically,since muscarine itself is totally inactive.It may be possible that these drugs interact directly with the mechanism of release itself ,which still remains a matter of conjecture.

ACKNOWLEDGEMENTS

This work was supported by the "Fonds National pour la Recherche

Scientifique"(grants No 3.341.0.78 and 3.675.0.80) and the Fondation
Schmidheiny.We are grateful to M. Fred Pillonel for illustrating assistance.

REFERENCES

Bourdois,P.S.,Mitchell,J.F.,Somogyi,G.T. and Szerb,J.C.,1974,The
output per stimulus of acetylcholine from cerebral cortical slices
in the presence or absence of cholinesterase inhibition,Br.J.
Pharmacol.,52:509.

Dunant,Y.,Eder,L. and Servetiadis-Hirt,L.,1980a, Acetylcholine release evoked by single or a few nerve impulses in the electric organ of
Torpedo,J. Physiol.(Lond.),298:185.

Dunant,Y.,Corthay,J.,Eder,L. and Loctin,F.,1980b, Acetylcholine
changes during nerve impulses transmission.Analysis with a rapid
freezing device,in"Ontogenesis and Functional Mechanisms of peripheral synapses,"INSERM Symposium No 13.J.Taxi,ed.,Elsevier/North-Hol-
land Biomedical Press,p.99.

Dunant,Y. and Walker,A.I.,1981,Presynaptic inhibition of acetylcholine release by oxotremorine and acetylcholinesterases in the electric organ of Torpedo,J. Physiol.(Lond.)(in press).

Eder, L., Dunant, Y. and Baumann, M., 1978, Localization of thiamine an
cholinergic nerve terminals:An histofluorescence study in the electric organ of Torpedo, J. Neurocytol. ,7 : 637.

Eder, L. and Dunant, Y., 1980a, Thiamine and cholinergic transmission
in the electric organ of Torpedo.I. Cellular localization and functional changes of thiamine and thiamine phosphate esters. J. Neurochem.,
35:1278

Eder,L.,Dunant,Y. and Loctin,F.,1980b,Thiamine and cholinergic
transmission in the electric organ of Torpedo.II.Effects of exogeneous thiamine analogues on acetylcholine release.J.Neurochem.,
35:1287.

Feldberg,W. and Fessard,A.,1942,The cholinergic nature of the nerves
to the elctric organ of the Torpedo(Torpedo marmorata),J.Physiol.,
101:200.

Ganguly,D.K. and Das,M.,1979,Effects of oxotremorine demonstrate
presynaptic muscarinic and dopaminergic receptors on motor nerve
terminals,Nature,278:645.

Gundersen,C.B. and Jenden,D.J.,1980,Oxotremorine does not enhance
acetylcholine release from rat diaphragm preparations,Br.J.
Pharmacol.,70:8.

Israël, M. and Tuček, S., 1974, Utilisation of acetate and pyruvate for the synthesis of "total","bound" and "free" acetylcholine in the electric organ of Torpedo, J. Neurochem., 22:487

Israël, M.,Lesbats,B.,Manaranche,R.,Meunier,F.M. and Frachon,P.,1980, Retrograde inhibition of transmitter release by ATP,J.Neurochem., 34:923.

Kilbinger,H.,1977,Modulation by oxotremorine and atropine of acetyl-choline release evoked by electrical stimulation of the myenteric plexus of the guines-pig ileum,Naunyn Schmiedebergs Arch.Pharmacol., 300:145..

Kloog,Y.,Michaelson,D.M. and Sokolovski,M.,1978,Identification of muscarinic receptors in the Torpedo electric organ.Evidence for their presynaptic localization,FEBS Lett.,95:331.

Meunier,F.M.,Israël,M. and Lesbats,B.,1975,Release of ATP from sti-mulated nerve electroplaque junction,Nature ,257:407.

Miledi,R.,Molenaar,P.C. and Polak,R.I.,1978, α-Bungarotoxin enhan-ces transmitter "released"at the neuromuscular junction,Nature, 272:641.

Michaelson,D.M.,Avissar,S.,Kloog,Y. and Sokolovsky,M.,1979,Mechanism of acetylcholine release:Possible involvement of presynaptic muscari-nic receptors in regulation of acetylcholine release and protein phosphorylation,Proc.Natl.Acad.Sci.USA,76:6336.

Szerb,J.C. and Somogyi,G.T.,1973,Depression of acetylcholine release from cerebral cortical slices by cholinesterase inhibition and by oxotremorine,Nature, 241:121.

THE UPTAKE AND METABOLISM OF CHOLINE ANALOGUES BY CHOLINERGIC NERVE TERMINALS

B. Collier and Y.N. Kwok

Department of Pharmacology and Therapeutics
McGill University, Montreal

INTRODUCTION

The purpose of this article is to review the contributions that studies with choline analogues can make to the understanding of events associated with the synthesis, compartmentation and release of the cholinergic neurotransmitter. It will concentrate on the analogues whose structure is shown in Fig. 1 because, as yet, most information of this kind has been obtained with those compounds.

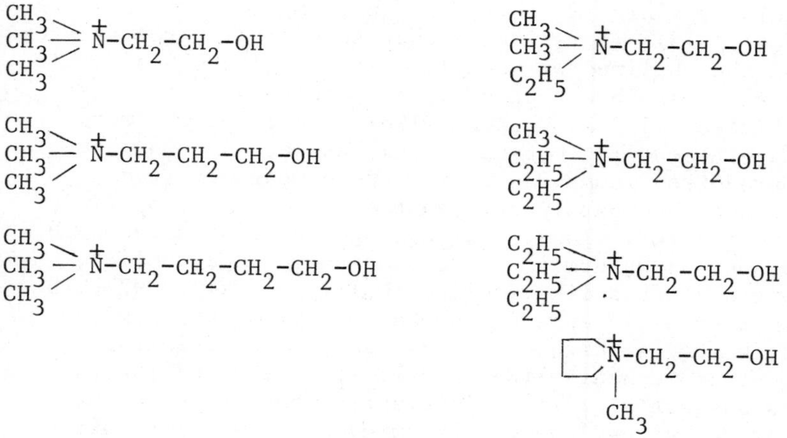

$$\begin{array}{l}CH_3 \\ CH_3 \\ CH_3\end{array} \!\!\!\diagdown\!\!\! \overset{+}{N}\text{-}CH_2\text{-}CH_2\text{-}OH$$

$$\begin{array}{l}CH_3 \\ CH_3 \\ C_2H_5\end{array} \!\!\!\diagdown\!\!\! \overset{+}{N}\text{-}CH_2\text{-}CH_2\text{-}OH$$

$$\begin{array}{l}CH_3 \\ CH_3 \\ CH_3\end{array} \!\!\!\diagdown\!\!\! \overset{+}{N}\text{-}CH_2\text{-}CH_2\text{-}CH_2\text{-}OH$$

$$\begin{array}{l}CH_3 \\ C_2H_5 \\ C_2H_5\end{array} \!\!\!\diagdown\!\!\! \overset{+}{N}\text{-}CH_2\text{-}CH_2\text{-}OH$$

$$\begin{array}{l}CH_3 \\ CH_3 \\ CH_3\end{array} \!\!\!\diagdown\!\!\! \overset{+}{N}\text{-}CH_2\text{-}CH_2\text{-}CH_2\text{-}CH_2\text{-}OH$$

$$\begin{array}{l}C_2H_5 \\ C_2H_5 \\ C_2H_5\end{array} \!\!\!\diagdown\!\!\! \overset{+}{N}\text{-}CH_2\text{-}CH_2\text{-}OH$$

$$\overset{+}{N}\text{-}CH_2\text{-}CH_2\text{-}OH$$
$$|$$
$$CH_3$$

Fig. 1. Structure of choline analogues compared to choline: left side, top to bottom – choline, homocholine, butylcholine; right side, top to bottom – monoethylcholine, diethylcholine, triethylcholine, pyrrolidinecholine.

191

Choline analogues were first used to define the structural specificity of choline's toxicity and vascular effects (Hunt and Taveau, 1909; 1911), and later in studies on the mechanism by which choline prevents fatty infiltration of the liver (Channon and Smith, 1936) or perosis in birds (Jukes and Welch, 1942). Such studies showing that the triethyl analogue of choline, hydroxyethyl triethylammonium or triethylcholine, could substitute for choline in metabolic functions prompted the suggestion (Keston and Wortis, 1946) that this analogue might be handled like choline at motor nerve terminals and, so, enter the terminal, be acetylated, and form a false neurotransmitter. It was almost 30 years later that final direct evidence was obtained to prove that hypothesis (Ilson and Collier, 1975). In retrospect, it appears that the first direct evidence showing a choline analogue to form a false transmitter was an experiment by Reitzel and Long (1959) which compared choline to the ethylcholines as antagonists of hemicholinium-induced neuromuscular blockade. Monoethylcholine was about 20% as effective as choline and the other analogues were ineffective; this was interpreted to indicate that the interaction required choline's quaternary head to fit a receptor site of specific volume not well satisfied by the ethylcholines; but it appears more likely that the ethyl analogues of choline formed false transmitters of which acetylmonoethylcholine was weakly active as a nicotinic agonist, and acetyldi- and acetyltri-ethylcholine were relatively inactive as agonists.

THE CHOLINE UPTAKE MECHANISM

Structural Specificity. Since about 10 years ago, it has been accepted by most cholinologists that choline enters cholinergic nerve terminals by a high affinity transport mechanism (see, e.g. review by Jope, 1979); it is likely that this uptake process provides most of the choline for acetylcholine (ACh) synthesis, although it remains possible that nerve terminals can synthesize some choline (Blusztajn and Wurtman, 1981). Much of the work characterizing the choline uptake system has been done on synaptosomes prepared from mammalian brain, and comparable studies with choline analogues have partly defined the structural specificity of the choline carrier. Thus, lengthening the amino alcohol chain of choline by one − CH_2 group yields a compound, homocholine, which can be transported like choline (Collier et al., 1977), but increasing that N-OH distance by another methylene group gives butylcholine, which is neither a substrate nor an inhibitor of the choline uptake mechanism (Batzold et al., 1980; Collier, 1981). These results suggest a critical interaction between substrate and carrier at two sites, one likely anionic to associate with the substrate's quaternary nitrogen and one possibly a hydrogen bonding site to interact with the −OH group; the optimal −N-to-OH distance for a substrate to fit these two sites is estimated to be between 3.1 and 3.3 Å (Batzold et al., 1980; Collier, 1981).

Much more variation of the structure of the substituents on the $\overset{+}{N}$ is possible without there being much loss of ability to be transported by the choline transport mechanism. Thus, successive replacement of methyl groups by ethyl groups to give mono-, di-, and tri-ethylcholine, or cyclization of two of the quaternary substituents as in pyrrolidinecholine, alters affinity for the choline carrier only modestly and changes the rate of transport hardly at all (Barker and Mittag, 1975; Barker et al., 1975).

The choline analogues mentioned above compete with choline for choline uptake sites; other analogues can do so without being transported (e.g. hemicholinium: Collier, 1973; Slater and Stonier, 1973); others inhibit choline transport but have not yet been tested as substrates for uptake (e.g. Simon et al., 1975; Batzold et al., 1980). The most interesting choline analogues yet to be completely characterized and exploited may be the nitrogen mustard analogues, which inhibit choline uptake irreversibly (Rylett and Colhoun, 1980a).

Regulation of Choline Transport. It is now clear that the rate of choline transport is regulated in some way by the functional activity of cholinergic nerve terminals. The mechanism(s) involved in this regulation remain largely unknown, and the functional relationship of this regulation to ACh synthesis rate is not always agreed upon. We consider there to be three types of regulatory phenomena: one revealed following transmitter depletion, one that is associated with an adaptive change in synaptic efficacy caused by conditioning, and one that occurs during more normal rates of transmitter turnover. Our own analysis of these phenomena has used cat sympathetic ganglia as the model cholinergic synapse, and the accumulation of the choline analogues, homocholine or triethylcholine, as indicators of choline transport activity. These analogues were used under conditions where they substitute for choline as substrate for uptake into nerve terminals but not as substrate for choline acetyltransferase once they are within the nerve terminals; thus, changes in accumulation as the result of altered transport can be distinguished readily from changes in accumulation as the result of increased metabolism.

(i) Regulation following transmitter depletion. This phenomenon as studied in ganglia probably bears most relationship to that discussed by Marchbanks (this volume) from studies upon synaptosomes. When ganglia are stimulated to release ACh by perfusion with a high K^+ medium, they do not maintain their full complement of transmitter and suffer ACh depletion. This is a somewhat artificial situation in sympathetic ganglia, for during neuronal stimulation, they maintain well their ACh store (Birks and MacIntosh, 1961; Collier and MacIntosh, 1969). Nevertheless, K^+-induced depletion of transmitter stores allows study of the choline transport activity following stimulation by K^+ during a phase of

increased ACh synthesis required to replenish ACh content. Following K$^+$ stimulation, ACh content returns to normal provided choline
is available, and measurement of choline uptake by homocholine
accumulation shows this process to be activated during that time
(Fig. 2).

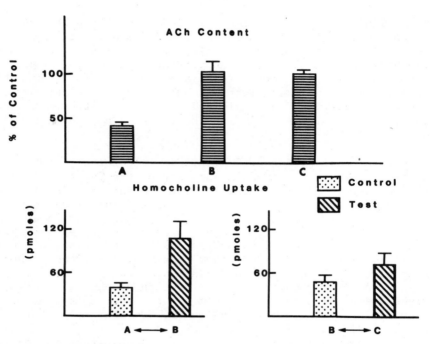

Fig. 2. Upper part shows the ACh content of ganglia after 60 min
exposure to K$^+$ (A), following such exposure followed by 15 min
perfusion (B) or 30 min perfusion (C) with normal medium. Lower
part shows homocholine uptake measured during the phase of ACh
repletion (A-B) and following that repletion (B-C).

     Analysis of a similar phenomenon in synaptosomes following ACh
depletion (e.g. Murrin and Kuhar, 1976; Roskoski, 1978; Weiler et
al., 1978; Marchbanks et al., 1981) has suggested the increased
choline transport to be responsible for the ACh repletion and most
of the evidence suggests the change in transport rate to be regulated by intraterminal ACh level; thus, lowered nerve terminal ACh
concentration enhances choline uptake which encourages ACh synthesis to replete transmitter store and turn off choline transport.
It is reasonable to suppose the same sequence of events might
occur in ganglia following K$^+$-induced depletion of ACh levels.

But, lowered intraterminal ACh is not the only stimulus for accelerated choline transport activity, and this is shown by:

(ii) Regulation following conditioning. As mentioned above, the ACh content of a sympathetic ganglion is well maintained during preganglionic nerve stimulation, so that at the end of, say, 60 min stimulation at 20 Hz it equals that of a resting ganglion. However, during rest following such or similar stimulation, ACh content increases above normal (Rosenblueth et al., 1939; Friesen and Khatter, 1971; Birks and Fitch, 1974; Bourdois et al., 1975; Birks, 1977 and 1978). This post-conditioning increase in ACh content is the result of increased ACh synthesis associated with increased choline uptake activity, as assessed by homocholine accumulation (Table I). Under all conditions so far studied, when post-stimulation choline analogue accumulation is enhanced, so too does ACh content increase, and when post-stimulation choline uptake is not activated, ACh content does not increase. Thus, as following K^+-stimulation, it seems reasonable to conclude that the increased choline delivery increases ACh synthesis and content; but in this situation, depleted intraterminal ACh level is not the trigger because the tissue store is not depleted.

TABLE I   INCREASED ACh CONTENT AND HOMOCHOLINE UPTAKE BY GANGLIA FOLLOWING PREGANGLIONIC CONDITIONING

Conditioning	Post-Conditioning	Homocholine Uptake	ACh Content
Normal medium	Normal medium	Increased	Increased
Ca^{++}-free medium	Normal medium	Not increased	Not increased
Tubocurarine medium	Normal medium	Increased	Increased
Normal medium	Na^+-free medium	Not increased	Not increased

(iii) Regulation during stimulation. Indirect evidence that the process of choline uptake into cholinergic nerve terminals is activated during stimulation was provided by experiments that studied choline recapture by sympathetic ganglia (Collier and Katz, 1974). During preganglionic nerve stimulation, choline derived from the hydrolysis of released transmitter was re-used for ACh synthesis, but during rest no such preferential uptake of choline by preganglionic terminals was evident, suggesting that activation of the nerve terminal's choline transport mechanism occurred during stimulation. This idea was tested using choline analogue accumulation as a measure of altered choline uptake activity (Collier and Ilson, 1977): preganglionic nerve stimulation increased the uptake of homocholine or triethylcholine under conditions where they were not acetylated to a significant extent. The physiological significance of this increased choline transport activity during stimulation is still a matter for conjecture. Clearly, in life, it must be conducive to the increased transmitter synthesis that occurs during synaptic activity, but altered choline transport, alone, appears to be an insufficient trigger for increased ACh synthesis during stimulation. Thus (Collier and Ilson, 1977; O'Regan and Collier, 1981), one can have increased choline uptake without proportional increased ACh synthesis, and one can have increased net synthesis of ACh without proportional increased choline uptake (Table II).

TABLE II   CHANGES OF CHOLINE ANALOGUE ACCUMULATION AND OF ACh
           SYNTHESIS BY GANGLIA DURING STIMULATION

Condition	Analogue Accumulation	ACh Synthesis
Normal	↑↑	↑↑
Ca^{++}-free	↔	↔
Increased Mg^{++}	↑↑	↑
Low Ca^{++}-high Mg^{++}	↑	↔
Ba^{++} instead of Ca^{++}	↑↑	↑
K^+ stimulation	↔	↑
Veratridine stimulation	↔	↑

It would appear that, in addition to choline uptake, some other factor(s) help regulate ACh synthesis during stimulation and we have some evidence that one of these other factors is an increased delivery of acetyl-CoA to choline acetyltransferase. This appears to occur during stimulation, where it might help regulate ACh synthesis, but not following stimulation, where ACh synthesis regulation seems to be accounted for by altered choline uptake.

THE ACETYLATION OF CHOLINE ANALOGUES

In vitro acetylation. The specificity of choline acetyltransferase for its acceptor substrate, choline, was studied first by Burgen et al. (1956) who established that several analogues of choline can be acetylated by the enzyme studied in a cell-free system; there have been many extensions and confirmations of this (e.g. Dauterman and Mehrotra, 1963; Hemsworth and Smith, 1970; Hemsworth, 1971; Currier and Mautner, 1974; Sollenberg et al., 1979). Overall, it appears that replacements of choline's N-methyl groups by N-alkyl groups reduces the affinity of the compounds for the enzyme with less change of Vmax; lengthening the amino alcohol chain even by one methylene group results in loss of affinity - thus homocholine is not acetylated in the cell-free system. It would appear that choline acetyltransferase in vitro shows somewhat greater substrate specificity than does the choline transport mechanism.

In situ acetylation. One might reasonably expect that the order of acetylation of choline analogues by choline acetyltransferase in a cell-free system would predict the order of their acetylation by intact tissues; but this appears not to be so. Thus Barker and Mittag (1975) found similar rates of acetylation of choline, monoethylcholine, diethylcholine and pyrrolidinecholine by intact synaptosomes, rather than an order of choline > monoethylcholine > diethylcholine = pyrrolidinecholine that might be predicted on the basis of studies with the cell-free system. An extreme example of this in situ - in vitro difference in choline analogue acetylation is homocholine, which is not acetylated in vitro, but can be acetylated by intact tissues (Barker and Mittag, 1976; Collier et al., 1977; von Schwarzenfeld, 1979; Luqmani et al., 1980; Nelson et al., 1980).

The reason for this difference between in vitro and in vivo rate of choline analogue acetylation is not yet clear. Barker and Mittag (1975) suggested it to reflect some sort of direct coupling between uptake and acetylating mechanisms, an idea supported by some (e.g. Rylett and Colhoun, 1980b; Weiler et al., 1981), but not all (Kessler and Marchbanks, 1979) experiments; certainly, in tissues other than synaptosomes from mammalian brain, there is little indication of tight coupling (e.g., Barker et al., 1975; Collier et al., 1977). An alternate explanation for the failure of cell-free acetylation to predict intact cell acetylation of choline analogues is that it reflects a unique property of membrane associated choline acetyltransferase not evident with soluble enzyme. When this idea was tested for homocholine by encouraging adsorption of soluble enzyme to membranes, the result was negative (Boksa and Collier, 1980a), but when membranes were washed and residual membrane-bound choline acetyltransferase was tested, the result was positive (Benishin and Carroll, 1981). If, indeed, membrane bound enzyme differs from soluble enzyme, this could be a very important consideration in understanding ACh turnover (see e.g., MacIntosh and Collier, 1976).

SUBCELLULAR STORAGE OF ACETYLATED CHOLINE ANALOGUES

Endogenous transmitter is considered to be synthesized in the nerve terminal cytoplasm and stored both in the cytoplasm and in synaptic vesicles; ACh being translocated from the former to the latter by some poorly-understood process. A major impetus to study

the subcellular distribution of acetylated choline analogues was
the hope that such might provide information about the process of
transmitter uptake into synaptic vesicles. A second hope of these
studies was that an analogue ester might be formed that would
localize uniquely to one subcellular storage site and, thus, provide information about the functional significance of cytoplasmic
and vesicle-bound transmitter. Neither of these ideals has yet
been realized, but some useful information has been gathered.

Mammalian Tissue. As indicated earlier, certain choline analogues
are transported by the choline transport mechanism and are acetylated by intact synaptosomes; of these, monoethylcholine, diethylcholine and homocholine have been compared to choline in measures
of the subcellular distribution of the acetyl esters. In these
experiments, isolated synaptosomes were incubated with radiolabelled
precursors; subsequently the synaptosomes were collected, burst,
and the proportion of acetylated compounds measured in cytoplasmic
and synaptic vesicle fractions (Fig. 3).

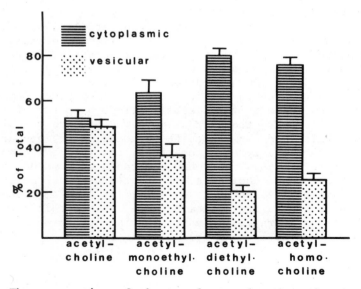

Fig. 3. The proportion of the total acetylated products of
choline or analogues measured in cytoplasmic (hatched) and vesicle
(dotted) fractions when synaptosomes were exposed to the precursors (10^{-6}M).

The choline analogues were acetylated and found in the same fractions as was ACh; thus, none of these esters uniquely localizes to any one transmitter compartment. But the analogue esters appear to show differences in the relative distribution between cytoplasmic and vesicle-bound stores, as if the mechanism responsible for translocating ACh from the cytoplasm into storage particles might show structural specificity, handling ACh better than acetylmonoethylcholine, better than diethylcholine or acetylhomocholine.

Unfortunately, these apparent differences in the ability of choline analogue esters to be translocated into ACh storage sites shown by studies with synaptosomes are less readily shown in more intact mammalian tissue such as slices of brain. The interest in working with more intact tissue, rather than with isolated synaptosomes is to extend comparisons of subcellular distribution of acetylated choline analogues to their relative releasability with the objective being a better characterization of the transmitter release mechanism in mammalian tissue (see next section); isolated synaptosomes are a poor model with which to study evoked transmitter release (see Jope, 1981). However, the subcellular distribution of acetyl products of the ethylcholine analogues formed in sliced brain exposed to the appropriate precursors is rather similar to that of ACh and did not significantly differ for mono-, di- or tri-ethylcholine (Boksa and Collier, 1981). The subcellular distribution of acetylhomocholine in this kind of experiment (Boksa and Collier, 1980a) showed some tendency toward the difference from that of ACh measured with synaptosomes, but was less so; indeed the results of Nelson et al. (1980) show no difference between relative amounts of ACh and acetylhomocholine in cytoplasmic and vesicle-bound stores.

The only study of the subcellular distribution of choline analogue esters formed in intact brain is that of von Schwarzenfeld (1979) who injected pyrrolidinecholine or homocholine together with choline directly to the brain and measured the acetylesters in subcellular fractions prepared from cerebral cortex. The acetylated choline analogues synthesized in situ appeared to distribute differently between subcellular stores than did the newly synthesized ACh: acetylhomocholine accumulated in a cytoplasmic fraction and appeared to poorly enter synaptic vesicles, whereas acetylpyrrolidinecholine was better able to enter vesicular transmitter stores.

Overall, these experiments with mammalian tissue have clearly demonstrated that acetylated choline analogues synthesized in situ are stored in the same subcellular fractions as is ACh: ultimately, these studies are likely to provide important information about the characteristics of the mechanism by which transmitter translocates from its site of synthesis to its site of storage, but this promise has not yet been fully realized.

Non-mammalian Tissue. The subcellular distribution of certain choline analogue esters has been studied with the electromotor system of Torpedo; in this tissue, also, ACh is stored in cytoplasmic and vesicle-bound compartments. All of the compounds studied so far can be shown present in both of these subcellular fractions and, as with mammalian tissue, no acetylated choline analogue uniquely localizes to any one compartment. When electric organ tissue was exposed to pyrrolidinecholine (Zimmermann and Dowdall, 1977), acetylated product appeared to have a similar distribution to that of ACh, but in similar studies, homocholine, after acetylation, was less well transferred to synaptic vesicles than was ACh (Luqmani et al., 1980); acetyltriethylcholine seems, also, to be a poor substrate for vesicular uptake in Torpedo (Whittaker and Luqmani, 1980). Thus, there is growing information about the specificity of the mechanism responsible for in situ transmitter entry to synaptic vesicles in Torpedo, and this information should be invaluable in studies in vitro which aim to measure ACh uptake by isolated vesicles (e.g. Carpenter et al., 1980; Koenigsberger and Parsons, 1980; Giompres and Luqmani, 1980).

RELEASE OF ACETYLATED CHOLINE ANALOGUES

As discussed already, certain choline analogues can enter cholinergic nerve terminals, be acetylated by choline acetyltransferase, and the acetyl esters are stored in the same subcellular stores as is ACh. This is so for the three ethylcholines, pyrrolidinecholine and homocholine. The release of these five choline analogue esters has been tested in a variety of tissue preparations. The results are consistent: in all tests, the acetylated choline analogues can be released from tissues containing cholinergic nerves by stimuli that are known to release ACh (Table III).

In all of these studies where the calcium-dependence of evoked release of the choline analogue esters was tested, the result was positive: analogue ester release required extracellular Ca^{++} in the same way as does ACh release. Thus, the five compounds can all be considered to be cholinergic false transmitters and studies of the release of these compounds should provide some information about the structural specificity of the transmitter release mechanisms. Except for one study, the release of false transmitter during stimulation appears not to be accompanied by the co-release of measurable amount of unacetylated choline analogue. The exception is the experiment of Luqmani et al. (1980) which showed the release of both unchanged homocholine as well as acetylhomocholine by the Torpedo electromotor system. At least in mammalian tissue, it appears that the release mechanism for evoked transmitter is absolutely specific for acetylated compounds, which could be a reflection of a specific transmitter release mechanism, or a reflection of a specificity of the transmitter uptake mechanism into synaptic vesicles prior to release.

TABLE III THE RELEASE OF CHOLINE ANALOGUE ESTERS BY STIMULI THAT
RELEASE ACh

Tissue	Analogue	Stimulus	Reference
1. Superior cervical ganglion	Acetylmono-ethylcholine	Preganglionic nerve	Collier et al. (1976)
Superior cervical ganglion	Acetyldi-ethylcholine	Preganglionic nerve	Boksa and Collier (1981)
Superior cervical ganglion	Acetyltri-ethylcholine	Preganglionic nerve	Ilson and Collier (1975)
Superior cervical ganglion	Acetylpyrro-lidinecholine	Preganglionic nerve	Collier et al. (1976)
Superior cervical ganglion	Acetylhomo-choline	Preganglionic nerve	Collier et al. (1977)
2. Cerebral cortex	Acetylmono-ethylcholine	Potassium	Boksa and Collier (1981)
Cerebral cortex	Acetyldi-ethylcholine	Potassium	Boksa and Collier (1981)
Cerebral cortex	Acetyltri-ethylcholine	Potassium	Ilson et al. (1977)
Cerebral cortex	Acetylpyrro-lidinecholine	Direct electrical	von Schwarzenfeld (1979)
Cerebral cortex	Acetylhomo-choline	Direct electrical	von Schwarzenfeld (1979)
Cerebral cortex	Acetylhomo-choline	Potassium	Boksa and Collier (1980b)
Cerebral cortex	Acetylhomo-choline	Potassium	Carroll and Aspry (1980)
3. Myenteric plexus	Acetylpyrro-lidinecholine	Field stimulation	Kilbinger (1977)
4. Skeletal muscle	Acetylmono-ethylcholine	Motor nerve	Colquhoun et al. (1977)
5. Torpedo electric organ	Acetyltri-ethylcholine	Field stimulation	Whittaker and Luqmani (1980)
Torpedo electric organ	Acetylpyrro-lidinecholine	Field stimulation	Zimmermann and Dowdall (1977)
Torpedo electric organ	Acetylhomo-choline	Field stimulation	Luquami et al. (1980)

The relative release of false transmitter compared to true transmitter in conjunction with similar information about the subcellular storage of false and true transmitter should, at least in principle, provide information about the site of storage of releasable transmitter. The main assumption in such studies is that the process of transmitter release per se will not distinguish a false transmitter from the true transmitter, so that any difference between the two in measured release reflects a difference in a compartment or store within the nerve terminal from which releasable transmitter originated. It is hard to test this assumption critically, but in sympathetic ganglia, where nothing is known about subcellular stores, all false transmitters measured as releasable appear to be equally available for release (Collier et al., 1979); similarly, in Torpedo electric organ under conditions where all subcellular stores appear to contain similar amounts of false (acetylpyrrolidinecholine) and true transmitter, similar amounts of each are released (Zimmermann and Dowdall, 1977). These pieces of evidence suggest, but do not prove, that the transmitter release mechanism per se does not distinguish one choline analogue ester from another.

The approach used most often to attempt to identify the subcellular origin of released transmitter with false transmitter involves pre-exposure of tissue to isotopically-labelled choline analogue as precursor to the false transmitter and a precursor to ACh labelled with a different isotope; the isotope ratio of transmitters synthesized is then compared to that of transmitters released. If a different isotope ratio for the transmitters can be obtained in the different subcellular fractions, released transmitters can be measured to test whether their isotope ratios match that of any subcellular store. From such a study that involved injecting the precursors, pyrrolidinecholine or homocholine, into mammalian brain, collecting transmitters from the surface of the brain, and analysing subcellular fractions prepared from cerebral cortex, von Schwarzenfeld (1979) concluded that evoked transmitters released had an isotope ratio similar to that contained in a particle-bound, likely synaptic vesicle, fraction and different from transmitters measured in a cytoplasmic fraction. A similar approach with homocholine on sliced brain was less conclusive (Boksa and Collier, 1980b) because isotope ratios for true : false transmitter in different subcellular fractions were not very different. This study, however, clearly differentiated Ca^{++}-independent spontaneous release from Ca^{++}-dependent evoked release by their true to false transmitter ratio, and showed that the Ca^{++}-independent release was unlikely to originate from synaptic vesicles, whereas the Ca^{++}-dependent release could have done so. A slightly different approach more clearly showed this last point (Carroll and Aspry, 1980). These investigators treated brain in vitro with a medium rich in K^+ free of Na^+ and containing

Li^+, a treatment that apparently depletes vesicle-bound ACh more completely than cytoplasmic ACh (Carroll and Nelson, 1978); subsequent exposure in normal medium to homocholine allows the synthesis of acetylhomocholine and measures of the ratio of newly synthesized acetylhomocholine to residual ACh provides a clear difference between cytoplasmic fraction (about 0.4) and vesicle-bound fraction (about 7). When transmitter release was measured from tissue loaded in that way, spontaneous Ca^{++}-independent release contained a ratio of false : true transmitter of about 0.6, and evoked Ca^{++}-dependent release was of ratio about 8. It must be acknowledged that this experiment uses unusual and unphysiological manipulations, but it would appear difficult to argue with the conclusion that the result shows vesicle-bound transmitter can be released in preference to cytoplasmic transmitter during evoked Ca^{++}-dependent release and the reverse can occur during spontaneous Ca^{++}-independent release.

Extension of the approach mentioned earlier upon Torpedo electric organ exposed to false transmitter precursors have also produced results consistent with vesicular storage of releasable transmitter. Thus, following preincubation with choline and homocholine under conditions where a cytoplasmic transmitter store had a true : false transmitter isotope ratio different from that in synaptic vesicle stores, subsequent stimulation released transmitters of a ratio consistent with a vesicular origin (Luqmani et al., 1980). This pattern of result was obtained also in experiments exposing electric tissue to triethylcholine and radiolabelled acetate: the acetate labelled false (acetyltriethylcholine) and true (ACh) transmitters, and the ratio of the two subsequently released resembled vesicle-bound stores rather than cytoplasmic transmitters (Whittaker and Luqmani, 1980).

Overall, these studies upon false transmitter release afford considerable biochemical evidence to support the morphological and electrophysiological evidence suggesting evoked transmitter release can be accounted for by release from synaptic vesicles. The biochemical studies can't distinguish between co-release of true and false transmitter from a single vesicle or from vesicles containing a single, but different ester. With monoethylcholine as precursor to the false transmitter, Large and Rang (1978) analysed by electrophysiology the release of quanta of true and false transmitter, making use of the shorter time constant of decay of synaptic current associated with the action at the neuromuscular junction of acetylmonoethylcholine than that of ACh. Their result was that quanta each appear to be composed of a mixture of true and false transmitters; they found no evidence for distinct populations of quanta containing one or the other. Thus, it appears that transmitter equilibration between stores is a prominent feature of intraterminal dynamics, at least in motor nerve terminals.

ACKNOWLEDGEMENT

We are grateful to M.R.C. of Canada for financial support.

REFERENCES

Barker, L.A. and Mittag, T.W., 1975. Comparative studies of substrates and inhibitors of choline transport and choline acetyltransferase. J. Pharmacol. exp. Ther. 192: 86–94.

Barker, L.A. and Mittag, T.W., 1976. Synaptosomal transport and acetylation of 3-trimethylamino-propan-1-ol. Biochem. Pharmacol. 25: 1931–1933.

Barker, L.A., Dowdall, M.J. and Mittag, T.W., 1975. Comparative studies on synaptosomes: high affinity uptake and acetylation of choline and pyrrolidinecholine. Brain Res. 86: 343–348.

Batzold, F., De Haven, R., Kuhar, M.J. and Birdsall, N., 1980. Inhibition of high affinity choline uptake: structure-activity studies. Biochem. Pharmacol. 29: 2413–2416.

Benishin, C.G. and Carroll, P.T., 1981. Acetylation of choline and homocholine by membrane-bound choline-0-acetyltransferase in mouse forebrain nerve endings. J. Neurochem. 36: 732–740.

Birks, R.I., 1977. A long-lasting potentiation of transmitter release related to an increase in transmitter stores in a sympathetic ganglion. J. Physiol. 271: 847–862.

Birks, R.I., 1978. Regulation by patterned preganglionic neural activity of transmitter stores in a sympathetic ganglion. J. Physiol. 280: 559–572.

Birks, R.I. and Fitch, S.J.G., 1974. Storage and release of acetylcholine in a sympathetic ganglion. J. Physiol. 240: 125–134.

Birks, R. and MacIntosh, F.C., 1961. Acetylcholine metabolism of a sympathetic ganglion. Canad. J. Biochem. Physiol. 39: 787–827.

Blusztajn, J.K. and Wurtman, R.J., 1981. Choline biosynthesis by a preparation enriched in synaptosomes from rat brain. Nature 290: 417–418.

Boksa, P. and Collier, B., 1980a. Acetylation of homocholine by rat brain: subcellular distribution of acetylhomocholine and studies on the ability of homocholine to serve as substrate for choline acetyltransferase in situ and in vitro. J. Neurochem. 34: 1470–1482.

Boksa, P. and Collier, B., 1980b. Spontaneous and evoked release of acetylcholine and a cholinergic false transmitter from brain slices: comparison to true and false transmitter in subcellular stores. Neuroscience 5: 1517-1532.

Boksa, P. and Collier, B., 1981. N-ethyl analogues of choline as precursors to cholinergic false transmitters. J. Neurochem. 35: 1099-1104.

Bourdois, P.S., McCandless, D.L. and MacIntosh, F.C., 1975. A prolonged effect of intense synaptic activity on acetylcholine in a sympathetic ganglion. Canad. J. Physiol. Pharmacol. 53: 155-165.

Burgen, A.S.V., Burke, G. and Desbarats-Schonbaum, M.L., 1956. The specificity of brain choline acetylase. Br. J. Pharmacol. 11: 308-312.

Carpenter, R.S., Koenigsberger, R. and Parsons, S.M., 1980. Passive uptake of acetylcholine and other organic cations by synaptic vesicles from Torpedo electric organ. Biochemistry 19: 4373-4379.

Carroll, P.T. and Aspry, J.M., 1980. Subcellular origin of cholinergic transmitter release from mouse brain. Science 210: 641-642.

Carroll, P.T. and Nelson, S.H., 1978. Cholinergic vesicles: ability to empty and refill independently of cytoplasmic acetylcholine. Science 199: 85-86.

Channon, H.J. and Smith, J.A.B., 1936. The dietary prevention of fatty livers. Triethyl-β-hydroxyethyl ammonium hydroxide. Biochem. J. 30: 115-120.

Collier, B., 1973. The accumulation of hemicholinium by tissues that transport choline. Canad. J. Physiol. Pharmacol. 51: 491-495.

Collier, B., 1981. The structural specificity of choline transport into cholinergic nerve terminals. J. Neurochem. 36: 1292-1294.

Collier, B. and Ilson, D., 1977. The effect of preganglionic nerve stimulation on the accumulation of certain analogues of choline by a sympathetic ganglion. J. Physiol. 264: 489-509.

Collier, B. and Katz, H.S., 1974. Acetylcholine synthesis from recaptured choline by a sympathetic ganglion. J. Physiol. 238: 639-655.

Collier, B. and MacIntosh, F.C., 1969. The source of choline for acetylcholine synthesis in a sympathetic ganglion. Canad. J. Physiol. Pharmacol. 47: 127-135.

Collier, B., Barker, L.A. and Mittag, T.W., 1976. The release of acetylated choline analogues by a sympathetic ganglion. Molec. Pharmacol. 12: 340-344.

Collier, B., Lovat, S., Ilson, D., Barker, L.A. and Mittag, T.W., 1977. The uptake, metabolism and release of homocholine: studies with rat brain synaptosomes and cat superior cervical ganglion. J. Neurochem. 28: 331-339.

Collier, B., Boksa, P. and Lovat, S., 1979. Cholinergic false transmitters. Progr. Brain. Res. 49: 107-121.

Colquhoun, D., Large, W.A. and Rang. H.P., 1977. An analysis of the action of a false transmitter at the neuromuscular junction. J. Physiol. 266: 361-395.

Currier, S.F. and Mautner, H.G., 1974. The mechanism of action of choline acetyltransferase. Proc. natn. Acad. Sci. 71: 3355-3358.

Dauterman, W.C. and Mehrotra, K.N., 1963. The N-alkyl group specificity of choline acetylase from rat brain. J. Neurochem. 10: 113-117.

Friesen, A.J.D. and Khatter, J.C., 1971. The effect of preganglionic stimulation on the acetylcholine and choline content of a sympathetic ganglion. Canad. J. Physiol. Pharmacol. 49: 375-381.

Giompres, P. and Luqmani, Y.A., 1980. Cholinergic synaptic vesicles isolated from Torpedo marmorata: demonstration of acetylcholine and choline uptake in an in vitro system. Neuroscience 5: 1041-1052.

Hemsworth, B.A., 1971. Effects of some polymethylene bis (hydroxyethyl) dimethylammonium compounds on acetylcholine synthesis. Br. J. Pharmacol. 42: 78-87.

Hemsworth, B.A. and Smith, J.C., 1970. Enzymic acetylation of the stereoisomers of α and β-methyl choline. Biochem. Pharmacol. 19: 2925-2927.

Hunt, R. and Taveau, R. de M., 1909. On the relation between the toxicity and chemical constitution of a number of derivatives of choline and analogous compounds. J. Pharmacol. exp. Ther. 1: 303-339.

Hunt, R. and Taveau, R. de M., 1911. The effects of a number of derivatives of choline and analogous compounds on the blood pressure. U.S. Hyg. Lab. Bull. 73: 1-136.

Ilson, D. and Collier, B., 1975. Triethylcholine as a precursor to a cholinergic false transmitter. Nature 254: 618-620.

Ilson, D., Collier, B. and Boksa, P., 1977. Acetyltriethylcholine: a cholinergic false transmitter in cat superior cervical ganglion and rat cerebral cortex. J. Neurochem. 28: 371-381.

Jope, R.S., 1979. High affinity choline transport and acetyl-CoA production in brain and their roles in the regulation of acetylcholine synthesis. Brain. Res. Rev. 1: 313-344.

Jope, R.S., 1981. Acetylcholine turnover and compartmentation in rat brain synaptosomes. J. Neurochem. 36: 1712-1721.

Jukes, T.H. and Welch, A.D., 1942. The effect of certain analogues of choline on perosis. J. biol. Chem. 146: 19-24.

Kessler, P.D. and Marchbanks, R.M., 1979. Choline transport is not coupled to acetylcholine synthesis. Nature 297: 542-544.

Keston, A.S. and Wortis, S.B., 1946. Antagonistic action of choline and its triethyl analogue. Proc. Soc. exp. Biol. Med. 61: 439-440.

Kilbinger, H., 1977. Formation and release of acetylpyrrolidine-choline as a false cholinergic transmitter in the myenteric plexus of the guinea-pig small intestine. Naunyn-Schmiedberg's Arch. Pharmacol. 295: 81-87.

Koenigsberger, R. and Parsons, S.M., 1980. Bicarbonate and magnesium ion-ATP dependent stimulation of acetylcholine uptake by Torpedo electric organ synaptic vesicles. Biochem. Biophys. Res. Commun. 94: 305-312.

Large, W.A. and Rang, H.P., 1978. Variability of transmitter quanta released during incorporation of a false transmitter into cholinergic nerve terminals. J. Physiol. 285: 25-34.

Luqmani, Y.A., Sudlow, G. and Whittaker, V.P., 1980. Homocholine and acetylhomocholine: false transmitters in the cholinergic electromotor system of Torpedo. Neuroscience 5: 153-160.

MacIntosh, F.C. and Collier, B., 1976. Neurochemistry of cholinergic terminals. Handb. exp. Pharmacol. 42: 99-228.

Marchbanks, R.M., Wonnacott, S. and Rubio, M.A., 1981. The effects of acetylcholine release on choline fluxes in isolated synaptic terminals. J. Neurochem. 36: 379-393.

Murrin, L.C. and Kuhar, M.J., 1976. Activation of high affinity choline uptake in vitro by depolarizing agents. Mol. Pharmacol. 12: 1082-1090.

Nelson, S.H., Benishin, C.G. and Carroll, P.T., 1980. Accumulation and metabolism of choline and homocholine by mouse brain subcellular fractions. Biochem. Pharmacol. 29: 1949-1957.

O'Regan, S. and Collier, B., 1981. Factors affecting choline transport by the cat superior cervical ganglion during and following stimulation, and the relationship between choline uptake and acetylcholine synthesis. Neuroscience 6: 511-520.

Reitzel, N.L. and Long, J.P., 1959. Hemicholinium antagonism by choline analogues. J. Pharmacol. exp. Ther. 127: 15-21.

Rosenblueth, A., Lissák, K. and Lanari, A., 1939. An explanation of the five stages of neuromuscular ganglionic synaptic transmission. Amer. J. Physiol. 128: 31-44.

Roskoski, R., 1978. Acceleration of choline uptake after depolarization induced acetylcholine release in rat cortical synaptosomes. J. Neurochem. 30: 1357-1361.

Rylett, B.J. and Colhoun, E.H., 1980a. Kinetic data on the inhibition of high-affinity choline transport into rat forebrain synaptosomes by choline-like compounds and nitrogen mustard analogues. J. Neurochem. 34: 713-719.

Rylett, B.J. and Colhoun, E.H., 1980b. Carrier-mediated inhibition of choline acetyltransferase. Life. Sci. 26: 909-914.

Simon, J.R., Mittag, T.W. and Kuhar, M.J., 1975. Inhibition of synaptosomal uptake of choline by various choline analogs. Biochem. Pharmacol. 24: 1139-1142.

Slater, P. and Stonier, P.D., 1973. The uptake of hemicholinium-3 by rat brain cortex slices. J. Neurochem. 20: 637-639.

Sollenberg, J., Stensiö, K-E. and Sörbo, B., 1979. N-substituted choline analogues as substrates for choline acetyltransferase. J. Neurochem. 32: 973-977.

Von Schwarzenfeld, I., 1979. Origin of transmitters released by electrical stimulation from a small, metabolically very active vesicular pool of cholinergic synapses in guinea-pig cerebral cortex. Neuroscience 4: 477-493.

Weiler, M.H., Jope, R.S. and Jenden, D.J., 1978. Effect of pretreatment under various cationic conditions on acetylcholine content and choline transport in rat whole brain synaptosomes. J.
Neurochem. 31: 789-796.

Weiler, M.H., Gundersen, C.B. and Jenden, D.J., 1981. Choline uptake and acetylcholine synthesis in synaptosomes: investigations
using two different labeled variants of choline. J. Neurochem.
36: 1802-1812.

Whittaker, V.P. and Luqmani, Y.A., 1980. False transmitters in
the cholinergic system: implications for the vesicle theory of
transmitter storage and release. Gen. Pharmacol. 11: 7-14.

Zimmermann, H. and Dowdall, M.J., 1977. Vesicular storage and
release of a false cholinergic transmitter (acetylpyrrolcholine)
in the Torpedo electric organ. Neuroscience 2: 731-739).

CHOLINE UPTAKE AND ACETYLCHOLINE RELEASE

R. M. Marchbanks

Department of Biochemistry
Institute of Psychiatry
London, SE5 8AF. UK

Among the first observations on the biochemistry of the cholinergic systems was the finding (Mann et al, 1939) that acetylcholine concentrations in tissue were sustained even though the release of substantial quantities had been elicited by depolarization. The biological necessity for such a rapid response is fairly obvious since otherwise the cholinergic synapse would fail under repeated stimulation. First thoughts on the mechanism involved choline acetyltransferase (Review Tuček, 1979 Ch.6) but this was never very plausible because the maximal activity of this enzyme considerably exceeds the rate of transmitter release in most tissues. As an illustration of this generality consider the mammalian cerebral cortex. The rate of acetylcholine release from constantly depolarized slices is about 2nmoles min^{-1}, g^{-1} (Richter and Marchbanks, 1971) whereas the maximal activity of the synthesising enzyme is about 100 nmoles $min^{-1}g$ (Hebb & Silver, 1956). Balancing the fact that normally release rates will be much lower than this with the probability that the concentration of choline and acetyl CoA in tissue is sub-optimal it is likely that the activity of enzyme can comfortably sustain the normal rates of release.

The control points of acetylcholine synthesis must therefore lie earlier in the biosynthetic sequence probably during provision of the precursors. There are good reasons for supposing that the control point does not lie in the supply of Acetyl CoA because this compound even in its extra mitochondrial location is the precursor of other compounds, and its turnover as a consequence of energy metabolism known to be much higher than that of ACh. This leaves events during the supply of choline to the brain as possible control points and the most likely, because it is the

slowest, would seem to be the trans-membrane passage of choline.
This is known to be mediated by a carrier system (Hodgkin & Martin,
1965, Schuberth et al, 1966) which is saturable, Na^+ dependent and
inhibited by the choline analogue Hemicholinium-3(HC-3). It has
been reported from several laboratories (Simon et al, 1976, Collier
& Ilson, 1977; Polak et al, 1977) that choline uptake in the
synaptic region is stimulated by acetylcholine release.

     Choline uptake seems therefore to respond to acetylcholine
release in a regulatory manner and the mechanism of this control
has been supposed (Simon et al, 1976) to lie in a close association
of the choline transport process with acetylcholine synthesis.
This association had been invoked and defined by Barker & Mittag
(1974) to explain their results on the transport and acetylation
of various analogues of choline. Barker and Mittag (1974) proposed
that 'transport and acetylation are coupled, i.e., choline transported into the synaptosome has no "free" existence and is
immediately acetylated by ChAC'. However this suggestion is not
consistent with the earlier evidence (Fonnum, 1967; Marchbanks &
Israel 1972) that at the high ionic strengths prevalent inside the
cell choline acetyltransferase is a soluble enzyme not associated
with any particulate or membranous material.

     An additional reason for discarding the coupling hypothesis
arises from a study of the mixing of extra and intra-terminal
choline. If only the choline that is transported is acetylated
(as the coupling hypothesis supposes) there should be a one to one
correspondence between the specific radioactivity of choline outside and that of the recently synthesised acetylcholine inside the
terminal (coupling ratio = 1). If however there is mixing with
intraterminal pools of choline the ratio of specific activities
$S_{ACh}/S_{(choline outside)}$ will be less than 1; the greater the
mixing, the smaller the ratio. This experiment gets over the
problem that not all synaptosomes are cholinergic; since only
choline that has entered cholinergic synaptosomes will affect the
results. The ratio of specific activities was found by two
different methods [using ^{14}C-glucose as precursor, Kessler &
Marchbanks, 1979; using ^{14}C-choline as precursor, Marchbanks,
1981] to be about 0.1 at choline concentrations of 10µM rising
to 0.2-0.6 at higher choline concentrations 10-50µM. This means
that recently transported choline has no privileged access to
choline acetyltransferase and appears to mix with the endogenous
choline pool. Indeed the extent of coupling appears to be roughly
equal to the contribution of transported choline to total endogenous choline as one would expect if transport and acetylation
are independent.

     Our own studies on the properties of the choline carrier have
suggested that acetylcholine release activates choline transport
by a different mechanism than the coupling of transport and

synthesis. Influx of ^{3}H-choline into synaptosomes was studied simultaneously with the efflux of ^{14}C-choline, our results (Marchbanks et al, 1981) may be summarised:

    (i)   Influx of choline is saturable and stimulated by high internal (trans) concentrations of choline

    (ii)   Efflux of choline is saturable and also stimulated by trans (outside) concentrations of choline

    (iii) Influx and efflux rates are not the same but at saturating trans concentrations approach a common maximal velocity.

The most likely explanation for these results is that the choline is transported inwards by a reciprocating carrier which must be returned to the outside (or its outside facing conformation) if influx is to proceed, and vice versa for efflux. Transport in the opposite direction is facilitated by combination with choline but since influx is not in general equal to efflux it is clear that the carrier can traverse the membrane either alone or in combination with some other substance, as yet unknown. It may also be that sodium co-transport is important in this respect.

    The kinetics of such a system will be rather complicated, it is clear that the simple application of the Michaelis-Menten treatment is quite incorrect. For example, consider the possible effects of compounds that compete for binding to the carrier site. If they are transported they will act as trans-activators as well as cis-inhibitors, but if they are not carried across the membrane they will inhibit from the cis side and also cause trans-inhibition of the oppositely directed flux. Trans-inhibition of the oppositely directed flux arises because a compound that binds to the carrier but it is not transported effectively prevents the carrier returning to its opposite conformation to mediate the oppositely directed flux.

    Acetylcholine is a weak competitor for the binding site that is itself hardly transported. In this respect is behaves similarly to the drug Hemicholinium-3. It would be predicted on this model that both compounds produce trans-inhibition of choline transport. This is demonstrated in Fig. 1 which shows the effect of outside concentrations of ACh and HC-3 on choline efflux. The left hand graph of Fig. 1 shows that 20μM choline (outside, i.e. trans) causes an increase in efflux from about 13 to 22 pmol.mg^{-1} min^{-1}. This increment is the carrier mediated component of efflux and as the adjacent bar shows it is inhibited by HC-3 in the trans position. The LHS curve shows that as the trans acetylcholine concentration is increased the carrier mediated component of efflux is inhibited so that at concentrations of 20mM it disappears completely. The RHS graph shows that increasing the choline concentration overcomes the trans-inhibition caused by 20mM

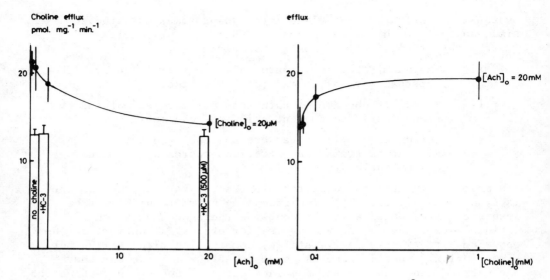

Fig. 1.   Synaptosomes (P_2B) were preincubated with ^{3}H-choline
           ($2\mu Ci/ml$) for 30 min at 37°C. They were then washed
           3 times and resuspended in a physiological medium
           containing $20\mu M$ choline in varying concentrations of
           acetylcholine (LHS) or $20\mu M$ acetylcholine in varying
           concentrations of choline (RHS). The results when HC-3
           ($500\mu M$) was added are shown in bars on the LHS. The
           ordinate shows the efflux of ^{3}H-choline measured over
           a 4 min period. The figures are the mean ± SEM of 4
           determinations.

acetylcholine, but because of the high affinity that choline has
for the carrier much lower concentrations are effective.

      Demonstration of the converse effect, i.e. trans-inhibition
of choline influx by internal acetylcholine is more difficult
because preloading with ACh results in high internal concentrations
of choline due to reversal of the reaction catalysed by choline
acetyltransferase. This swamps the effect of acetylcholine,

nevertheless a statistical analysis (Marchbanks, et al, 1981) of the effects of increased internal acetylcholine concentration show that it does indeed inhibit choline influx.

It is suggested therefore that depolarization induced activation of choline uptake is mediated by the acetylcholine concentration within synaptosomes. The binding of acetylcholine without concomitant transport has the effect of immobilising the carrier on the side of the high acetylcholine concentration. It will not therefore be available for choline transport from the other side of the membrane. If the acetylcholine concentration is reduced by the release process the immobilisation of the carrier will be relieved thus enabling it to return to the outside of the membrane and mediate choline influx. The mechanism would work as well whatever was the immediate source of released ACh provided the cytoplasmic concentration was eventually lowered.

Synaptosomes are artificial particles and it is pertinent to ask how relevant the phenomena is to the physiological control of acetylcholine levels in vivo, particularly since the concentrations of acetylcholine required to show trans-inhibition are rather high. Where it has been measured (in the neuromuscular junction, Katz & Miledi, 1977) the cytoplasmic concentrations of ACh is found to be in the mM range. Furthermore there is an artefactual rapid break-down of phospholipids in synaptosomes that leads to intra-terminal concentrations of choline considerably higher than in vivo. This will tend to nullify (by competition) the effect of acetylcholine in inhibiting influx. The lower tissue choline concentrations found in vivo will therefore allow a much more dramatic activation of transport as a result of acetylcholine release than is discernable in the synaptosome preparation.

ACKNOWLEDGEMENT

I am grateful to the MRC for support for these studies (Grants G974/907/N, G976/298/N and G979/507/N).

REFERENCES

Barker, L. A. and Mittag, T. W. 1974. Comparative studies of
substrates and inhibitors of choline transport and choline
acetyltransferase. J.Pharmacol.Exptl.Therap. 192: 86-94.

Collier, B. and Ilson, D. 1977. The effect of preganglionic
nerve stimulation on the accumulation of certain analogues of
choline by a sympathetic ganglion. J.Physiol. 264: 489-509.

Hebb, C. O. and Silver, A. 1956. Choline acetylase in the central
nervous system of man and some other mammals. J.Physiol. 134:
718-728.

Hodgkin, A. L. and Martin, K. 1965. Choline uptake by giant
axons of Loligo. J.Physiol(Lond). 179: 26-27.

Katz, B. and Miledi, R. 1977. Transmitter leakage from motor
nerve endings. Proc.R.Soc.Lond. 196: 59-72.

Kessler, P. D. and Marchbanks, R. M. 1979. Choline transport is
not coupled to acetylcholine synthesis. Nature 279: 542-544.

Mann, P. J. G., Tennenbaum, M. and Quastel, J. H. 1939.
Acetylcholine metabolism in the central nervous system. The
effects of potassium and other cations on acetylcholine liberation.
Biochem.J. 33: 822-835.

Marchbanks, R. M. 1981. 'Interaction of choline transport with
acetylcholine release and synthesis' in: Cholinergic Mechanisms,
G. Pepeu and H. Ladinsky, eds. Plenum, New York.

Marchbanks, R. M. Wonnacott, S. and Rubio, M. A. 1981. The effect
of acetylcholine release on choline fluxes in isolated synaptic
terminals. J.Neurochem. 36: 379-393.

Polak, R. L., Molenaar, P. C. and van Gelder, M. 1977. Acetylcholine metabolism and choline uptake in cortical slices.
J.Neurochem. 29: 477-485.

Richter, J. A. and Marchbanks, R. M. 1971. Synthesis of radioactive acetylcholine from [3H]choline and its release from cerebral
cortex slices in vitro. J.Neurochem. 18: 691-703.

Schuberth, J., Sundwall, A., Sorbo, B. and Lindell, J-O. 1966.
Uptake of choline by mouse brain slices. J.Neurochem. 13: 343-352.

Simon, J. R., Atweh, S. and Kuhar, M. 1976. Sodium-dependent high affinity uptake: a regulatory step in the synthesis of acetyl-choline. J.Neurochem. 26: 909-922.

Tuček, S. 1978. Acetylcholine synthesis in neurons. Chapman & Hall, London.

IN VIVO REGULATION OF NIGRO-STRIATAL AND MESOCORTICO-PREFRONTAL

DOPAMINERGIC NEURONS

Jacques Glowinski

Groupe NB, INSERM U.114, Collège de France
75231 Paris cedex 05, France

INTRODUCTION

Two main problems will be discussed : the first one is concerned with the mechanisms involved in the reciprocal regulation of the two nigrostriatal dopaminergic (DA) pathways. I will describe and summarize experiments which reveal the role of DA released from dendrites in this phenomenon. The second problem is related to some specific properties of the mesocortico-prefrontal DA neurons. Particularly, I intend to show that these neurons are distinct from those of the mesolimbic DA system which innervate subcortical structures and also originate from the ventro-tegmental area (VTA). The role of the mesocortico-prefrontal DA neurons in the regulation of DA transmission in subcortical structures through cortical efferent pathways will also be briefly discussed.

Interactions of nigrostriatal DA neurons with other neuronal pathways of the basal ganglia can be determined with electrophysiological methods by measuring changes in activity of pars compacta DA cells induced by selective stimulation of various nigral afferent pathways. Microiontophoretic electrophysiological investigations may facilitate the identification of the transmitters involved. A second approach, selected in our own studies, consists in the estimation of changes in the in vivo release of DA from nerve terminals induced by physiological or pharmacological treatments which modify the activity of striatal or nigral afferent pathways. An isotopic method which allowed the continuous delivery of ^{3}H-tyrosine to a push-pull cannula implanted in the cat caudate nucleus and the measurement of ^{3}H-DA released in successive superfusate fractions (10 min) was used for this purpose. We could thus show that ^{3}H-DA release from nerve terminals was dependent on nerve activity and

219

also modulated by presynaptic influences. Moreover, animals implanted
with several push-pull cannulae could be successfully used to study
simultaneously the effects of various treatments on DA release from
nerve terminals and dendrites of the two nigrostriatal DA pathways
(see review Chéramy et al., 1981a). The effects of the unilateral
nigral application of transmitters, their agonists or antagonists
on ^{3}H-DA release in both caudate nuclei and both substantiae nigrae
(SN) were particularly examined. This led to the discovery of the
reciprocal regulation of the two nigrostriatal DA pathways and to
investigations on the interneuronal processes involved in this
phenomenon.

Our interest in the mesocortico-prefrontal DA neurons originated in 1973 when we detected the presence of DA nerve terminals
in the rat cerebral cortex (Thierry et al., 1973). Curiously, this
discovery was made with biochemical methods by measuring cortical
DA levels and ^{3}H-DA synthesis in synaptosomes after the 6-hydroxy-
dopamine (6-OHDA) induced degeneration of the ascending noradrenergic neurons. Thereafter histochemical and lesion studies made by
other workers rapidly indicated that the cortical DA innervation
was restricted to the prefrontal medial cortex, the suprarhinal,
cingular and entorhinal cortices and that these DA nerve terminals
originated from neurons located both in the VTA and the SN. The
well known role of the frontal cortex in cognitive processes and
the localization in the VTA of DA cells innervating this cortical
area led particularly to investigate the properties of the DA
neurons projecting to the prefrontal cortex. This in fact was a
joint effort since we highly benefited from contributions of the
groups of B. Berger, J. Bockaert and M. LeMoal with respective
competences in the field of neuroanatomy, receptor and behavioural
researches. These were of great value.

RECIPROCAL REGULATION OF THE TWO NIGROSTRIATAL DA PATHWAYS

For several years it has been assumed that the two nigrostriatal DA pathways were independent. In various studies, one
pathway was even used as a control for examining the effects of
specific treatments on the other. A first series of experiments led
us to demonstrate that this was not the case and to propose that DA
released from dendrites in one SN was involved in the regulation of
the activity of the contralateral DA neurons.

Asymmetric modifications of the activity of the two DA pathways
induced by various unilateral treatments

Asymmetric changes in ^{3}H-DA release in the two caudate nuclei
of halothane anaesthetized cats were observed for the first time
when we examined the effects of the unilateral electrocoagulation
of the SN (Nieoullon et al., 1977a). Confirming that the spontaneous

release of newly synthesized ^{3}H-DA from nerve terminals was dependent on nerve impulse flow this lesion markedly reduced ^{3}H-DA release in the ipsilateral caudate nucleus. Surprisingly, this effect was associated with an enhanced release of ^{3}H-DA in the contralateral structure which lasted for two hours at least. We also noted that the slight variations in ^{3}H-DA spontaneous release seen from one fraction to another in both caudate nuclei of the control cats were in opposite directions : the oscillations in ^{3}H-DA spontaneous release in both structures were asymmetric. This first study indicated that messages originating in one SN could influence the activity of the contralateral DA neurons.

The effects of the unilateral electrical stimulation of deep cerebellar nuclei (Nieoullon et al., 1978) and the delivery of unilateral sensory stimuli (Nieoullon et al., 1977b) on the activity of the two DA pathways further revealed bilateral asymmetric changes in ^{3}H-DA release in both caudate nuclei. THe electrical stimulation of the right cerebellar dentate nucleus enhanced ^{3}H-DA release in the contralateral caudate nucleus while it induced an opposite effect on the ipsilateral side. Reverse asymmetric responses were observed under unilateral sensory stimuli. These asymmetric changes in ^{3}H-DA release could be dependent on messages reaching the contralateral SN. Indeed, the dentate nucleus sends a projection to the contralateral SN and evoked potentials were only observed in the contralateral SN of halothane-anaesthetized cats under unilateral delivery of sensory stimuli (Leviel et al., 1981). In these experiments asymmetric changes in the dendritic release of ^{3}H-DA were also seen in the two SN. These responses, in directions opposite to those intervening in corresponding caudate nuclei, were of similar duration exceeding the period of the stimulations and were even more pronounced than those observed at the nerve terminals level.

The results just described led to several conclusions : 1) DA dendritic release can be modulated when neuronal pathways involved in motor or sensory processes are stimulated ; 2) DA released in the SN originates from dendrites and not from collaterals of the DA cells since changes in DA release in the SN and in the ipsilateral caudate nucleus were in opposite directions ; 3) finally, changes in ^{3}H-DA dendritic release seen in the contralateral SN under the various treatments made could contribute to the asymmetric modifications of the activity of the two nigrostriatal DA pathways.

Role of DA released from dendrites in the reciprocal regulation of the two nigrostriatal DA pathways

The role of DA released from dendrites in the reciprocal regulation of the activity of the two nigrostriatal DA pathways was demonstrated when we investigated the effects induced by unilateral

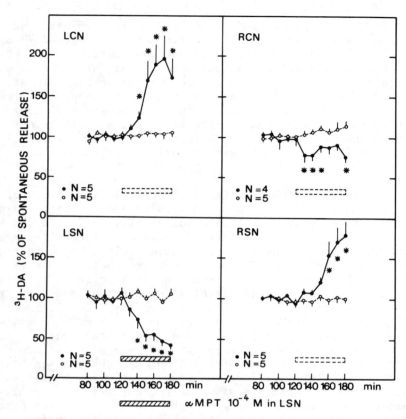

Fig. 1. Effects of α-MpT application into the left SN on the release
of ^{3}H-DA from the two caudate nuclei and the two SN. Four
push-pull cannulae were simultaneously implanted in the left
(LCN) and the right (RCN) caudate nuclei and in the left
(LSN) and the right (RSN) SN in anaesthetized cats. The
four structures were perfused with an artificial CSF
containing L(3,5-^{3}H)tyrosine (50 Cimmol^{-1}, 50 μCiml^{-1},
1 ml h^{-1}). ^{3}H-DA was estimated in 10 min successive superfusate fractions. The average quantities of ^{3}H-DA released
in superfusate fractions of the SN (0.4 nCi) and the CN
(0.6 nCi) were respectively 20 and 30 times the blank value.
α-MpT (10^{-4}M) was introduced for 60 min into the CSF superfusing the LSN (hatched bar). In each animal and for each
cannula, ^{3}H-DA in each successive fraction was expressed
as a percentage of an average spontaneous release calculated
from the five fractions collected before the treatment.
Data are the mean ± s.e.m. of results obtained with five
animals (---•---). * P<0.05 when compared with correspond-
ding control values obtained in five untreated animals
(---○---), ▨ α-MpT application.

modifications of nigral DA transmission on ^{3}H-DA release in both caudate nuclei and SN. The facilitation of nigral DA transmission was induced by adding in one SN, DA or drugs such as benztropine or D-amphetamine which enhance the local release of DA (Nieoullon et al., 1979 ; Leviel et al., 1979). In all cases, ^{3}H-DA release was reduced in the ipsilateral caudate nucleus but enhanced in the contralateral structure. The reverse asymmetric changes in ^{3}H-DA release were observed in both caudate nuclei when DA transmission was interrupted in one SN by α-methyl-paratyrosine (α-MpT) or neuroleptics (Nieoullon et al., 1979 ; Leviel et al., 1979). Moreover, amphetamine and α-MpT which enhanced and decreased respectively the local release of ^{3}H-DA induced asymmetric changes in ^{3}H-DA release in the contralateral SN. Therefore, as in our previous studies, changes in ^{3}H-DA dendrite release induced in both SN were in directions opposite to those seen in corresponding caudate nuclei. Moreover, additional experiments indicated that the unilateral facilitation or interruption of DA transmission in one caudate nucleus were without effect on DA release in the contralateral caudate nucleus or SN (Leviel et al., 1979).

This series of results obtained in studies made by A. Chéramy, A. Nieoullon and V. Leviel first provided further evidence for the critical role of DA released from dendrites in the control of the activity of the ipsilateral DA neurons since a reduction of DA release from nerve terminals was associated to an increased release of the transmitter from dendrites and vice versa. They thus completed the electrophysiological studies of Bunney and Aghajanian (1973) and Groves and his coworkers (1975) which led to the concept of self- or lateral-inhibition of the DA neurons, a process mediated by the action of DA on DA autoreceptors located on parent or adjacent DA cells or their dendrites. The changes in the activity of the contralateral DA neurons induced by the unilateral nigral facilitation of interruption of DA transmission also indicated that DA released from dendrites in one SN was involved in the regulation of the contralateral DA pathway. No direct connection being known between the two SN we suggested that DA released from dendrites in one SN was influencing contralateral DA neurons through a polysynaptic pathway involving nigral efferent non DA neurons.

Role of the nigro-thalamic neurons in the reciprocal regulation of the nigrostriatal DA pathways

The role of the nigro-thalamic neurons in the transfer of messages from one SN to the contralateral DA neurons was demonstrated by analyzing the effects of various sagittal sections on the asymmetric changes in ^{3}H-DA release induced in both caudate nuclei and SN by the unilateral nigral application of D-amphetamine or α-MpT (Chéramy et al., 1981b) or by the unilateral delivery of mild electric shocks to the forelimb (Leviel et al., 1981).

Among all sagittal sections made, the only one which could prevent the changes in ^{3}H-DA release in the contralateral caudate nucleus and SN induced by the unilateral nigral application of D-amphetamine or α-MpT was a transection which interrupted the midline thalamic nuclear mass. This section was also the only one which abolished the changes in ^{3}H-DA release from nerve terminals and dendrites of the ipsilateral DA neurons induced by the unilateral delivery of sensory stimuli although it did not suppressed the evoked potentials and the increased dendritic release of ^{3}H-DA in the contralateral SN. Therefore, in these lesioned cats, modifications of DA release induced in one SN were without influence on the activity of the contralateral DA neurons.

These results obtained mainly by A. Chéramy, V. Leviel and M.F. Giorguieff-Chesselet, led us to conclude that the interruption (α-MpT) or the facilitation (D-amphetamine, sensory stimuli) of DA release in one SN of unlesioned cats affect the activity of nigral efferent neurons projecting to several thalamic nuclei including the motor and intralaminar nuclei and that messages are then transferred to the contralateral side through connections between paired thalamic nuclei. Various projections could then be involved in the delivery of signals to the contralateral DA neurons. Signals may reach the contralateral SN through thalamo-nigral fibres or various neuronal loops including the thalamo-striato-nigral or thalamo-cortico-nigral polysynaptic pathways. Changes in ^{3}H-DA release in the contralateral caudate nucleus could also be induced by thalamo-striatal or thalamo-cortico-striatal projections exerting directly or indirectly a presynaptic control on ^{3}H-DA release from nerve terminals. Experiments are in progress to determine the role of these various connections in the effects observed in the contralateral side.

In conclusion, it appears that messages which reach some thalamic nuclei on one side of the brain via the nigro-thalamic neurons (ipsi-lateral application of α-MpT or of D-amphetamine in the SN, sensory stimuli applied to the contralateral forelimb) or more directly through ascending somesthesic pathways (sensory stimuli applied to the contralateral forelimb) play a critical role in the regulation of the activity of the contralateral DA neurons. Electrophysiological studies are also in favor of an action of DA released from dendrites on nigro-thalamic neurons since Ruffieux and Schultz (1980) have reported that DA exerts an excitatory effect on numerous cells in the SN pars reticularis. Some of these cells, identified by antidromic activation correspond to the nigro-thalamic neurons and these authors also indicated that the DA excitatory effect on these cells was antagonized by neuroleptics. It should be added that recent studies have indicated that some of these nigro-thalamic GABAergic neurons are branched neurons which also innervate the superior colliculus or the striatum (Deniau et al., 1978). Therefore, through DA released from dendrites, the nigrostriatal DA neurons may influence various structures involved in sensory motor processes. This should be taken into account in further investigations made to study the functional role of the nigrostriatal DA neurons.

THE MESOCORTICO-PREFRONTAL DA NEURONS, A PATHWAY DISTINCT FROM THE MESOLIMBIC DA SYSTEM

The discovery of the cortical DA innervation has aroused a broad interest, particularly among researchers working on the DA hypothesis of schizophrenia, since neuroleptics could exert their antipsychotic effects by interrupting excessive DA transmission in some cortical areas. However, although DA cells involved in the DA innervation of distinct cortical areas are not homogeneously distributed in the mesencephalon (Lindvall and Björklund, 1978) numerous workers concluded taht the mesocortical DA neurons were part of the mesolimbic DA system. Rapidly, we reach the conclusion that this was not the case since in various situations the mesocortico-prefrontal DA neurons were shown to react in a different way than VTA DA cells innervating subcortical structures.

Difference in the reactivity of DA neurons innervating the prefrontal cortex and subcortical structures

In the rat, as in other species, the DA innervation of the prefrontal cortex is not as dense as that of the nucleus accumbens or the striatum. Therefore, in our experiments microdiscs of tissues were punched out from coronal slices of the rat brain in areas rich in DA nerve terminals and DA levels and those of dihydroxyphenyl acetic acid (DOPAC), one of the main DA metabolite, were estimated by sensitive radioenzymatic methods after separation of catechol derivatives. In most cases, changes in DA utilization were determined by calculating the ratio of the DOPAC and DA levels found in each sample. This ratio is a good index of the transmitter rate of utilization since DOPAC and DA levels are increased and decreased respectively under activation of DA neurons and the reverse occurred when the firing rate of the DA cells is reduced. With this method marked differences in DA utilization were found in the prefrontal cortex and the nucleus accumbens in various situations, the nucleus accumbens being used as a reference for subcortical limbic areas innervated by mesolimbic DA neurons.

1. In control rats, the DOPAC/DA ratio as well as the DA decline after α-MpT treatment were higher in the prefrontal cortex than in the nucleus accumbens or the striatum. This indicated that DA utilization was more pronounced in the prefrontal cortex and suggested that VTA DA cells innervating the prefrontal cortex and the nucleus accumbens were different.

2. Self-stimulation can be induced in the rat by electrodes implanted in the VTA. DA neurons are involved since self-stimulation is reduced by α-MpT pretreatment. When electrical stimulation of the VTA was performed with parameters identical to those inducing self-stimulation behavior the DOPAC/DA ratio was markedly increased in the prefrontal cortex but the effect was much less pronounced in the nucleus accumbens (Simon et al., 1979b). This suggested that the parameters for the electrical activation of DA cells innervating the prefrontal cortex and the nucleus accumbens were different.

3. When rats were stressed by intermittent electric foot-shocks (20 min) the DOPAC/DA ratio (Lavielle et al., 1979) or the DA decline after α-MpT treatment (Thierry et al., 1976) were markedly increased in the prefrontal and cingular cortices. DA turnover was only slightly enhanced in the nucleus accumbens and no effect occurred in the olfactory tubercles, the septum the amygdala or the striatum. This further revealed that the mesocortical DA neurons were submitted to interneuronal regulatory processes distinct from those of other ascending DA neurons. Interestingly, the stimulatory effect of the stress on the activity of the mesocortico-prefrontal DA neurons was prevented by benzodiazepines suggesting that inhibitory GABA neurons were involved in the regulation of these DA cells (Lavielle et al., 1979). More recently, we have also shown that this stress reduced substance P levels in the VTA but not in the SN (Lisoprawski et al., 1981). Since striato-nigral substance P neurons exert a tonic excitatory effect on nigrostriatal DA neurons, substance P neurons which originate in the habenula and project into the VTA may regulate in a similar way DA cells innervating the prefrontal cortex. The stresss-induced activation of the mesocortico-prefrontal DA neurons could depend on the activation of the habenula-VTA substance P pathway.

4. Finally, differences in the reactivity of the DA neurons innervating the frontal cortex and limbic structures such as the nucleus accumbens and the olfactory tubercules were also seen under acute or chronic neuroleptic treatments (Scatton et al., 1976).

Direct evidence for the distinction between mesocortico-prefrontal and mesolimbic DA neurons

To further demonstrate that the VTA DA cells are distributed in specific DA systems these cells were identified by antidromic activation of their fibres in various target areas. Secondly, changes in DA utilization were determined in the prefrontal cortex and the nucleus accumbens after chemical or electrolytic lesions of neuronal pathways projecting to the VTA.

The electrophysiological study of Deniau et al.(1980) first

indicated that distinct VTA cells were involved in the innervation
of the prefrontal cortex, the septum, the nucleus accumbens and the
head of the striatum. In few cases, only a VTA cell was shown to
send axon branches to two different structures such as the septum
and the cortex or the septum and the nucleus accumbens. Moreover,
from the conduction velocity of the VTA cells, it was concluded
that two types of VTA cells at least were projecting to each structure. One type of these cells which exhibited a slow axonal conduction velocity corresponded to the DA neurons. Indeed, their number
was markedly reduced after the 6-OHDA-induced degeneration of the
DA neurons (Thierry et al., 1980). This dual innervation of each
structure by DA and non-DA neurons (which have still to be identified) has been confirmed by combined visualization of the DA
cells by histochemistry and of the non-DA cells by retrograde transport of horseradish peroxidase or dyes injected in the nucleus
accumbens (Berger et al., 1978) or in the prefrontal cortex
(Albanese and Bentivoglio, 1981). The respective contributions of
these two types of cells in the regulation of the activity of target
neurons in corresponding structures has still to be determined.

Neuronal pathways originating from the VTA can be distinguished
not only by their target structures but also by their regulation
through VTA afferences. Anatomical studies have indicated that the
VTA is mainly innervated by neurons from the habenula, the dorsal
and median raphe, the deep nuclei of the cerebellum and the locus
coeruleus (Philipson, 1979 ; Simon et al., 1979a). The effects
induced by electrolytic or chemical lesion of these structures on
the activity of DA neurons innervating the prefrontal cortex and
the nucleus accumbens were thus determined in biochemical studies.
Three patterns of responses were obtained in the lesioned rats.
1) Some lesions affected only DA utilization in the prefrontal
cortex : the bilateral electrolytic lesions of the habenula
increased the DOPAC/DA ratio only in the prefrontal cortex
(Lisoprawski et al., 1980) while a reduction of DA utilisation
only occurred in this structure after the electrlytic lesion of the
interposate nucleus of the cerebellum (unpublished observations)
or the chemical lesion of ascending noradrenergic neurons (Tassin
et al., 1979 ; Hervé et al., 1981a). 2) The electrolytic lesion of
the dorsal raphe was the only one which did not affect the DOPAC/
DA ratio in the prefrontal cortex but which selectively influenced
the activity of DA cells innervating the nucleus accumbens since
the DOPAC/DA ratio was enhanced in this structure a few days after
the lesion (Hervé et al., 1979). 3) In contrast to other lesions,
the electrolytic lesion of the median raphe led to changes in
activity of DA cells projecting to both structures. However, the
effect observed were in opposite direction since the DOPAC/DA ratio
was enhanced in the nucleus accumbens and reduced in the prefrontal
cortex (Hervé et al., 1981b).

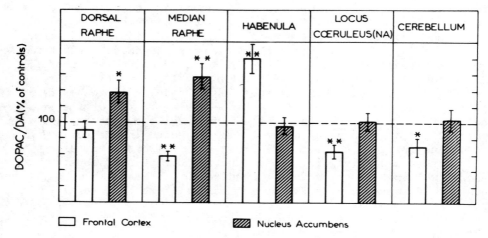

Fig.2   Effects of destruction of various pathways projecting into
        the VTA on DA utilization in the prefrontal cortex and the
        nucleus accumbens of the rat. VTA afferences were destroyed
        either by electrolytic lesions of various nuclei or by a
        6-OHDA microinjection made to induce the degeneration of
        the NA pathway originating from the locus coeruleus.

        Five to seven days after the lesion, rats were sacrificed
        and samples of tissue were punched out from the prefrontal
        cortex and the nucleus accumbens (720 and 64 μg of protein
        respectively). After homogeneization, DA and DOPAC were
        estimated and the DOPAC/DA ratios were calculated and
        compared to those of sham-operated animals. Values for DA
        and DOPAC levels and DOPAC/DA ratios in the sham-operated
        animals were respectively in the prefrontal cortex and the
        nucleus accumbens : 1.1 $\pm$ 0.1 and 85 $\pm$ 8 ng/mg protein (DA),
        0.52 $\pm$ 0.04 and 28 $\pm$ 2.5 ng/ml protein (DOPAC) and
        0.5 $\pm$ 0.04 and 0.25 $\pm$ 0.02 (DOPAC/DA). Results are the mean
        $\pm$ s.e.m. of data obtained with groups of 8 animals at least.
        * P <0.05 and ** P < 0.01 when compared with respective
        values in sham-operated animals. Electrolytic lesions of
        the cerebellum were placed in the interposate nucleus.

Some remarks should be made. The destruction of the VTA noradrenergic innervation was the only one which induced an effect on the activity of the mesocortico-prefrontal DA neurons which lasted for several weeks. The changes induced by other lesions were of shorter duration. The electrolytic lesions may destroy various types of neurons exerting different effect on DA cells. It will be important to know whether or not the specific chemical destruction of serotoninergic neurons from the dorsal and median raphe induced effects similar to those of the electrolytic lesions. In any cases, these results indicated that the VTA DA neurons which project to the prefrontal cortex or to the nucleus accumbens were submitted to distinct regulatory processes. This explains the difference in the reactivity of these two populations of VTA DA neurons.

Involvement of the mesocortico-prefrontal DA neurons in the control of the activity of other ascending DA neurons

Anatomical studies have indicated that neurons originating from the prefrontal cortex project to various subcortical structures innervated by DA neurons such as the septum, the nucleus accumbens, the striatum, etc(Beckstead, 1979). Moroever, projections to mesencephalic areas which contain the cell bodies of the various ascending DA systems have also been described. Recently, A.M. Thierry, A. Ferron and G. Chevalier have observed that most of these cortical neurons were branched neurons (unpublished observations). Neurons originating from the prefrontal cortex and exerting a facilitatory or inhibitory control on VTA cells projecting to some limbic subcortical structures including the nucleus accumbens were also identified through their action on cortical efferent pathways. The mesocortico-prefrontal DA neurons could thus be involved in the regulation of DA release in subcortical limbic structures. These regulations may involve projections reaching DA cell bodies or their dendrites in the VTA and the SN or connections exerting a presynaptic control on DA release in target areas innervated by DA neurons.

The involvement of the mesocortico-prefrontal DA neurons in the control of the activity of other DA neurons was suggested by recent experiments made by Pycock et al. (1980). These authors demonstrated that 6-OHDA microinjections made in the frontal cortex of rats pretreated with desmethylimipramine in order to prevent the destruction of noradrenergic terminals increase DA utilization in the nucleus accumbens and the striatum. Therefore, the mesocortico-prefrontal DA neurons could exert an inhibitory influence on DA transmission in subcortical structures. It has still to be demonstrated that such regulatory processes may intervene in physiological states.

Interestingly in rats isolated during several weeks from their partners we observed that the DOPAC/DA ratio was decreased in the prefrontal cortex and enhanced in the nucleus accumbens and the striatum when compared to results obtained in animals housed in groups (Blanc et al., 1980). Since similar opposite changes in the activity of DA neurons projecting to the prefrontal cortex or to the nucleus accumbens have also been seen after electrolytic lesion of the median raphe it remains to determine whether the reduction of the cortical DA utilization in the isolated rats is directly responsible for the increased DA transmission intervening in subcortical structures. Whatever are the mechanisms involved these asymmetric changes in the activity of the DA neurons projecting either to the prefrontal cortex or to the nucleus accumbens may contribute to the control of a given function. Indeed, it has been shown that locomotor activity in rats is enhanced either by facilitation of DA transmission in the nucleus accumbens (Kelly et al., 1975) or by interruption of cortical DA transmission (Pycock et al., 1980 ; Tassin et al., 1978). Moreover, locomotor activity is increased both in rats submitted to prolonged isolation and in animals with median raphe lesions (Jacobs et al., 1974),two situations in which as previously described, DA utilization is reduced in the prefrontal cortex and enhanced in the nucleus accumbens.

CONCLUDING REMARKS

Numerous studies have been made to investigate the role of various identified pathways which project into the SN in the control of the activity of the nigrostriatal DA neurons. This is particularly the case for the striato-nigral GABA or substance P neurons and for the serotoninergic neurons which originate from the dorsal and median raphe. The present report indicates that the VTA DA neurons which innervate the prefrontal cortex and the nucleus accumbens are submitted to different regulations by pathways or fibres originating or passing through structures such as the habenula, the raphe nuclei, the locus coeruleus or the deep decebellar nuclei. Most of the neuronal pathways involved in these regulations have still to be identified. It remains also to establish whether or not subpopulations of DA cells located both in the VTA and the SN and which innervate structures other than the prefrontal cortex, the nucleus accumbens and the striatum are also under the control of specific pathways. For instance, it will be of particular interest to know whether DA neurons projecting to the cingular or enhorhinal cortices share properties similar to those detected for the mesocortico-prefrontal DA neurons. Are they or not indirectly involved in the regulation of DA transmission in some subcortical structures? Studies similar to those described in this review could help to clarify these questions Interactions between DA systems can also be mediated by DA release from the dendrites of the DA cells. This has particularly been shown

for the reciprocal regulation of the two nigrostriatal DA systems.
It remains to determine whether DA released in the SN is also
involved in the regulation of the activity of nigral DA cells innervating the cerebral cortex.

REFERENCES

Albanese, A., and Bentivoglio, M., 1981, Dopaminergic and non-
    dopaminergic mesocortical neurons in the rat, Neurosci.
    Lett. suppl., 7 S 397
Beckstead, R.M., 1979, An autoradiographic examination of cortico-
    cortical and subcortical projections of the mediodorsal
    projection (prefrontal) cortex in the rat,J. Comp.Neur.,
    184: 43
Blanc, G., Hervé, D., Simon, H., Lisoprawski, A., Glowinski, J.,
    and Tassin, J.P., 1980, Response to stress of mesocortico-
    frontal dopaminergic neurons in rats after long-term
    isolation, Nature, 284: 265
Berger, B., Nguyen-Legros, J., and Thierry, A.M., 1978, Demonstra-
    tion of horseradish peroxidase and fluorescent catechola-
    mines in the same neuron, Neurosci. Lett., 9: 297
Bunney, B.S., Aghajanian, G.K., and Roth, R.H., 1973, Comparison of
    the effects of L-DOPA,amphetamine and apomorphine on firing
    rate of rat dopaminergic neurons, Nature New Biol.,245:123
Chéramy, A., Leviel, V.,and Glowinski, J., 1981a, Dendritic release
    of dopamine in the substantai nigra, Nature, 289: 537
Chéramy, A., Leviel, V., Daudet, F., Guibert, B., Chesselet, M.F.,
    and Glowinski, J., 1981b, Involvement of the thalamus in the
    reciprocal regulation of the two nigrostriatal dopaminergic
    pathways, Neuroscience (in press)
Deniau, J.M., Hammond, C., Riszk, A., and Féger, J., 1978, Electro-
    physiological properties of identified output neurons of the
    rat substantia nigra (pars compacta and pars reticulata):
    evidences for the existence of branched neurons, Exp.Brain
    Res., 32:409
Deniau, J.M., Thierry, A.M., and Féger, J., 1980, Electrophysiolo-
    gical identifications of mesencephalic ventromedial tegmen-
    tal (VMT) neurons projecting to the frontal cortex, septum
    and nucleus accumbens, Brain Research, 189: 315
Groves, P.M., Wilson, C.J., Young, S.J., and Rebec, G.V.,1975, Self-
    inhibition by dopaminergic neurons: an alternative to the
    "Neuronal feedback loop" hypothesis for the mode of action
    of certain psychotropic drugs, Science, 190: 522
Hervé, D., Blanc, G., Glowinski, J.,and Tassin, J.P., 1981a, Reduc-
    tion of dopamine utilization in the prefrontal cortex but
    not in the nucleus accumbens after selective destruction of
    noradrenergic fibers innervating the ventral tegmental area
    in the rat, Brain Research (in press)

Hervé, D., Simon, H., Blanc, G., LeMoal, M., Glowinski, J., and
    Tassin, J.P., 1981b, Opposite changes in dopamine utiliza-
    tion in the nucleus accumbens and the frontal cortex after
    electrolytic lesion of the median raphe in the rat,
    Brain Research, 216 n°2: 422
Hervé, D., Simon, H., Blanc, G., Lisoprawski, A., LeMoal, M.,
    Glowinski, J.,and Tassin, J.P., 1979, Increased utilization
    of dopamine in the nucleus accumbens but not in the cerebral
    cortex after dorsal and raphe lesion in the rat, Neurosci.
    Lett., 15 n°2-3:127
Jacobs, B.L., Wisen, W.D., and Taylor,K.M., 1974, Differential
    behavioral and neurochemical effects following lesions of
    the dorsal or median raphe nucleus in rats, Brain Research,
    79:353
Kelly, P.H., Seviour, P.W., and Iversen, S.D., 1975, Amphetamine
    and apomorphine responses in the rat following 6-OHDA
    lesions of the nucleus accumbens septi and corpus striatum,
    Brain Research, 94: 507
Lavielle, S., Tassin, J.P., Thierry, A.M., Blanc, G., Hervé, D.,
    Barthelemy, C.,and Glowinski, J.,1979, Blockade by benzodia-
    zepines of the selective high increase in dopamine turnover
    induced by stress in mesocortical dopaminergic neurons of
    the rat, Brain Research, 168 n°3: 585
Leviel, V., Chéramy, A., and Glowinski, J., 1979, Role of the
    dendritic release of dopamine in the reciprocal control of
    the two nigrostriatal dopaminergic pathways, Nature, 280:
    236
Leviel, V., Chesselet, M.F., Glowinski, J.,and Chéramy, A., 1981,
    Involvement of the thalamus in the asymmetric effect of
    dopaminergic pathways in the cat, Brain Research, 226
    (in press)
Lindvall, D., and Björklund, A, 1978, Organization of catechola-
    mine neurons in the rat central neurons system, in:
    "Handbook of Psychopharmacology", L.L.Iversen, S.D. Iversen,
    & S.H. Snyder, eds.,vol.3, 139, Plenum
Lisoprawski, A., Blanc, G., and Glowinski, J., 1981, Activation by
    stress of the habenulo-interpeduncular substance P neurons
    in the rat, Neurosci. Lett., 25: 47
Lisoprawski, A., Hervé, D., Blanc, G., Glowinski, J., and Tassin,
    J.P., 1980, Selective activation of the mesocortico-frontal
    dopaminergic neurons induced by lesion of the habenula in
    the rat, Brain Research, 183 n°1: 229
Nieoullon, A., Chéramy, A., and Glowinski, J., 1977a, Interdepen-
    dence of the nigrostriatal dopaminergic systems on the two
    sides of the brain in the cat, Science, 198: 416
Nieoullon, A., Chéramy, A., and Glowinski, J., 1977b, Nigral and
    striatal dopamine release under sensory stimuli, Nature,
    269: 340

Nieoullon, A., Chéramy, A., and Glowinski, J., 1978, Release of dopamine in both caudate nuclei and both substantiae nigrae in response to unilateral stimulation of cerebellar nuclei in the cat, Brain Research, 148:143

Nieoullon, A., Chéramy, A., Leviel, V., and Glowinski, J., 1979, Effects of the unilateral nigral application of dopaminergic drugs on the in vivo release of dopamine in the two caudate nuclei of the cat, Europ.J.Pharmacol., 53: 289

Phillipson, O.T., 1979, Afferent projections to the ventral tegmental area of Tsai and interfascicular nucleus: a horseradish peroxydase study in the rat, J.Comp.Neurol., 187: 117

Pycock, C.J., Carter, C.J., and Kerwin, P.W., 1980, Effect of 6-hydroxydopamine lesion in the medial prefrontal cortex on neurotransmitter systems in subcortical sites in the rat, J. Neurochem., 34: 91

Ruffieux, A., and Schultz, W., 1980, Dopaminergic activation of reticulata neurons in the substantia nigra, Nature, 285:240

Scatton, B., Glowinski, J., and Julou, L., 1976, Dopamine metabolism in the mesolimbic and mesocortical dopaminergic systems after single or repeated administrations of neuroleptics, Brain Research, 109: 184

Simon, H., LeMoal, M., and Calas, A., 1979a, Efferents and afferents of the ventral tegmental A10 region studies after local injection of ^{3}H-leucine and horseradish peroxydase, Brain Research, 178:17

Simon, H., Stinus, L., Tassin, J.P., Lavielle, S., Blanc, G., Thierry, A.M., Glowinski, J., and LeMoal, M., 1979b, Is the dopaminergic mesocortico-limbic system necessary for intracranial self-stimulation ? Behavioral & Neural Biol. 27:125

Tassin, J.P., Lavielle, S., Hervé, D., Blanc, G., Thierry, A.M., Alvarez, C., Berger, B.,and Glowinski, J.,1979, Collateral sprouting and reduced activity of the rat mesocortical dopaminergic neurons after selective destruction of the ascending noradrenergic bundles, Neuroscience,4:1569

Tassin, J.P., Stinus, L., Simon, H., Blanc, G., Thierry, A.M., LeMoal, M., Cardo, B.,and Glowinski,J.,1978, Relationships between the locomotor hyperactivity induced by A10 lesions had the destruction of the frontocortical dopaminergic innervation in the rat, Brain Research, 141 n°2: 267

Thierry, A.M., Blanc, G., Sobel, A., Stinus, L., and Glowinski, J., 1973, Dopaminergic terminals in the rat cortex, Science, 182: 499

Thierry, A.M., Deniau, J.M., Hervé, D., and Chevalier, G., 1980, Electrophysiological evidence for non-DA mesocortical neurons in the rat, Brain Research, 201: 210

Thierry, A.M., Tassin, J.P., Blanc, G., and Glowinski, J., 1976, Selective activation of the mesocortical DA system by stress, Nature, 263: 242

ACETYLCHOLINE-DOPAMINE INTERACTIONS IN THE CORPUS STRIATUM AND

NUCLEUS ACCUMBENS

J. S. de Belleroche

Departments of Neurology and Biochemistry
Charing Cross Hospital and Medical School
London, W6 8RF, U.K.

INTRODUCTION

It has been recognised for a number of years that there are interactions between the cholinergic and dopaminergic systems of the brain. Maintenance of the correct balance between these transmitters is, for example, important in the central regulation of motor activity and is impaired in a number of neurological disorders. Thus, anticholinergic drugs are a beneficial adjunct in the treatment of Parkinson's disease, suppression of the cholinergic system in line with the deficient dopaminergic system leads to some improvement in the symptoms. It has also recently been confirmed that the use of anticholinergic drugs such as procyclidine in schizophrenia, where there is an apparent overactivity of dopaminergic transmission, has the opposite effect of exacerbating the symptoms of this condition (Singh and Kaye, 1975; Crow *et al.*, 1980).

The present discussion concerns these interactions in two of the main dopaminergically innervated structures in the brain, the corpus striatum and nucleus accumbens. The role of the nucleus accumbens in man has received little attention, unlike the striatum, but recently Price *et al.* (1978) have shown from post mortem analysis that there is a considerable reduction in the dopamine levels of this region in Parkinson's disease. This deficit (a 60% decrease) which is of the same order as that occurring in the caudate (a 65% decrease in this study) is likely to be of considerable importance, and may give rise to the akinesia occurring in Parkinson's disease, since animal studies indicate that this region is responsible for promoting locomotor activity (Pijnenburg and van Rossum, 1973). It will also emerge in this discussion that in addition to the conventional postsynaptic site of transmitter action, that presynaptic

235

modulation of transmitter release and synthesis is commonly
detected.

Organisation of the corpus striatum and nucleus accumbens
_____

      The corpus striatum and nucleus accumbens have a number of
common features in their organisation (reviewed by Nauta and
Domesick, 19·79; Nauta *et al.*, 1978). Both receive a dopaminergic
input from the mesencephalon, the ventral tegmental area (A10) serving the nucleus accumbens and the zona compacta of substantia nigra
(A9) serving the corpus striatum. Both regions also receive serotonergic afferents from the dorsal raphé and projections from the
thalamus. Different regions of the thalamus serve the caudate/
putamen and nucleus accumbens, for example, the parafasciculus
nucleus projects to the caudate/putamen and the more medial thalamic structures, e.g. nucleus paraventricularis project to nucleus
accumbens. A major innervation of the striatum is also received
from the cerebral cortex, mainly the neocortex, i.e. sensory, motor
and association areas, although all regions appear to be involved,
including limbic structures such as cingulate cortex. The analogous structures innervating the nucleus accumbens are mainly parts
of the limbic system such as allocortex and hippocampus, although
structures outside the limbic system such as the motor cortex also
project to the nucleus accumbens. Both the frontal cortex projection to the striatum and the allocortex projection to the nucleus
accumbens appear to use glutamate as a transmitter since frontal
decortication and fornix transection significantly reduce (by
approximately half) glutamate uptake in the striatum and nucleus
accumbens respectively (Walaas, 1981; McGeer *et al.*, 1977).

      The efferent systems are once again similar, both having a
major pathway to the globus pallidus, the ventral pallidum in the
case of the nucleus accumbens and the main regions of the internal
and external segments of the globus pallidus for striatum. A transmitter in each of these efferents has been identified as GABA (Dray
and Oakley, 1978; Jones and Mogenson, 1980). Other striatal efferents pass directly to the substantia nigra, whereas the remaining
efferents from the nucleus accumbens are more widely distributed,
and pass to the preoptic area, hypothalanus, A10, A8, substantia
innominata, central grey as well as the zona reticulata of the substantia nigra. From this outline of the regions and pathways linked
to the striatum and accumbens, it can be seen that they both are
important in motor control through their efferent pathways to globus
pallidus and the mesencephalon, the striatum integrating the neocortical influences and the nucleus accumbens integrating mainly
limbic influences.

      As mentioned above, dopamine, serotonin and glutamate are
afferent transmitters of both the striatum and nucleus accumbens.

The peptide cholecystokinin is also present in afferents from the
mesencephalon (Hökfelt *et al.*, 1980), and other peptides such as
substance P may also be present in afferents, as well as cell body
populations in these regions (Ljungdahl *et al.*, 1978). A considerable proportion of the acetylcholine and GABA in these regions, both
of which contain high levels of these transmitters, is found in
interneurones. Thus, lesions which were used as described above to
reduce glutamate uptake in striatum and accumbens had little effect
on the activity of choline acetyltransferase and glutamic acid decarboxylase or on GABA uptake (Schwartz and Coyle, 1977; Walaas and
Fonnum, 1979). On the other hand, destruction of the interneurones
with kainic acid injection into the nucleus accumbens significantly
reduced the activity of choline acetyltransferase, GABA uptake and
glutamic acid decarboxylase activity in this region (Walaas and
Fonnum, 1979). Like acetylcholine, dopamine and 5-hydroxytryptamine,
the peptide, enkephalin, shows a fairly even distribution in both
striatum and accumbens. However, other peptides such as cholecystokinin (Hökfelt *et al.*, 1980) and neurotensin (Uhl *et al.*, 1977)
are most abundant in the nucleus accumbens, which may form the basis
of a significant difference between these regions.

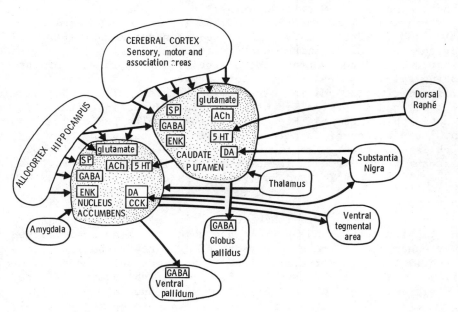

Fig. 1.   Afferent and efferent connections of nucleus accumbens and
corpus striatum and some associated transmitter systems.
SP, Substance P; ENK, enkephalin; ACh, acetylcholine; DA,
dopamine; 5HT, 5-hydroxytryptamine; GABA, γ-aminobutyric
acid; CCK, cholecystokinin.

The connections and transmitters of corpus striatum and nucleus accumbens are summarised in Fig. 1.

Biochemical analysis of transmitter interactions in the striatum and nucleus accumbens

The aim of this study was to examine transmitter interactions in these regions by measuring the action of one transmitter system on the release of another transmitter, using predominantly *in vitro* methods such as tissue slices and synaptosomes. The principle transmitters under consideration being dopamine and acetylcholine.

DOPAMINE ACTION ON CHOLINERGIC CELLS

The action of dopamine in the corpus striatum

The release of acetylcholine from rat striatal slices was measured by bioassay using the guinea-pig ileum. Both 56 mM K^+ and 75 μM veratrine cause a substantial enhancement (3-4 fold increases) of acetylcholine release from striatal slices, the veratrine effect being blocked by 1 μM tetrodotoxin (Fig. 2a). Dopamine depressed the K^+-evoked release of acetylcholine (de Belleroche *et al.*, 1980; Miller and Friedhoff, 1979) in a dose-dependent manner (Fig. 2b) over the range of dopamine concentrations used (10^{-7}-10^{-3}M). At the higher dopamine concentrations, a significant depression of the resting release was also seen, for example, 1 mM dopamine (Fig. 2c). Chlorpromazine (20 μM) largely abolished this action of dopamine (Fig. 2c) and also significantly antagonised the inhibitory action of apomorphine (20 μM) (Fig. 2d). These results indicate a clear inhibitory action of dopamine on cholinergic cells in the striatum which is consistent with the *in vivo* actions of dopamine agonists on acetylcholine release (Stadler *et al.*, 1973), turnover (Trabucchi *et al.*, 1975; Consolo *et al.*, 1975) and steady state levels (McGeer *et al.*, 1974a).

In contrast to this inhibitory action of dopamine agonists, neuroleptics such as haloperidol and chlorpromazine administered *in vivo*, enhance the K^+-evoked release of $[^3H]$-acetylcholine from subsequently prepared striatal slices (Fig. 3, de Belleroche and Neal, 1981). This action is marked, a doubling of the evoked release occurring with both haloperidol (2 mg kg^{-1}) and chlorpromazine (25 mg kg^{-1}). The mechanism of action of neuroleptics is likely to be due to a blocking of dopamine mediated inhibition, since the neuroleptics themselves do not elevate acetylcholine release and the elevated extracellular K^+ promotes enhanced dopamine release which would inhibit acetylcholine release. No change in this response to haloperidol occurred with chronic treatment up to 25 days which

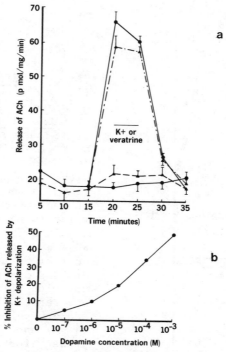

Fig. 2a. <u>Effect of 56 mM K⁺ and 75 µM veratrine on the release of
acetylcholine from striatal slices</u>. Tissue slices were
transferred to fresh incubation medium at 5 min intervals
after an initial 20 min preincubation period. K⁺ or veratrine were present for two successive periods only, ie the
4th and 5th collection periods, as indicated by the bar.
Values are means (p mol/mg wet wt/min) ± SEMs for the number of experiments indicated in brackets. Control incubation (12) throughout and control with K⁺ (56 mM) present
in collection periods 4 and 5, ●———●; veratrine (75 µM)
present (5), ▲–·–·–▲; veratrine (75 µM) and tetrodotoxin
(1 µM) present (3), ▲————▲.

Fig. 2b. <u>Effect of dopamine on the K⁺-evoked release of acetylcholine
from striatal slices</u>. Tissue slices were incubated as described in Fig. 2a. Dopamine at various concentrations
(10⁻⁷–10⁻³M), was present for the 2nd, 3rd, 4th and 5th
incubation period. To determine the amount of K⁺-evoked
release of acetylcholine, the base line level of release
was subtracted from each value (K⁺ present) and related to
the value of K⁺-evoked release of acetylcholine in the absence of dopamine, as a percentage. Each concentration is
a mean from 6 experiments. Data from de Belleroche *et al*.
(1981b).

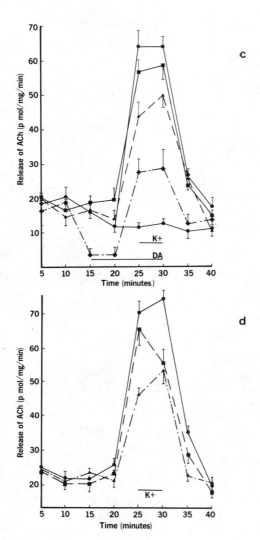

Fig. 2c. <u>Effect of 1 mM dopamine and 20 μM chlorpromazine
on acetylcholine release from
striatal slices.</u> Striatal
slices were incubated in control
or K⁺ (56 mM) containing medium
(4th and 5th period) together
with dopamine and/or chlorpromazine (in the 2nd, 3rd, 4th and
5th periods) as indicated. Each
value (p mol/mg wet wt/min) is
a mean ± SEM from 6 experiments.
●———●, control throughout, and
control, 56 mM K⁺ present in the
4th and 5th period; ◆–·–·–◆ ,
dopamine (1 mM) present for 2nd-
5th period, K⁺ present in 4th
and 5th period; ▲----▲, dopamine
(1 mM) and chlorpromazine (20 μM)
present for 2nd-5th period, K⁺
present in 4th and 5th periods;
■———■ , chlorpromazine (20 μM)
present for 2nd-5th period,
56 mM K⁺ present in the 4th and
5th periods.

Fig. 2d.   <u>Effect of apomorphine (20 μM) and chlorpromazine (20 μM)
on the release of acetylcholine from striatal slices.</u>
Striatal slices were incubated as described above. Values
are means ± SEMs for 2-4 experiments. ●———●, control
incubation, 56 mM K⁺ present in the 4th and 5th incubation
periods. ▲–·–·–▲, Apomorphine (20 μM) present in the 2nd-
5th incubation periods, 56 mM K⁺ also present in the 4th
and 5th incubation periods. ■----■ apomorphine (20 μM)
and chlorpromazine (20 μM) both present in the 2nd-5th
incubation periods, 56 mM K⁺ present in the 4th and 5th
incubation periods. Data from de Belleroche *et al.* (1981b).

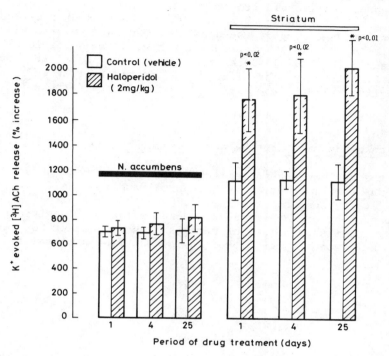

Fig. 3. Effect of haloperidol treatment on the K⁺-evoked release of [³H]-acetylcholine synthesised from exogenous [³H]-choline from tissue slices of nucleus accumbens and corpus striatum. Haloperidol (2 mg.kg⁻¹) or vehicle injections were given i.p. (hatched and clear histograms respectively) for 1, 4 or 25 days as indicated. After 90 min, tissue slices were prepared, in Krebs bicarbonate medium containing [³H]-choline at 37°C for 30 min and were then continuously superfused. Samples were collected after an initial period of 30 min. The 34 mM K⁺-evoked release (fractional rate coefficient, min⁻¹) of [³H]-acetylcholine is expressed as a percentage of the control release in the sample immediately prior to the K⁺ pulse. The values are means ± SEM for 4–6 experiments. *Indicates that haloperidol treatment significantly enhanced the evoked release of [³H]-acetylcholine student's unpaired t-test. Data is taken from de Belleroche and Neal (1981).

indicated that this action of neuroleptics could be a significant
factor in man where continuous drug treatment is in use. A drug
with low incidence of extrapyramidal side effects such as clozapine
only enhanced cholinergic transmission to a small degree even with
a considerable drug dose, eg 50 mg kg^{-1}. The lack of a marked effect
in response to neuroleptics such as clozapine and thioridazine was
unlikely to be due to their relatively high antimuscarinic activity
(Miller and Hiley, 1974) since high concentrations of atropine were
not able to antagonise the effect of haloperidol (1 mg kg^{-1}) on
acetylcholine release from striatal slices (de Belleroche and Neal,
1981).

The action of dopamine in the nucleus accumbens

In the nucleus accumbens, the action of dopamine on acetylcholine was very much attenuated (approximately by half) by comparison with its action in the striatum (Fig. 4). Neuroleptic treatment
had no enhancing effect on the K$^+$-evoked release of acetylcholine
(Fig. 3) from tissue slices of nucleus accumbens under the same conditions that promoted acetylcholine release from striatal slices.

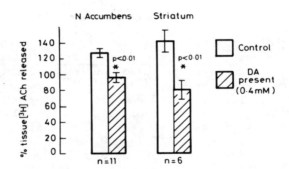

Fig. 4. Effect of dopamine (*in vitro*) on the resting release of
         [^{3}H]-acetylcholine from nucleus accumbens and striatum.
         Tissue slices of nucleus accumbens and corpus striatum were
         superfused with Krebs bicarbonate medium, a steady rate of
         resting release of [^{3}H]-acetylcholine was obtained and a
         pulse of dopamine was applied. Values, % [^{3}H]-acetylcho-
         line released.min^{-1} x 10^3 are means ± SEM for n experiments
         (as indicated). *Indicates that release (%[^{3}H]-acetylcho-
         line released.min^{-1} x 10^{-3}) was significantly decreased by
         dopamine (p < 0.01: paired student's t-test). Data is taken
         from de Belleroche and Neal (1981).

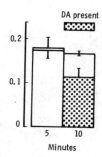

Fig. 5a. <u>Effect of dopamine on the release of acetylcholine from striatal synaptosome beds</u>. Striatal synaptosome 'beds' were transferred at 5 min intervals after an initial 20 min preincubation period. Each synaptosome preparation was used to make two synaptosome 'beds', one of which was used as a control and the other was used for dopamine application. Values (p mol/mg protein/min) are means for 4 experiments. Dopamine significantly depressed the release of acetylcholine (p < 0.05).

Thus a clear difference emerges in the organisation of striatum and nucleus accumbens, whereas dopamine has a marked inhibitory action on cholinergic cells in the striatum, a post-synaptic cholinergic cell is not directly affected by dopamine in the n.accumbens. The latter conclusion is also borne out by the observation that atropine does not enhance or block intra-accumbens dopamine induced locomotor activity (Costall *et al*., 1980) and hence does not require a cholinergic cell distal to the site of dopamine action for expression of this activity.

Presynaptic action of dopamine in the corpus striatum

In order to investigate whether a component of the inhibitory action of dopamine was mediated through presynaptic receptors, the effect of dopamine was studied on a striatal synaptosome preparation. The synaptosomes were used in the form of a deposit between nylon

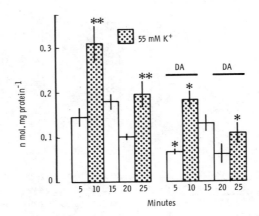

Fig. 5b. Effect of dopamine on the release of acetylcholine from
cerebral cortex synaptosome beds. Cerebral cortex synaptosome beds were transferred at 5 min intervals after an
initial 20 min incubation period. Each synaptosome preparation was used to make two synaptosome beds, one of which
was used as a control and the other was used for dopamine
application. 56 mM K$^+$ stimulation was carried out in each
group as indicated by the shaded histograms. Values (p mol/
mg protein/min) are means ± SEMs for the number of 4-5 experiments. Data is taken from de Belleroche *et al.* (1981b).

gauzes (de Belleroche and Bradford, 1972) which can easily be ma-
nipulated by means of a McIlwain Quick Transfer Holder, and the
synaptosome bed transferred at 5 minute intervals using the same
method as employed in the tissue slice experiment. Using this preparation, dopamine was found to significantly reduce the resting release of acetylcholine (Fig. 5a) by approximately 30% The effect
was smaller than was obtained with similar concentrations of dopamine
on striatal slices (an 80% reduction). However, synaptosome preparations take several hours for their completion and these results
would therefore underestimate the response *in vivo*.

Presynaptic action of dopamine in cerebral cortex

A presynaptic action of dopamine on acetylcholine release is also seen in cerebral cortex synaptosomes (Fig. 5b) where both the resting and K^+-evoked release of acetylcholine are clearly reduced as in striatum. Although both cholinergic and dopaminergic innervations are present in the cerebral cortex, it is not yet known whether the terminal fields would overlap. The cholinergic terminal fields are restricted to specific cortical layers (McGeer et al., 1974b), whereas the dopaminergic terminals are found in well-defined regions such as prefrontal and entorhinal cortex (Lindvall et al.. 1974; Thierry et al., 1973). As with the striatum it still remains to be demonstrated whether a strict synaptic connection exists, e.g. axo-axonic, of a dopamine terminal onto a cholinergic terminal or whether presynaptic receptors respond to transmitter which diffuses outside the synaptic cleft.

CHOLINERGIC ACTION ON DOPAMINERGIC NERVE TERMINALS

Cholinergic agents have been shown to affect dopamine turnover in vivo, for example, physostigmine and oxotremorine elevate homovanillic acid levels (Andén and Bedard, 1971; Bartholini et al., 1975). A direct action of the cholinergic agents in the region of the dopamine terminal is indicated from both in vivo striatal superfusion and striatal slice experiments (Giorgiueff et al., 1976), where the local application of cholinergic agents enhances the release of dopamine. The specific localisation of this interaction to the dopamine nerve terminal itself is supported by experiments carried out using striatal synaptosomes where a similar action of cholinergic agents on dopamine release is shown, both nicotinic and muscarinic mechanisms being involved (de Belleroche and Bradford, 1978). Both the nicotinic and muscarinic receptor concentration, assayed by the specific binding of α-bungarotoxin and N-methylatropine respectively, are in fact depleted at 7-14 days in the striatal synaptosome fraction following 6-hydroxydopamine lesion, which reduced the striatal tyrosine hydroxylase activity by 70% but did not affect the GABA levels (de Belleroche et al., 1979). Other studies on whole tissue concentrations of muscarinic receptors in striatum following 6-hydroxydopamine lesion similarly show a reduction in receptor concentration in the striatum (Kato et al., 1978; Gurwitz et al., 1980).

Cholinergic action on dopamine release in the nucleus accumbens

Although dopamine has little effect on acetylcholine release in the nucleus accumbens, a considerable reciprocal activity is seen, as occurs in striatum. The cholinergic agonist, oxotremorine and acetylcholine itself enhance the K^+-evoked release of [^{14}C]-dopamine (de Belleroche and Gardiner, 1981). The EC_{50} for the oxotremorine enhancement is $1.5 \times 10^{-7}M$, the maximal stimulation was reached at $2 \times 10^{-7}M$ oxotremorine. No further enhancement of $[^{14}C]$-dopamine release occurred until concentrations of oxotremorine of $10^{-3}M$ were reached. The oxotremorine enhancement of the K^+-evoked release of $[^{14}C]$-dopamine was abolished both by atropine and by incubation in high K^+ medium in the absence of calcium. These results indicated that the elevation of the K^+-evoked release of $[^{14}C]$-dopamine by oxotremorine was through a muscarinic receptor dependent on the operation of a calcium current. This action of oxotremorine on dopamine release contrasted sharply with its effect on the release of acetylcholine. Oxotremorine inhibited acetylcholine release, the IC_{50} for this effect being $4.3 \times 10^{-5}M$. This action appeared to be independent of the low and high concentration effects of oxotremorine as it occurred at oxotremorine concentrations more than one order of magnitude different. Acetylcholine similarly inhibited the release of $[^3H]$-acetylcholine synthesised from $[^3H]$-choline. These results indicated that acetylcholine could modulate dopamine release in the accumbens by a mechanism which was apparently indpendent of the autoregulatory process operating on the cholinergic terminals. The more precise localisation of the receptors to the presynaptic terminal membrane was determined by lesion studies using two further approaches, firstly by meausrement of receptor concentrations and secondly by behaviour studies.

Muscarinic receptors on dopamine terminals in the nucleus accumbens

In order to determine whether muscarinic receptors resided on the dopamine terminals in the nucleus accumbens, the dopaminergic cell bodies in the ventral tegmental area were destroyed using 6-hydroxydopamine and receptor concentration subsequently examined in the nucleus accumbens. A small volume (0.2 µl) of 6-hydroxydopamine (0.8 µg) was used to ensure a reasonably specific lesion and histological verification of the site of injection was carried out in all cases. At 7 days after the lesion, the level of dopamine in the nucleus accumbens ipsilateral to the lesion side was reduced by 83% compared to the control side. This loss of dopamine was accompanied by a significant decrease in the concentration of muscarinic receptors (Table 1) at both 7 and 14 days (de Belleroche *et al.*, 1981a). No loss of muscarinic receptors occurred on the lesion side, when artificial csf was injected into the ventral tegmental area or when the site of injection was just outside the ventral tegmental area. No change in the antagonist affinity constant occurred with lesion. However, further examination of the three agonist binding sites, ie the 'super high', 'high' and 'low' affinity binding sites using the methods of Birdsall *et al.* (1978, 1980) and Hulme *et al.* (1978), clearly showed that there was a selective loss of the highest affinity binding sites, ie the 'super high' affinity binding sites. This is the first observation that a

Table 1. Effect of unilateral 6-hydroxydopamine lesion in the ventral tegmental area on muscarinic receptor concentration and dopamine levels in nucleus accumbens.

Days after lesion	6-Hydroxydopamine lesion in A-10				Lesion outside A-10	
	7		14		14	
	Unlesioned side	Lesioned side	Unlesioned side	Lesioned side	Unlesioned side	Lesioned side
Muscarinic receptor concentration						
Specific binding of N-methylscopoloamine p.mol g.wet wt^{-1}	111.20±5.70 (6)	101.20±2.4*	105.20±5.7 (12)	89.80±6.9*	105.1±8.7 (10)	105.5±3.2
Specific binding of 3 nM oxotremorine-M p.mol.g^{-1}	2.01±0.22 (4)	1.66±0.1*	2.20±0.3 (7)	1.66±0.45*		
Super high affinity binding site: percentage occupancy of total receptor population	2.14±0.10 (4)	1.64±0.11**	2.12±0.19 (9)	1.81±0.16**		
Dopamine n mol.g^{-1}	34.60±0.3 (7)	5.90±0.9**				

*Indicates that value is significantly decreased on the lesioned side compared to the unlesioned side, p < 0.05, paired t-test.
**Indicates a significant decrease p < 0.01. Data from de Belleroche *et al.* (1981a).

selective loss of one class of muscarinic receptor can occur, which
may provide some insight into the functional role of different
agonist binding sites.

The role of presynaptic muscarinic receptors in regulating dopamine mediated behaviour

The study of a class of receptors is in the long term of little
interest unless a function can be attributed to them in the intact
animal. This was examined by testing whether intra-accumbens injections of cholinergic agonists affected the enhanced locomotor activity
induced by bilateral injection of dopamine into the nucleus accumbens
of rat. A rapid enhancement of dopamine-induced locomotor activity
was indeed stimulated by bilateral injections of oxotremorine into
the nucleus accumbens (de Belleroche et al., 1981c) and has also
been shown in response to carbachol (Jones et al., 1981). This
effect was consistent with the action of oxotremorine in vitro, to
elevate the K^+-evoked release of dopamine, described above. Similar
injections of oxotremorine into animals previously treated with
6-hydroxydopamine caused no stimulation of locomotor activity and
even reduced the level of dopamine-induced activity to a low level.
Thus, destruction of the dopamine terminal completely abolished the
stimulatory effect of oxotremorine. A delayed inhibitory action of
cholinergic agents such as eserine and arecoline has already been
reported after 1-2 hours in unlesioned animals (Costall et al., 1980)
and this action may be equivalent to that seen in the 6-hydroxydopa-
mine treated animals. This excitatory behavioural measure seen above
may give some indication of a possible role of one type of presynaptic receptor in the intact animal.

CONCLUSIONS

Studies on transmitter release in the corpus striatum and
nucleus accumbens clearly show regional differences in their transmitter organisation. A number of examples indicate that receptor
mediated modulation of release may occur directly at the level of
the presynaptic terminal. Dopamine modulates acetylcholine release
through presynaptic receptors in striatum and acetylcholine modulates
dopamine release through muscarinic and probably nicotinic receptors
in both striatum and accumbens. In addition to these interactions,
5HT has also been shown to act presynaptically on striatal nerve
terminals through its inhibitory action on dopamine synthesis in
striatal synaptosomes, which process is methysergide sensitive (de
Belleroche and Bradford, 1980). Presynaptic peptide actions on dopamine synthesis and release have also been demonstrated for substance
P and cholecystokinin. This approach therefore opens up a diverse
field of transmitter interactions.

ACKNOWLEDGEMENTS

This work was financially supported by the Mental Health Fund. I would like to thank the following people for their help and co-operation in carrying out the work described in this chapter: H.F. Bradford, J. Coutinho-Netto, M.J. Neal, N.J. Birdsall, E.C. Hulme, I.C. Kilpatrick, I.M. Gardiner and H.J. Herberg. I am also grateful to Pergamon and Raven Press, who gave permission for re-production of Figures 2, 3, 4 and 5.

REFERENCES

Andén, N.-E., and Bedard, P., 1981, Influences of cholinergic mech-anisms on the function and turnover of brain dopamine, J. Pharm. Pharmacol., 23: 460.

Bartholini, G., Keller, H.H., and Pletcher, A., 1975, Drug-induced changes in dopamine turnover in striatum and limbic system of the rat, J. Pharm. Pharmacol., 27: 439.

Birdsall, N.J.M., Burgen, A.S.V., and Hulme, E.C., 1978, The binding of agonists to brain muscarinic receptors, Molec. Pharmacol., 14: 723.

Birdsall, N.J.M., Hulme, E.C., and Burgen, A.S.V., 1980, The charac-ter of muscarinic receptors in different regions of the rat brain, Proc. R. Soc. Lond. B., 207: 1.

Costall, B., Hui, S.C.G., and Naylor, R.J., 1980, Hyperactivity in-duced by intra-accumbens dopamine: Actions and interactions of neuroleptic, cholinomimetic and cholinolytic agents, Neuro-pharmacology, 18: 661.

Consolo, S., Ladinsky, H., and Bianchi, S., 1975, Decrease in rat striatal acetylcholine levels by some direct and indirect-acting dopaminergic antagonists, Europ. J. Pharmacol., 33: 345.

Crow, T.J., Firth, C.D., Johnstone, E.C., and Owens, D.V.C., 1980, Extrapyramidal and antipsychotic effects of neuroleptic drugs in acute schizophrenia and their response in anticholinergic medication, XXIIth CINP Congress, Abstract No. 150, Prog. Neuro-psychopharmacol. Suppl., 118.

de Belleroche, J., and Bradford, H.F., 1972, Metabolism of beds of mammalian cortical synaptosomes: response to depolarizing influ-ences, J. Neurochem., 19: 585.

de Belleroche, J.S., and Bradford, H.F., 1978, Biochemical evidence for the presence of presynaptic receptors on dopaminergic nerve terminals, Brain Res., 142: 53.

de Belleroche, H.S., and Bradford, H.F., 1980, Presynaptic control of the synthesis and release of dopamine from striatal synapto-somes: a comparison between the effects of 5-hydroxytryptamine, acetylcholine and glutamate, J. Neurochem., 35: 1227.

de Belleroche, J., and Gardiner, I.M., 1981, Cholinergic action in the nucleus accumbens: modulation of dopamine and acetylcholine release. Submitted to Br. J. Pharmacol.

de Belleroche, J.S., and Neal, N.J., 1981, The contrasting effects
    of neuroleptics on transmitter release from the nucleus accumbens
    and corpus striatum. Submitted to Neuropharmacology.
de Belleroche, J.S., Coutinho-Netto, J., and Bradford, H.F., 1980,
    Presynaptic receptors on striatal cholinergic nerve terminals,
    Neurosci. Lett. Suppl. 5: 360.
de Belleroche, J., Kilpatrick, I.C., Birdsall, N.J.M., and Hulme, E.C.,
    1981a, Presynaptic muscarinic receptors on dopaminergic terminals
    in the nucleus accumbens, Brain Res., in press.
de Belleroche, J., Coutinho-Netto, J., and Bradford, H.F., 1981b,
    Dopamine inhibits the release of endogenous acetylcholine from
    corpus striatum and cerebral cortex in tissue slices and synapto-
    somes: A presynaptic response. In press to J. Neurochem.
de Belleroche, J., Herberg, J., Winn, P., Murzi, E., and Williams, S.
    1981c, Modulation of dopaminergic activity in the nucleus accum-
    bens by oxotremorine, in preparation, Proc. Int. Soc. Neurochem.
de Belleroche, J.S., Luqmani, Y., and Bradford, H.F., 1979, Evidence
    for presynaptic cholinergic receptors on dopaminergic terminals:
    degeneration studies with 6-hydroxydopamine, Neurosci. Lett.,
    11: 209.
Dray, A., and Oakley, N.R., 1978, Projections from the nucleus accum-
    bens to globus pallidus and substantia nigra in the rat.
    Experientia, 34: 68.
Giorguieff, M.F., Le Floc'h, M.L., Westfall, T.C., Glowinski, J.,
    and Beeson, M.-J., 1976, Nicotinic effect of acetylcholine on
    the release of newly synthesised [^{3}H]-dopamine on rat striatal
    slices and cat caudate nucleus, Brain Res., 106: 117.
Gurwitz, D., Kloogg, Y., Yaakov, E., and Sokolovsky, M., 1980, Central
    muscarinic degeneration following 6-hydroxydopamine lesion in
    mice, Life Sci., 26: 79.
Hökfelt, T., Skirbool, L., Rehfeld, J.F., Goldstein, M., Markey, K.,
    and Dann, O., 1980, A subpopulation of mesencephalic dopamine
    neurones projecting to limbic areas contains a cholecystokinin-
    like peptide: evidence from immunohistochemistry combined with
    retrograde tracing, Neuroscience, 5: 2093.
Hulme, E.C., Birdsall, N.J.M., Burgen, A.S.V., and Mehta, P., 1978,
    The binding of antagonists to brain muscarinic receptors, Molec.
    Pharmacol., 14: 737.
Jones, D.L., Mogenson, G.J., and Wu, M., 1981, Injections of dopa-
    minergic, cholinergic, serotinergic and GABAergic drugs into
    nucleus accumbes: effects on locomotor activity in the rat,
    Neuropharmacology, 20: 29.
Jones, D.L., and Mogenson, G.J., 1980, Nucleus accumbens to globus
    pallidus GABA projection: electrophysiological and ionophoretic
    investigations, Brain Res., 188: 93.
Kato, G., Carson, S., Kemel, M.L., Glowinski, J., and Giorguieff,
    M.F., 1978, Changes in striatal specific [^{3}H]-atropine binding
    after unilateral 6-hydroxydopamine lesions of nigrostrial dopa-
    minergic neurones, Life Sci., 22: 1607.

Lindvall, O., Björklund, A., Moore, R.Y., and Stenevi, U., 1974, Mesencephalic dopamine neurones projecting to neocortex, Brain Res., 81: 325.

Ljungdahl, A., Hökfelt, T., and Nilsson, G., 1978, Distribution of substance P-like immunoreactivity in the central nervous system of the rat. I. Cell bodies and nerve terminals, Neuroscience 3: 861.

McGeer, P.L., Grewaal, D.S., and McGeer, E.G., 1974a, Influences of noncholinergic drugs on rat striatal acetylcholine levels, Brain Res., 80: 211.

McGeer, P.L., McGeer, E.G., Scherer, U., and Singh, K., 1977, A glutamate corticostriatal path? Brain Res., 128: 369.

McGeer, P.L., McGeer, E.G., Singh, V.K., and Chase, W.H., 1974b, Choline acetyltransferase localization in the central nervous system by immunohistochemistry, Brain Res., 81: 373.

Miller, J.C., and Friedhoff, A.J., 1979, Dopamine receptor coupled modulation of the K^+-depolarized overflow of ^{3}H-acetylcholine from rat striatal slices: alteration after chronic haloperidol and alpha-methyl-p-tyrosine pretreatment, Life Sci., 25: 1249.

Miller, R.J., and Hiley, C.R., 1974, Antimuscarinic properties of neuroleptics and drug-induced Parkinsonism, Nature, 248: 596.

Nauta, W.J.H., and Domesick, V.B., 1979, Anatomy of the extra-pyramidal system, in "Dopaminergic Ergot Derivatives and Motor Function", K. Fuxe and D. Calne, eds., Pergamon Press, Oxford, p. 3.

Nauta, W.J.H., Smith, J.P., Faull, R.L.M., and Domesick, V.B., 1978, Efferent connections and nigral afferents of the nucleus accumbens septic in the rat, Neuroscience, 3: 385.

Pijnenburg, A.J.J., and Van Rossum, J.M., 1973, Stimulation of loco-motor activity following injections of dopamine into the nucleus accumbens, J. Pharm. Pharmacol., 25: 1003.

Price, K.S., Farley, I.J., and Hornykiewicz, O., 1978, Neurochemistry of Parkinson's disease: relation between striatal and limbic dopamine, Adv. Biochem. Psychopharmacol., 19: 293.

Schwartz, R., and Coyle, J.T., 1977, Striatal lesions with kainic acid: neurochemical characteristics, Brain Res., 120: 379.

Singh, M.M., and Kay, S.R., 1975, A comparative study of haloperidol and chlorpromazine in terms of clinical effects and therapeutic reversal with benztropine in schizophrenia, Psychopharmacologia 43: 103.

Stadler, H., Lloyd, K.G., Gadea-Ciria, M., and Bartholini, G., 1973, Enhanced striatal acetylcholine release by chlorpromazine and its reversal by apomorphine, Brain Res., 55: 476.

Thierry, A.M., Blanc, G., Sobel, A., Stinus, L., and Glowinski, T., 1973, Dopamine terminals in the rat cortex, Science, 182: 499.

Trabucchi, M., Cheney, D.L., Racaghi, G., and Costa, E., 1975, In vivo inhibition of striatal acetylcholine turnover by L-DOPA, apomorphine and (+) amphetamine, Brain Res., 85: 130.

Uhl, G.R., Kuhar, M.J. and Snyder, S.H., 1977, Neurotensin: Immunohistochemical localization in rat central nervous system. Proc. Natl. Acad. Sci. USA, 74: 4059.
Walaas, I., 1981, Biochemical evidence for overlapping neocortical and allocortical glutamate projections to the nucleus accumbens and rostral caudatoputamen in the rat brain, Neuroscience, 6:399.
Walaas, I., and Fonnum, F., 1979, The effects of surgical and chemical lesions on neurotransmitter candidates in the nucleus accumbens of rat, Neuroscience, 4: 209.

CHOLINERGIC SYSTEMS IN THE CNS

P.L. McGeer, H. Kimura, E.G. McGeer and J.H. Peng

Kinsmen Laboratory of Neurological Research
Department of Psychiatry, U. of British Columbia
Vancouver, B.C. Canada V6T 1W5   253

INTRODUCTION

Considerable progress has been made in recent years in
determining the precise nature of cholinergic systems in the
central nervous system. This has come about as a result of
substantial improvements in the basic techniques necessary for
gathering data with respect to these systems. The techniques are
the following: a) immunohistochemistry of choline acetyltransferase (ChAT); b) histochemistry of acetycholinesterase (AChE) following administration of the irreversible cholinesterase inhibitor
diisopropylfluorophosphate (DFP); c) lesioning of suspected cholinergic pathways in the CNS, particularly with kainic acid which
destroys cells but spares terminals and axons of passages. Ancil-
lary techniques include autoradiographic localization of receptors
using labelled ligands presumed to be specific for cholinergic
receptors, high affinity choline uptake, and ACh release.

Since each of these principal techniques has its limitations,
extensive confirmation of all data is necessary for there to be
firm confidence in the results. Because no histochemical method
for ACh exists at present, the only true marker for cholinergic
systems is ChAT, the synthesizing enzyme for ACh. While in theory
the localization of this enzyme at the cellular and subcellular
level by immunohistochemistry should be the definitive way of
establishing the nature and presence of cholinergic systems, in
practice the technique has imperfections. The immunohistochemical
method is fraught with difficulties, and these seem to apply
particularly to ChAT. Good immunohistochemical localization must
be performed on fixed tissue. The fixation process obviously can
alter the nature of the recognition sites on the enzyme that forms

253

the basis of the antigen-antibody reaction, thus reducing its intensity. For specific staining to be detected there must be a relatively strong reaction to overcome the non-specific staining introduced by the complicated sandwich technique which marks the reaction. That this is a particular problem with ChAT is evidenced by several reports from laboratories that have been successful in raising monospecific antibodies to ChAT only to have weak or negative immunohistochemical results. Some reports have even suggested that the specific staining that has been achieved has resulted from impure antigen (Rossier, 1976). Some highly satis-factory results have, however, been obtained using Fab fragments of high titer rabbit antibodies against human ChAT. Cells bodies, some axonal tracts and dense concentrations of terminals were observed (Kimura et al., 1980, 1981). However, an additional difficulty with ChAT was that many cells receive high concentra-tions of cholinergic terminals in the cell body region, making it difficult in some cases to determine whether the cell is choliner-gic, or merely one which receives dense quantities of terminals on the soma (See Figs. 3 and 4).

Next to ChAT, the most valuable marker for establishing cholinergic systems is AChE. AChE is an enzyme with activity generally two orders of magnitude higher than ChAT. It is stable, permitting reliable assay of its presence at the cellular level using histochemical, as opposed to immunohistochemical, methods.

AChE cannot be regarded as a definitive marker for cholin-ergic neurons. In most regions there is an excellent correlation between AChE and ChAT activity (Table 1), but in some areas, as for example the substantia nigra and the cerebellum, the ratio between the two is radically different. Some neurons, such as dopaminergic neurons of the substantia nigra and noradrenergic neurons of the locus coeruleus, are not only non-cholinergic but are not even thought to be highly cholinoceptive. Yet they contain considerable AChE. On the other hand, all neurons that have been proven beyond reasonable doubt to be cholinergic have high levels of AChE. It may be, therefore, that high AChE activity is a necessary, but not sufficient, characteristic of a cholinergic neuron. The intensity of AChE activity can best be determined by using the technique of AChE regeneration after irreversible inhibition with DFP. Used in this fashion, AChE activity can be valuable in confirming the existence of cholinergic neurons when other evidence suggests their presence and, in addition, can provide useful clues for systems that are still in doubt.

The technique of lesioning is a classical one for establish-ing specific biochemical neuronal pathways in brain. It is the use of this technique which helped establish the presence of the first known cholinergic pathway in brain from the septum to the hippo-campus (McGeer et al., 1969; Fonnum, 1970). However, a problem with this technique is the possibility of interrupting fibers of passage. Thus, the early suggestion that a cholinergic tract extended from the habenula to the interpeduncular nucleus has needed to be revised on the basis that cholinergic fibers emanating from the medial basal forebrain were apparently interrupted (Gottesfeld and Jacobowitz, 1979). The use of kainic acid as a lesioning tool has helped to alleviate potential problems with this technique, and has allowed resolution of some doubtful data on pathways.

The main features of the map of Kimura et al. (1981) will form the principal basis of this paper, with data from other techniques being used to consolidate the information where possible.

This mapping followed upon a number of earlier and incomplete studies from several laboratories which demonstrated the potential of the immunohistochemical technique for ChAT (Eng et al., 1974; McGeer et al., 1974; Cozzari and Hartman, 1977; Kan et al., 1978) The sensitivity and resolution achieved by the most recent study of Kimura et al. (1981) depended upon using Fab fragments of a high titer anti-ChAT antibody. Examples of this staining are shown in Figures 1-4. Figure 1 is a photomicrograph of a cholinergic cell taken from the insterstitial nucleus of the anterior commissure. Figure 2 is a terminal field in the superficial molecular layer of the cerebral cortex. Figures 3 and 4 represent the kinds of cells which have produced some problems in mapping. Figure 3 is an example of a pure cholinoceptive cell with heavy terminal densities around the cell soma observed in the presubicular cortex. No diffuse staining is seen in this cell. Figure 4 is a cholinergic-cholinoceptive cell from a magnocellular field. It shows both smooth staining of the cytoplasm and the intense dots of terminal boutons. Detecting differences between the cell types illustrated in Figures 3 and 4 obviously requires excellent fixation. Diffusion in the terminal fields or poor fixation of tissues could easily cause a cholinoceptive cell to appear cholinergic. This is a major difficulty with the method and one of the main reasons for uncertainties with respect to certain cholinergic cell types in the brain.

CHOLINERGIC CELL BODIES AND CHOLINOCEPTIVE STRUCTURES

At least five major cholinergic cellular systems have been shown to exist in brain. In all cases, the cholinergic cells are large to giant cells. The systems are the following: 1) The medial basal forebrain system which serves the cerebral cortex and limbic system. This includes cell groups in the olfactory tubercle, medial septum, the nucleus of the diagonal band of Broca, and the substantia innominata complex. 2) The large cells of the caudate, putamen and nucleus accumbens which serve the extrapyramidal system. 3) The large motor neurons of the cranial nerve nuclei which send fibers to either the voluntary or parasympathe-

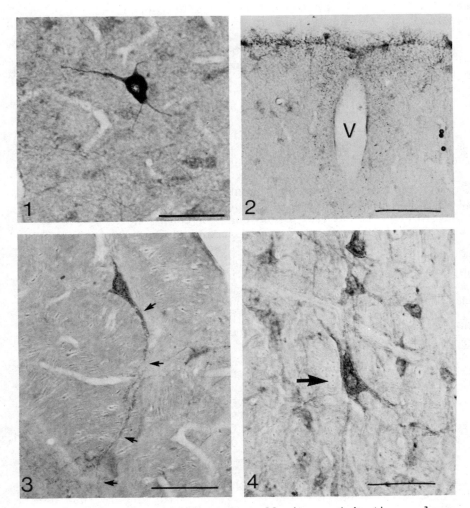

Figs. 1-4. (1) A pure cholinergic cell observed in the nucleus
interstitialis commissurae anterioris. Note the dense and even
stain throughout the cytoplasm extending into the fine processes.
A few, short stained fibers from other cholinergic neurons can
also be seen in the field. (2) An example of a terminal field
observed in the superficial molecular layer of the cerebral cortex
characterized by fine dots (probably nerve terminals). Such fine
dots can also be seen around the blood vessel (v). (3) A pure
cholinoceptive cell observed in the presubicular cortex. Note
that the surface of the long process (arrows) is contacted by tiny
dots (probably nerve terminals) while no diffuse staining product
is seen. (4) A cholinergic-cholinoceptive cell (arrow) seen in the
magnocellular terminal field. In each case the bar indicates 100 μm.

tic systems. 4) The parabrachial nuclear complex. 5) The giganto and magnocellular elements of the tegmental fields of the pons and medulla. The systems served by the last two groups are unknown. Other cholinergic cell clusters are found in the red nucleus, superior olivary complex, some vestibular nuclei and a few other areas where they probably serve a more restricted function.

Representative photomicrographs for the first four of these major groups are shown in Figures 5-8. It should be noted that all of these areas had been described previously as staining intensely for AChE (Koelle, 1963; Shute and Lewis, 1967; Palkovits and Jacobowitz, 1974). In particular, large to giant cells in some of these areas had been noted to stain for AChE following in vivo DFP administration prior to sacrifice so that the AChE would only be observed in the cell bodies of those neurons possessing high AChE turnover (Butcher et al., 1975; Mesulam et al., 1977; Lehmann et al., 1980). As previously mentioned, this is now considered to be a necessary, but not sufficient condition for a cholinergic cell.

As might be judged from the ubiquitous nature of acetylcholine (ACh), ChAT and AChE in the nervous system (Table 1), coupled with the limited sources of cholinergic cell bodies, the occurrence of cholinoceptive cells and terminal fields is much broader than the cell bodies themselves. This means that cholinergic cells must have axons which diverge, thereby serving many other cells. No area of the brain has been found which is totally devoid of cholinergic innervation. However, some areas are more richly served than others and an indication of this can be found in Table 1.

In the olfactory bulb, there are no cholinergic cells. Fibers have been observed entering the bulb from the lateral olfactory tract (Kimura et al., 1980, 1981). Terminations are found in the mitral cell area and more intensely in the glomerular area. A number of mitral, tufted and periglomerular cholinoceptive cells are seen, but most of the innervation is in dense terminal fields.

Dense terminal fields, and some cholinoceptive cells are found in the field of the olfactory tubercle. It is here that the most rostrally located cholinergic cells in the brain are found (Fig. 9). The lateral extent of cholinergic cells in the olfactory tubercle area is clearly demarcated by the lateral olfactory tract from the area prepyriformis which contains no ChAT reactive cells. The cholinergic cell group in the olfactory tubercle merges with those belonging to the nucleus of the substantia innominata ventrolaterally, the accumbens, caudate and putamen dorsolaterally and the medial septum and diagonal band dorsomedially (Fig. 9).

The techniques used by Kimura et al. (1981) revealed no cholinergic cells in the neocortex but significant numbers of cholino-

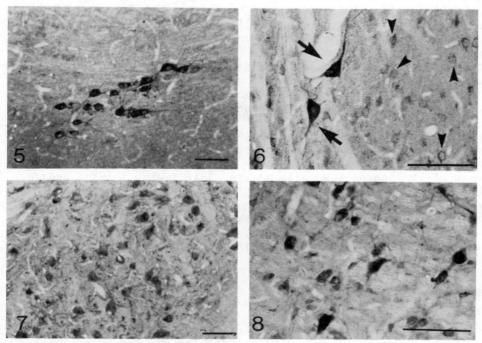

Figs. 5-8. Examples of some major ChAT-containing cell systems in brain. (5) Olfactory tubercle. (6) Putamen. Arrows indicate cholinergic cells and arrowheads cholinoceptive cells. (7) Nucleus motorius originis n. trigmemini. (8) Parabrachial nucleus. In each case the bar indicates 100 μm.

TABLE I. LEVELS OF ChAT, AChE and [^{3}H]QNB (MUSCARINIC) BINDING IN SOME HUMAN AND RAT BRAIN REGIONS*

Area	Human			Rat		
	ChAT	AChE	QNB	ChAT	AChE	QNB
Putamen	114	16	472	{51	{30	{625
Caudate	107	15	480			
N. accumbens	83	14	-	32	33	503
Olfactory tubercle	59	8.6	-	61	41	484
Amygdala	21	3.9	297	28	6.7	280
Preoptic area	16	5.5	-	7.4	3.4	216
Septal area	14	2.5	-	12	3.5	205
Int. globus pallidus	7.4	5.1	{60	{16	{8	{11
Ext. globus pallidus	19	5.0				
Hippocampus	8.7	2.2	196	20	4.0	508
Cortex	5.7	1.5	294	9	-	518
Thalamus	7.1	1.8	182	25	5.9	269
Hypothalamus	7.8	3.5	49	8.9	3.6	170
Substantia nigra	4.3	3.9	18	3.0	-	116
Cerebellar cortex	3.6	3.9	N.D.	-	-	55
Medial habenula	-	-	-	69	6.1	87
Lateral habenula	-	-	-	15	11	160
Interpeduncular nucleus	-	-	-	240	-	160
Locus coeruleus	15	3.5	-	-	-	-

*ChAT (nmoles/mg protein-hr) and AChE (μmoles/mg protein-hr) for the human are from McGeer and McGeer (1976); rat data are for ChAT from Brownstein et al. (1975) and for AChE from Hoover et al. (1978). [^{3}H]QNB binding data (fmoles/mg protein-hr) are from Wastek et al. (1976) for humans and from Kobayashi et al. (1978) for rats. More detailed data are available in the references given.

ceptive cells as well as dense terminal fields. As will be described later, this cannot be taken as firm evidence for the absence of cholinergic cells in the neocortex, but does indicate that the predominant source of innervation is external. The localization of cholinergic terminals shows some variation according to the particular cortical gyrus, but in general the densest area is in layers five and six. From layer four extending superficially, cholinoceptive cells gradually decrease in number as does the density of terminal boutons contacting the somatic surfaces. However, dense terminal fields are found in a thin layer which occupies about one-third of the molecular layer just beneath the cortical surface (Fig. 2).

The pattern of staining in the caudate, putamen and nucleus

accumbens is highly similar. There are large, loosely distributed multipolar ChAT-containing cells throughout the three nuclei. Long axonal fibers are occasionally traced from the cells. The cholinoceptive cells are much more densely distributed and are of medium size, the most predominant cell type in the neostriatum.

The similarity between cholinergic cells and densely cholinoceptive cells presents a difficulty for the immunohistochemical method, and probably accounts for the earlier report of medium sized cholinergic neurons in the striatum (Hattori et al., 1976). It is a source of difficulty which may necessitate future revisions in current assignments of cholinergic structures in the CNS.

Following DFP administration, it is only the large sized cells which stain intensely for AChE (Butcher et al., 1975). Thus, the combination of ChAT staining by the more refined technique involving Fab fragments and careful fixation, coupled with the data on AChE levels following DFP administration confirms this assignment as cholinergic interneurons (McGeer et al., 1971). These amount to only about one percent of the total cells in the neostriatum.

The basal and lateral nuclei of the amygdala contain high concentrations of cholinoceptive neurons. The densest cluster, predominantly of large size, is situated in the lateral, or magnocellular division, of the basal nucleus. The central nucleus also contains cholinoceptive cells, but these are of the medium size, and may be closely related to the contiguous putamen cells. A loosely packed cholinoceptive cell cluster is found in the anterior amygdala. Laterally, they merge with those in the deep layer of the pyriform cortex. Cholinoceptive structures in the cortical and medial nuclei are sparse (Figs. 10, 11).

The hippocampus contains dense terminal staining and typical cholinoceptive cell staining in the stratum oriens. The highest density is in the pyramidal cell layer corresponding to the basal pyramidal dendritic zone. Terminal staining decreases in density from the pyramidal cell layer to the stratum radiatum. Low density staining is found in the stratum lacunosum-moleculare gyrus. In the dentate gyrus, the granular layer has the most densely staining terminal fields with the molecular and polymorphic layers showing relatively low density.

The nucleus of the diagonal band of Broca contains the most striking group of ChAT positive cells in the brain. It can be divided into a ventral part, or horizontal limb, and a septal part, or vertical limb. Rostro-medially, the cells merge with the cells in the olfactory tubercle, and caudo-laterally with those of the substantia innominata complex. They are large sized, oblong, (> 40 μm), multipolar, and are cholinergic-cholinoceptive, i.e.

they receive many cholinergic terminals as well as being cholinergic themselves. Rostro-medially, this group is also continuous
with the positively staining cell mass in the medial septal area
which forms a narrow band close to the midline. More laterally in
the septum, cholinergic and cholinoceptive cells are not found,
but dense ChAT positive dots are seen among the fibers forming the
columns of the fornix in the septal area.

     The cholinergic cell group near the ventral surface of the
brain ventral to the anterior commissure and lateral to the hypothalamus extending caudally through the full extent of the globus
pallidus has so far been referred to as the substantia innominata
complex. It is an ill-defined region containing clusters of large
sized, intensely staining, cholinergic and cholinergic-cholinoceptive cells arranged in a disk-like fashion throughout this region.
For convenience, we have refined the terminology of this area
(Kimura et al., 1981), dividing it into the following regions:
the interstitial nucleus of the anterior commissure; the interstitial nucleus of the stria terminalis; the nucleus of the substantia innominata; the interstitial nucleus of the ansae lenticularis; and the medullary stria between the putamen and pallidum.

     The large cells of the interstitial nucleus of the anterior
commissure and the stria terminalis are pure cholinergic neurons
(Fig. 10). The nucleus of the substantia innominata refers to
the gray matter ventral to the putamen lying between the interstitial nucleus of the anterior commissure and the interstitial
nucleus of the ansae lenticularis (Figs. 10, 11). This area is
often referred to as the nucleus basalis of Meynert, although the
exact demarcation has not been well defined. The cells of this
nucleus are large, multipolar, intercalated with ChAT fibers, and
exclusively cholinoceptive-cholinergic. In addition, there are
many cholinoceptive cells of various types distributed throughout
this region. This cell group merges with the olfactory tubercle
group anteriorly, the horizonal limb of the diagonal band medially, and the putamen dorsally. It also moves caudally to merge with
ChAT cells of the globus pallidus and the interstitial nucleus of
the ansae lenticularis (Fig. 11). The interstitial nucleus of the
ansae lenticularis contains large, multipolar cholinoceptive-
cholinergic neurons which are continuous with those in the globus
pallidus and the medullary stria separating the putamen from the
pallidum. ChAT cells can be seen streaming in the ansae lenticularis in the medial direction between the optic tract and the
internal capsule. In this region they are mixed with numerous
fibers and axonal cell processes. Many long, ovoid cholinoceptive
cells are also scattered among the cholinergic cells throughout
the entire extent of this nucleus (Fig. 11). A striking ChAT cell
group is found in the white matter between the putamen and
pallidum (Fig. 11).

The lateral aspect of the globus pallidus contains vast numbers of exclusively medium sized cholinoceptive neurons. In the ventral medial portion, however, large sized, ovoid or spindle shaped ChAT-containing cells can be found. ChAT-containing cells are aggregated in a cluster which increases caudally and extends in both dorsal and ventral directions uniting with the ChAT cell groups of the medullary stria of the pallidum and the interstitial nucleus of the ansae lenticularis. The entopeduncular nucleus, which corresponds to the internal globus pallidus in primates, contains only a sparse representation of ChAT cells. The few that occur are situated adjacent to the ansae lenticularis. It is not clear whether these are displaced neurons of this latter nucleus or genuinely belong to the nucleus entopeduncularis.

With the techniques employed by Kimura et al. (1981), cholinergic neurons could not be positively identified in any diencephalic structure although many areas are strongly cholinoceptive. In the thalamus, the most prominent cholinoceptive group can be found in the reticular nucleus. Caudally, these cells divide into separate dorsal and ventral clusters with the caudoventral part of the group intermingling with a large group in the nucleus peripeduncularis. Another prominent cholinoceptive cell mass is found in the pulvinar. All other thalamic nuclei contain moderate numbers of cholinoceptive cells.

Intensely stained terminal dots can be observed in the neuropile of the parafascicular nucleus. Prominent cholinoceptive cells can be found in the lateral geniculate nucleus in all layers but only in uneven fashion in the medial geniculate body.

Cholinoceptive cells are sprinkled throughout the entire region of the hypothalamus. The most prominent clusters are found in the lateral hypothalamic area, the nucleus paraventricularis, the supraoptic nucleus, the ventromedial nucleus, and the dorsal nucleus. The anterior hypothalamic area contains few cholinoceptive neurons. The arcuate nucleus and the infundibulum contain dense terminal fields. The supramammillary nucleus, the medial mammillary nucleus, and the posterior hypothalamic area contain numerous cholinoceptive neurons.

The techniques of Kimura et al. (1981) in the cat failed to reveal cholinergic neurons in either the medial or lateral habenular nuclei. On the other hand, the medial nucleus contains a dense terminal field, while the lateral contains only a few cholinoceptive cells. The fasciculus retroflexus contains intensely stained fibers which can be followed from the medial habenular nucleus to the interpeduncular nucleus.

The subthalamic nucleus contains densely packed cholinoceptive cell clusters, while irregularly scattered cholinoceptive cells are found in the zona incerta and Forel's field.

Relatively few cholinergic cells are seen in the mesencephalon except in the cranial motor nuclei and the red nucleus. Very
large, loosely packed ChAT cells are found in the caudal magnocellular division of the nucleus (Fig. 12). These cells have no
cholinoceptive features, in common with ChAT cell clusters of most
motor nuclei of the cranial nerves. There are irregularly
scattered, smaller cholinoceptive neurons in the parvocellular
division of the nucleus.

The motor nucleus of the third nerve contains typical cholinergic motor neuron type cells. The fibers of the third cranial
nerve are also stained well for ChAT. These cells cannot be
clearly differentiated from those in the posterior portion of the
Edinger-Westphal nucleus. Throughout the extent of the Edinger-
Westphal nucleus there are cholinoceptive-cholinergic neurons of
somewhat smaller size than in the motor nucleus.

No cholinergic neurons are found in the substantia nigra or
the ventral tegmental area of Tsai. Thus, the regions of the A8,
A9 and A10 dopaminergic cell groups are free of cholinergic
neurons. However there are numerous cholinoceptive neurons in
these regions, particularly in the ventral tegmental area. A
second prominent cholinoceptive cell cluster is found in the pars
compacta of the substantia nigra and another prominent group is
found in the lateral division of the nucleus (Fig. 12).

Cholinoceptive cells are found in the nucleus linearis, the
nucleus brachii colliculi inferioris of Berman, the central tegmental field, the nucleus of Darkschewitsch and the interstitial
nucleus of Cajal. The periaqueductal gray contains a dense cholinergic terminal field throughout its longitudinal extent (Fig. 12).

The most intensely staining area of the midbrain is the
interpeduncular nucleus which can be seen as a dense terminal
field with the exception of a few cholinoceptive cells which can
be distinguished in the outer division of the posterior portion.

Both cholinoceptive cells and dense terminal fields can be
seen in the superior colliculus. Terminal staining gradually decreases in density in the deeper layers. A number of large size,
prominent cholinoceptive cells, heavily contacted by terminal boutons, are arranged between the intermediate and deep layers of the
colliculus (Fig. 12).

In contrast to the superior colliculus, the inferior colliculus contains only a few cholinoceptive cells. These are only
poorly contacted by faintly staining terminal boutons.

A densely packed, medium sized cholinoceptive cell cluster is found in an area identical to the parabigeminal nucleus. It seems to fuse with that in the rostral part of the nucleus sagulum which contains many small sized cholinoceptive cells (Fig. 13).

In the pons, a vast number of cholinoceptive cells are enbedded in the diffusely stained pontine gray, giving the appearance of a dense terminal field. They are so densely punctated by intense ChAT-positive terminal boutons that they almost appear to be cholinergic. Again, this represents a problem area in assignment, although, at the present time, these are regarded as purely cholinoceptive cells (Fig. 13).

The most prominent ChAT staining cell group in the pons is the nucleus parabrachialis, dorsal and ventral divisions. This complex occupies a considerable and continuous longitudinal extent of the pons in and around the brachium conjunctivum. The group is generally made of intensely stained, irregularly arranged, large multi-polar cholinergic cells. Medially, the cell group extends into the periaqueductal gray and fuses laterally with some ChAT positive cells in the nucleus of the lateral lemniscus. This group is of a somewhat indefinite configuration as is the ventral forebrain ChAT cell mass. Nevertheless, the cell group is made up of highly similar, if not identical, neurons which are predominantly cholinoceptive-cholinergic with only a sprinkling of pure cholinergic neurons (Figs. 13, 14, 15). Beneath the floor of the fourth ventricle, the cholinergic cells embedded in the periaqueductal gray matter are loosely packed and are situated more medially than the cells of the locus coeruleus. The cells of the area are thus distinct from the noradrenergic cell system of the locus coeruleus but there may be a relationship between these two prominent systems. Cholinoceptive cells are also scattered in the same areas as the cholinergic ones. A few faintly cholinoceptive cells are scattered in the nucleus cuneiformis but there are no cholinergic cells and the nucleus can easily be discerned from the dorsal division of the parabrachial nucleus (Fig. 13).

No cholinergic cells are found in the raphe nuclei that give rise to serotonergic systems. Intensely stained cholinoceptive cells are, however, aggregated in this region, particularly in the medial part of the dorsal raphe nucleus.

Large sized cholinergic cells and variously shaped cholinoceptive cells, mostly medium size, are irregularly scattered throughout the paralemniscal tegmental field and the ventral division of the parabrachial nucleus (Figs. 13 and 14).

A conspicuous cholinoceptive cell cluster is found in both the central and pericentral divisions of the reticular tegmental nucleus of Bechterew. The cholinergic cells which are loosely distributed throughout the extent of the lateral lemniscal nucleus may be displaced cells of the nucleus parabrachialis. They are cholinoceptive cells which resemble the latter cellular group. The lateral lemniscus also contains a vast number of medium size cholinoceptive cells densely packed in both the ventral and dorsal divisions (Fig. 14).

Large ovoid and well stained cholinoceptive-cholinergic cells are sparsely distributed in the Kolliker-Fuse nucleus. Again, the morphological features resemble those seen in the parabrachial and lateral lemniscal regions.

Very large and intensely stained giant cells (> 65 μm) of a cholinoceptive-cholinergic nature are scattered throughout the gigantocellular and magnocellular tegmental fields of the reticular formation. Caudally, the giant and magnocellular ChAT-containing neurons are gradually aggregated medially towards the granular layer of the raphe and ventrally to the area just about the inferior olivary nucleus. Thus, these cells extend continuously from the pons into the medulla oblongata as a longitudinally oriented cluster (Figs. 14-17).

The gray matter of the superior olivary complex stains as a dense terminal field. Only a few cholinoceptive neurons can be definitely identified. All of the four closely grouped nuclei of the superior olivary complex contain ChAT-positive cells. In contrast to the majority of cholinergic cell clusters, these are mostly medium to small sized. In addition, these cells stain relatively faintly making it difficult to assign them as cholinergic with absolute certainty. These cells appear to have fewer, if any, terminal boutons, although there is dense and diffuse ChAT terminal staining in the neuropile where they are embedded (Fig. 16).

The motor nucleus of the 5th nerve contains large motor neuron type ChAT cells (Fig. 15). Numerous cholinoceptive cells with distinctly stained terminal boutons can be observed throughout the entire cochlear nucleus complex. Almost all of the neuronal somata appear cholinoceptive. Fairly large to medium sized cells can be found in the cranial motor nuclei of the abducens nerve. Some may be cholinergic-cholinoceptive.

Among the four nuclei of the vestibular complex, lateral, medial, superior and inferior nuclei, Deiter's nucleus appears to be the only component which contains cholinergic cells. Large or giant multipolar cholinergic cells are loosely arranged within the nucleus and some are also found scattered among the afferent fibers of the vestibular nerve. The cells appear to be cholinoceptive-cholinergic, although the terminal boutons are very much smaller in diameter (approximately 0.5 μm as compared with the usual 2-3 μm) than those found in other cholinoceptive clusters.

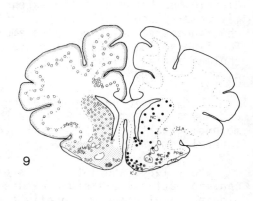

9

Figs. 9-19.
Cross-sectional diagrams of
cat brain proceeding caudally
from the olfactory tubercle
to the cervical cord.
Cholinergic cell bodies (●),
or cholinoceptive-cholinergic
(◉), are indicated on the
right hand side of the diagrams. Cholinoceptive cells
(○) or terminal fields are
indicated on the left.
Relative intensity of terminal fields (·∵· low, ░░ high)
is also indicated. Abbreviations are listed in Table III.

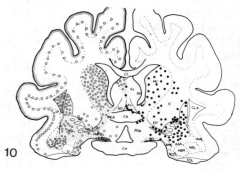

10

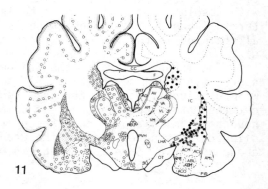

11

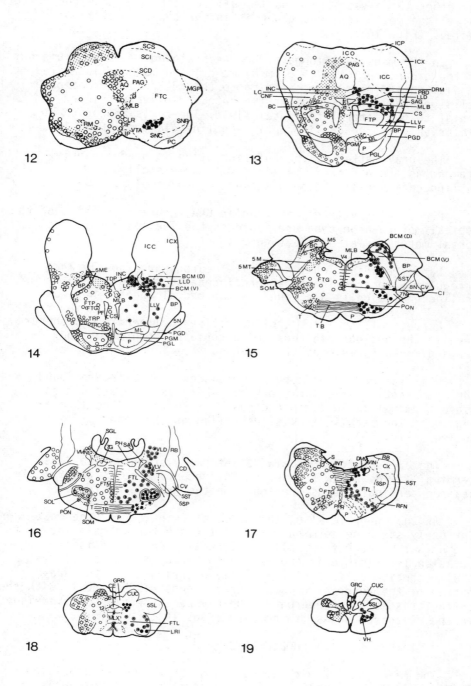

The other three vestibular nuclei all contain some cholinoceptive cells; the most prominent group is in the superior vestibular nucleus (Fig. 16).

In the medulla oblongata, ChAT-containing cells are numerous in the gigantocellular (>65 μm diameter) and magnocellular (ca 50 μm diameter) fields corresponding to the reticular formation. The cells generally lie dorsal to the anterior olivary complex and medial to the lateral tegmental field. The cells appear to be exclusively of the cholinoceptive-cholinergic type (Fig. 17).

The gray matter of the inferior olive is predominantly stained as a dense terminal field with some small sized cholinoceptive cells being observed in the complex.

Predominantly large, multipolar ChAT-containing cells of the typical motorneuron type are found in the facial, hypoglossal and dorsal motor nuclei of the vagus.

Large, distinct cholinoceptive neurons are loosely and irregularly located in the external cuneate nucleus and a few cholinoceptive cells are found in the medial cuneate nucleus.

Large, well stained, cholinoceptive-cholinergic neurons are seen in the nucleus ambiguus which contains both motor and preganglionic parasympathetic neurons.

Well stained, cholinergic-cholinoceptive cells are found in the "substantia reticularis grisea" which is also stained as a dense terminal field. This nucleus is situated in the lateral region of the medulla and is identified as the lateral reticular nucleus (Fig. 18).

The area postrema is always intensely stained as a dense terminal field. A few scattered cholinoceptive cells and faintly stained terminal fields are found in the gracile nucleus.

At the upper level of the cervical spinal cord, the most intensely staining terminal area is the substantia gelatinosa of the dorsal horn. A few small sized cholinoceptive cells are occasionally visible in and around the area. Medium and large cholinoceptive cells are irregularly distributed in the gray matter of the anterior column. Three groups of ChAT cells with the characteristic motor neuron morphology can be easily distinguished in the classical areas of the cord (Fig. 19).

CHOLINERGIC PATHWAYS

The main cholinergic pathways and the evidence supporting them are listed in Table II. Establishment of these pathways

requires synthesis of information obtained from immunohistochemical staining for ChAT, histochemical staining for AChE, biochemical measurements of ChAT and AChE following electrolytic or
kainic acid lesioning, plus other techniques, such as the effects
of lesions on uptake or ACh release.

TABLE II PROBABLE (AND SUGGESTED) CHOLINERGIC PATHWAYS

Olfactory tubercle to olfactory bulb
Diagonal band and substantia innominata to olfactory bulb
Medial septum and diagonal band to hippocampus
Medial septum and diagonal band to cingulate gyrus
Diagonal band to interpeduncular nucleus
(Habenular-interpeduncular tract)
Substantia innominata complex to cortex
(Cortical interneurons)
(Lateral preoptic area to amygdala)
Neostriatal interneurons
Nucleus accumbens interneurons
(Thalamo-striatal tract)
(Lateral tegmental nucleus to anteroventral thalamus)
(Hypothalamic interneurons)
(Olivocochlear efferents)
Some mossy fiber efferents to the cerebellum
Motor nuclei of cranial nerves III-VII, IX-XII
Anterior horn cells to all voluntary muscles
Lateral horn cells to all autonomic ganglia
Postganglionic parasympathetic fibers
Some postganglionic sympathetic fibers
Some retinal amacrine cells

Innervation of the Cortex: The presence of cholinoceptive cells in
the cerebral cortex and the release of acetylcholine from the
cortex have long been established (Phillis, 1975) but there is
still considerable doubt as to the nature of the afferent cholinergic systems. Reductions of about 65 to 80 percent in ChAT and
AChE staining have been reported in isolated cortical slabs (Green
et al., 1970; Hebb et al., 1963; Shute and Lewis, 1963) and in the
anterior and middle portion of the cortex in rats with large lesions of the globus pallidus (Kelly and Moore, 1978; Hartgraves et
al., 1979) or substantia innominata (Johnston and Coyle, 1979a).
However, Ulman et al. (1975) found only a 45% decrease in AChE and
a 10% decrease in ChAT after undercutting the rat cerebral cortex.
Shute and Lewis (1967) originally proposed a projection to the
neocortex from the globus pallidus on the basis that AChE rich
axons projecting to the cortex appear to originate from this area.
Others (Divac, 1975; Jones et al., 1976; Lehmann et al., 1980;

Mesulam and Van Hoesen, 1976) demonstrated that horseradish peroxidase was transported from the cortex to AChE-rich neurons of the nucleus basalis of the substantia innominata. Lesions of the basalis neurons sparing the globus pallidus brought about drops in cortical ChAT indicating that this area, and not the globus pallidus, was the source of the major afferent connection to the cortex (Johnston and Coyle, 1979a; Lehmann et al., 1980). However, it is equally clear that this is not the sole source of cholinergic afferents to the cortex. Following extensive lesions to the basal forebrain, ChAT activity still persists in the cortex in an amount approximating at least 30% of the total activity and possibly much higher depending somewhat upon the time between lesioning and sacrifice (Ulman et al., 1975). This means that either cortical cholinergic interneurons exist or that some unidentified subcortical system also supplies afferents to the neocortex. ChAT-containing cortical interneurons have been observed (McGeer et al., 1974) but, as mentioned previously, this may represent merely intensely cholinoceptive neurons. Johnston and Coyle (1979b) provided new evidence for the existence of neocortical cholinergic interneurons by examining changes in the activities of AChE and ChAT in cortical layers following either lesions to the nucleus basalis cortical cholinergic pathway or induced cortical hypoplasia through fetal administration of methylazoxymethanol acetate. Lesions of the nucleus basalis produced marked reductions in the activities of cholinergic markers in all cortical layers plus an elimination of the uneven distribution of these markers within the cortex. On the other hand fetally induced hypoplasia of the cortex produced enrichment in all layers. These data are interpreted as being consistent with the existence of cholinergic interneurons. Further, more exact experiments will be required to determine the exact nature of cholinergic cortical innervation not associated with the magnocellular basal forebrain region.

Innervation of the Olfactory Bulb: Lesions caudal to the olfactory bulb lead to almost complete loss of ChAT activity in the bulb according to Ross et al. (1978) and we have found in unpublished work decreases of 71% in ChAT and 86% in AChE with an insignifichange in GAD. Youngs et al. (1979) showed decreases of from 22-65% in ChAT in olfactory bulbs contralateral to lesions placed in the magnocellular preoptic area (nucleus of the horizontal limb of the diagonal band) in the hamster, suggesting this is one source of cholinergic innervation. De Olmos et al. (1978) reported, following HRP studies, that the afferent connections to the olfactory bulb originated in the nucleus of the horizontal limb of the diagonal band, the vertical limb and the substantia innominata amongst other areas. These areas all contain cholinergic cell bodies (Kimura et al., 1980). Thus it seems likely that these areas innervate the olfactory bulb via the olfactory tract.

Innervation of the Extrapyramidal System: The caudate and putamen are extremely rich in all cholinergic indices and the evidence is convincing that all, or almost all, of the activity is in intrinsic neurons. Initial evidence for such intrinsic neurons came from experiments showing that lesioning the known afferents and efferents did not cause any significant decrease in ACh, ChAT or AChE activities in the caudate-putamen (McGeer et al., 1971; Butcher and Butcher, 1974). A cholinergic input from the thalamus to the head of the striatum has been suggested on the basis of local changes in AChE, ChAT, and ACh following lesions of the parafascicular nucleus of the thalamus (Wagner et al., 1975; Simke and Saelens, 1977; Saelens et al., 1979), but this cannot be confirmed in our laboratory. Simke and Saelens (1977) have reported a decrease in only the anterolateral tip of the caudate nucleus involving less than 15% of the tissue. Since the thalamo-striatal tract is a massive projection, it would certainly appear that the bulk of the fibers must be served by some other trans-mitters. Moreover, no evidence of neurons staining for ChAT (Kimura et al., 1981) or intensely staining for AChE (Jacobowitz and Palkovits, 1974) has been seen in the parafascicular nucleus or other nuclei of the thalamus from which striatal afferents might originate.

Immunohistochemical studies of ChAT in the cat neostriatum have, however, provided morphological evidence of large sized cholinergic neurons in the striatum which is consistent with previous indications from AChE studies (Butcher et al., 1975; Lehmann and Fibiger, 1979). This type of neuron is thought to com-prise less than 1% of the total neuronal population of the neo-striatum (Kemp and Powell, 1971) and whether this is sufficient to account for the extremely high levels of ChAT and AChE cannot yet be regarded as a certainty. However, while this large aspiny neuron was once considered to be the sole source of descending projections from the striatum, this view has been revised since it has been shown through HRP studies that at least 50% of the medium spiny neurons have descending projections (Graybiel et al., 1979). It seems probable now that the large aspiny neuron does not project significantly beyond the neostriatum but the extent to which it ramifies within the neostriatum is not yet established. Lesions to the substantia innominata region which cause sharp decreases in ChAT in the cortex do not affect levels in the neostriatum, indicating that the projection field passes through, but does not terminate in this region.

The nucleus accumbens resembles the caudate-putamen in its high concentration of ChAT, AChE, ACh and muscarinic binding sites. As in the caudate-putamen, ChAT activity in the accumbens is seriously depleted following local injections of kainic acid but is not affected by hemitransections or other lesions which

would influence extrinsic afferents (Fonnum et al., 1977; Walaas
and Fonnum, 1979). Since the accumbens possesses similar large
sized cholinergic neurons to the caudate and putamen, it is
provisionally assumed that the cholinergic innervation is the same
as in the neostriatum.

The globus pallidus and entopeduncular nucleus contain only
about 20-30% of the levels of ChAT and AChE found in the striatum
(see Table I). Nevertheless, they contain high levels of cholinoceptive neurons and terminal fields as previously mentioned. They
also contain some intrinsic cholinergic neurons in their medial
aspects and have large size cholinergic neurons around their
margins (Kimura et al., 1981). These adjacent neurons are obviously candidates for innervation of the globus pallidus as are the
large neurons of the neostriatum. Unfortunately, the exact source
is not yet known.

The substantia nigra (SN) has relatively high AChE compared
to ChAT activity (McGeer and McGeer, 1976). Histochemical studies
on AChE in normal and lesioned cats and monkeys led to the suggestion of the possible existence of striatopallidal and striato-
nigral cholinergic systems with the latter constituting a massive
indirect feedback to the dopaminergic system (Olivier et al.,
1970). Studies in rats with hemitransections between the caudate
and globus pallidus (anterior lesions) or SN (posterior lesions)
indicated no significant decreases of ChAT in either the pallidum
or the SN (McGeer et al., 1973). Confirmatory reports have come
from several laboratories working with rats, cats and baboons
(Fonnum et al., 1978; McGeer et al., 1971; Kataoka et al., 1974).
These data make it seem unlikely that the striatopallidal and the
striatonigral tracts contain significant cholinergic components.
Other evidence indicates that a major problem in using AChE data
in this system is that there is considerable AChE activity in dopaminergic neurons (Butcher and Butcher, 1974; Lehmann and Fibiger,
1978). Nigral injections of kainic acid that caused extensive destruction of neuronal cell bodies in the SN, as evidenced by both
histological examination and by losses of up to 50% in SN GAD and
up to 95% in striatal tyrosine hydroxylase activity, had no significant effect on ChAT activity in the nigra, but did decrease AChE
activity by about 50% (Nagy et al., 1978). These data argue in
favor of much of the ChAT activity in the substantia nigra being
in afferents but hemitransection data suggest they could not come
from a rostro-lateral direction. As yet the source is unknown.

Innervation of the Limbic System: The septo-hippocampal pathway
was the first cholinergic path to be reasonably well established
and has been the most widely investigated by electrophysiological
and chemical techniques (Kuhar, 1976). Lesions of the septal area
cause large decreases of ACh, AChE, ACh turnover, ChAT and high

affinity choline uptake in the hippocampus on the operated side (Fonnum, 1970; Kuhar et al., 1973; Lewis and Shute, 1967; McGeer et al., 1969; Marshall et al., 1980; Pepeu et al., 1971; Sethy et al., 1973). It has also been shown that the turnover and release of ACh in the hippocampus are increased by septal stimulation (Atwah and Kuhar, 1976; Dudar, 1975; Smith, 1974) and the excitatory action of such stimulation on dentate granule cells is blocked by atropine (Wheal and Miller, 1980). Results obtained using kainic acid are consistent with the localization of all or almost all of the ChAT activity in the hippocampus in afferent neurons. Injections of kainic acid into the hippocampus lead to decreases of at least 70% in hippocampal glutamate decarboxylase (GAD) but cause no significant change in hippocampal ChAT activity (Fonnum and Walaas, 1978; Schwarcz et al., 1978).

The probability that a substantial portion of the AChE activity in the hippocampus is located within processes of cholinergic neurons is indicated by the parallel decreases in the two enzymes in lesion experiments (Oderfeld-Nowak et al., 1974) and by the remarkably constant ratio between AChE and ChAT activities in various regions of the hippocampus (Fonnum, 1970). Thus, in this instance, AChE histochemistry is probably a reliable tool and has given considerable information as to the precise localization of the cholinergic neuronal elements in the septo-hippocampal system. Lewis and Shute (1967) found that AChE-containing afferents to the hippocampus appeared to arise from the medial septal nucleus and the nucleus of the diagonal band and travel via the medial supra-callosal stria of Lancisi, the dorsal fornix, the alveus and the fimbria. Within the hippocampus itself, AChE staining was shown by Storm-Mathisen (1970) to be localized to very discrete bands. The staining seen agrees with the finding of Fonnum (1970) that the regions of the hippocampus with the highest AChE and ChAT activities are the narrow, infrapyramidal zone of the striatum oriens, which contains the basal dendrites of the pyramidal cells, and the supragranular and hilus fasciae dentatae of the area dentata. In light microscopic studies of the autoradiographic localization of tentative cholinergic muscarinic receptors in the hippocampus, very high grain densities have been observed in regions that contain the dendrites of pyramidal and granule cells (Kuhar and Yamamura, 1976). Electrophysiological studies have been consistent in that they have indicated excitation of both pyramidal and (more strongly) granule cells by iontophoretically applied ACh (Bland et al., 1974). Studies of the regional distribution of grains in the hippocampus following injections of radioactive leucine into the medial septal nucleus have also been generally consistent (Rose et al., 1976).

The source of cholinergic efferents to the amygdala has been suggested to be the lateral preoptic area (Emson et al., 1979). No cholinergic cells intrinsic to the amygdala have yet been found.

The interpedunclar nucleus (IPN) has the highest concentration of ChAT thus far found in brain. It is known to receive a massive input from the habenula via the fasciculus retrofluexus. The cholinergic nature of many neurons in the habenulo-interpeduncular tract was initially indicated by the sharp fall of ChAT activity in the IPN following lesions of this tract (Kataoka et al., 1973) and was subsequently confirmed by further measurements of ChAT, choline uptake and other cholinergic markers in the IPN in lesioned animals (Kuhar et al., 1975; Leranth et al., 1975; Mata et al., 1977; Sorimachi and Kataoka, 1974). Cuello et al.(1978) and Emson et al. (1977) suggested that the cholinergic innervation of the IPN originated in the lateral habenula and that this also sent cholinergic fibers to the medial habenula. Others have argued in favor of the medial habenula being the principal source of the IPN cholinergic afferents on the basis of the higher ChAT activity and much more intense immunohistochemical staining in the medial as compared to the lateral habenula. More recent lesion and histo-chemical evidence suggests that much -if not all - of the cholin-ergic input to the IPN arises in areas such as the stria terminal-is or the nucleus of the diagonal band of Broca (NDB) with the axons passing through and innervating the habenula before descend-ing through the fasciculus retroflexus to the IPN. Electrolytic or surgical lesions of the stria medullaris or NDB cause drops of 45-52% in ChAT activity in the IPN (Gottesfeld and Jacobowitz, 1978, 1979). Kainic acid injections into the habenula cause much smaller drops in ChAT activity in the IPN than do electrolytic lesions of the same nucleus (McGeer et al., 1979; Vincent et al., 1980). An early report of positive immunohistochemical localiza-tion of ChAT to the medial habenula may reflect the intensely cholinoceptive nature of those neurons (Hattori et al., 1977). At this stage it must be concluded that some, but not necessarily all, cholinergic innervation of the interpeduncular nucleus comes from forebrain cholinergic neurons in the diagonal band area.

On the basis of AChE staining, Wilson and Watson (1980) suggested that the interpedunculotegmental tract might be cholinergic. Kimura et al. (1981) saw no cholinergic cells in the interpeduncular nucleus but the strong terminal field staining in that area may have made detection of positive cells difficult.

Innervation of the Diencephalon: At present, there are no known cholinergic cell bodies in the thalamus, but there are extensive and widely distributed terminal fields and cholinoceptive neurons. The source of these might be complex, and at this stage little information exists with respect to the afferent cholinergic input to any part of the thalamus. Hoover and Baisden (1979) have reported an AChE-rich tract from the lateral tegmental nucleus of the rat to the anteroventral thalamic nucleus.

Within the hypothalamus of rats, Walaas and Fonnum (1979) have reported that AChE staining and ChAT activity are concentrated in the median eminence and the arcuate nucleus with relatively little in the ventromedial nucleus. Intermediate amounts are found in the dorsomedial nucleus. Other authors (Brownstein et al., 1975; Hoover et al., 1978), using different dissection techniques, have not found such high activities in the arcuate nucleus but all agree on the relatively high concentration of ChAT in the median eminence. When neurons of the arcuate nucleus are destroyed by neonatal administration of sodium glutamate, significant decreases in ChAT activity and AChE staining in both the median eminence and the arcuate nucleus were found (Carson et al., 1977; Nemeroff et al., 1978; Walaas and Fonnum, 1978). There were no significant changes in other hypothalamic regions examined, in the amygdala or in the habenula. These results are interpreted as indicating the existence of cholinergic fibers in the tuberoinfundibular tract. Meyer and Brownstein (1980) measured the concentration of ChAT in the supraoptic nucleus after a variety of lesions. Only lesions that separated the nucleus from the posterior part of the lateral hypothalamus slightly decreased its concentration of ChAT. They concluded that the bulk of cholinergic neurons innervating that structure are either in the nucleus itself or in its immediate vicinity.

All of these data suggest the possibility of intrinsic cholinergic neurons in the hypothalamus, despite the fact that they have not been identified by immunohistochemistry. The alternative seems to be innervation of these hypothalamic regions by the areas immediately adjacent to the lateral hypothalamus.

Innervation of the Cerebellum: Kan et al. (1978, 1980) have reported the specific immunohistochemical localization of ChAT to the mossy fibers and the glomeruli of rabbit and human cerebellar folia, but not all mossy fibers are cholinergic. This immunohistochemical finding is consistent with previous reports that ChAT occurs in the white matter and in the granular cell layer but not in the molecular layer of the rabbit cerebellum (McCaman and Hunt, 1965), that AChE staining is dense in glomeruli of the granular layer (Csillik et al., 1965; Friede and Fleming, 1964; Kasa et al., 1965; Shute and Lewis, 1965), and that mossy fiber- and glomeruli-enriched fractions of the cerebellum have relatively high concentrations of ACh (Israel and Whittaker, 1965) and ChAT (Balasz et al., 1975). The cholinergic mossy fibers presumably originate outside of the cerebellum, since ChAT levels drop sharply in the cerebellar folia after transection of the cerebral peduncles (Fonnum, 1972) or surgical isolation of the vermis (Kasa and Silver, 1969). As yet the source of these mossy fiber cholinergic inputs is unknown.

It has been suggested on the basis of AChE staining that Golgi cells of the cerebellum may be cholinergic (Kasa and Silver, 1969; Shute and Lewis, 1965). However, these cells do not stain for ChAT, and present evidence would suggest that they are cholinoceptive, GABAergic cells that receive an input from the mossy fibers (Eccles et al., 1967). The presence of AChE in cholinoceptive as well as cholinergic cells is not unexpected, particularly in view of the unusually high ratio of AChE to ChAT activity in the cerebellum (McGeer and McGeer, 1976).

Innervation of the Retina: Physiological evidence suggests the presence of cholinergic neurons in the retina (Ross and McDougall, 1976; Braughman and Bader, 1977). Within the retina both ChAT and AChE are believed to be in a population of amacrine cells (Braughman, 1979; Graham, 1974; Hayashi, 1980; Nichols and Koelle, 1968; Ross and McDougall, 1976) that symmetrically line both margins of this layer (Masland, 1980). Autoradiographic studies on [^{3}H]choline uptake support this localization (Braughman and Bader, 1977), as do studies in rats treated with sodium glutamate in the neonatal period (Karlsen and Fonnum, 1976) or in chicks injected intraocularly with kainic acid (Morgan and Ingham, 1981; Schwarcz and Coyle, 1977). Almost no ChAT activity was found in the lesioned retinas and there is considerable morphological evidence that these treatments preferentially destroy retinal ganglion cells and interneurons while leaving the photoreceptor and Müller cells intact. Uptake and lesion studies argue against cholinergic ganglion cells; the scattered cells in the ganglionic cell layer which take up [^{3}H]choline are believed to be displaced amacrine cells (Hayden et al., 1980).

CONCLUSIONS

The foregoing discussion indicates that much has recently been learned regarding the nature of cholinergic systems in the central nervous system. Although doubt still exists regarding the presence or absence of cholinergic cell bodies in a few areas of brain, it seems probable that most have been located and assigned. Considerable information is available about the intensity and distribution of terminal fields throughout the brain. However, much information is needed about the precise connections between the cell body groups and the terminal fields. A few of the major pathways have been well defined, but much work obviously remains to be done. So far, little information is available regarding the ultrastructural details of the terminals.

With respect to the physiological function of the various pathways which have been identified, even less is known. However, cholinergic function has been implicated in some of the most fundamental aspects of brain physiology. It has prominently been associated with cognitive, extrapyramidal motor, emotional, and memory functions. The balance of cholinergic and dopaminergic function in extrapyramidal disorders has long been noted (McGeer et al., 1961), along with the loss of cholinergic striatal cells in Huntington's disease (McGeer et al., 1973). More recently, the loss of cognitive function and memory in Alzheimer's disease has been attributed to specific drops in cholinergic function in the hippocampus and cerebral cortex (Perry et al., 1977; Davies et al., 1978). Janowsky et al. (1973) found that stimulation of central cholinergic systems will suppress mania but increase depression and psychomotor retardation.

All of this suggests that there is much significant work to be done in the cholinergic field in the future, and that the ground work for this will be laid by more detailed knowledge of the anatomical systems which underlie these functions.

TABLE III   ABBREVIATIONS USED IN FIGURES

ABL, M	nucleus amygdalae basalis; lateralis, medialis
ACO	nucleus amygdalae corticalis
AD	nucleus anterior dorsalis thalami
AM	nucleus anterior medialis thalami
AME	nucleus amygdalae medialis
AML	nucleus amygdalae lateralis
AQ	aqueductus cerebri
AV	nucleus anterior ventralis thalami
BC	brachium conjunctivum (pedunculus cerebellaris)
BCM(D,V)	marginal n., brachium conjunctivum (dorsal, ventral)
BP	brachium pontis
CA	commissura anterior
CC	corpus callosum
CD	nucleus cochlearis dorsalis
CE	canalis centralis
CH	chiasma opticum
CI	nucleus centralis inferior (raphe)
CLA	claustrum
CLR	nucleus linearis centralis (raphe)
CNF	nucleus cuneiformis
CS	nucleus centralis superioris
CUC	nucleus cuneatus, caudal division
CV	nucleus cochlearis ventralis
CX	nucleus cuneatus externus (accessorius)
D	nucleus Darkschewitsch
DMV	nucleus originis dorsalis n. vagi
DRM	nucleus raphe dorsalis
EP	nucleus entopeduncularis

Table III (continued).

F	corpus fornicis
FTC	central tegmental field
FTG	gigantocellular tegmental field
FTL	lateral tegmental field
FTM	magnocellular tegmental field
FTP	paralemniscal tegmental field
FX	columna fornicis
GP	globus pallidus
GRC, R	nucleus gracilis; caudal, rostral
IC	capsula interna
ICC	insulae Callejae
ICO	commissura colliculi inferioris
ICP	pericentral nucleus of the inferior colliculus
ICX	external nucleus of the inferior colliculus
INC	nucleus incertus
INCA	nucleus interstitialis commissura anterioris
INT	nucleus intercalatus
IP	nucleus interpeduncularis
IST	nucleus interstitialis striae terminalis
LC	locus coeruleus
LD	nucleus lateralis dorsalis thalami
LHA	area hypothalami lateralis
LLD, V	nucleus lemnisci lateralis; dorsalis, ventralis
LML, M	lamina medullaris; lateralis, medialis
LR	nucleus linealis rostralis
LRI	nucleus reticularis lateralis; internal division
M5	tractus mesencephalicus nervi trigemini
MFB	fasciculus medialis prosencephali
MGP	principal nucleus of the medial geniculate body
ML	lemniscus medialis
MLB	fasciculus longitudinalis medialis
MLX	decussatio lemnisci medialis
NAL	nucleus interstitialis ansae lenticularis
NC	nucleus caudatus
NSI	substantia innominata
OT	tractus opticus
P	tractus corticospinalis
PAG	substantia grisea centralis (periaqueductal gray)
PBD	nucleus parabrachialis dorsalis
PC	crus cerebri
PF	nucleus parafascicularis
PGD,L,M	nuclei pontis; dorsolateral, lateral, medial
PH	nucleus prepositus hypoglossi
PIR	cortex pyriformis
POA	area preoptica
PON	nucleus preolivalis
PPIR	area prepyriformis
PPR	postpyramidal nucleus of the raphe

Table III (continued).

PT	nucleus paraventricularis thalami
PV	nucleus periventricularis thalami
PVH	nucleus periventricularis hypothalami
PX	decussatio pyramidum
RB	corpus restiforme
RE	nucleus reticularis thalami
REU	nucleus reuniens
RFN	nucleus retrofacialis
RM	nucleus ruber, pars magnocellularis
S	tractus solitarius
SA	striae acusticae
SAG	nucleus sagulum
SCI,D,S	colliculus superior; intermediate, deep, superficial
SGL	subependymal granular layer
SMT	stria medullaris thalami
SNC,R	substantia nigra;zona compacta, reticularis
SO	nucleus supraopticus
SOL,M	superior olive; lateral, medial
SP	area septalis
ST	stria terminalis
T	nucleus corporis trapezoidei
TB	corpus trapezoideum
TDP	n. tegmenti dorsalis (Gudden);pericentral division
TOL	tractus olfactorius lateralis
TRC,P	nucleus reticularis tegmenti; central, pericentral
TUO	tuberculum olfactorium
V4	fourth ventricle
VA	nucleus ventralis anterior
VH	ventral horn
VIN	nucleus vestibularis inferior
VL	nucleus ventralis lateralis
VLD,V	nucleus vestibularis lateralis; dorsal, ventral
VM	nucleus ventralis medialis
VMN	nucleus vestibularis medialis
VTA	area tegmentalis ventralis Tsai
5M	nucleus motorius n. trigemini
5ME.	nucleus tractus mesencephali n. trigemini
5MT	motor trigeminal tract
5N	nervus trigeminus
5SL	nucleus tractus spinalis n. trigemini, laminar division
5SP	nucleus tractus spinalis n. trigemini, alaminar division
5ST	tractus spinalis n. trigemini
7G	genu n. facialis
7N	nervus facialis
8N	nervus vestibulocochlearis
12	nucleus originis n. hypoglossi

REFERENCES

Atwah, S.T. and Kuhar, M.J., 1976. Effects of anesthetics and septal lesions and stimulation on ^{3}H-acetylcholine formation in rat hippocampus. Eur. J. Pharmacol. 37: 311-319.

Balazs, R., Hajos, F., Johnson, A.L., Reynierse, G.L.A., Tapia, R. and Wilkin, G.P., 1975. Subcellular fractionation of rat cerebellum: An electron microscopic and biochemical investigation. III. Isolation of large fragments of the cerebellar glomeruli. Brain Research 86: 17-30.

Baughman, R.W.,1979. The cholinergic system in the chicken retina: cellular localization and development, in "Developmental Neurobiology of Vision", (R.D. Freeman, ed.), pp. 421-432, Plenum Press, New York.

Bland, B.H., Kostopoulos, G.K., and Phillis, J.W., 1974. Acetylcholine sensitivity of hippocampal formation neurons. Can. J. Physiol. Pharmacol. 52: 966-971.

Braughman, R.W. and Bader, C.R., 1977. Biochemical characterization and cellular localization of the cholinergic system in the chick retina. Brain Research 138: 469-485.

Brownstein, M., Kobayashi, R., Palkovira, M. and Saavedra, J.M., 1975. Choline acetyltransferase levels in diencephalic nuclei of the rat. J. Neurochem. 24: 35-38.

Butcher, S.G. and Butcher, L.L., 1974. Origin and modulation of acetylcholine activity in the neostriatum. Brain Research 71: 167-171.

Butcher, L.L., Talbot, K. and Bilezikjian, L., 1975. Acetylcholinesterase neurons in dopamine-containing regions of the brain. J. Neural. Transm. 37: 127-153.

Carson, K.A., Nemeroff, C.B., Rone, M.S., Youngblood, W.W., Prange, A.J. Jr., Hanker, J.S. and Kizer, J.S., 1977. Biochemical and histochemical evidence for the existence of a tuberoinfundibular cholinergic pathway in the rat. Brain Research 129: 169-173.

Cozzari, C. and Hartman, B.K., 1977. Purification and preparation of antibodies to choline acetyltransferase from beef caudate nucleus, Proc. Intl. Soc. Neurochem. 6: 140.

Csillik, B., Joo, F. and Kasa, P., 1963. Cholinesterase activity of archicerebellar mossy fiber apparatuses. J. Histochem. Cytochem. 11: 113-114.

Cuello, A.C., Emson, P.C., Paxinos, T. and Jessell, T., 1978. Substance P containing and cholinergic projections from the habenula. Brain Research 149: 413-423.

Davies, P., 1978. Studies in the neurochemistry of central cholinergic systems in Alzheimer's disease, in "Aging", (R. Katzman, R.D. Terry and K.L. Bick, eds.), pp. 453-468, Raven Press, New York.

Divac, I., 1975. Magnocellular nuclei of the basal forebrain project to neocortex, brain stem and olfactory bulb. Review of some functional correlates. Brain Research 9: 385-398.

De Olmos, J.,Hardy, H. and Heimer, L., 1978. The afferent connect-ions of the main and the accessory olfactory bulb formations in the rat: An experimental HRP-study. J. Comp. Neurol. 181: 213-244.

Dudar, J.D., 1975. The effect of septal nuclei stimulation on the release of acetylcholine from the rabbit hippocampus. Brain Research 83: 123-133.

Eccles, J.C., Ito, M. and Szentagothai, J., 1967. The Cerebellum as a Neuronal Machine. Springer-Verlag, New York.

Emson, P.C., Cuello, A.C., Paxinos, G., Jessel, T. and Iversen, L.L., 1977. The origin of Substance P and acetylcholine projections to the ventral tegmental area and interpeduncular nucleus in the rat. Acta Physiol. Scand. [Suppl.] 452: 43-46.

Emson, P.C., Paxinos, G., Le Gal La Salle, G., Ben-Ari, Y. and Silver, A., 1979. Choline acetyltransferase and acetylcholinester-ase containing projections from the basal forebrain to the amygdaloid complex of the rat. Brain Research 165: 271-282.

Eng, L.F., Uyeda, C.T., Chao, L.P. and Wolfgram, F., 1974. Anti-body to bovine choline acetyltransferase and immunofluorescent localization of the enzyme in neurons. Nature 250: 243-245.

Fex, J. and Adams, J.C., 1979. α-Bungarotoxin blocks reversibly cholinergic inhibition in the cochlea. Brain Research 159: 440-444

Fonnum, F., 1970. Topographical and subcellular localization of choline acetyltransferase in rat hippocampal region. J. Neurochem. 17: 1029-1037.

Fonnum, F., 1972. Application of microchemical analysis and sub-cellular fractionation technique to the study of neurotransmitters in discrete areas of mammalian brain. Adv. Biochem. Psychopharm-acol. 6: 75-88.

Fonnum, F., Gottesfeld, Z. and Grofova, I., 1978. Distribution of glutamate decarboxylase, choline acetyltransferase and aromatic amino acid decarboxylase in the basal ganglia of normal and operated rats. Evidence for striatopallidal, striatoentopeduncular and striatonigral GABAergic fibers. Brain Research 143: 125-128.

Fonnum, F. and Walaas, I., 1978. The effect of intrahippocampal kainic acid injections and surgical lesions on neurotransmitters in hippocampus and septum. J. Neurochem. 31: 1173-1181.

Fonnum, F., Walaas, I. and Iversen, E., 1977. Localization of GABAergic, cholinergic and aminergic structures in the mesolimbic system. J. Neurochem. 29: 221-230.

Friede, R.L. and Fleming, L.M., 1964. A comparison of cholinesterase distribution in the cerebellum of several species. J. Neurochem. 11: 1-17.

Gottesfeld, Z. and Jacobowitz, D.M., 1978. Cholinergic projection of the diagonal band to the interpeduncular nucleus of the rat brain. Brain Research 156: 329-332.

Gottesfeld, Z. and Jacobowitz, D.M., 1979. Cholinergic projections from the septal-diagonal band area to the habenular nuclei. Brain Research 176: 391-394.

Graham, L.T., 1974. Comparative aspects of neurotransmitters in the retina, in "The Eye", Vol. 6 (H. Davson and L.T. Graham, eds.), pp. 283-342, Academic Press, New York.
Graybiel, A.M., Ragsdale, C.W. and Edley, S.M., 1979. Compartments in the striatum of the cat observed by retrograde cell labelling. Exp. Brain Res. 34: 189-195.

Green, J.R., Halpern, L.M. and Van Niel, S., 1970. Alterations in the activity of selected enzymes in chronic isolated cerebral cortex of the rat. Brain 93: 57-64.

Hartgraves, S.L., Mensah, P.L. and Kelly, P.H., 1979. Effects of subcortical lesions on neocortical cholinergic markers. Soc. Neurosci. 5: 590.

Hattori, T., McGeer, E.G., Singh, V.K. and McGeer, P.L., 1977. Cholinergic synapse of the interpeduncular nucleus. Exp. Neurol. 55: 666-679.

Hattori, T., Singh, V.K., McGeer, E.G. and McGeer, P.L., 1976. Immunohistochemical localization of choline acetyltrtansferase containing neostriatal neurons and their relationship with dopaminergic synapses. Brain Research 102: 164-173.

Hayden, J., Mills, J.W. and Masland, R.M., 1980. Acetylcholine synthesis in displaced amacrine cells. Science 210: 435-437.

Hayashi, T., 1980. Histochemical localization of dopamine and acetylcholinesterase activity in the carp retina. Acta Histochem. Cytochem. 13: 330-342.

Hebb, C.O., Krnjevic, K. and Silver, A., 1963. Effect of undercutting on the acetylcholinesterase and choline acetyltransferase activity in the cat's cerebral cortex. Nature 198: 692.

Hoover, D.B. and Baisden, R.H., 1980. Localization of putative cholinergic neurons innervating the anteroventral thalamus. Brain Res. Bull. 5: 519-524.

Hoover, D.B., Muth, E.A. and Jacobowitz, D.M., 1978. A mapping of the distribution of acetylcholine, choline acetyltransferase and acetylcholinesterase in discrete areas of rat brain. Brain Research 153: 295-306.

Israel, M. and Whittaker, V.P., 1965. The isolation of mossy fiber endings from the granular layer of the cerebellar cortex. Experientia (Basel) 21: 325-326.

Jacobowitz, D.M. and Palkovits, M., 1974. Topographic atlas of catecholamine and acetylcholinesterase-containing neurons in the rat brain. 1. Forebrain (telencephalon, diencephalon). J. Comp. Neurol. 157: 13-28.

Johnston, M.V. and Coyle, J.T., 1979a. Laminar distribution of cholinergic innervation in rat neocortex: lesions of extrinsic and intrinsic components. Soc. Neurosci. 5: 116.

Johnston, M.V. and Coyle, J.T., 1979b. Histological and neurochemical effects of fetal treatment with methylazoxymethanol on rat neocortex. Brain Research 170: 135-155.

Jones E.G., Burton, H., Saper, C.B. and Swanson, L.W., 1976. Midbrain, diencephalic and cortical relationships of the basal nucleus of Meynert and associated structures in primates. J. Comp. Neurol. 167: 385-420.

Kan, K.S.K., Chao, L.P. and Eng, L.F., 1978. Immunohistochemical localization of choline acetyltransferase in rabbit spinal cord and cerebellum. Brain Research 146: 221-230.

Kan, K.S.K., Chao, L-P. and Forno, L.S., 1980. Immunohistochemical localization of choline acetyltransferase in the human cerebellum. Brain Research 193: 165-171.

Karlsen, R.L. and Fonnum, F., 1976. The toxic effect of sodium glutamate on rat retina: changes in putative transmitters and their corresponding enzymes. J. Neurochem. 27: 1437-1441.

Kasa, P., Joo, F. and Csillik, B., 1965. Histochemical localization of acetylcholinesterase in the cat cerebellaar cortex. J. Neurochem. 12: 31-35.

Kasa, P. and Silver, A., 1969. The correlation between choline acetyltransferase and acetylcholinesterase activity in different areas of the cerebellum of rat and guinea pig. J. Neurochem. 16: 389-396.

Kataoka, K., Bak, I.J., Hassler, R., Kim, J.S., and Wagner, A., 1974. L-Glutamate decarboxylase and choline acetyltransferase activity in the substantia nigra and the striatum after surgical interruption of the strio-nigral fibers of the baboon. Exp. Brain Res. 19: 217-227.

Kataoka, K., Nakamura, Y. and Hassler, R., 1973. Habenulo-interpeduncular tract: a possible cholinergic neuron in rat brain, Brain Research 62: 264-267.

Kataoka, K., Sorimachi, M., Okuno, S. and Mizuno, N., 1977. Cholinergic and GABAergic fibers in the stria medullaris of the rabbit. Brain Res. Bull. 2: 461-464.

Kelly, P.H. and Moore, K.E., 1978. Decrease of neocortical choline acetyltransferase after lesion of the globus pallidus in the rat. Exp. Neurol. 61: 479-484.

Kemp, J.M. and Powell, T.P.S., 1971. The structure of the caudate nucleus of the cat: light and electron microscopy, Phil. Trans. B, 262: 383-401.

Kimura, H., McGeer, P.L., Peng, F. and McGeer, E.G., 1980. Choline acetyltransferase-containing neurons in rodent brain demonstrated by immunohistochemistry. Science 208: 1057-1059.

Kimura, H., McGeer, P.L., Peng, J.H. and McGeer, E.G., 1981. The central cholinergic system studied by choline acetyltransferase immunohistochemistry in the cat. J. Comp. Neurol. (in press).

Kobayashi, R.M., Palkovits, M., Hruska, R.E., Rothschild, R. and Yamamura, H.I., 1978. Regional distribution of muscarinic cholinergic receptors in rat brain. Brain Research 154: 13-24.

Koelle, G.B., 1963. Cytological distributions and physiological functions of cholinesterase, in "Handbuch der Experimentellen

Pharmacologie, Vol. 15, (O. Eichler and A. Farah, eds.), pp. 187-298, Springer, Berlin.

Kuhar, M.J., 1976. Cholinergic Neurons: Septal-hippocampal relationships, in: "The Hippocampus", Vol. 1, (R.L. Isaacson and K.H. Pribram, eds.), pp. 269-284, Plenum Press, New York.

Kuhar, M.J., DeHaven, R.N., Yamamura, H.I., Rommelspacher, H. and Simon, J.R., 1975. Further evidence for cholinergic habenulo-interpeduncular neurons: pharmacologic and functional character-istics. Brain Research 97: 265-275.

Kuhar, M.J., Sethy, V.H., Roth, R.H. and Aghajanian, G.K., 1973. Choline: Selective accumulation by central cholinergic neurons. J. Neurochem. 20: 581-593.

Kuhar, M.J. and Yamamura, H.I., 1976. Localization of cholinergic muscarinic receptors in rat brain by light microscopic radioautography. Brain Research 110: 229-243.

Lehmann, J. and Fibiger, H.C., 1979. Minireview: Acetylcholinest-erase and the cholinergic neuron. Life Sciences 25: 1939-1947.

Lehmann, J. and Fibiger, H.C., 1978. Acetylcholinesterase in the substantia nigra and caudate-putamen of the rat: properties and localization in dopaminergic neurons. J. Neurochem. 30: 615-624.

Lehmann, J.C., Nagy, J.I., Atmadja, S. and Fibiger, H.C., 1980. The nucleus basalis magnocellularis: the origin of a cholinergic projection to the neocortex of the rat. Neuroscience 5: 1161-1174.

Leranth, C.S., Brownstein, M., Zaborsky, L., Jaranyi, Z.S. and Palkovits, M., 1975. Morphological and biochemical changes in the rat interpeduncular nucleus following the transection of the habenulo-interpeduncular tract. Brain Research 99: 124-128.

Lewis, P.R. and Shute, C.C.D., 1967. The cholinergic limbic system: Projections to hippocampal formation, medial cortex, nuclei of the ascending cholinergic reticular system, and the subfornical organ and supraoptic crest. Brain 90: 521-542.

McCaman, R.E. and Hunt, J.M., 1965. Microdetermination of choline acetylase in nervous tissue. J. Neurochem. 12: 253-259.

McGeer, E.G., Fibiger, H.C., McGeer, P.L. and Brooke, S., 1973. Temporal changes in amine synthesizing enzymes of rat extrapyram-idal structures after hemitransections or 6-hydroxydopamine administration. Brain Research 52: 289-300.

McGeer, E.G., Scherer-Singler, U. and Singh, E.A., 1979. Confirm-atory data on habenular projections. Brain Research 168: 375-376.

McGeer, E.G., Wada, J.A., Terao, A. and Jung, E., 1969. Amine synthesis in various brain regions with caudate or septal lesions. Exp. Neurol. 24: 277-284.

McGeer, P.L., Boulding, J.C., Gibson, W.C. and Foulkes, R.G., 1961. Drug-induced extrapyramidal reactions. J.A.M.A. 177: 665-670

McGeer, P.L. and McGeer, E.G., 1976. Enzymes associated with the metabolism of catecholamines, acetylcholine and GABA in human controls and patients with Parkinson's disease and Huntington's chorea. J. Neurochem. 26: 65-76.

McGeer, P.L., McGeer, E.G and Fibiger, H.C., 1973. Choline acetylase and glutamic acid decarboxylase in Huntington's chorea. Neurology 23: 912-917.

McGeer, P.L., McGeer, E.G., Fibiger, H.C. and Wickson, V., 1971. Neostriatal choline acetylase and cholinesterase following selective brain lesions. Brain Research 35: 308-314.

McGeer, P.L., McGeer, E.G., Singh, V.K. and Chase, W.H., 1974. Choline acetyltransferase localization in the central nervous system by immunohistochemistry. Brain Research 81: 373-379.

Marshall, K.C., Flumerfelt, B.A. and Gwyn, D.G., 1980. Acetylchol-inesterase activity and acetylcholine effects in the cerebello-rubro-thalamic pathway of the cat. Brain Research 190: 493-504.

Masland, R.H., 1980, Acetylcholine in the retina. Neurochem. Int. 1: 501-518.

Mata. M. M., Schrier, B.K. and Moore, R.Y., 1977. Interpeduncular nucleus: differential effects of habenula lesions on choline acetyltransferase and glutamic acid decarboxylase. Exp. Neurol. 57: 913-921.

Mesulam, M.M. and Van Hoesen, G.W., 1976. Acetylcholinesterase-rich projections from the basal forebrain of the rhesus monkey to neocortex. Brain Research 109: 152-157.

Mesulam, M.M., Van Hoesen, G.W. and Rosene, D.L., 1977. Substantia innominata, septal area and nuclei of the diagonal band in the rhesus monkey: Organization of efferents and their acetylcholin-esterase histochemistry. Soc. Neurosci. 3: 202.

Meyer, D.K. and Brownstein, M.J., 1980. Effect of surgical deafferentation of the supraoptic nucleus on its choline acetyltransferase content. Brain Research 193: 566-569.

Morgan, I.G. and Ingham, C.A., 1981. Kainic acid affects both plexiform layers of chicken retina. Neurosci. Lett. 21: 275-280.

Nagy, J.I., Vincent, S.R., Lehmann, J., Fibiger, H.C. and McGeer, E.G., 1978. The use of kainic acid in the localization of enzymes in the substantia nigra. Brain Research 149: 431-441.

Neal, M.J., 1976. Acetylcholine as a retinal transmitter substance, in: "Transmitters in the Visual Process", (S.J. Bonting, ed.), pp. 126-143, Pergamon Press, Oxford.

Nemeroff, C.B., Lipton, M.A. and Kizer, J.S., 1978. Models of neuroendocrine regulation: use of monosodium glutamate as an investigational tool. Dev. Neurosci. 1: 102-109.

Nichols, C.W. and Koelle, G.B., 1968. Comparison of the localization of acetylcholinesterase and non-specific cholinesterase activities in mammalian and avian retinas. J. Comp. Neurol. 133: 1-15

Oderfeld-Nowak, B., Narkiewicz, O., Bialowas, J., Dabrowska, J., Wieraszko, A and Gradkowska, M., 1974. The influence of septal nuclei lesions on activity of acetylcholinesterase and choline acetyltransferase in the hippocampus of the rat. Acta Neurobiol. Exp. 34: 583-6.

Olivier, A., Parent, A., Simard, H. and Poirier, L.J. (1970). Cholinesterasic striatopallidal and striatonigral efferents in the cat and the monkey. Brain Research 18: 273-282.

Palkovits, M. and Jacobowitz, D.M., 1977. Topographic atlas of catecholamine and acetylcholinesterase-containing neurons in the rat brain. J. Comp. Neurol. 157: 29-42.

Palkovits, M., Saavedra, J.M., Kobayashi, R.M. and Brownstein, M., 1974. Choline acetyltransferase content of limbic nuclei of the rat. Brain Research 79: 443-450.

Pepeu, G., Mulas, A., Ruffi, A. and Sotgiu, P., 1971. Brain acetylcholine levels in rats with septal lesions. Life Sciences 10: 181-184.

Phillis, J.W., 1975. Evidence for cholinergic transmission in the cerebral cortex, in: "Neurohumoral Coding of Brain Function", (R. D. Myers and R.R. Druker-Colin, eds.), pp. 55-77.

Rose, A.M., Hattori, T. and Fibiger, H.C., 1976. Analysis of the septo-hippocampal pathway by light and electron microscopic autoradiography. Brain Research 108: 170-174.

Ross, C.D., Godfrey, D.A., Williams, A.D. and Matschinsky, F.M., 1978. Evidence for a central origin of cholinergic structures in the olfactory bulb. Soc. Neurosci. 4: 264.

Ross, C.D. and McDougall, D.B., 1976. The distribution of choline acetyltransferase in vertebrate retina. J. Neurochem. 26: 521-526.

Rossier, J., 1976. Immunological properties of rat brain choline acetyltransferase. J. Neurochem. 26: 549-553.

Saelens, J.K., Edwards-Neale, S. and Simke, J.P., 1979, Further evidence for cholinergic thalamo-striatal neurons. J. Neurochem. 32: 1093-1094.

Schwarcz, R. and Coyle, J.T., 1977. Kainic acid: neurotoxic effects after intraocular injection. Invest. Ophthalmol. Visual Sci. 16: 141-148.

Schwarcz, R., Zaczek, R. and Coyle, J.T., 1978. Microinjections of kainic acid into the hippocampus. Eur. J. Pharmacol. 50: 209-220.

Sethy, V.H., Roth, R.H., Kuhar, M.J. and Van Woert, M.H., 1973. Choline and acetylcholine: Regional distribution and effect of degeneration of cholinergic nerve terminals in the rat hippocampus. Neuropharmacology 12: 819-823.

Shute, C.C.D. and Lewis, P.R., 1963. Cholinesterase-containing systems of the brain of the rat. Nature 199: 1160-1164.

Shute, C.C.D. and Lewis, P.R., 1965. Cholinesterase-containing pathways of the hindbrain: afferent cerebellar and centrifugal cochlear fibres. Nature 205: 242-246.

Shute, C.C.D. and Lewis, P.R., 1967. The ascending cholinergic reticular system: neocortical, olfactory and subcortical projections. Brain 90: 497-522.

Simke, J.P. and Saelens, J.K., 1977. Evidence for a cholinergic fiber tract connecting the thalamus with the head of the striatum of the rat. Brain Research 126: 487-495.

Smith, C.M., 1974. Acetylcholine release from the cholinergic septo-hippocampal pathway. Life Sciences 14: 2159-2166.

Sorimachi, M. and Kataoka, K., 1974. Choline uptake by nerve terminals: a sensitive and a specific marker of cholinergic innervation. Brain Research 72: 350-353.

Storm-Mathisen, J., 1970. Quantitative histochemistry of acetylcholinesterase in rat hippocampal region correlated to histochemical staining. J. Neurochem. 17: 739-750.

Ulmar, G., Ljungdahl, A. and Hokfelt, T., 1975. Enzyme changes after undercutting of cerebral cortex in the rat. Exp. Neurology 46: 199-208.

Vincent, S.R., Staines, W.A., McGeer, E.G. and Fibiger, H.C., 1980. Transmitters contained in the efferents of the habenula. Brain Research 195: 479-484.

Vizi, S.E. and Palkovits, M., 1978. Acetylcholine in different regions of the rat brain. Brain Res. Bull. 3: 93-96.

Wagner, A., Hassler, R. and Kim, J.S., 1975. Striatal cholinergic enzyme activities following discrete centromedian nucleus lesions in cat thalamus. Proc. Int. Soc. Neurochem. 5: 116.

Walaas, I. and Fonnum, F., 1978. The effect of parenteral glutamate treatment on the localization of neurotransmitters in the mediobasal hypothalamus. Brain Research 153: 549-562.

Walaas, I. and Fonnum, F., 1979. The distribution and origin of glutamate decarboxylase and choline acetyltransferase in ventral pallidum and other basal forebrain regions. Brain Research 177: 325-336.

Wastek, G.J., Stern, L.Z., Johnson, P.C. and Yamamura, H.I., 1976. Huntington's disease: regional alteration in muscarinic cholinergic receptor binding in human brain. Life Sciences 19: 1033-1040.

Wheal, H.V. and Miller, J.J., 1980. Pharmacological identification of acetylcholine and glutamate excitatory systems in the dentate gyrus of the rat. Brain Research 182: 145-155.

Wilson, P.W. and Watson, C., 1980. Acetylthiocholinesterase staining in an interpedunculotegmental pathway in four species: Procavia capensis (dassie), Cavia procellus (guinea-pig), Trichosurus vulpecula (brush-tail possum) and Rattus rattus (hooded rat). Brain Research 201: 418-422.

Youngs, W.M., Nadi, N.S., Davis, B.J., Margolis, F.L. and Macrides, F., 1979. Evidence for a cholinergic projection to the olfactory bulb from the magnocellular preoptic area. Soc. Neurosci. 5: 36.

DISTRIBUTION AND NATURE OF SUBPOPULATIONS OF MUSCARINIC RECEPTORS IN THE CNS AS JUDGED BY RECEPTOR BINDING

N.J.M. Birdsall

Division of Molecular Pharmacology
National Institute for Medical Research
Mill Hill, London NW7 1AA, U.K.

With the development of receptor-specific ligands, radio-labelled to high specific activity, it has become feasible to study <u>directly</u> the binding of drugs to their receptors. This approach can be used to measure the detailed binding properties of receptors in whole tissue as well as in membrane preparations. In particular it is possible to determine both the number and the localisation of receptor binding sites in the nervous system. These results complement information regarding the distribution of receptors as assessed by electrophysiological and other histochemical techniques. The muscarinic acetylcholine receptor is one example in which biochemical and histochemical approaches are being used to further characterise a neurotransmitter receptor system.

BINDING STUDIES

The radioligands most commonly used to study muscarinic receptors are the potent reversible antagonists [^{3}H]-3-quinuclidinyl-benzilate (QNB), [^{3}H]-N-methylscopolamine (NMS), the agonist [^{3}H]-oxotremorine-M and the irreversible antagonist [^{3}H]-N-2'-chloro-ethyl-N-propyl-2-aminoethylbenzilate (PrBCM). In subcellular preparations the binding properties of the muscarinic receptors are, in general, in accord with the binding properties measured in whole tissue as well as those estimated in pharmacological assays. Initial studies indicated that the binding of agonists showed complexities which were not apparent in the binding of antagonists. The binding data could be explained by the presence of three populations of agonist binding sites which have the same affinity constant for antagonists but up to 3000 fold different affinities for potent agonists. The proportions of these subpopulations have been shown to vary in different brain regions. More recently,

291

binding studies have indicated that a selective antagonist, pirenzepine, can also distinguish between subclasses of muscarinic receptors, which are present in both the central and peripheral nervous system. Besides this heterogeneity of binding of agonists and antagonists, there are regional differences in the complex modulation of the agonist binding properties of the receptors by magnesium ions and guanine nucleotides.

AUTORADIOGRAPHIC STUDIES

To date, it has been possible to localise muscarinic receptors at the light microscope level using both reversible and irreversible antagonists and to monitor changes in receptors during development and after various lesions. The autoradiographic localisation at the electron microscope level has been shown to be of limited usefulness but did indicate that a significant fraction of the receptors was associated with synapses. Further studies require a technique with higher resolving power.

The subpopulations of agonist binding sites have been localised at the light microscope level and, in principle, it is possible to localise subpopulations of receptors distinguished by pirenzepine as well as those whose agonist binding properties are regulated by magnesium ions and guanine nucleotides. Autoradiographic studies have also demonstrated that there appears to be differential axonal transport of the subpopulations of muscarinic agonist binding sites.

The anatomical information, obtained in such studies, will need to be integrated with the electrophysiological data, the binding data and molecular characterisation studies of the receptor in order to form a picture of the number of receptor subtypes and their physiological roles.

REFERENCES

Berrie, C.P., Birdsall, N.J.M., Burgen, A.S.V. and Hulme, E.C., 1979, Guanine nucleotides modulate muscarinic receptor binding in the heart. Biochem. Biophys. Res. Commun., 87:1000-1005.

Birdsall, N.J.M., Berrie, C.P., Burgen, A.S.V. and Hulme, E.C., 1980. Modulation of the binding properties of muscarinic receptors and evidence for receptor-effector coupling, in: "Receptors for neurotransmitters and peptide hormones" G. Pepeu, M.J. Kuhar and S. Enna, eds., pp 107-116, Raven Press, New York.

Birdsall, N.J.M., Burgen, A.S.V. and Hulme, E.C., 1978. Correlation between the binding properties and pharmacological responses of muscarinic receptors, in: "Cholinergic Mechanisms and

Psychopharmacology", D.J. Jenden, ed., pp.25-33, Plenum
  Press, New York.

Birdsall, N.J.M., Burgen, A.S.V., and Hulme, E.C., 1978. The binding
  of agonists to brain muscarinic receptors, Mol. Pharmacol.,
  14:723-736.

Birdsall, N.J.M., Burgen, A.S.V., and Hulme, E.C., 1979. A study of
  muscarinic receptor by gel electrophoresis, Brit. J.
  Pharmacol., 66:337-342.

Birdsall, N.J.M., Hulme, E.C., and Burgen, A.S.V., 1980. The
  character of muscarinic receptors in different regions of
  the rat brain. Proceedings of the Royal Society of London.B,
  207:1-12.

Birdsall, N.J.M., Hulme, E.C., Hammer, R., and Stockton, J., 1980.
  Subclasses of muscarinic receptors, in: "Psychopharmacology
  and biochemistry of neurotransmitter receptors", R. Olsen,
  E. Usdin and H.I. Yamamura, eds., pp.97-100, Elsevier,
  New York.

Burgen, A.S.V., Hiley, C.R., and Young, J.M., 1974. The properties
  of muscarinic receptors in mammalian cerebral cortex,
  Brit. J. Pharmacol., 51:279-285.

Ehlert, F.J., Roeske, W.R., and Yamamura, H.I., 1981. Muscarinic
  receptor: regulation by guanine nucleotides, ions and N-
  ethylmaleimide. Federation Proceedings, 40:153-159.

Gurwitz, D., and Sokolovsky, M., 1980. Agonist specific reverse
  regulation of muscarinic receptors by transitional metal
  ions and guanine nucleotides, Biochem. Biophys. Res.
  Commun., 96:1296-1304.

Hulme, E.C., Birdsall, N.J.M., Berrie, C.P., and Burgen, A.S.V.,
  1980. Muscarinic receptor binding: modulation by ions and
  nucleotides, in: "Neurotransmitters and their Receptors",
  U.Z. Littauer, Y. Dudai, I. Silman, U.I. Teichberg and
  Z. Vogel, eds., pp.241-250, J. Wiley & Sons, Chichester.

Hulme, E.C., Birdsall, N.J.M., Berrie, C.P., and Burgen, A.S.V.,
  1981. Interactions of muscarinic receptors with guanine
  nucleotides and adenylate cyclase, in: "Drug Receptors and
  their Effectors", N.J.M. Birdsall, ed., pp.23-34,
  MacMillan, London.

Hulme, E.C., Birdsall, N.J.M., Burgen, A.S.V., and Mehta, P.,
  1978. The binding of antagonists to brain muscarinic
  receptors, Molec. Pharmacol., 14:737-750.

Kloog, Y., Egozi, Y., and Sokolovsky, M., 1979. Regional heterogeneity of muscarinic receptors of mouse brains. FEBS
  Lett., 97:265-268.

Kobayashi, R.M., Palkovits, M., Hruska, R.E., Rothschild, R., and
  Yamamura, H.I., 1978. Regional distribution of muscarinic
  cholinergic receptors in rat brain, Brain Research,
  154:13-23.

Krnjevic, K., 1974. Chemical nature of synaptic transmission in
  vertebrates. Physiol. Rev., 54:418-540.

Kuhar, M.J., 1976. in: "Biology of Cholinergic Function" , A.M.
        Goldberg and I. Hanin, eds., pp.3-28, Raven Press, New York.
Kuhar, M.J., Birdsall, N.J.M., Burgen, A.S.V., and Hulme, E.C.,
        1980. Ontogeny of muscarinic receptors in rat brain.
        Brain Res., 184:375-383.
Kuhar, M.J., Taylor, N., Birdsall, N.J.M., and Hulme, E.C., 1981.
        Muscarinic cholinergic receptor localization in brain by
        electron microscope autoradiography. Brain Res., 216:1-10.
Kuhar, M.J., and Yamamura, H.I., 1976. Localization of cholinergic
        muscarinic receptors in rat brain by light microscopic
        radioautography. Brain Res., 110:229-243.
Laduron, P., 1980. Axoplasmic transport of muscarinic receptors,
        Nature (Lond.), 286:287-288.
Rotter, A., Birdsall, N.J.M., Burgen, A.S.V., Field, P.M., Hulme,
        E.C., and Raisman, G., 1979. Muscarinic receptors in the
        central nervous system of the rat. I. Technique for auto-
        radiographic localisation of the binding of [^{3}H]propyl-
        benzilylcholine mustard and its distribution in the fore-
        brain. Brain Research Reviews, 1:141-166.
Rotter, A., Birdsall, N.J.M., Burgen, A.S.V., Field, P.M., Smolen, A.,
        and Raisman, G., 1979. Muscarinic receptors in the central
        nervous system of the rat. IV. A comparison of the effects
        of axotomy and deafferentation on the binding of [^{3}H]-
        propylbenzilylcholine mustard and associated synaptic changes
        in the hypoglossal and pontine nuclei, Brain Research
        Reviews, 1:207-224.
Rotter, A., Birdsall, N.J.M., Field, P.M., and Raisman, G., 1979.
        Muscarinic receptors in the central nervous system of the
        rat. II. Distribution of binding of [^{3}H]propylbenzilyl-
        choline mustard in the midbrain and hindbrain, Brain
        Research Reviews, 1:167-184.
Rotter, A., Field, P.M., and Raisman, G., 1979. Muscarinic receptors
        in the central nervous system of the rat. III. Postnatal
        development of binding of [^{3}H]propylbenzilylcholine
        mustard, Brain Research Reviews, 1:185-206.
Sokolovsky, M., Gurwitz, D., and Galvon, R., 1980. Muscarinic
        receptor binding in mouse brain: regulation by guanine
        nucleotides, Biochem. Biophys. Res. Commun., 94:487-492.
Wamsley, J.K., Zarbin, M.A., Birdsall, N.J.M., and Kuhar, M.J.,
        1980. Muscarinic cholinergic receptors: autoradiographic
        localization of high and low affinity agonist binding sites.
        Brain Research, 200:1-12.
Wamsley, J.K., Lewis, M.L., Young, W.S., and Kuhar, M.J., 1981.
        Autoradiographic localization of muscarinic cholinergic
        receptors in rat brainstem. J. Neurosci., 1:176-191.
Wamsley, J.K., Zarbin, M.A., and Kuhar, M.J., 1981. Muscarinic
        cholinergic receptors flow in the sciatic nerve. Brain
        Research, 217:155-162.

Yamamura, H.I., Kuhar, M.J., and Snyder, S.H., 1974. In vivo
    identification of muscarinic cholinergic receptor binding
    in rat brain, Brain Research, 80:170-176.
Yamamura, H.I., and Snyder, S.H., 1974. Muscarinic cholinergic
    binding in rat brain, Proc. Nat. Acad. Sci. (USA),
    71:1725-1729.

REGULATION OF ANTAGONIST AND AGONIST BINDING TO THE MUSCARINIC

ACETYLCHOLINE RECEPTOR BY PROTEIN PHOSPHORYLATION

Robert D. Burgoyne

National Institute for Medical Research
The Ridgeway, Mill Hill
London NW7 1AA

The mechanisms by which receptors for neurotransmitters and hormones are regulated are largely unknown. Recently, however, I have suggested that muscarinic cholinergic receptors of rat brain synaptic membranes may be regulated by a protein phosphorylation mechanism (Burgoyne, 1980, 1981). This suggestion stemmed from the two observations. First, that incubation of synaptic membranes under protein phosphorylating conditions led to a calmodulin-dependent, cAMP-stimulated loss in ^{3}H-QNB binding. Second, that exposure of primary cultures of rat cerebellum to the agonist carbachol led to an increase in membrane protein phosphorylation concomitant with agonist-induced receptor loss.

Incubation under phosphorylating conditions not only results in a loss in antagonist binding but also brings about an alteration in the relative proportions of the super-high (SH), high (H), and low (L) affinity agonist binding sites. Phosphorylation results in a loss in total binding sites and a further apparent conversion of H into SH sites. Furthermore, phosphorylation results in a partial inhibition of the guanyl nucleotide-mediated conversion of SH and H sites into L sites. The interpretation of these findings is that phosphorylation blocks the agonist and guanyl nucleotide driven interconversion of agonist states from SH to H to L; the three agonist states representing differences in the coupling of the receptor with a guanyl nucleotide binding protein and an effector protein. Such an inhibition in the interconversion of receptor states would result in a functional uncoupling of the receptor as is seen in the rapid desensitisation to muscarinic agonists.

297

REFERENCES

Burgoyne, R.D., 1980, A possible role of synaptic membrane protein
        phosphorylation in the regulation of muscarinic acetylcholine
        receptors, FEBS Letts. 122: 288.
Burgoyne, R.D., 1981, The loss of muscarinic acetylcholine receptors
        in synaptic membranes under phosphorylating conditions is
        dependent on calmodulin, FEBS Letts. 127: 144.

GABA ENZYMES AND PATHWAYS

E.G. McGeer, P.L. McGeer and S.R. Vincent

Kinsmen Laboratory of Neurological Research
Department of Psychiatry, U. of British Columbia
Vancouver, Canada

INTRODUCTION

Since Eugene Roberts and Jorge Awapara independently discovered the presence of GABA in brain tissue in 1950, an enormous amount of work has been done on GABA enzymes and pathways. There are still many questions unanswered, however, particularly with regard to pathways.

The anatomy of the GABA systems in brain is extremely difficult to sort out because of an embarrassment of riches. The same difficulty probably exists with regard to glutamate-aspartate systems but here the problem is not even well defined because of the lack of good chemical indices.

The multiplicity of GABA systems was first indicated by the very high concentrations of GABA in brain relative to other then known neurotransmitters, such as acetylcholine, dopamine, noradrenaline or serotonin. As indicated in Table I, the putative peptide neurotransmitters, which have created such excitement in the past few years, are present in brain in even smaller overall concentrations. GABA has a uniquely high concentration level among the transmitter candidates believed to be limited to neurons: in fact, this relatively high concentration in brain led many to argue for years against the hypothesis--now well accepted--that GABA was a neurotransmitter. It is hard for most neuroscientists working today to realize how vehement and recent those arguments were but it may be salutory to remember that one of the people attending the 1959 Conference on GABA remarked ruefully that GABA had gone into the conference as a rich neurotransmitter and had emerged as a poor metabolite.

TABLE I. APPROXIMATE LEVELS IN RAT BRAIN OF VARIOUS PROPOSED
TRANSMITTERS

Range 1-15 μmoles per gram		Range 1-25 nmoles per gram	
Glutamate	14**	Acetylcholine	25
(Taurine)	5**	Dopamine	6.5
Aspartate	4**	Noradrenaline	2.5
GABA	2.5	Serotonin	2.5
Glycine	2**	Histamine	1**

Range 1-500 pmoles per gram		Range < 1 pmole per gram	
CCK	470	ACTH	< 1
Met-enkephalin	350	α-MSH	< 1
Substance P	100	TRH	< 0.3
VIP	40	Bombesin	< 0.2
Somatostatin	30	(Angiotensin II)	0-78 ?
LHRH	7		
Vasopressin	2.5	** Also in non-transmitter	
Neurotensin	1.5	pools.	
		() Doubt transmitter role.	

Those days are gone and GABA is now recognized as the
inhibitory "work horse" of the mammalian brain. GABA and its
key synthetic enzyme, glutamate decarboxylase (GAD), are rather
evenly distributed in brain, as might be anticipated for a
transmitter suspected of serving the inhibitory interneurons found
in almost all regions. Uptake studies with labelled GABA suggest
that 25-45% of nerve endings, depending on the brain area, may
contain this neurotransmitter (Table II). It should be pointed
out, however, that GABA is certainly taken up into glia as well as
neurons and may be taken up also by some non-GABAergic nerve
endings (Belin et al., 1980). GABA may also be stored in non-
GABAergic cells (Tappaz et al., 1977). Hence, uptake and levels
of the amino acid are not as specific indices as is the synthetic
enzyme.

GABA ENZYMES

The routes of synthesis and metabolism of GABA through the
so-called "GABA shunt" are well established (equation 1) but there
are still some questions relating to the localization of some of
the enzymes.

TABLE II. LOCALIZATION OF [³H]-GABA UPTAKE IN NERVE TERMINALS OF
          RAT BRAIN*

Area	% total terminals labeled
In vitro	
Cerebral cortex	27
Cerebellum	
Molecular layer	14
Granular layer	46
Substantia nigra	51
In vivo	
Locus coeruleus	44
Hypothalamus	39
Caudate	27

*From Iversen and Schon, 1973

Equation 1:

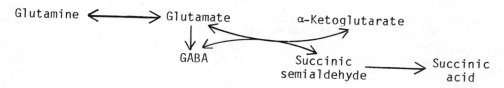

GAD: This synthetic enzyme is specific to GABAergic neurons and
is probably the most widely used index of the integrity of such
neurons. It is apparently rapidly transported from the cell
bodies and much of the total GAD activity is found in nerve
terminals (Ribak et al., 1978) where it occurs in the cytoplasm.
GAD has been purified by several laboratories and immunohistochemical work with GAD antibodies is yielding valuable information
on the anatomy and morphology of central GABAergic systems.

Glutaminase: GABA neurons do not apparently take up glutamate but
rather take up glutamine which is transformed within the nerve
ending into glutamate by the cytoplasmic enzyme glutaminase. This
enzyme is found in glia as well as in GABAergic neurons. It has
been hypothesized that glutaminase might also occur in glutamate
neurons but experiments in the striatum of lesioned rats yielded
no support for this hypothesis. The striatum contains many GABA-
ergic neurons which are destroyed by local injections of kainic
acid; such injections do not decrease glutamate uptake in the

striatum. This index of glutamate neurons is, however, decreased
in the striatum by lesions of the corticostriatal tract. No significant decrease in striatal glutaminase activity was found in rats
with unilateral lesions of the corticostriatal tract (Table III).
There were, on the other hand, significant decreases in glutaminase activity in the neostriata of rats which had received intrastriatal injections of kainic acid. There was furthermore a highly
significant correlation between the glutaminase and GAD activities
in the neostriata of rats injected locally with 0-10 nmol of
kainic acid either 7-10 or 60 days before killing. The position
of the line of correlation suggested that some 60% of the glutaminase activity in the neostriatum is located in GABAergic structures (or at least in some structures destroyed by the kainic acid
injections) while about 40% is in some unaffected compartment
(McGeer & McGeer, 1979). Such kainic acid injections into the
neostriatum are known to destroy systems containing GABA, acetylcholine, substance P, enkephalin, choleocystokinin, and
angiotensin converting enzyme (Coyle et al., 1978; Emson et al.,
1980). Of those systems presently known to be affected, only the
GABAergic system would appear likely to contain glutaminase. A
weakness in the interpretation of kainic acid lesion data is that
it is by no means established that all the glia existing in the
intact striatum remain after injections of kainic acid. In kainic
acid lesioned tissue there are abundant glia but these may not
have the same chemical characteristics as the glia which normally
exist in close association with nerve endings. This possibility is
strengthened by the reports of different chemical characteristics
in glia obtained from different regions of brain (Henn, 1976;
Shousboe and Divac, 1979). The probable association of much of the
glutaminase activity in brain with GABAergic systems is, however,
also indicated by the fact that glutaminase decreased in parallel

TABLE III. GLUTAMINE, GAD AND GLUTAMATE UPTAKE (AS PERCENT OF
          CONTROL) IN THE NEOSTRIATA OF RATS AFTER LESIONS OF
          THE CORTICOSTRIATAL TRACT OR INTRASTRIATAL INJECTIONS
          OF KAINIC ACID

Lesion of:	Glutamate Uptake	GAD	Glutaminase
Corticostriatal tract	50±17%*	104±12%	91±12%
Kainic acid - 4 nm	119±11%	43±13%*	67±11%*
- 10 nm	112±14%	23±12%*	56± 9%*

*Significantly different from control

with GAD in the substantia nigra of rats following striatal injections of kainic acid (McGeer and McGeer, 1979).

GABA Transaminase: The key enzyme for metabolism of GABA is GABA transaminase (GABA-T) which is attached to mitochondria. This enzyme, like acetylcholinesterase in the cholinergic system, is not completely specific to GABAergic neurons and may also occur in other kinds of neurons as well as in glia. Nevertheless, some recent studies indicate that histochemical work with GABA-T may provide some clues to the anatomy of GABAergic systems. This would again be analogous to acetylcholinesterase which has been a very valuable, if not completely definitive, tool in studying cholinergic systems. After kainic acid injections into the striatum, which are known to destroy some of the GABAergic neurons projecting to the substantia nigra, GABA-T staining was markedly reduced in both the injected striatum and the ipsilateral substantia nigra. Similarly, following lesions of the entopeduncular nucleus (EP), decreased staining was seen in the habenula which is known to receive a GABAergic projection from the EP (Vincent et al., 1981).

The procedure for the histochemical demonstration of GABA-T activity was introduced by van Gelder (1965). Numerous improvements of this technique have been reported, allowing visualization of the enzyme activity in aldehyde fixed tissue both at the light and electron microscopic level (Hyde and Robinson, 1976a,b). A problem with the technique has been the intense and diffuse staining of the neuropile which obscures the identification of reactive elements. Thus it is often difficult to differentiate between stained glia or neurons, and between cell bodies or nerve terminals in juxtaposition with them (Hyde and Robinson, 1974). A similar difficulty occurs in the histochemical procedure for acetylcholinesterase and has been alleviated to some extent by the use of the irreversible cholinesterase inhibitor, diisopropyl fluorophosphate (DFP) (Butcher et al., 1975; Lynch et al., 1972). Recently ethanolamine-O-sulfate (EOS), a specific and irreversible inhibitor of GABA-T, has become available and has been applied to the histochemical localization of GABA-T in a manner analogous to the use of DFP for acetylcholinesterase. Within 17 hours after an intraventricular injection of EOS in the rat, sufficient new GABA-T has been synthesized to allow histochemical visualization of positive soma against unstained neuropile. In studies of the cerebellar cortex, for example, GABA-T staining following EOS treatment is most intense in Purkinje cells but some stellate, Golgi and basket cells are also stained (Vincent et al., 1980a). All of these types of cerebellar cells are believed to be GABAergic.

Chemical measurements can also be used to study the localization of GABA-T and, as in so many investigations, the extrapyramidal system is convenient because there is considerable
information available on its biochemical neuroanatomy. Following
striatal injections of kainic acid (KA) there were parallel
decreases of GAD and GABA-T in the striatum (Table IV; cf. Kurihara et al., 1980) indicating the localization of most of the
GABA-T in this structure in elements destroyed by such kainic acid
injections. If the kainic acid were injected into the striatum of
10-day-old rats, rather than adult animals, choline acetyltransferase (ChAT) in the striatum was still markedly affected but
there was no significant decrease in either GAD or GABA-T, suggesting that there are not large amounts of GABA-T in cholinergic
neurons of the striatum (Table IV).

TABLE IV. SOME ENZYME ACTIVITIES AS PERCENT OF CONTROLS IN THE
           STRIATUM AND SUBSTANTIA OF RATS AFTER VARIOUS LESIONS

Area and Enzyme	Intrastrial Injections of KA			6-OHDA Area Lesions
	Adult		10-day-old	
	5 nm	10 nm	20 nm	
Striatum				
Tyrosine hydroxylase	112%	109%	-	48%**
ChAT	55%**	18%	43%**	101%
GAD	64%**	25%**	93%	113%
GABA-T	62%**	34%**	110%	101%
Substantia nigra				
GAD	74%*	33%**	-	86%
GABA-T	100%	89%	-	98%

*$p < 0.01$,   **$p < 0.001$.

A surprising aspect of these data is the indication of relatively little GABA-T activity in glial cells of the striatum. As
mentioned in connection with glutaminase, however, such an interpretation would be dangerous since kainic acid may affect particular types of glia cells. Studies with the gliatoxic D,L-α-
aminoadipic acid in the retina have also been interpreted as indicating a neuronal localization for GABA-T in that region (Linser
and Moscona, 1981).

In the adult rats given striatal kainic acid injections, the decrease of GABA-T in the ipsilateral substantia nigra was much less than the decrease in GAD (Table IV) suggesting that a high GAD to GABA-T ratio may exist in GABA terminals but not in GABA cell bodies (Vincent et al., 1980b). A slight decrease in nigral GABA-T was previously reported in hemitransected rats showing more than 70% loss of nigral GAD (Kataoka et al., 1974).

Injections of 6-hydroxydopamine into the nigro-striatal bundle, which selectively destroy the nigrostriatal dopaminergic projection, were found to have no effect on either GAD or GABA-T activity in the striatum or the substantia nigra (Table IV). It had previously been suggested that GABA released at the synapses is taken up and catabolized in the post-synaptic neuron and in surrounding glial elements since these were the structures thought to contain most of the GABA-T (Baxter, 1976). However, this experiment indicated that the dopamine neurons of the substantia nigra do not contain much GABA-T, although they are thought to be postsynaptic to a major GABAergic system. This observation suggests that all neurons which receive GABAergic synapses do not necessarily contain GABA-T.

From all these data it would appear that GABA-T may be a useful adjunct in the study of GABA systems although it certainly cannot be regarded as definitive.

Succinic Semialdehyde and Glutamate Synthetase: The metabolism of GABA by GABA-T results in the formation of one molecule of succinic semialdehyde and one of glutamate. The succinic semialdehyde may be oxidized by succinic dehydrogenase (SSDH) to succinic acid which is returned to the Kreb's cycle. If the glutamate is formed from GABA-T within the GABA nerve ending, it may be decarboxylated by GAD to GABA. If, on the other hand, the glutamate is formed in glial cells, it is apparently transformed by glutamine synthetase into glutamine before being returned to the GABAergic nerve ending. Glutamine synthetase is a cytoplasmic enzyme restricted to glia (Norenberg and Martin-Hernandez, 1979) while SSDH is attached to mitochondria in both neurons and glia. Neither of these enzymes appears of use in studying the anatomy of GABAergic systems.

GABA PATHWAYS

As indicated in the introduction, the high levels of GABA in brain and its relatively even distribution, as well as uptake studies with labelled GABA, suggest that a significant proportion of all CNS neurons may use GABA as their neurotransmitter. Where are these GABA neurons located?

Figure 1 gives a diagram of most of the long axoned GABA
pathways on which there is literature. Not shown in Fig. 1 is the
proposed path from the amygdala to the bed nucleus of the stria
terminalis. In addition, there is evidence supporting the
existence of GABAergic interneurons in the cerebellum,
hippocampus, striatum, nucleus accumbens, olfactory system, spinal
cord, retina, lateral geniculate, cochlear nucleus, inferior
colliculus, raphe, hypothalamus, septal area and cortex. This is
obviously a far from complete list of GABAergic systems and it is
based upon only partially adequate methodology. It can be
anticipated that there will be many additions and probably some
deletions in future years.

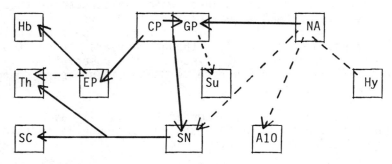

(Hb, habenular; CP, caudate-putamen; GP, globus pallidus; NA,
nucleus accumbens; Th, thalamus; EP, entopeduncular nucleus; Su,
subthalamus; Hy, hypothalamus; SC, superior colliculus; SN,
substantia nigra; A10, ventral tegmental area of Tsai.)

Fig. 1. Diagram of some probable (⎯⎯►) and suggested, but contro-
        versial (----►), GABAergic pathways.

Cerebellum: The cerebellar Purkinje cell is the classical example
of a cell that has been proved to exert an inhibitory action by
release of GABA. A review of the evidence gives a good idea of
the various techniques used to identify presumptive GABAergic
systems as well as the postsynaptic actions of GABA:

      1. Stimulation of Purkinje cells results in hyperpolari-
zation of postsynaptic cells in the deep cerebellar nuclei and
Deiters nuclei. This hyperpolarization is reversed when the
resting membrane potential of the postsynaptic cell is increased
beyond the equilibrium potential for the IPSP.

      2. The postsynaptic membrane is permeable to chloride and
other anions of comparably small size during transmitter action.

3. Picrotoxin and bicuculline, which are classical GABA antagonists, block the effect of stimulation while strychnine, which is not a GABA blocker, is ineffective.

4. Iontophoretic application of GABA on single Deiters neurons mimics Purkinje cell stimulation. The effect is blocked by picrotoxin and bicuculline but not by strychnine (Ito and Yoshida, 1964).

5. There is a large difference in GABA concentration in different neuronal groups in Deiters nucleus. Those in the dorsal part, that receive nerve endings from Purkinje cell neurons, have much higher GABA concentrations than cells in the ventral part of the nucleus.

6. When the cerebellar cortex is removed by suction, or the axons undercut, there is a decrease in GABA and GAD content in the dorsal, but not the ventral part of Deiters nucleus (Fonnum et al., 1970).

7. Stimulation of Purkinje cells results in the release of detectable amounts of GABA into the perfusion fluid of the fourth ventricle or into the output fluid of a push-pull cannula inserted into the area of the deep cere-bellar nuclei (Obata and Takeda, 1969).

8. GAD has been detected by immunohistochemistry in Purkinje cell terminals in the deep cerebellar nuclei. This is the most convincing evidence of all (McLaughlin et al., 1974; Saito et al., 1974).

9. Purkinje cells show intense staining for GABA-T after EDS treatment (Vincent et al., 1980a) and can be stained for GAD after colchicine treatment (Ribak et al., 1978).

10. Radioactive GABA is conveyed by specific axonal transport processes from the Purkinje cell bodies to nerve terminals in Deiters nucleus (McGeer et al., 1975).

11. Retrograde and anterograde transport of antibodies to GAD occurs in the Purkinje cell - deep nuclei connections (Chan-Palay et al., 1979).

Other cells in the cerebellum, beside the Purkinje cells, also appear to use GABA as a transmitter substance. The most obvious of these are the basket cells. Basket cells lie close to the Purkinje cell layer. They are excited by granule cell para-llel fibers just as are Purkinje cells, and act to inhibit rows of Purkinje cells which lie parallel to the row being primarily excited. The basket cells accomplish this action by clustering

their terminals in a pouchlike fashion around the axon hillocks of
the Purkinje cells (Ito and Yoshida, 1964). Basket cells in the
cerebellum have been stained by the immunohistochemical method for
GAD, take up radioactive GABA and, as previously mentioned, also
stain for GABA-T (Hokfelt and Ljungdahl, 1970, 1972; Ljundahl et
al., 1973; McLaughlin et al., 1974; Ribak et al., 1978; Saito et
al., 1974; Vincent et al., 1980a).

Very similar evidence from the same laboratories indicates
that cerebellar Golgi cells and cerebellar stellate cells are also
GABAergic. Lesion studies with kainic acid are consistent since
local injections into the cerebellum which selectively destroy
Purkinje, basket, Golgi and stellate cells cause large drops in
GAD and in GABA uptake (Foster and Roberts, 1980).

Chan-Palay et al. (1979) suggest their work on transport of
GAD antibodies provides new evidence for a GABA component in part
of the nucleocortical cerebellar pathway.

Hippocampus: The hippocampus is a layered structure which in some
respect parallels the cerebellum. The most prominent feature is a
layer of large pyramidal cells lying in a sheet approximately 0.5
mm deep to the surface. Stimulation of the known inputs to the
hippocampus, i.e., from the hippocampal commissure and the septum,
as well as local stimulation, produce identical inhibitory
effects. Such a physiological action could take place only if
special inhibitory interneurons were excited by all three inputs,
with these interneurons ramifying broadly to the pyramidal cells.
Basket cells, lying just superficial to the pyramidal cells (i.e.,
in the region of the basal dendrites) fulfill these criteria. They
are activated by all of the inputs to the hippocampus and
discharge just prior to the onset of the inhibition of pyramidal
cells. The basket cells are also driven by axon collaterals of pyramidal cells, which in turn inhibit surrounding pyramidal cells.

Storm-Mathisen and Fonnum (1971, 1972) studied the GAD
activity in the various layers of the hippocampus and found the
activity to be highest in the area of the pyramidal cells. Okada
and Shimada (1975) confirmed this result by finding a high
concentration of GABA in the pyramidal cell layer. Hippocampal
GAD was not altered by lesioning any of the known hippocampal
afferents (Storm-Mathisen, 1975) but was markedly decreased by
local injections of kainic acid (Schwarcz et al. 1978). These
data are consistent with its associated with interneurons. The
high concentration in the molecular and pyramidal cell layers
would be consistent with GAD being contained in basket
cell terminals. In physiological studies GABA has been found to
inhibit pyramidal cells in the hippocampus, an effect which is
blocked by bicuculline (Anderson et al. 1964). Iversen and Schon
(1973) found 42% of the terminals were labeled when slices of

hippocampus were incubated with [^{3}H]-GABA, the highest percentage of terminals so labeled in the six areas of the brain that they studied. Finally, immunohistochemistry for GAD has shown localization to nerve terminals around the somata of pyramidal cells in keeping with the localization of basket cell terminals (Wood et al. 1976) and to basket cell soma following colchicine injections (Ribak et al. 1978).

Basal ganglia: Some of the highest levels of GAD and GABA are found in the basal ganglia, particularly in the globus pallidus (GP) and substantia nigra (SN). Electrolytic lesions of the globus pallidus, hemitransections of the brain at the level of the subthalamus, or destruction of the striatum by suction produced significant decreases in GABA, GAD and GABA uptake in the substantia nigra (SN). This suggests that long GAD-containing neurons extend from the basal ganglia to the SN. The supposition that the substantia nigra has such GAD-containing nerve endings is greatly strengthened by experiments showing that GABA is avidly taken up by slices of SN and is highly localized to nerve endings (Hattori et al., 1973). Many of these nerve endings have been shown by immunohistochemistry to contain GAD (Ribak et al., 1979). There has been considerable controversy as to whether the projections from the striatum to the SN arise in the caudate or in the globus pallidus. The problem has been complicated because of the existence of striato-nigral projections using other neurotransmitters, such as substance P. The weight of evidence from lesion experiments now indicates that the GABA projection to the SN probably arises in a small region at the border of the caudate and the globus pallidus and passes through the latter (Brownstein et al., 1977; Di Chiara et al., 1980; Fonnum et al., 1974; Hattori et al., 1973; Jessell et al., 1978; Kataoka et al., 1974; Kim et al., 1971; Kurihara et al., 1980; Nagy and Fibiger, 1980; Okada et al., 1971; Porceddu et al., 1980; Staines et al., 1980; Storm-Mathisen, 1975; Taniyama et al., 1980).

The existence of such a pathway gains addional support from evidence that GABA is released in the SN following stimulation of the striatum (Kondo and Iwatsubo, 1978; van der Heyden et al., 1979) and that the inhibitory effect of such stimulation in the SN is blocked by GABA antagonists (Crossman et al., 1973; Goswell et al., 1971; Obata and Yoshida, 1973). The path has been studied by axonal transport of radioactive GABA (McGeer et al., 1974; Streit et al., 1979). Ribak et al. (1977b) showed that many nerve endings in the SN stained for GAD by immunohistochemistry.

There are several other GABAergic efferents from nuclei of the extrapyramidal system which seem probable on the basis of available evidence. The most thoroughly studied of these is the projection from the SN to the superior colliculus and, by

collaterals, to the ventromedial nucleus of the thalamus. This
path is supported by considerable lesion (DiChiara et al., 1979;
Kilpatrick et al., 1980; Vincent et al., 1978) and physiological
(Anderson and Yoshida, 1977; Deniau et al., 1978a,b; MacLeod et
al., 1980; Yoshida and Omata, 1979) data. The nerve endings in
the thalamus have been studied by immunohistochemistry (Houser et
al., 1980; Ribak et al., 1980) and those in the tectum by
electron microscopic autoradiography following axonal transport of
^{3}H-leucine-labeled protein in the tract (Vincent et al., 1978).

A projection from the caudate-putamen to the globus pallidus
(GP) and entopeduncular nucleus (EP) is evidenced by both lesion
(Fonnum et al., 1978a; Hattori et al. 1973; Kurihara et al., 1980;
Nagy et al., 1978; Staines et al., 1980; Taniyama et al., 1980)
and physiological (Obata and Yoshida, 1973) data.

A projection from the EP to the habenula is fairly well
established by lesion (Gottesfeld and Jacobowitz, 1978; McGeer
et al., 1978; Nagy et al., 1978; Kataoka et al., 1977) and
physiological (Jones and Mogenson, 1980a) evidence.
Immunohistochemical evidence has also been adduced for this
projection (Gottesfeld et al., 1981).

Some measurements on GAD and GABA uptake following lesions
have suggested projections from the EP to the ventroanterolateral
nucleus of the thalamus (Penney and Young, 1981) and from the GP
to the subthalamus (Fonnum et al. 1978). The former study was
done with kainic acid and thus avoids the difficulty of axons of
passage. The latter, however, involved multiple stereotaxic
lesions and the interpretation may be in error since van der Kooy
et al. (1981), using kainic acid lesions in the rat, found no
evidence of a GABAergic component in the pallido-subthalamic
tract. On the other hand, Rouzaire-Dubois et al. (1980) found that
iontophoretically applied bicuculline or picrotoxin reversibly
blocked GP-evoked inhibition in the subthalamus, a finding
consistent with the hypothesis that GABA is the transmitter
released by the inhibitory pallido-subthalamic pathway. In view
of the controversial data, however, this hypothesis must be
regarded as doubtful.

In addition to these long-axonal tracts the nuclei of the
extrapyramidal system probably all contain some GABAergic
interneurons. The existence of many such neurons in the caudate-
putamen-globus pallidus system has been evidenced by physiological
(Spehlmann et al., 1977) and uptake (Hattori et al., 1973) data as
well as by the repeated findings of no large change in GABAergic
indices in the neostriatum as a whole following lesions of known
afferents and efferents (McGeer and McGeer, 1975; Nagy et al.,
1980). The very large decreases in the GABAergic indices in the

neostriatum following local injections of kainic acid provide
further support for the existence of such interneurons (Coyle et
al., 1975).

Nucleus Accumbens: The nucleus accumbens resembles the caudate-
putamen in having a high density of GABAergic interneurons,
evidenced by lesion data (Walaas and Fonnum, 1979; Waddington and
Cross, 1978), as well as sending long axon GABAergic projections
to other regions. The best established such projection is that
from the accumbens to the globus pallidus which is evidenced by
extensive lesion and some physiological data (Dray and Oakley,
1978; Jones and Mogenson 1980a,b; Walaas and Fonnum, 1979b).
Lesioning data have also suggested GABAergic projections to the
supraoptic nucleus (Mayer et al. 1980), the substantia
innominata (Walaas and Fonnum 1979b) and to both the medial
portion of the SN and the A10 (Walaas and Fonnum, 1980;
Waddington and Cross, 1978). Others have found no decrease in the
SN as a whole following lesions of the accumbens and believe the
path may be excitatory (Dray and Oakley, 1978). Some have also
reported no drop in GAD in the A10 area following hemitransections
between the accumbens and A10 (Fonnum et al.,1977; McGeer et al.,
1977). The very limited decreases which are reported in the later
papers suggest there is no massive GABAergic component in the
accumbens to A10 projection although stimulation of the accumbens
produces strong inhibition in A10 which is blocked by picrotoxin
(Wolf et al. 1978; Yim and Mogensen, 1980); this may, however, be
indirect.

Amygdala: Studies of the distribution and lesion-induced changes
in GAD and GABA in the amygdaloid complex and the stria terminalis
system of the rat have suggested a GABAergic projection from the
amygdala to the bed nucleus of the stria terminalis as well as
amygdaloid interneurons (Ben Ari et al., 1976; Le Gal La Salle
et al., 1978).

Olfactory System: Rall and his colleagues (1966) and Nicoll (1969)
have provided convincing evidence, both physiological and
histological, that in the olfactory bulb the granule cells inhibit
mitral cells by quite a unique reciprocal synaptic arrangement.
GAD has been identified by immunohistochemistry in the granule
cells and in the gemmules of their dendrites, establishing that
these unusual inhibitory interneurons are GABAergic (Ribak et al.,
1977a). Distribution (Graham, 1973), uptake (Halasz et al., 1979)
and lesion (Hirsch, 1980; Hirsch and Margolis, 1980; McGeer, et
al., unpublished data) evidence is all consistent.

    A limited amount of lesion data also suggest that most of the
GAD in the olfactory tubercle is probably in interneurons (Gilad
and Reis, 1979).

Spinal Cord: Presynaptic inhibition in the spinal cord plays a role in negative feedback control of sensory pathways (Eccles et al., 1963). Immunohistochemical work has shown that the interneurons responsible for this effect are GABAergic (Barber et al. 1978; Wood et al., 1976). Again, uptake (Iversen and Bloom, 1972; Ribeiro-da-Silva and Coimbra, 1980) and a limited amount of lesion (Homma et al., 1979; Miyata and Otsuka, 1971, 1975) data are in keeping with such localization.

Visual System: GABA inhibits the firing of retinal ganglion cells (Noell, 1959; Straschell and Perwein, 1969). GABA and GAD have been detected in the retina but not in the optic nerve, iris, or ciliary body of the eye. The retina is a layered structure, and the content of the GABA system varies widely according to which layer is investigated. By far the highest levels are found in the areas near ganglion cells (Graham, 1972). Since the optic nerve is deficient in GABA, it seems unlikely tht the origin of the high activity could be the ganglion cells themselves, or their projections to the optic nerve. It is also unlikely that any excitatory interneurons would be GABA-containing since, in the majority of systems, GABA is inhibitory. Amacrine cells are appropriately located, however, and have the correct physiological action. They can form multiple synapses with ganglion and bipolar cells. They are morphologically similar to basket cells in the cerebellum. Uptake (Iversen and Schon, 1973; Brandon et al. 1979; Marc et al. 1978; Marshall and Voaden 1975; Pourcho, 1980) and immunohistochemical (Brandon et al., 1979; Lam et al., 1979; Wood et al., 1976) studies, as well as lesion work with neurotoxins (Lund Karlsen, 1978; Guarneri et al., 1981; Goto et al., 1981; Morgan and Ingram, 1981), suggest one population of amacrine cells is probably GABA-containing; other populations may use glycine, dopamine or one of various peptides as the transmitter. There is some indication that some of the horizontal cells in some species may also use GABA (Lam et al., 1980; Wu and Dowling, 1980).

     Selective accumulation of radioactive GABA by small neurons in the cat lateral geniculate body indicates that GABA may be the transmitter for these small interneurons which appear to mediate a feed-forward inhibition (Sterling and Davis, 1980).

     Following lesions of the superior vestibular nucleus, GAD levels decrease in the ipsilateral trochlear nucleus with no change in the oculomotor nucleus (Roffler-Taplov and Taplov, 1975).

Auditory System: The spiral ganglion cell layer of the inner ear contains high levels of GABA (Tachibana and Kuriyama, 1974). This is in sharp contrast to the outer hair cell and inner hair cell layers, as well as the spiral ligament and vascular stria. Since spiral ganglion cells are excitatory in nature there is speculation that the GABA may be due to interneurons in the area (Fisher and Davies, 1976). The auditory nerve is low in GAD and lesions do not change GAD levels in the cochlear nucleus (Wenthold, 1979). It is believed that, while GABA may be a mediator of some of the centrifugal fibers coursing in the dorsal acoustic stria, most of the GABA in the cochlear nucleus is in an intrinsic network (Davis, 1977). Some physiological evidence supports this position (Evans and Nelson, 1973).

The lack of change in GAD in the inferior colliculus after lesioning of inputs from the cortex and cochlear nucleus also suggests the presence of large numbers of GABAergic interneurons (Adams and Wenthold, 1979).

Raphe: Physiological studies of inhibition in the raphe following stimulation of the habenula were initially interpreted as indicating a direct GABAergic tract but were later thought to involve excitation of inhibitory interneurons in the raphe. Lesioning of the fasciculus retroflexus does not cause decreases of GAD in either the interpeduncular nucleus or the raphe (Belin et al., 1979; Gottesfeld et al., 1978; McGeer et al., 1979; Mata et al., 1977) which argues against descending GABAergic fibers. Moreover, studies on ^{3}H-GABA uptake in the raphe (Belin et al., 1979; Gamrani et al., 1979) and marked decreases in GAD activity following local injections of kainic acid (McGeer et al., 1979) are consistent with the existence of an extensive system of GABAergic interneurons.

Other interneurons: Similar lesion and uptake studies have suggested intrinsic GABAergic systems in the hypothalamus (Tappaz et al., 1977; Makara et al. 1975), septal area (Malthe-Sorenssen et al., 1980) and cortex (Bloom and Iversen, 1971; Johnston and Coyle, 1979; Collins, 1979). The existence of such cortical neurons is supported as well by physiological data (Krnjevic and Schwartz, 166) and demonstrated by immunohistochemical work (Ribak, 1978).

GABA BINDING SITES

A great deal of work is appearing on the distribution of GABA binding sites in brain but such work offers little definitive information on GABA pathways. The distribution of GABA binding sites seems to differ from the distribution of GAD and [^{3}H]GABA uptake (Chan-Palay, 1978) and there may be binding sites on glia as well as neurons.

An interesting aspect of the GABA story is that both physiological and binding studies indicate the existence of more

than one type of GABA receptor. Some - but not all - GABA binding
sites seem to be coupled to a benzodiazepine recognition site
which allows modulatory interactions between GABA and benzodiazepines (and presumably, the so far unidentified endogenous ligand
for the benzodiazepine receptor (Placheta and Karobath, 1979;
Squires et al., 1980). The identification of the endogenous
ligand(s) for the benzodiazepine binding sites will therefore cast
new light on the actions of GABA. The problem is made more complex
by the recent evidence that there are at least two different types
of benzodiazepine binding sites in brain which can be distinguished by certain ⁻carbolines which act as powerful agonists or
antagonists of benzodiazepine effects (Nielsen and Braestrup,
1980; Oakley and Jones, 1980).

CONCLUSIONS

    The elucidation of the anatomy of the GABAergic systems in
the CNS is far from complete, but is sufficient to suggest that
such systems will be found important in every central function.
Particular attention has been given to involvement of GABA in
convulsive phenomena and movement disorders. It is clear that
convulsions can be evoked by depression of GABAergic activity and
the widely used benzodiazepines probably exert their anti-
epileptic activity by modulation of GABA systems. It is also
clear that movement disorders can be induced by injection of GABA
agonists and antagonists into extrapyramidal nuclei and that GABA
systems in such nuclei are abnormal in Huntington's disease and
Parkinsonism. The exact role of GABA systems in these (and other)
functions is, however, far from clear. The very prolixity of
GABAergic neurons suggests that clarification of their functional
roles will be slow.

REFERENCES

Adams, J.C. and Wenthold, R.J., 1979. Distribution of putative
amino acid transmitters, choline acetyltransferase and glutamate
decarboxylase in the inferior colliculus. Neuroscience 4: 1947-
1951.

Anderson, M. and Yoshida, M., 1977. Electrophysiological evidence
for branching nigral projection to the thalamus and the superior
colliculus. Brain Research 137: 361-364.

Anderson, P., Eccles, J.C. and Loyning, Y., 1964. Location of
postsynaptic inhibitory synapses on hippocampal pyramids. J.
Neurophysiol. 27: 592-607.

Barber, R.P., Vaughn, J.E., Saito, K., McLaughlin, B.J. and Roberts, E., 1978. GABAergic terminals are presynaptic to primary afferent terminals in the substantia gelatinosa of the rat spinal cord. Brain Research 141: 35-55

Baxter, C.F., 1976. Some recent advances in studies of GABA metabolism and compartmentation, in "GABA in Nervous System Function" (E. Roberts, T.N. Chase and D.B. Tower, eds.), pp. 61-87, Raven Press, New York.

Belin, M.F., Aguera, M., Tappaz, M., McRae-Degueurce, A., Bobillier, P. and Pujol, J.F., 1979. GABA-accumulating neurons in the nucleus raphe dorsalis and periaqueductal gray in the rat: a biochemical and radioautographic study. Brain Research 170: 279-297.

Belin, M.F., Gamrani, H., Aguera, M., Calas, A. and Pujol, J.F., 1980. Selective uptake of [^{3}H]gamma-aminobutyrate by rat supra- and subependymal nerve fibers, histological and high resolution radioautographic studies. Neuroscience 5:241-254.

Ben-Ari, Y., Kanazawa, I. and Zigmond, R.E. 1976. Regional distribution of glutamate decarboxylase and GABA within the amygdaloid complex and stria terminalis system of the rat. J. Neurochem. 26: 1279-1283.

Bloom, F.E. and Iversen, L.L., 1971. Localizing [^{3}H]-GABA in nerve terminals of rat cerebral cortex by electron microscopic auto-radiography. Nature 229: 628-630.

Brandon, C., Lam, D.M.K. and Wu, J.Y., 1979. The gamma-aminobutyric acid system in rabbit retina: Localization by immunocyto-chemistry and autoradiography. Proc. Natl. Acad. Sci. U.S.A. 76: 3557-3561.

Brownstein, M.J., Mroz, E.A., Tappaz, M.L. and Leeman, S.E., 1967. On the origin of substance P and glutamic acid decarboxylase (GAD) in the substantia nigra. Brain Research 135: 315-323.

Butcher, L.L., Talbot, K. and Bilezikjian, L., 1975. Acetylcholin-esterase neurons in dopamine-containing regions of the brain. J. Neurol. Trans. 37: 127-153.

Chan-Palay, V., 1978. Autoradiographic localization of gamma-aminobutyric acid receptors in the rat central nervous system by using [^{3}H]muscimol. Proc. Natl. Acad. Sci. U.S.A. 75: 1024-1028.

Chan-Palay, V., Palay, S.L. and Wu, J.Y., 1979. γ-Aminobutyric acid pathways in the cerebellum studied by retrograde and antero-grade transport of glutamic acid decarboxylase antibody after in vivo injections. Anat. Embryol. (Berl.) 157: 1-14.

Collins, G.G.S., 1979. Effect of chronic bulbectomy on the depth distribution of amino acid transmitter candidates in rat olfactory cortex. Brain Research 171: 552-555.

Coyle, J.T., McGeer, E.G., McGeer, P.L. and Schwarcz, R., 1978. Neostriatal injections: A model for Huntington's chorea, in "Kainic Acid as a Tool in Neurobiology" (E.G. McGeer, J.W. Olney and P.L. McGeer, eds), pp.139-160, Raven Press, New York.

Crossman, A.R., Walker, R.J. and Woodruff, G.N., 1973. Picrotoxin antagonism of gamma-aminobutyric acid inhibitory responses and synaptic inhibition in the rat substantia nigra. Brit. J. Pharmacol. 49: 696-698.

Davis, W.E., 1977. GABAergic innervation of the mammalian cochlear nucleus, in "Inner Ear Biology" (M. Portmann and J.-M. Aran, eds.), pp. 155-164, INSERM. Paris.

Deniau, J.M., Chevalier, G. and Feger, J., 1978a. Electrophysio-logical study of the nigrotectal pathway in the rat. Neurosci. Lett. 10: 215-220.

Deniau, J.M., Hammond, C., Riszk, A. and Feger, J., 1978b. Electrophysiological properties of identified output neurons of the rat substantia nigra (pars compacta and pars reticulata): evidence for the existence of branched neurons. Exp. Brain Res. 32: 409-422.

Di Chiara, G., Porceddu, M.L., Morelli, M., Mulas, M.L. and Gessa, G.L., 1979. Evidence for a GABAergic projection from the substan-tia nigra to the ventromedial thalamus and to the superior colli-culus of the rat. Brain Research 176: 273-284.

Di Chiara, G., Morelli, M., Porceddu, M.L., Mulas, M. and Del Fiacco, M., 1980. Effect of discrete kainic acid-induced lesions of corpus caudatus and globus pallidus on glutamic acid decarboxy-lase of rat substantia nigra. Brain Research 189: 193-208.

Dray, A. and Oakley, N.R., 1978. Projections from nucleus accumbens to globus pallidus and substantia nigra in the rat. Experientia 34:68-70.

Eccles, J.C., Schmidt, R.F. and Willis, W.D., 1963. Inhibition of discharges into the dorsal and ventral spinocerebellar tracts. J. Neurophysiol. 26: 635-645.

Emson, P.C., Rehfeld, J.F., Langevin, H. and Rossor, M., 1980. Reduction in cholecystokinin-like immunoreactivity in the basal ganglia in Huntington's disease. Brain Research 198: 497-500.

Evans, E.F. and Nelson, P.G., 1973. On the functional relationship between the dorsal and ventral divisions of the cochlear
nucleus of the cat. Exp. Brain Res. 17: 428-442.

Fisher, S.K. and Davies, W.E., 1976. GABA and its related enzymes
in the lower auditory system of the guinea pig. J. Neurochem. 27:
1145-1155.

Fonnum, F., Storm-Mathisen, J. and Walberg, F., 1970. Glutamate
decarboxylase in inhibitory neurons. A study of the enzyme in
Purkinje cell axons and boutons in the cat. Brain Research 20:
259-275.

Fonnum, F., Grofova, I., Rinvik, E., Storm-Mathisen, J. and Wald-
berg, F., 1974. Origin and distribution of glutamate decarboxylase
in substantia nigra of the cat. Brain Research 71: 77-92.

Fonnum, F., Walaas, I. and Iversen, E., 1977. Localization of
GABAergic, cholinergic and aminergic structures in the mesolimbic
system. J. Neurochem. 29: 221-230.

Fonnum, F., Gottesfield, Z. and Grofova, I., 1978a. Distribution
of glutamate decarboxylase, choline acetyltransferase and aromatic
amino acid decarboxylase in the basal ganglia of normal and operated rats. Evidence for striatopallidol, striatoentopeduncular and
striatonigral gabaergic fibers. Brain Research 143: 125-128.

Fonnum, F., Grofova, I. and Rinvik, E., 1978b. Origin and distribution of glutamate decarboxylase in the nucleus subthalamicus of
the cat. Brain Research 153: 370-374.

Foster, A.C. and Roberts, P.J., 1980. Morphological and biochemical changes in the cerebellum induced by kainic acid in vivo. J.
Neurochem. 34: 1191-1200.

Gamrani, C.A.H., Belin, M.F., Aguera, M. and Pujol, J.F., 1979.
High resolution radioautographic identification of [^{3}H]GABA
labeled neurons in the rat nucleus raphe dorsalis. Neurosci. Lett.
15:43-48.

Gilad, G.M. and Reis, D.J., 1979. Transneuronal effects of olfactory bulb removal on choline acetyltransferase and glutamic acid
decarboxylase activities in the olfactory tubercle. Brain Research
178: 185-190.

Goswell, M.J. and Sedgwell, E.M., 1971. Inhibition in the substantia nigra following stimlation of the caudate nucleus. J. Physiol
(London) 218: 84P-85P.

Goto, M., Inomata, N., Ono, H., Saito, K. and Fukuda, H., 1981. Changes of electroretinogram and neurochemical aspects of gaba-ergic neurons of retina after intraocular injection of kainic acid in rats. Brain Research 211: 305-314.

Gottesfeld, Z. and Jacobowitz, D.M., 1978. Further evidence for GABAergic afferents to the lateral habenula. Brain Research 152: 609-613.

Gottesfeld, Z., Hoover, D.B., Muth, E.A. and Jakobowitz, D.M., 1978. Lack of biochemical evidence for a direct habenulo-raphe GABAergic pathway. Brain Research 141: 353-356.

Gottesfeld, Z., Brandon, C. and Wu, J-Y., 1981. Immunocytochemistry of glutamate decarboxylase in the deafferented habenula. Brain Research 208: 181-186.

Graham, L.T. Jr., 1972. Intraretinal distribution of GABA content and GAD activity. Brain Research 36: 476-479.

Graham, L.T., 1973. Distribution of glutamic acid decarboxylase activity and GABA content in the olfactory bulb. Life Sci. 12: 443-447.

Guarneri, P., Corda, M.G., Concas, A. and Biggio, G., 1981. Kainic acid-induced lesion of rat retina: differential effect on cyclic GMP and benzodiazepine and GABA receptors. Brain Research 209: 216-220.

Halasz, N., Ljungdahl, A. and Hokfelt, T., 1979. Transmitter histochemistry of the rat olfactory bulb. III. Autoradiographic localization of [^{3}H]GABA. Brain Research 167: 221-240.

Hattori, T., McGeer, P.L., Fibiger, H.C. and McGeer, E.G., 1973. On the source of GABA-containing terminals in the substantia nigra. Electron microsopic autoradiograph and biochemical studies. Brain Research 54: 103-114.

Henn, F.A., 1976. Neurotransmission and glial cells. A functional relationship? J. Neurosci. Res. 2: 271-282.

Hirsch, J.D., 1980. Opiate and muscarinic ligand binding in five limbic areas after bilateral olfactory bulbectomy. Brain Research 195: 271-283.

Hirsch, J.D. and Margolis, F.L., 1980. Influence of unilateral olfactory bulbectomy on opiate and other binding sites in the contralateral bulb. Brain Research 199: 39-47.

Hokfelt, T. and Ljungdahl, A., 1970. Cellular localization of

labeled gamma-aminobutyric acid (^{3}H-GABA) in rat cerebellar
cortex: an autoradiographic study. Brain Research 22: 391-396.

Hokfelt, T. and Ljungdahl, A., 1972. Autoradiographic identification of cerebral and cerebellar cortical neurons accumulating
labeled gamma-aminobutyric acid (^{3}H-GABA). Exp. Brain Res. 14:
331-353.

Homma, S, Suzuki, T., Murayama, S. and Otsuka, M., 1979. Amino
acid and substance P contents in spinal cord of rats with
experimental hind-limb rigidity produced by occlusion of spinal
cord blood supply. J. Neurochem. 32: 691-698.

Houser, C.R., Vaughn, J.E., Barber, R.P. and Roberts, E., 1980.
GABA neurons are the major cell type of the nucleus reticularis
thalami. Brain Research 200: 341-354.

Hyde, J.C. and Robinson, N., 1974. Gamma-aminobutyrate transaminase activity in rat cerebellar cortex: a histochemical study.
Brain Research 82: 109-116.

Hyde, J.C. and Robinson, N., 1976a. Improved histological localization of GABA-transaminase in rat cerebellar cortex after aldehyde fixation. Histochemistry 46: 261-268.

Hyde, J.C. and Robinson, N., 1976b. Electron cytochemical localization of gamma-aminobutyric acid in rat cerebellar cortex.
Histochemistry 49: 51-65.

Ito, M. and Yoshida, M., 1964. The cerebellar-evoked monosynaptic
inhibition of Deiters neurons. Experientia 20: 515-516. 1-396.

Iverson, L.L. and Bloom, F.E., 1972. Studies of the uptake of ^{3}H-
Gaba in homogenates of rat brain and spinal cord by electron
microscopic autoradiography. Brain Research 41: 131-143.

Iverson, L.L. and Schon, F.E., 1973. The use of autoradiographic
techniques for the identification and mapping of transmitter
specific neurons in CNS, in "New Concepts in Neurotransmitter
Mechanisms", (A.J. Mandell, ed.), pp. 153-193, Plenum Press, New
York.

Jessell, T.M., Emson, P.C., Paxinos, G. and Cuello, A.C., 1978.
Topographic projections of substance P and GABA pathways in the
striato- and pallido-nigral system: a biochemical and immunohistochemical study. Brain Research 152: 487-498.

Johnston, M.V. and Coyle, J.T., 1979. Histological and neurochemical effects of fetal treatment with methylazoxymethanol on rat
neocortex in adulthood. Brain Research 170: 135-155.

Jones, D.L. and Mogenson, G.J., 1980a. Nucleus accumbens to globus pallidus GABA projection subserving ambulatory activity. Am. J. Physiology 238: R65-69.

Jones, D.L. and Mogensen, G.J., 1980. Nucleus accumbens to globus pallidus GABA projection: electrophysiological and iontophoretic investigations. Brain Research 188: 93-105.

Kataoka, K., Bak, I.K., Hassler, R., Kim, J.S. and Wagner, A., 1974. L-Glutamate decarboxylase and choline acetyltransferase activity in the substantia nigra after surgical interruption of the strio-nigral fibres of the baboon. Exp. Brain Res. 19: 217-227.

Kataoka, K., Sorimachi, M., Okuno, S. and Mizuno, N., 1977. Cholinergic and Gabaergic fibers in the stria medullaris of the rabbits. Brain Res. Bull: 2: 461-464.

Kilpatrick, I.C., Starr, M.S., Fletcher, A., James, T.A. and MacLeod, N.K., 1980. Evidence for a GABAergic nigrothalamic pathway in the rat. I. Behavioural and biochemical studies. Exp. Brain Res. 40: 45-54.

Kim, J.S., Bak, I.J., Hassler, R. and Okada, Y., 1971. Role of γ-aminobutyric acid (gaba) in the extrapyramidal motor system. Exp. Brain Res. 14: 95-140.

Kondo, Y. and Iwatsubo, K., 1978. Increased release of preloaded [^{3}H]GABA from substantia nigra in vivo following stimulation of caudate nucleus and globus pallidus. Brain Research 154: 395-400.

Krnjevic, K. and Schwartz, S., 1966. Is γ-aminobutyric acid an inhibitory transmitter? Nature 211: 1372-1374.

Kurihara, E., Kuriyama, K. and Yoneda, Y., 1980. Interconnection of GABAergic neurons in rat extrapyramidal tract: analysis using intracerebral microinjection of kainic acid. Exp. Neurology 68: 12-26.

Lam, D.M.K., Su, Y.Y.T., Swain, L., Marc, R.E., Brandon, C. and Wu, J.Y., 1979. Immunocytochemical localization of L-glutamic acid decarboxylase in the goldfish retina. Nature 278: 565-567.

Lam, D.M.K., Marc, R.E., Sarthy, P.V. et al., 1980. Retinal organization: neurotransmitters as physiological probes. Neurochem. Int. 1: 183-190.

Le Gal La Salle, G., Paxinos, G., Emson, P. and Ben-Ari, Y., 1978.

Neurochemical mapping of GABAergic systems in the amygdaloid complex and bed nucleus of the stria terminalis. Brain Research 155: 397-403.

Linser, P.J. and Moscona, A.A., 1981. Induction of glutamine synthetase in embryonic neural retina: Its suppression by the gliatoxic agent α-aminoadipic acid. Devel. Brain Res. 1:103-119.

Lund-Karlsen, R., 1978. The toxic effect of sodium glutamate and DL-α-aminoadipic acid on rat retina: changes in high affinity uptake of putative transmitters. J. Neurochem. 31: 1055-1061.

Ljungdahl, A., Seiger, A., Hokfelt, T. and Olson, L., 1973. [^{3}H]GABA uptake in growing cerebellar tissue: Autoradiography of intraocular transplants. Brain Research 61: 379-381.

Lynch, G., Lucas, P.A. and Deadwyler, S.A., 1972. The demonstration of acetylcholinesterase containing neurons within the caudate nucleus of the rat. Brain Research 45: 617-621.

MacLeod, N.K., James, T.A., Kilpatrick, I.C. and Starr, M.S., 1980. Evidence for a GABAergic nigrothalamic pathway in the rat. II. Electrophysiological studies. Exp. Brain Res. 40: 55-61.

McGeer, E.G., Scherer-Singler, U. and Singh, E.A., 1979. Confirmatory data on habenular projections. Brain Research 168: 375-376.

McGeer, E.G. and McGeer, P.L., 1978. Localization of glutaminase in the rat neostriatum. J. Neurochem. 32: 1071-1075.

McGeer, P.L. and McGeer, E.G., 1975. Evidence for glutamic acid decarboxylase containing interneurons in the neostriatum. Brain Research 91: 331-335.

McGeer, P.L., Fibiger, H.C., Hattori, T., Singh, V.K., McGeer, E.G. and Maler, L., 1974. Biochemical neuroanatomy of the basal ganglia. Adv. Biochem. Biol. 10: 27-47.

McGeer, P.L., Hattori, T. and McGeer, E.G., 1975. Chemical and autoradiographic analysis of γ-aminobutyric acid transport in Purkinje cells of the cerebellum. Exp. Neurol. 47: 26-41.

McGeer, P.L., McGeer, E.G. and Hattori, T., 1977. Dopamine-acetylcholine-GABA neuronal linkages in the extrapyramidal and limbic systems, in "Nonstriatal Dopaminergic Neurons", (E. Costa and G.L. Gessa, eds.), pp. 397-402, Raven Press, New York.

McGeer, P.L., McGeer, E.G. and Hattori, T., 1978. Transmitters in the basal ganglia, in "Amino Acids as Chemical Transmitters", (F. Fonnum, ed.), pp. 123-141, Raven Press, New York.

McLaughlin, B.J., Wood, J.G., Saito, K., Barber, R., Vaughn, J.E., Roberts, E. and Wu, J.Y., 1974. The fine structural localization of glutamate decarboxylase in synaptic terminals of rodent cerebellum. Brain Research 76: 377-391.

Makara, G.B., Rappay, G. and Stark, E., 1975. Autoradiographic localization of ^{3}H-gamma-aminobutyric acid in the medial hypothalamus, Exp. Brain Res. 22: 449-455.

Malthe-Sorenssen, D., Odden, E. and Walaas, I., 1980. Selective destruction by kainic acid of neurons innervated by putative glutamergic afferents in septum and diagonal band. Brain Research 182: 461-465.

Marc, R.E., Stell, W.K., Bok, D. and Lam, D.M., 1978. GABA-ergic pathways in the goldfish retina, J. Comp. Neurol. 182: 221-245.

Marshall, J. and Voaden, M., 1975. Autoradiographic identification of the cells accumulating ^{3}H gamma-aminobutyric acid in mammalian retina: a species comparison, Vision Res. 15: 459-461.

Mata, M.M., Schrier, B.K. and Moore, R.Y., 1977. Interpeduncular nucleus: differential effects of habenula lesions on choline acetyltransferase and glutamic acid decarboxylase. Exp. Neurol. 57: 913-921.

Meyers, D., Oertel, W. and Brownstein, M., 1980. Deafferentation studies on the glutamic acid decarboxylase content of the supra-optic nucleus of the rat. Brain Research 200: 165-168.

Miyata, Y. and Otsuka, M., 1972. Distribution of γ-aminobutyric acid in cat spinal cord and the alteration produced by local ischemia, J. Neurochem. 19: 1833-1834.

Miyata, Y. and Otsuka, M., 1975. Quantitative histochemistry of γ-aminobutyric acid in cat spinal cord with special reference to presynaptic inhibition, J. Neurochem. 25: 239-244.

Morgan I.G. and Ingram, C.A., 1981. Kainic acid affects both plexiform layers of chicken retina. Neurosci. Lett. 21: 275-280.

Nagy, J.I., Carter, D.A., Lehmann, J. and Fibiger, H.C., 1978. Evidence for a GABA-containing projection from the entopeduncular nucleus to the lateral habenula in the rat. Brain Research 145: 360-364.

Nagy, J.I. and Fibiger, H.C., 1980. A striatal source of glutamic acid decarboxylase activity in the substantia nigra. Brain Research 187: 237-242

Nicoll, R.A., 1969. Inhibitory mechanisms in the rabbit olfactory bulb: dendro-dendritic mechanisms. Brain Research 14: 157-172.

Nielson, M. and Braestrup, C., 1980. Ethyl β-carboline-3-carboxylate shows differential benzodiazepine receptor interaction. Nature 286: 606-607.

Noell, W.K., 1959. The visual cell: electric and metabolic manifestations of its life processes. Am. J. Ophthalmol. 48: 347-370.

Norenberg, M.D. and Martin-Hernandez, A., 1979. Fine structural localization of glutamine synthetase in astrocytes of rat brain. Brain Research 161: 303-310.

Oakley, N.R. and Jones, B.J., 1980. The proconvulsant and diazepam-reversing effects of ethyl β-carboline-3-carboxylate. Eur. J. Pharmacol. 68: 381-382.

Obata, K. and Takeda, K., 1969. Release of GABA into the fourth ventricle induced by stimulation of the cat cerebellum. J. Neurochem. 16: 1043-1047.

Obata, K. and Yoshida, M., 1973. Caudate-evoked inhibition and actions of GABA and other substances on cat pallidal neurons. Brain Research 65: 455-459.

Okada, Y., Nitsch-Hassler, C., Kim, J.S., Bak, I.J. and Hassler, R., 1971. The role of γ-aminobutyric acid (GABA) in the extra-pyramidal motor system. Exp. Brain Res. 13: 514-518.

Okada, Y. and Shimada, C., 1975. Intrahippocampal distribution of γ-aminobutyric acid (GABA) in the guinea pig, in "GABA and Nervous System Function" (E. Roberts, T.N. Chase and D.B. Towers, eds.), pp. 223-228, Raven Press, New York.

Penney, Jr., J.B. and Young, A.B., 1981. GABA as the pallido-thalamic neurotransmitter: implications for basal ganglia function. Brain Research 207: 195-199.

Placheta, P. and Karobath, M., 1979. Regional distribution of Na^+-dependent GABA and benzodiazepine binding sites in rat CNS. Brain Research 178: 580-583.

Porceddu, M.L., Morelli, M., Del Fiacco, M. and Di Chiara, G., 1980. Origin of GABA-ergic strio-nigral neurons as studied by kainate-induced lesions. Pharmacol. Res. Communication 12: 695-698.

Pourcho, R.G., 1980. Uptake of [^{3}H]glycine and [^{3}H]GABA by amacrine cells in the cat retina. Brain Research 198: 333-346.

Rall, W., Shepherd, G.M., Reese, T.S. and Brightman, M.W., 1966. Dendrodendritiic synaptic pathway for inhibition in the olfactory bulb. Exp. Neurol. 14: 44-56.

Ribak, C.E., 1978. Aspinous and sparsely-spinous stellate neurons in visual cortex of rats contain glutamic acid decarboxylase. J. Neurocytology 7: 461-478.

Ribak, C.E., Vaughn, J.E., Saito, K., Barber, R. and Roberts, E., 1977a. Glutamate decarboxylase localization in neurons of the olfactory bulb. Brain Research 126: 1-18.

Ribak, C.E., Vaughn, J.E., Saito, K., Barber, R. and Roberts, E., 1977b. Immunohistochemical localization of glutamate decarboxylase in rat substantia nigra. Brain Research 116: 287-298.

Ribak, C.E., Vaughn, J.E. and Saito, K., 1978. Immunocytochemical localization of glutamic acid decarboxylase in neuronal somata following colchicine inhibition of axonal transport. Brain Research 140: 315-332.

Ribak, C.E., Vaughn, J.E. and Roberts, E., 1979. The GABA neurons and their axon terminals in rat corpus striatum as demonstrated by GAD immunocytochemistry. J. Comp. Neurol. 187: 261-283.

Ribak, C.E., Vaughn, J.E. and Roberts, E., 1980. GABAergic nerve terminals decrease in the substantia nigra following hemitransect-ionsof the striato-nigral and pallidonigral pathways. Brain Research 192: 413-420.

Ribeiro, A., da Silva and Coimbra, A., 1980. Neuronal uptake of [^{3}H]GABA and [^{3}H]glycine in laminal 1-111 (Substantia gelatinosa rolandi) of the rat spinal cord: an autoradiographic study. Brain Research 188: 449-464.

Roffler-Taplov, S. and Taplov, E., 1975. Studies of suspected neurotransmitters in the vestibuloocular pathways. Brain Research 95: 303-304.

Rouzaire-Dubois, B., Hammond, C., Hamon, B. and Feger, J., 1980. Pharmacological blockade of the GABA-induced inhibitory response of subthalamic cells in the rat. Brain Research 200: 321-329.

Saito, K., Barber, R., Wu, J., Matsuda, T., Roberts, E. and Vaughn, J.E., 1974. Immunohistochemical localization of glutamate decarboxylase in rat cerebellum. Proc. Natl. Acad. Sci. U.S.A. 71: 269-277.

Schousboe, A. and Divac, I., 1979. Differences in glutamate uptake in astrocytes cultures from different brain regions. Brain Research 177: 407-409.

Schwarcz, R. Zaszek. R and Coyle, J.T., 1978.Microinjection of kainic acid into the rat hippocampus. Eur. J. Pharmacol. 50: 209-220.

Spehlmann, R., Norcross, K. and Grimmer, E.J., 1977. GABA in the caudate nucleus: a possible synaptic transmitter of interneurons. Experientia 33: 623-625.

Squires, R.F., Klepner, C.A. and Benson, D.I., 1980. Multiple benzodiazepine receptor complexes: some benzodiazepine recognition sites are coupled to GABA receptors and ionophors, in "Receptors for Neurotransmitters and Peptide Hormones", (G. Pepeu and M.J. Kuhar, eds.), pp. 285-293, Raven Press, New York.

Staines, W.A., Nagy, J.I., Vincent, S.R. and Fibiger, H.C., 1980. Neurotransmitters contained in the efferents of the striatum. Brain Research 194: 391-402.

Sterling, P. and Davis, T.L., 1980. Neurons in cat lateral geniculate nucleus that concentrate exogenous [^{3}H]-γ-aminobutyric acid (GABA). J. Comp. Neurology 192: 737-749.

Straschell, M. and Perwein, J., 1969. The inhibition of retinal ganglion cells by catecholamines and γ-aminobutyric acid. Pfluegers Arch. 312: 45-54.

Streit, P., Knecht, E. and Cuenod, M., 1979, Transmitter-specific retrograde labeling in the striato-nigral and raphe-nigral pathways, Science 205:306-308.

Storm-Mathisen, J., 1975. High affinity uptake of GABA in presymed GABA-ergic nerve endings in rat brain. Brain Research 84: 409-427.

Storm-Mathisen, J. and Fonnum, F., 1971. Quantitative histochemistry of glutamate decarboxylase in the rat hippocampal region. J. Neurochem. 18: 1105-1111.

Storm-Mathisen, J. and Fonnum, F., 1972. Localization of transmitter candidates in the hippocampal region. Progr. Brain Res. 36: 40-57.

Tachibana, M. and Kuriyama, K., 1974. Gamma-amminobutyric acid in the lower auditory pathway of the guinea pig. Brain Research 69: 370-374.

Taniyama, K., Nitsch, C., Wagner, A. and Hassler, R., 1980. Aspartate, glutamate and GABA levels in pallidum, substantia

nigra, center median and dorsal raphe nuclei after cylindric
lesion of caudate nucleus in cat. Neurosci. Lett. 16: 155-160.

Tappaz, M.L., Brownstein, M.J. and Kopin, I.J., 1977. Glutamate
decarboxylase (GAD) and gamma-aminobutyric acid (GABA) in discrete
nuclei of hypothalamus and substantia nigra. Brain Research 125:
109-121.

van der Heyden, J.A., Venema, K. and Korf, J., 1979. In vivo
release of endogenous GABA from rat substantia nigra measured by a
novel method. J. Neurochem. 32: 469-476.

van der Kooy, D., Hattori, T., Shannak, K. and Hornykiewicz, O.,
1981. The pallido-subthalamic projection in rat: anatomical
and biochemical studies. Brain Research 199: 466-472.

van Gelder, N.M., 1965. The histochemical demonstration of γ-
aminobutyric acid metabolism by reduction of a tetrazolium salt.
J. Neurochem. 12: 231-237.

Vincent, S.R., Hattori, T. and McGeer, E.G., 1978. The nigrotectal projection: a biochemical and ultrastructural characterization. Brain Research 151: 159-164.

Vincent, S.R. Kimura, H. and McGeer, E.G., 1980a. The pharmaco-
histochemical demonstration of gaba-transaminase. Neurosci. Lett.
16: 345-348.

Vincent, S.R., Lehmann, J. and McGeer, E.G., 1980b. The localization of GABA-transaminase in the striato-nigral system. Life
Sci. 27: 595-601.

Vincent, S.R., Kimura, H. and McGeer, E.G., 1981. The histochemical localization of GABA transaminase. Brain Research, in press.

Waddington, J.L. and Cross, A.J., 1978. Neurochemical changes
following kainic acid lesions of nucleus accumbens - implications
for a gabaergic accumbal-ventral tegmental pathway. Life Sci. 22:
1011-1014.

Waddington, J.L. and Cross, A.J., 1980. The striatonigral GABA
pathway: functional and neurochemical characteristics in rats with
unilateral striatal kainic acid lesions. Eur. J. Pharmacol. 67:
27-32.

Walaas, I. and Fonnum, F., 1979. The distribution and origin of
of glutamate decarboxylase and choline acetyltransferase in ventral pallidum and other basal forebrain regions. Brain Research
177: 325-336.

Walaas, I. and Fonnum, F., 1979. Biochemical evidence for gamma-aminobutyrate containing fibres from the nucleus accumbens to the substantia nigra and ventral tegmental area in the rat. Neuroscience 5: 63-72.

Wenthold, R.J., 1979. Release of endogenous glutamic acid, aspartic acid and GABA from cochlear nucleus slices. Brain Research 162: 338-343.

Wolf, P., Olpe, H.R., Avrith, D. and Haas, H.L., 1978. GABAergic inhibition of neurons in the ventral tegmental area. Experientia 34: 73-74.

Wood, J.G., McLaughlin, B.J. and Vaughn, J.E., 1976. Immunocytochemical localization of glutamate decarboxylase in electron microscopic preparations of rodent CNS, in "GABA in Nervous System Function" (E. Roberts, T.N. Chase and D.B. Tower, eds.), pp. 133-148, Raven Press, New York.

Wu, S.M. and Dowling, J.E., 1981. Effects of GABA and glycine on the distal cell of the cyprinia retina. Brain Research 199: 401-414.

Yim, C.Y. and Mogensen, G.J., 1980. Effects of picrotoxin and nipecotic acid on inhibitory reesponse of dopaminergic neurons in the ventral tegmental area to stimulation of the nucleus accumbens. Brain Research 199: 466-472.

Yoshida, M. and Omata, S., 1979. Blocking by picrotoxin of nigra-evoked inhibition of neurons of ventromedial nucleus of the thalamus. Experientia 35:794-795.

GABA-TRANSAMINASE INHIBITORS AND NEURONAL FUNCTION

Michel J. Jung

Centre de Recherche Merrell International
16, rue d'Ankara
67084, Strasbourg cedex, France

The immunocytochemical localisation of the GABA-synthetic enzyme, glutamate decarboxylase (GAD), allows distinction of two types of GABA-containing neurons (Pérez de la Mora et al., 1981). The first type, with long projections which makes axo-somatic and axo-dentritic contacts, has a high density in the substantia nigra, the globus pallidus and some cerebellar nuclei. This type forms the specialized tracts previously recognized by other methods and may possibly mediate postsynaptic inhibition. In contrast, the second class consists of short interneurons, is diffusely spread over the whole brain, makes axo-dendritic, axo-somatic and axo-axonic synapses, and mediates both presynaptic and postsynaptic inhibition. This wide distribution of GABA-containing neurons reflects the important role of GABA as a major inhibitory neurotransmitter in the mammalian CNS (Roberts, 1974).

A GABA-ergic synapse is shown schematically in Figure 1. GABA is synthesized by GAD in the afferent neuron by decarboxylation of L-glutamate. It is not known whether GABA is stored in a free or bound form in nerve endings. However, it has been calculated that the local concentration can be as high as 100-150 mM (Fonnum and Walberg, 1973). The question whether GABA is metabolized presynaptically, will be dealt with later. On nerve stimulation, a quantum of GABA is released into the synaptic cleft to bind to its receptor site. Binding and receptor activation can be facilitated or impeded by a regulatory subunit, one of the presumed sites of action of the benzodiazepines (see Karobath, 1979 for review). In invertebrates, the interaction of GABA with its receptor results in increased membrane conductance to chloride ions with little change in the resting potential. In mammalian CNS, the ionic basis of GABA neurotrans-

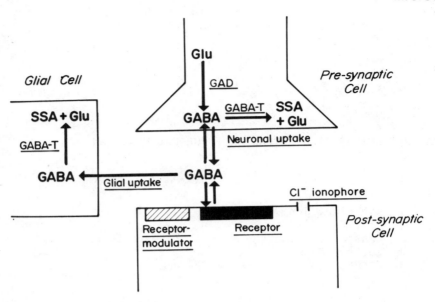

FIGURE 1.   Scheme of a GABA-ergic synapse.

mission is probably more complex (see Roberts, 1974 for review).
Termination of action, i.e., removal of GABA from the synapse is
accomplished by glial or neuronal uptake. The GABA captured in
glial cells is then metabolized by GABA-transaminase. The presence of an auto-receptor for GABA, regulating the release of the
neurotransmitter, is too new a concept to be firmly established
(Bowery et al., 1980). All the above mechanisms have been considered possible targets for increasing the availability of GABA at
its receptor site in order to enhance GABA-ergic neurotransmission.

    An increase in the presynaptic pool of GABA could result in
an augmented quantal release. The resultant enhanced GABA-ergic
action would be dependent on nerve stimulation and should be more
selective than generalized GABA receptor activation by a GABA
agonist. The purpose of this presentation is to demonstrate that
inhibition of GABA-T is presently the only practical way to
increase the presynaptic pool of GABA, to review the status of
GABA-T inhibitors, and to present some biochemical evidence that
elevation of whole-brain GABA through GABA-T inhibition does
indeed result in enhanced GABA-ergic functions.

SUBCELLULAR LOCALISATION OF GAD AND GABA-T

While it was readily accepted that the GABA-synthetic enzyme is localized mainly, if not exclusively, in nerve endings,
it was questioned for some time whether GABA-T, a mitochondrial
enzyme was present in this subcellular fraction (Reijnierse et
al., 1975). There is now enough cytochemical evidence to state
that the GABA metabolic enzyme is indeed present there (Barber
and Saito, 1976). In addition, there is biochemical evidence.
After loading a highly purified preparation of brain synaptosomes
with [^{3}H]-GABA, a significant portion of the radioactivity is
recovered as ^3H_2O. This metabolism can be prevented by addition
of a GABA-T inhibitor (Gardner and Richards, 1981).

The presynaptic pool of GABA could be increased by augmenting its production or by inhibiting its degradation. To increase
the production of GABA one would have to increase the concentration of GAD, to stimulate its activity, or, if the enzyme is not
already saturated, to augment the pool of glutamate accessible to
it. The regulation of GAD is poorly understood and the origin of
the glutamate which serves as substrate for GAD is unknown.
Hence, at present there is no rational approach to increased
production of GABA. It should be mentioned, however, that dipro-
pylacetate, which has a pharmacologic action out of proportion to
its potency as a GABA-T inhibitor in vivo, has been claimed to
act by stimulating GAD (Löscher and Frey, 1977).

Inhibition of degradation of GABA is conceptually simple.
However, at least two groups have reported that there are two
forms of GABA-T in the brain (Ngo and Tunnicliff, 1978; Bloch-
Tardy et al., 1980) and it has been suggested that one might be
selectively associated with nerve terminals (Bloch-Tardy et al.,
1980). Unfortunately, the physical and kinetic differences of the
two forms are so tenuous that exploitation of these differences
in designing inhibitors specific for either species seems utopic.

GABA-T INHIBITORS

The structures of GABA-T inhibitors to be discussed are
shown in Table 1. The upper part of the table lists those which
are either pyridoxal scavengers, such as hydroxylamine, aminooxyacetic acid (AOAA), γ-glutamyl hydrazide and isonicotinic hydrazide (INH), or weak competitive inhibitors, such as dipropylace-
tate (DPA). The second class of GABA-T inhibitors are the enzyme-
activated or suicide inhibitors developed during the last decade:
ethanolamine-O-sulphate (EOS), γ-acetylenic GABA (GAG), γ-Vinyl
GABA (GVG), the natural product, gabaculine (GBL), its synthetic
isomer, isogabaculine (IGBL), and the fluoromethyl derivatives of
β-alanine. Suicide inhibitors inhibit irreversibly those enzymes

TABLE 1. Structure of GABA-T inhibitors discussed in the text.

NAME	STRUCTURE	LITERATURE REFERENCE	
		IN VITRO	IN VIVO
HYDROXYL AMINE	H_2N-OH	BAXTER/ROBERTS, 1961	ID.
AOAA	H_2N-O COOH	WALLACH, 1961	
γ-GLUTAMYL HYDRAZIDE	H_2NHNOC — NH_2 COOH	-	WALTERS ET AL., 1977
INH	CONHNH$_2$ (pyridine)	-	WOOD & PEESKER, 1974
DPA	COOH	MAITRE ET AL., 1976	SIMLER ET AL., 1976
EOS	$O-SO_3^-$ NH_3^+	FOWLER & JOHN, 1972	FOWLER, 1973
GAG	COO$^-$ NH_3^+	JUNG & METCALF, 1975	JUNG ET AL., 1977A
GVG	COO$^-$ NH_3^+	LIPPERT ET AL., 1977	JUNG ET AL., 1977B
GBL	COO$^-$ NH_3^+	RANDO & BANGERTER, 1976	RANDO & BANGERTER, 1977
IGBL	COO$^-$ NH_3^+	METCALF & JUNG, 1979	ID.
DFM-β-ALA	F_2CH COOH NH_3^+ / FCH_2 F COO$^-$ NH_3^+	BEY ET AL., IN PRESS	ID.

which are able to activate them chemically. In this list, the
most selective inhibitors for GABA-T are EOS, GVG and the fluori-
nated compounds. GAG inhibit also glutamic acid decarboxylase and
other transaminases, such as ornithine-δ-aminotransferase. The
latter action is also shared by the gabaculines (see Jung, 1978
for review).

All the compounds, even EOS, when given systemically to rats
or mice in large enough doses inhibit brain GABA-T and cause an
increase in whole brain GABA levels. Their potency in vivo does
not correlate with the in vitro affinity for the enzyme, presumably due to pharmacokinetic factors especially differences in permeability of the blood-brain barrier. The most potent of these
compounds are difluoromethyl-β-alanine and its analogue,
3-amino,2,4-difluorobutanoic acid. GVG and EOS which are equally
selective in vitro and in vivo are 100-200 times less potent on a

mg/kg basis. The former two compounds are mentioned here only to update the list, since they have been little studied in relation to the present topic.

INFLUENCE OF GABA-T INHIBITORS ON THE PRESYNAPTIC POOL OF GABA

It was realized long ago that total brain GABA correlates poorly with anticonvulsant properties of GABA-elevating drugs (Wood and Peesker, 1974) and that the correlation might be improved if one could estimate the concentration of GABA in nerve endings. Unfortunately, it is technically impossible to separate quantitatively the different cellular and subcellular fractions in which GABA is present: glial cells, nerve cell bodies and nerve terminals.

One approach used to estimate the pool of GABA which is most likely to function as neurotransmitter is to measure GABA in synaptosomes. The results of two recently published studies using different inhibitors have been recalculated in Table 2. Wood et al. (1980) took whole mouse brains as the source of synaptosomes and expressed the data as nmoles/mg/protein in the synaptosomal fraction assuming that the recovery was the same in treated and control animals. Sarhan and Seiler, (1979) used rat cortex as the source of synaptosomes and attempted to correct for the yield of synaptosome recovery by measuring presumed marker enzymes of nerve endings (GAD and aromatic amino acid decarboxylase) in the synaptosomal and supernatant fractions. All GABA-T inhibitors cause an increase in the synaptosomal content of GABA; however,

TABLE 2. Effect of GABA-T inhibitors on total and synaptosomal GABA.

INHIBITOR	DOSE (MMOLE/KG)	% CONTROL			REFERENCE
		TOTAL (A) GABA	SYNAPTOSOMAL (B)	RATIO B/A	
AOAA	0.23	410	220	0.53	WOOD ET AL.,
GBL	0.58	670	293	0.43	1980
GAG	0.79	300	272	0.91	SAHRAN & SEILER,
GVG	5.8	200	290	1.45	1979

the ratios of increase of synaptosomal to total content are different. This ratio is greater than one for GVG and lowest for gabaculine even though the latter compound produces the greatest absolute elevations of synaptosomal GABA. Gabaculine is a poor anticonvulsant in a variety of seizure models (Schechter and Tranier, 1978). It is possible therefore, as suggested by Sarhan and Seiler (1979), that an increase of GABA in the glial pool might have a negative effect on the GABA release from nerve terminals. In this respect, a compound which would only inhibit GABA-T presynaptically would be highly desirable.

In both studies, the relation between synaptosomal and total GABA was studied for the first six hours after drug adminis- tration. However, brain GABA elevations usually last much longer and the anticonvulsant effects usually disappear before GABA levels have returned to normal. These studies should, therefore, be extended for longer time periods to determine if there is a re- equilibration of the two pools. The intriguing observation has been made that 60 hr after its administration, GVG protects against seizures induced by bicuculline, pentylenetetrazole or electroshock (Gale and Iadarola, 1980), while at earlier time points there was no effect (Schechter and Tranier, 1978). In order to explain these discrepancies, Gale and Iadarola tried to estimate the increase in the neurotransmitter GABA pool at differ- ent time points. Their method consisted of causing an unilateral degeneration of GABA afferents to the substantia nigra by surgi- cal transsection of the striato-nigral pathway. The difference in GABA increase between the lesioned and unlesioned sides after GABA-T inhibition is attributed to the neuronal pool. Indeed, the difference is maximum at 60 hr at the time of highest anticonvul- sant activity and nil at shorter time points (Gale and Iadarola, 1980). This could mean that the GABA pools are affected different- ly in different brain regions.

DOES THE INCREASE OF GABA IN NERVE ENDINGS RESULT IN AN AUGMENTED QUANTAL RELEASE?

The development of simple and extremely sensitive methods of measuring picomole amounts of GABA made possible an evaluation of the release of endogenous GABA from brain synaptosomes, brain slices or even from whole brain cortex.

In synaptosomes prepared from rat cortices treated with a dose of 750 mg/kg of GVG, 18 hours before death, the K^+-stimu- lated GABA release is increased 3-fold over that found in control animals, i.e., to the same extent as the synaptosomal GABA content (Gardner et al., in preparation). It seems, therefore, that all or almost all of the accumulated GABA can be released.

However, the objection can be raised that the kind of stimulation used was not physiological and that in the synaptosomal preparation the interaction between glial cells and nerve endings has been disrupted.

Bradford and collaborators have developed a technique for superfusing small areas of exposed brain cortex in anaesthetized rats (Dodd et al., 1974). Combining the superfusion technique with sensitive amino acid analysis, this group was able to show that GABA appeared in the superfusate after administration of GABA-T inhibitors, GAG (100 mg/kg) or GVG (1500 mg/kg), (Abdul-Ghani et al., 1980 and 1981). Contralateral stimulations of the brachial plexus increased the amount of GABA in the superfusate significantly, while ipsilateral stimulation had no effect. Upon cessation of the stimulus, GABA release returned to prestimulation levels. Apart from glutamic acid, no other amino acid present in the superfusate was affected by administration of the GABA-T inhibitors. It is questionable whether this increase of GABA in the superfusate is due to synaptic release only and the authors do not reject the possibility of a GABA-releasing action of the GABA-T inhibitors from glial or neuronal cells. Indeed, when GVG (100 μM) was added to artificial CSF used for the superfusion, a small but significant amount of GABA appeared in the superfusate after about 20 min. However, no biochemical determinations of GABA metabolism have been carried out in this experiment and it is conceivable that during the lag-time of 20 min, there was enough GABA-T inhibition and accumulation of GABA in superficial layers of the cortex to explain the appearance of GABA in the superfusate.

Both free and conjugated GABA are increased in the CSF of animals or humans treated with GVG (Böhlen et al., 1979; Grove et al., 1981). However, it is not known if this GABA is of glial or neuronal origin. The question could be answered, as in Obata's classical experiment (1976), by showing that cerebellar stimulation results in increased amounts of GABA in the CSF of animals treated with GABA-T inhibitors.

GABA-T inhibitors have also been studied in a number of electrophysiological experiments. Hydroxylamine and AOAA increase the primary afferent depolarization in amphibian spinal cord preparations (Davidoff et al., 1973). GAG augments the height of a segmentally evoked dorsal root potential in spinally transsected cats (Larson and Anderson, 1979). Both GAG and GVG produce hypersynchronisation of EEG in rats (Myslobodsky and Mansour, 1979). Unfortunately, none of these experiments implies unequivocally enhanced neuronal GABA release to explain the effects of the GABA-T inhibitors.

EFFECTS OF GABA-T INHIBITORS ON OTHER NEUROTRANSMITTER SYSTEMS

In the preceding sections, it has been established that GABA-T inhibitors cause an increase of the nerve-ending pool of GABA and that this results in an augmented release of GABA upon adequate stimulation. The GABA neurons are not isolated in the CNS, and it becomes important to know whether the functional state of other neurotransmitters is changed concomitantly. Acutely or chronically increased GABA levels could influence the basal level of other neurotransmitters, their turnover, the density or kinetic properties of their receptors or the activity of the enzymes involved in their synthesis.

a.)   Effects on the Concentrations:

AOAA elevates brain GABA levels several-fold at a dose of 50 mg/kg, but does not change the concentrations of dopamine and noradrenaline in rat brain (Andén, 1974). EOS given intracerebrally (100 µg) multiplies the concentration of GABA by four in seven regions of the brain without affecting the concentrations of dopamine, noradrenaline or serotonin in any of these regions (Pycock and Horton, 1978). γ-Acetylenic GABA, however, increased the concentration of dopamine significantly in the striatum and olfactory tubercles, 4 hr after a dose of 100 mg/kg, at a time when GABA levels were 400% of control (Palfreyman et al., 1978). The concentrations of dopamine, noradrenaline and serotonin were unchanged in whole rat brain after single or subacute administration of GVG at a dose of 250 mg/kg/day. In the same animals the brain GABA concentration was multiplied by 3 at the end of the two week treatment (Jung, unpublished).

b.)   Effects on Neurotransmitter Turnover:

The concentration of metabolites of biogenic amines and the rate of disappearance after inhibition of synthesis are better indices for neurotransmitter activity than the concentration of the transmitter. AOAA decreases the rate of disappearance of dopamine in the striatum and limbic system and accelerates the decrease of noradrenaline in the brains of rats treated with the tyrosine hydroxylase inhibitor, α-methyl p-tyrosine (Andén, 1974). EOS, given by the intracerebroventricular route (i.c.v.) decreased significantly the concentration of DOPAC, a dopamine metabolite, in the limbic system, but did not change the level of the noradrenaline metabolite, MOPEG-sulphate, in any of the regions examined. 5-HIAA, a serotonin metabolite, was increased in the cortex, pons and mid-brain (Pycock and Horton, 1978). γ-Acetylenic GABA decreased the concentration of DOPAC significantly in the substantia nigra and ventral tegmentum, but the effect in the nucleus accumbens was less significant (Gundlach and Beart,

1980). In another study (Palfreyman et al., 1978), it was shown that GAG, given systemically, decreased the rate of depletion of dopamine after α-methyl p-tyrosine in the striatum and olfactory tubercle but increased it significantly in the hypothalamus. In accordance with this finding, the concentration of HVA, another dopamine metabolite was diminished in the first two regions and increased in the hypothalamus.

<u>c.)</u> <u>Receptor Binding</u>:

The studies mentioned previously demonstrate that elevation of GABA by means of a GABA-T inhibitor decreases the dopamine turnover in extrapyramidal structures. This could result, after long-term treatment, in supersensitivity of postsynaptic dopamine receptors as in the case of chronic administration of receptor blockers. Such a phenomenon was reported for AOAA, GAG and isonicotinic hydrazide (Enna et al., 1980). The neuroleptic, haloperidol, was included for comparison. All compounds were given daily for 2 weeks at doses showing biochemical or pharmacological effects. The density of dopamine receptors (^{3}H-spiroperidol binding), muscarinic cholinergic receptor (^{3}H-QNB) and GABA receptors (^{3}H-muscimol) was determined in the corpus striatum and the frontal cortex. The results for the striatum have been recalculated in Table 3.

TABLE 3. Effects of chronic administration of GABA-T inhibitors on receptor sensitivity for Dopamine, GABA and acetylcholine in rat striatum.

INHIBITOR	DOSE (MG/KG)	GABA % CONTROL	STRIATAL BINDING (% CONTROL)		
			^{3}H-SPIROPERIDOL	^{3}H-MUSCINOL	^{3}H-QNB
AOAA	10	182	128*	51*	104
INH	20	227	170*	60*	122
GAG	10	164	123*	71*	-
HALOPERIDOL	2	88	133*	83	93

* $P < 0.05$ ENNA ET AL., 1980

All three GABA-T inhibitors produce significant increases in spiroperidol binding at doses giving comparable elevations of whole-brain GABA. GABA binding is reduced to various extents and the cholinergic system appears to be essentially unaffected. Thus, in chronic treatment a GABA-T inhibitor is equivalent to a dopamine receptor antagonist in inducing supersensitivity of dopamine receptors in the striatum.

d.) Effects on Enzymic Activity or Inducibility:

It is well established that acute administration of a dopamine receptor blocker, such as haloperidol, increases tyrosine hydroxylase activity in dopaminergic nerve terminals. The actual mechanism is still controversial although the biochemical basis seems to be an increased affinity of the enzyme for its tetrahydropteridine cofactor (Lerner et al., 1977). Microinjection of GVG into the substantia nigra prevents tyrosine hydroxylase activation by haloperidol (Casu and Gale, 1981). Conversely, tyrosine hydroxylase activity is decreased in the neostriatum after chronic administration of amphetamines. AOAA and GAG given at the same time as the amphetamine block the depression of enzyme activity (Hotchkiss and Gibb, 1980). Both studies lend support to the conclusion that GABA elevation can dampen the metabolic alterations at dopaminergic synapses due to pharmacophores leading either to an increase or a decrease of this function.

GABA-T INHIBITORS AND RELEASE OF PITUITARY HORMONES

The release of pituitary hormones is controlled by the hypothalamus which is one of the brain regions with the highest GABA concentration (Fahn, 1976) and the highest synaptosomal uptake of GABA (Young et al., 1976). GABA neurons in the hypothalamus may play an important role in controlling hunger and satiety centers (Kuriyama and Kimura, 1976), but they may also have other functions such as direct or indirect control of pituitary hormone release. GABA itself inhibits the release of prolactin in vitro and in vivo (Schally et al., 1977). EOS given i.c.v. to male rats, in a dose which doubles the hypothalamic GABA concentration, reduces the basal levels of plasma prolactin by 50% (Locatelli et al., 1978). AOAA, given by i.v. infusion over a period of 2 hr (60 mg/kg total dose), had no effect on basal prolactin levels but reduced the hyperprolactinemia produced by sulpiride, a potent dopamine antagonist (Debeljuk et al., 1980). Similarly, GAG inhibits, in a dose-dependent fashion, the hypersecretion of prolactin due either to inhibition of catecholamine biosynthesis (α-methyl p-tyrosine) or to dopamine receptor blockade with pimozide (Fuxe et al., 1979). This finding is in agreement with the increase of the dopamine metabolite HVA in the hypothalamus after GAG administration to rats (Palfreyman et al., 1978).

Both AOAA and GVG prevent the increase in plasma levels of vasopressin due to polyethylene glycol administration to rats, while mercaptopropionic acid, a GABA-synthesis inhibitor, produces a dose-dependent increase of vasopressin release (Knepel et al., 1980). These studies suggest that control of pituitary hormone release by GABA can be reinforced by GABA-T inhibitors.

PHARMACOLOGICAL AND CLINICAL PROPERTIES OF GABA-T INHIBITORS

So far it has been shown that GABA-T inhibitors can increase GABA-ergic functions in a variety of more or less isolated systems. This section will be devoted to the effects of GABA-T inhibitors at a more integrated level. The pharmacology of GABA-T inhibitors in laboratory animals has been recently reviewed (Palfreyman et al., 1981). In rodents they all produce a dose-related sedation and, at high doses, ataxia, lacrymation and catatonia. Upon chronic administration of the more selective compounds, there is a lesser gain of body weight than in controls due to a reduction of food consumption. No appreciable cardiovascular effects have been reported and analgesic actions are weak. Of more importance, they act as anticonvulsants in a variety of chemically-induced seizures with some differences in effectivity among the compounds, which are not readily explained.

The only compounds which have undergone clinical evaluation are INH, AOAA, DPA, GAG and GVG. The first four compounds are not effective in correcting the motor disability in Huntington's disease (see Grove et al., 1981 for references; Tell et al., 1981a). GVG increases the CSF concentration of free and conjugated GABA (Grove et al., 1981). Its effect in Huntington's chorea has not yet been reported.

In agreement with the ability of GABA-T inhibitors to reduce the turnover of dopamine in the extrapyramidal system demonstrated in animals, GAG and GVG were found to reduce the dyskinetic movements in patients suffering from tardive dyskinesia (Casey et al., 1980; Tell et al., 1981b). GABA-T inhibitors also reduced the turnover of dopamine in the limbic system, it remains to be seen if a similar effect in man can be beneficial in the treatment of schizophrenia. Finally the anticonvulsant activities found in various animal models could indicate some anti-epileptic properties in man.

CONCLUSIONS

Compounds are now available which inhibit GABA-T selectively and cause elevation of brain GABA when given systemically. The design of inhibitors acting selectively on the enzyme in nerve endings seems beyond reach at the present time. However, the imperfect compounds at hand produce an increase of the presynaptic GABA pool in parallel with other pools. The additionally accumulated GABA can be released and enhances GABA-ergic neurotransmission as demonstrated indirectly in a variety of experimental models.

Due to the ubiquity of GABA containing neurons throughout the brain, it was difficult to foresee what the clinical end result of a general increase of GABA-ergic neurotransmission could be. Therefore, the improvement of dyskinetic movements in patients, in agreement with the results of biochemical studies in animals, has been most rewarding.

REFERENCES

Abdul-Ghani, A.-S., Coutinho-Netto, J. and Bradford, H.F., 1980. The action of γ-vinyl-GABA and γ-acetylenic-GABA on the resting and stimulated release of GABA in vivo. Brain Res. 191: 471-481.

Abdul-Ghani, A.-S., Coutinho-Netto, J., Druce, D. and Bradford, H.F., 1981. Effects of anticonvulsants on the in vivo and in vitro release of GABA. Biochem. Pharmacol. 30: 363-368.

Andén, N.-E., 1974. Inhibition of the turnover of the brain dopamine after treatment with the gammaaminobutyrate: 2-oxyglutarate transaminase inhibitor aminooxyacetic acid. Naunyn-Schmiedeberg's Arch. Pharmacol. 283: 419-424.

Barber, R. & Saito, K., 1976. Light microscopic visualization of GAD and GABA-T in immunocytochemical preparations of rodent CNS, in "GABA in nervous system function" (Roberts, E., Chase, T.N. and Tower, D.B. eds.) pp. 113-132, Raven Press, New York.

Bey, P., Jung, M.J., Gerhart, F., Schirlin D., Van Dorsselau, V. and Casara, P., ω-Fluoromethyl analogues of ω-amino acids as irreversible inhibitors of 4-aminobutyrate-2-oxoglutarate aminotransferase. J. Neurochem. in press.

Bloch-Tardy, M., Buzenet, A., Fages, C., Rolland, B. and Gonnard, P., 1980. Two forms of GABA transaminase in pig brain. Neurochem. Res. 5: 1147-1154.

Böhlen, P., Huot, S. and Palfreyman, M.G., 1979. The relationship between GABA concentrations in brain and cerebrospinal fluid. Brain Res. 167: 297-305.

Bowery, N.G., Hill, D.R. and Hudson, A.L., 1980. (-)Baclofen decreases neurotransmitter release in the mammalian CNS by an action at a novel GABA receptor. Nature 283: 92-93.

Casey, D.E., Gerlach, J., Magelund, G. and Christensen, T.R., 1980. γ-Acetylenic GABA in tardive dyskinesia, in "Long-term effects of neuroleptics" (Adv. Biochem. Psychopharmacol, Vol. 27), (Cattabeni et al. eds.) pp. 577-580, Raven Press, New York.

Casu, M. & Gale, K., 1981. Effects of gamma-vinyl-GABA on dopamine neurons: relationship between elevation of GABA in nerve-terminals and change in tyrosine hydroxylase activity. Fed. Proc. 40: 314.

Davidoff, R.A., Grayson, V. and Adair, R., 1973. GABA-transaminase inhibitors and presynaptic inhibition in the amphibian spinal cord. Am. J. Physiol. 224: 1230-1234.

Debeljuk, L., Goijman, S., Seilicovich, A. Diaz, M.C. and Rettori, V.B., 1980. Current concepts: II. Effect of aminooxyacetic acid and bicuculline on prolactin release in castrated male rats. Life Sci. 27: 2025-2029.

Dodd, P.R., Pritchard, M.J., Adams, R.C.F., Bradford, H.F., Hicks, G. and Blanshard, K.C., 1974. A method for the continuous long-term superfusion of the cerebral cortex of unanaesthetised unrestrained rats. J. scient. Instr. E7: 897-901.

Enna, S.J., Ferkany, J.W. and Strong, R., 1980. Drug-induced alterations in neurotransmitter receptor binding and function, in "Receptors for neurotransmitters and peptide hormones" (Pepeu, G., Kuhar, M.J. and Enna, S.J. eds.) pp. 253-263, Raven Press, New York.

Fahn, S., 1976. Regional distribution studies of GABA and other putative neurotransmitters and their enzymes, in "GABA in nervous system function (Roberts, E., Chase, T.N. and Tower, D.B. eds.) pp. 169-186, Raven Press, New York.

Fonnum, F. & Walberg, F., 1973. The concentration of GABA within inhibitory nerve terminals. Brain Res. 62: 577-579.

Fowler, L.J. & John, R.A., 1972. Acitve-site-directed irreversible inhibition of rat brain 4-aminobutyrate aminotransferase by ethanolamine O-sulphate in vitro and in vivo. Biochem. J. 130: 569-573.

Fowler, L.J., 1973. Analysis of the major amino acids of rat brain after in vivo inhibition of GABA transaminase by ethanolamine O-sulphate. J. Neurochem. 21: 437-440.

Fuxe, K., Andersson, K. Ogren, S.-O., Pérez De La Mora, M., Schwarcz, R., Hökfelt, T., Eneroth, P., Gustafsson, J.-A. and Skett, P., 1979. GABA Neurons and their interaction with monoamine neurons. An anatomical, pharmacological and functional analysis, in "GABA-neurotransmitters" (Krogsgaard-Larsen, P., Scheel-Krüger, J. and Kofod, H. eds.) pp. 74-94, Munksgaard, Copenhagen.

Gale, K. & Iadarola, M.J., 1980. Seizure protection and increased nerve-terminal GABA: Delayed effects of GABA transaminase inhibition, Science 208: 288-291.

Gardner, C.R. & Richards, M.H., 1981. Presence of radiolabelled metabolites in release studies using [^{3}H]γ-aminobutyric acid. J. Neurochem. 36(4): 1590-1593.

Grove, J., Schechter, P.J., Tell, G., Koch-Weser, J., Sjoerdsma, A., Warter, J.-M., Marescaux, C. and Rumbach, L., 1981. Increased gamma-aminobutyric acid (GABA), homocarnosine and β-alanine in cerebrospinal fluid of patients treated with γ-vinyl GABA (4-amino-hex-5-ynoic acid). Life Sci. 28: 2431-2439.

Gundlach, A.L. & Beart, P.M., 1981. Effect of GABAergic drugs on
    dopamine catabolism in the nigrostriatal and mesolimbic dopa-
    minergic pathways of the rat. J. Pharm. Pharmacol. 33: 41–43.
Hotchkiss, D. & Gibb, J.W., 1980. Blockade of methamphetamine-
    induced depression of tyrosine hydroxylase by GABA transami-
    nase inhibitors. Eur. J. Pharmacol. 66: 201–205.
Jung, M.J., 1978. In vivo biochemistry of GABA transaminase
    inhibition, in "Enzyme-activated irreversible inhibitors"
    (Seiler, N., Jung, M.J. and Koch-Weser, J. eds.) pp.
    135–148, Elsevier/North-Holland Biomedical Press.
Jung, M.J. Lippert, B., Metcalf, B.W., Böhlen, P. and Schechter,
    P.J., 1977a. γ-Vinyl GABA (4-amino-hex-5-enoic acid), a new
    selective irreversible inhibitor of GABA-T: effects on brain
    GABA metabolism in mice. J. Neurochem. 29: 797–802.
Jung, M.J., Lippert, B., Metcalf, B.W., Schechter, P.J., Böhlen,
    P. and Sjoerdsma, A., 1977b. The effect of 4-amino-hex-5-
    ynoic acid (γ-acetylenic GABA, γ-ethynyl GABA) a catalytic
    inhibitor of GABA transaminase, on brain GABA metabolism
    in vivo. J. Neurochem. 28: 717–723.
Jung, M.J. & Metcalf, B.W., 1975. Catalytic inhibition of γ-amino-
    butyric acid α-ketoglutarate transaminase of bacterial ori-
    gin by 4-amino-hex-5-ynoic acid, a substrate analog. Biochem.
    Biophys. Res. Commun. 67: 301–306.
Karobath, M., 1979. Molecular basis of benzodiazepine actions,
    Trends in Neurosciences pp. 166–168.
Knepel, W., Nutto, D. and Hertting, G., 1980. Evidence for the
    involvement of a GABA-mediated inhibition in the hypovolae-
    mia-induced vasopressin release. Eur. J. Physiol. 388: 177–
    183.
Kuriyama, K. & Kimura, H., 1976. Distribution and possible func-
    tional roles of GABA in the retina, lower auditory pathway,
    and hypothalamus, in "GABA in nervous system function"
    (Roberts, E., Chase, T.N. and Tower, D.B. eds.) pp. 203–216,
    Raven Press, New York.
Larson, A.A. & Anderson, E.G., 1979. Changes in primary afferent
    depolarization after administration of γ-acetylenic γ-amino-
    butyric acid (GAG), a γ-aminobutyric acid (GABA) transami-
    nase inhibitor. J. Pharmacol. Exp. Ther. 211: 326–330.
Lerner, P., Nose, P., Gordon, E.K. and Lovenberg, W., 1977. Halo-
    peridol: Effect of long-term treatment on rat striatal dopa-
    mine synthesis and turnover. Science 197: 181–183.
Lippert, B., Metcalf, B.W., Jung, M.J. and Casara, P., 1977.
    4-Aminohex-5-enoic acid, a selective catalytic inhibitor of
    4-aminobutyric amino-transferase in mammalian brain. Eur. J.
    Biochem. 74: 441–445.
Locatelli, V., Cocchi, D., Racagni, G., Cattabeni, F., Maggi, A.,
    Krogsgaard-Larsen, P. and Müller, E.E., 1978. Prolactin-
    inhibiting activity of gamma-aminobutyric acid-mimetic drugs
    in the male rat. Brain Res. 145: 173–179.

Löscher, W. & Frey, H.-H., 1977. Zum Wirkungsmechanismus Von Valproinsäure. Arzneim.-Forsch./Drug Res. 27: 1081-1082.

Maitre, M., Ossola, L. and Mandel, P., 1976. In vitro studies into the effect of inhibition of rat brain succinic semialdehyde dehydrogenase on GABA synthesis and degradation. FEBS Lett. 72: 53-57.

Metcalf, B.W. & Jung, M.J., 1979. Molecular basis for the irreversible inhibition of 4-aminobutyric acid:2-oxoglutarate and L-ornithine:2-oxoacid aminotransferases by 3-amino-1,5-cyclohexadienyl carboxylic acid (isogabaculine). Mol. Pharmacol. 16: 539-545.

Myslobodsky, M.S. & Mansour, R., 1979. Hypersynchronisation and sedation produced by GABA-transaminase inhibitors and picrotoxin: does GABA participate in sleep control? Waking and Sleeping 3: 245-254.

Ngo, T.T. & Tunnicliff, G., 1978. Further evidence for the existence of isozymes of brain γ-aminobutyrate aminotransferase. Comp. Biochem. Physiol. 59C: 101-104.

Palfreyman, M.G., Huot, S., Lippert, B. and Schechter, P.J., 1978. The effect of γ-acetylenic GABA, an enzyme-activated irreversible inhibitor of GABA-transaminase, on dopamine pathways of the extrapyramidal and limbic systems. Eur. J. Pharmacol. 50: 325-336.

Palfreyman, M.G., Schechter, P.J., Buckett, W.R., Tell, G.P. and Koch-Weser, J., 1981. The pharmacology of GABA-transaminase inhibitors. Biochem. Pharmacol. 30: 817-824.

Pérez de la Mora, M., Possani, L.D., Tapia, R., Teran, L., Palacios, R., Fuxe, K., Hökfelt, T. and Ljungdahl, A., 1981. Demonstration of central γ-aminobutyrate-containing nerve terminals by means of antibodies against glutamate decarboxylase. Neuroscience 6: 875-895.

Pycock, C. & Horton, R., 1978. Regional changes in the concentrations of cerebral monoamines and their metabolites after ethanolamine-O-sulphate induced elevation of brain γ-aminobutyric acid concentrations. Biochem. Pharmacol. 27: 1827-1830.

Rando, R.R., & Bangerter, F.W., 1976. The irreversible inhibition of mouse brain γ-aminobutyric acid (GABA)-α-ketoglutaric acid transaminase by gabaculine. J. Amer. Chem. Soc. 98: 6762-6764.

Rando, R.R. & Bangerter, F.W., 1977. The in vivo inhibition of GABA-transaminase by gabaculine. Biochem. Biophys. Res. Commun. 76: 1276-1281.

Reijnierse, G.L.A., Veldstra, H. and Van den Berg, C.J., 1975. Subcellular localization of γ-aminobutyrate transaminase and glutamate dehydrogenase in adult rat brain. Biochem. J. 152: 469-475.

Roberts, E., 1974. γ-aminobutyric acid and nervous system function – a perspective. Biochem. Pharmacol. 23: 2637-2649.

Sarhan, S. & Seiler, N., 1979. Metabolic inhibitors and subcellular distribution of GABA. J. Neurosci. Res. 4: 399-421.

Schally, A.V., Redding, T.W., Arimura, A., Dupont, A. and Linthi-
    cum, G.L., 1977. Isolation of gamma-amino butyric acid from
    pig hypothalami and demonstration of its prolactin release-
    inhibiting (PIF) activity in vivo and in vitro. Endocrinolo-
    gy 100: 681-691.
Schechter, P.J. & Tranier, Y., 1978. The pharmacology of enzyme-
    activated inhibitors of GABA-transaminase, in "Enzyme-activa-
    ted irreversible inhibitors" (Seiler, N., Jung, M.J. and
    Koch-Weser, J. eds.) pp. 149-162, Elsevier/North-Holland
    Biomedical Press.
Simler, S., Gensburger, C., Ciesielski, L. and Mandel, P., 1976.
    Effets du n-dipropylacétate de sodium sur le taux de GABA de
    certaines zones du cerveau de la Souris. Comptes rendus
    176: 1285-1288.
Tell, G., Böhlen, P., Schechter, P.J., Koch-Weser, J., Agid, Y.,
    Bonnet, A.M., Coquillat, G., Chazot, G. and Fischer, C.,
    1981a. Treatment of Huntington disease with γ-acetylenic
    GABA, an irreversible inhibitor of GABA-transaminase: In-
    creased CSF GABA and homocarnosine without clinical ameliora-
    tion. Neurology 31: 207-211.
Tell, G., Schechter, P.J., Koch-Weser, J., Cantiniaux, P., Chaban-
    nes, J.P. and Lambert, P., 1981b. γ-Vinyl GABA, an irrevers-
    ible, enzyme-activated GABA-transaminase inhibitor: Prelimi-
    nary open study in tardive dyskinesia. Abstract presented at
    IIIrd World Congress on Biological Psychiatry (Stockholm,
    June 28th - July 3rd).
Wallach, D.P. & Crittenden, N.J., 1961. Studies on the GABA
    pathway-I. The inhibition of γ-aminobutyric acid-α-ketogluta-
    ric acid transaminase in vitro and in vivo by U-7524 (amino-
    oxyacetic acid). Biochem. Pharmacol. 5: 323-331.
Walters, J.R., Eng, N. Pericic, D. and Miller, L.P., 1978.
    Effects of aminooxyacetic acid and L-glutamic acid-α-hydra-
    zide on GABA metabolism in specific brain regions. J. Neuro-
    chem. 30: 759-766.
Wood, J.D. & Peesker, S.J., 1974. Development of an expression
    which relates the excitable state of the brain to the level
    of GAD activity and GABA content, with particular reference
    to the action of hydrazine and its derivatives. J. Neuro-
    chem. 23: 703-712.
Wood, J.D., Russell, M.P. and Kurylo, E., 1980. The γ-aminobuty-
    rate content of nerve endings (synaptosomes) in mice after
    the intramuscular injection of γ-aminobutyrate-elevating
    agents: A possible role in anticonvulsant activity. J. Neuro-
    chem. 35: 125-130.
Young, A.B., Enna, S.J., Zukin, S.R. and Snyder, S.H., 1976.
    Synaptic GABA receptor in mammalian CNS, in "GABA in nervous
    system function" (Roberts, E., Chase, T.N. and Tower, D.B.
    eds.) pp. 305-317, Raven Press, New York.

GABA SYNTHESIS: ITS DYNAMICS IN RELATION

TO GLUTAMATE AND GLUTAMINE METABOLISM

Cees J. Van den Berg, Dugald F. Matheson, Mieke C.
Nijenmanting and Roel Bruntink

Studygroup Inborn Errors and Brain, Department of
Psychiatry, Faculty of Medicine, University of Groningen
Oostersingel 59, Groningen, The Netherlands

Since 1950 we know that the brains of mammals contain about
$2\mu mol/gram$ wet weight of γ-aminobutyrate (GABA), and very soon
afterwards it was shown that this GABA was formed from glutamate by
the action of glutamate decarboxylase (GAD) and degraded into
succinate by the combined action of γ-aminobutyrate transaminase
(GABAT) and succinic semialdehyde dehydrogenase. But, while since
the early fifties an enormous mass of data on GABA has been
published, there is still a considerable uncertainty on the precise
amounts of GABA formed during normal or abnormal conditions. Many
attempts have been made to measure the rate of synthesis or degradation of GABA, but in all those attempts assumptions had to be
made to arrive at an estimate of those rates.

In this paper we will review a number of published data related to this question, and present a number of still unpublished
data which may bring this whole question a bit further to a solution.
However, no definite solutions will be offered, the complexities of
the metabolic pathways of which GABA is a part are evidently such,
that it will be very difficult to find a simple, unique and definite
method for the measurement of the rate of GABA synthesis, or for
the measurement of changes in the rate of GABA synthesis, due to
natural or unnatural stimuli. Nevertheless, the analysis presented
may shed some light on current attempts to relate changes in GABA
metabolism to changes in brain function.

The cellular and subcellular localization of GAD and GABAT

Most of the GAD does occur in presynaptic nerve terminals:
this has been shown by density gradient fractionation studies

345

(Salganicoff & De Robertis, 1965; Van Kempen et al., 1965), by
direct visualization of GAD by immunocytochemical techniques
(McLaughlin et al., 1974) and by degeneration studies (Storm-
Mathisen, 1976). Those methods have also shown that some GAD does
occur in axons and the cell bodies of neurons of which those GAD
containing terminals form a part; but this amount of GAD is only
a small fraction of the total amount of GAD. While these enzyme
distribution studies cannot be used to establish the sites where
most of the GABA is synthesized, we will assume that most of the
GABA in the brain is indeed synthesized within GAD containing nerve
terminals, but it is well to realise that no convincing prove for
this assumption has been provided.

     Those GAD containing nerve-terminals contain little or no
GABAT; this follows from the results of studies with density
gradients, where GABAT containing mitochondria were found to sediment to higher densities than the GAD containing nerve-terminals
(Salganicoff & De Robertis, 1965; Van Kempen et al., 1965) and
from studies with cytochemical techniques at the electron microscopical level, in which very little GABAT could be seen in presynaptic
nerve-terminals (Hyde & Robinson, 1976). At a cruder level, histochemical studies have shown GABAT to be present in glia cells and
neuronal perikarya (Hyde and Robinson, 1974). It is therefore very
likely that most or all of the GABAT is located in neuronal and
glial structures, situated around GAD containing nerve-terminals;
and one may therefore assume that most or all of the GABA is
synthesized within GAD containing nerve-terminals, that this GABA
moves out of those terminals, possibly when action potentials arrive
in those terminals, and that this GABA, after having acted as an
inhibitory transmitter is taken up by structures surrounding those
sites of GABA action, where this GABA is then degraded by GABAT.
Some GABA may return to the presynaptic sites from which it
originated, but despite much speculation no definite prove for this
return of GABA (known as reuptake) has as yet been provided. We
also do not know whether GABA is only released when action potentials
arrive within the nerve-terminals: there may be spontaneous release.
We only know that the GABA which is synthesized and degraded, in
short, which shows "turnover", has to pass membranes to move from
the site (or sites) of synthesis to the site (or sites) where it is
degraded. And although one may assume that this GABA flux is
directly related to the rate of utilization of GABA as neurotransmitter, we should realise that no direct or indirect evidence
for this assumption is available.

Synthesis of GABA

     When labelled glucose is administered to experimental animals,
there is a very quick labelling of GABA and other amino acids in
the brain (Gaitonde et al., 1965; Cremer et al., 1978), indicating
a high rate of GABA synthesis. From those incorporation data

calculations of this rate have been made, assuming the label from glucose to arrive into GABA via pyruvate, acetyl-CoA, α-oxoglutarate and glutamate. Cremer and coworkers (Cremer et al., 1978) arrived at a figure of 0.76μmol/min. per gram wet weight; Costa and coworkers (Bertilsson et al., 1977) arrived at even higher figures for a number of brain regions of the rat. It is generally agreed that the rate of glucose utilization in the rat brain is about 0.8μmol/min. per gram wet weight, which results in a rate of acetyl-CoA utilization of about 1.6μmol/min. per gram wet weight. Comparing those values, it is evident that roughly 50% of acetyl-CoA entering the tricarboxylic acid cycle would be involved in GABA metabolism, or expressed in other terms that roughly 50% of the mitochondria would be involved in GABA synthesis and therefore be present within GAD containing nerve-terminals: an impossibly high number.

To arrive at these high values for the rate of synthesis of· GABA these authors assumed GABA to be formed from the total glutamate pool, the specific radioactivity of this pool being used to calculate the rate of GABA synthesis. If the specific radio-activity of the actual glutamate precursor pool of GABA was higher than the measured specific radioactivity of the total glutamate pool, the calculated rate of GABA synthesis would be lower in direct proportion to this higher specific radioactivity of the actual glutamate precursor pool of GABA. But, we cannot measure this pool directly; there is no way of isolating this pool, separate from all the other glutamate pools in the brain. Nevertheless, an estimate of the maximal specific radioactivity of a small glutamate pool, which could be the precursor pool of GABA, may be made, using the specific radioactivity of glucose and assuming this glucose to be converted into glutamate without dilution. Using the data of Cremer et al. (1978) one arrives at a figure of about 4 times that of the total glutamate pool. Using this number for the calculation of the rate of GABA synthesis, one then arrives at a number of about 0.19μmol/ min. per gram wet weight. How real is this value?

The rate of GABA synthesis obtained by GABAT inhibition

During normal steady-state conditions the rate of GABA synthesis will be the same as the rate of GABA degradation, provided no GABA leaves the brain. Assuming that all (or most) of the GABA is degraded by the transaminase pathway, inhibitors of GABAT may be used to obtain information on the rate of GABA degradation, and thus of GABA synthesis. A great many inhibitors of GABAT have been used: aminooxyacetic acid, cycloserine, gabaculine, γ-vinyl-GABA or γ-acetylenic-GABA. In Table 1 a number of rates of GABA accumulation in mice brain after injection of these inhibitors have been summarized.

It may be seen from Table 1 that the rates of GABA accumulation are all around 0.06μmol/min., only one being higher than 0.1μmol/min.

Table 1.   Rate of GABA synthesis in mice. Studies with GABAT-
           inhibitors

µmol/min. per gram wet wt.

AMINOOXYACETIC ACID		
25-50 mg/kg	0.02	Kuriyama et al. (1966)
	0.08	Van Gelder (1966)
	0.03	Löscher and Frey (1978)
	0.03-0.05	Wood and Peesker (1975)
	0.05-0.07	Van den Berg et al., unpublished
GABACULINE	0.03/0.08	Rando and Bangerter (1977); Matsui and Deguchi (1977)
γ-VINYL-GABA	0.11	Jung et al. (1977b)
γ-ACETYLENIC-GABA	0.07	Jung et al. (1977a)
CYCLOSERINE	0.05	Wood et al. (1978)

These values are considerably lower than 0.19µmol/min. calculated
on the basis of the highest possible specific radioactivity of
glutamate. What could be the source of this discrepancy? There may
be something wrong with the assumptions made in those calculations,
or on the other hand the GABAT inhibitors may inhibit GABA synthesis
besides many other reactions. There is indeed convincing evidence
that aminooxyacetic acid in vitro has powerful inhibitory actions
on a great many reactions (Berl et al., 1970; Starr, 1975).

It is widely believed that aminooxyacetic acid is inhibiting
besides GABAT many other reactions in the intact brain, but
surprisingly enough there is as yet no evidence to support this
believe. Accordingly, we studied the rate of incorporation of
labelled acetate and glucose into brain amino acids in animals given
aminooxyacetic acid (25 mg/kg) 60 min. earlier. The results presented
in Table 2 clearly show that there was no effect on the rate of
incorporation of both acetate and glucose into GABA, indicating that
the rate of synthesis of GABA was not affected. There was a decrease
in the rate of acetate and glucose incorporation into glutamine;
it should be of interest to know why.

While there was no effect at 60 min. after the administration
of AOAA, there were some effects in some experiments at earlier
times after the administration of AOAA. In one experiment we did
observe a decrease of about 25% in the incorporation of acetate
into GABA at 10 min. after the administration of AOAA (25 mg/kg)
but in another experiment no such decrease was noted. The striking
observation was that in the one experiment there was much less

Table 2.   Incorporation of $(2-^{14}C)$glucose or (^3H)acetate in a
10 min. period in mice given aminooxyacetic acid
(25 mg/kg) 60 min. earlier. GABA increased from 1.78
to 5.93 µmol/gram

| | dpm x 10^{-3} in amino acid/gram wet wt. | | | |
	glutamate	glutamine	aspartate	GABA
^3H-acetate				
Control	44+9	47+5	–	6.6+1.7
AOAA	42+6	35+6	–	5.8+0.5
$(2-^{14}C)$glucose				
Control	1045+99	225+9	227+21	82+8
AOAA	765+99	130+26	178+22	84+9

GABA accumulation than in the other experiment. Evidently, there
are some conditions where GAD may indeed be inhibited by AOAA
but we have no idea which conditions that are. We always use mice
from the same source; and the experiment with the low rate of GABA
accumulation was done with animals from the same group, as was the
experiment with a normal rate of GABA accumulation after AOAA,
and without an inhibition of the rate of GABA formation ascertained
by isotopic methods.

We conclude that AOAA gives rates of GABA accumulation of
about 0.06µmol/min.; it is unlikely that an inhibition of GABA
synthesis has played a measurable role in producing this low
number. But, we cannot exclude the possibility that AOAA has very
specific influences on the glutamate precursor pool of GABA, which
may have very special kinetic properties.

Excluding for the moment the possibility that AOAA gives an
underestimate of the rate of GABA synthesis in the brain, we will
have to ask whether there were still some hidden assumptions in the
calculations based on the isotope kinetic data.

A suggestion to solve the discrepancies between the rates of GABA
synthesis obtained by the labelling method and the GABAT-
inhibition method

The calculation of the rate of GABA synthesis from the
incorporation was based on the assumption that the labelled carbon
from glucose entered glutamate and GABA by the direct route via

acetyl-CoA, and that these amino acids were only labelled once.
By assuming glucose to label a small glutamate pool without
dilution, the rate of GABA formation could be brought down from
about 0.76μmol/min. to 0.19μmol/min., but this last number is still
higher than that observed with GABAT-inhibitors. Could the specific
radioactivity of the glutamate precursor pool still be higher?
There is one simple mechanism by which this could happen: if
pyruvate is carboxylated to oxaloacetate, there will be two pathways from glucose to glutamate/GABA; the maximal specific
radioactivity of the glutamate precursor pool of GABA will then
be even higher by a factor of about two and the corresponding rate
of GABA formation will be half that calculated earlier. If we make
these assumptions, the two procedures lead to roughly the same
rate of GABA synthesis, between 0.06 and 0.09μmol/min.

Carboxylation of pyruvate certainly does occur in the brain
(Berl et al., 1962, Salganicoff & Koeppe, 1968), we have however
no direct data on the role of this carboxylation reaction in the
synthesis of GABA, with one exception. Costa and coworkers
(Bertilsson and Costa, 1976, Bertilsson et al., 1977) have used
masspectophotometric methods to study the rate of incorporation of
(^{13}C)-glucose into glutamate and GABA. They have reported that
the GABA molecule was not doubly labelled; something which can be
ascertained easily with those methods. However, the enrichment of
^{13}C in GABA was around 4% in those experiments; the chances of
double labelling would therefore be less than 1%, not much above
the natural background. Analysis and identification of the
various mass-fragments of GABA, will certainly settle this question
in the future.

Although this analysis is somewhat hypothetical, it certainly
solves some discrepancies, and we hope that future experimentation
will bring this problem to a final solution. If this analysis is
correct, it does mean that there is within the GAD terminals a
highly active mechanism for the continuous synthesis of
tricarboxylic acid cycle intermediates, needed for the continuous
synthesis of GABA which leaves those terminals. In addition, it
does seem that there may be within those terminals very little
dilution of glucose, or: the overall concentration of glycolytic
and tricarboxylic acid cycle intermediates is very small. There
certainly is therefore a high dependency on the continuous
availability of glucose, it almost seems to be a very explosive
situation.

Sources of glutamate for GABA synthesis

Although we have argued that the glutamate which is converted
into GABA does originate directly from α-oxoglutarate from the
tricarboxylic acid cycle, there is much evidence that other
sources of glutamate may also be of importance. It is well known

that labelled glutamine injected into the brain is rapidly converted into glutamate and GABA (Berl et al., 1961). Brain slices or crude synaptosomal preparations do also convert rapidly added glutamine into GABA (Reubi et al., 1978, Tapia and González, 1978, Bradford et al., 1978). As most or all of the glutamine synthase is present in astroglia cells (Nörenberg and Martinez-Hernandez, 1979) these data in combination with earlier schemes of glutamate comparti-mentation have led to the suggestion that this movement of glutamine from the astroglia cells is of great importance for the continuous supply of glutamate for GABA synthesis (Van den Berg and Garfinkel, 1971, Van den Berg et al., 1978).

Although it is currently generally assumed that the carbon-skeletons of GABA, glutamate and glutamine may move hence and forwards between nerve-terminals and surrounding neuronal or glia structures, most of the evidence provided is still very indirect; we have therefore tried to find more direct evidence. The in vivo study of movements of small molecules between cells is of course extremely difficult, but in some instances isotopes may offer unusual opportunities. In our earlier studies in this area we used the fact that the fate of a particularly labelled carbon is dependent in its position; this allowed us to establish with a fairly great deal of certainty that glutamine was synthesized at another cellular site than where it was degraded, moving very likely from one site (later shown to be the astroglia cells) to a site -among others- where GABA is made (Van den Berg et al., 1969, Van den Berg and Garfinkel, 1971). But, the evidence provided was highly indirect.

We will now present a few data which take this analysis a small step further. We have used doubly labelled glutamine and GABA, both compounds labelled with ^{14}C and ^3H. When these two amino acids are metabolised, α-oxoglutarate and succinate are formed respectively. During the further metabolism of these two tricarboxylic acid cycle intermediates tritium will be lost at a number of steps, while a fair amount of the labelled carbon (present in all carbon atoms of these two intermediates) will be retained and eventually arrive via α-oxoglutarate into glutamate. From this glutamate GABA and/or glutamine may be formed again. Therefore if the carbon skeletons of GABA and glutamine move around, this will show itself in a decrease of the (^3H, ^{14}C) ratio of the GABA and glutamine isolated after various times from the brain. This we did in fact observe (Table 3).

These data are entirely consistent with the schemes proposing the movements of these carbon-skeletons, but it should be realised that they do not settle this question for once and all. The data show that the carbon skeleton of GABA is again used for the synthesis of GABA, following a route which passes through a large segment of a tricarboxylic acid cycle, but they do not prove that

Table 4.   The fate of $(^3H,U-^{14}C)$-glutamine after intracerebral injection in mice

		$(^3H)/(^{14}C)$-ratio			
Time (min.)	n	glutamine	glutamate	GABA	"GABA" [x)
5	6	1.02+0.01	0.93+0.02	1.11+0.11	(0.89)
10	7	0.90+0.02	0.74+0.02	0.88+0.10	(0.70)
15	3	0.88+0.01	0.71+0.02	0.89+0.02	(0.71)
20	5	0.83+0.004	0.64+0.02	0.85 (1)	(0.68)

[x) corrected with factor 0.8 for loss one C-atom

Having brought the story of the sources of glutamate for GABA synthesis a little further, the data given by no means tell us something about the quantitative importance of those sources of glutamate coming from structures situated around the GAD nerve-terminals.

Ammonia and GABA synthesis

Some years ago we published a small note (Matheson and Van den Berg, 1975, for review: Van den Berg et al., 1978) showing that the acute administration of ammonium chloride to mice resulted in a quick rise of brain glutamine. This increase of glutamine was the direct result of an inhibition of glutamine degradation, rather than of an increased rate of glutamine synthesis as commonly assumed. This led us to study the effect of acute ammonium chloride administration on the rate of incorporation of a variety of labelled precursors into GABA.We did indeed observe a striking decrease of the rate of labelled acetate and not of 3-hydroxybutyrate incorporation into GABA (Table 5). Those data strongly suggest that the conversion of glutamine into GABA may indeed be of some quantitative importance; it may even be that the toxic effects of ammonia may be the direct result of an inhibition of GABA synthesis. There is however one disturbing observation: we never found a decrease in GABA levels (Table 6). In a few experiments a small decrease was observed, but when extending the series of experiments to more than 40 animals, it became very clear that no decrease of GABA did occur, despite an inhibition of about 30% of the rate of (^3H)-acetate incorporation!

Table 3.   Recycling of the carbon skeletons of GABA and glutamine: $(2,3-{}^3H, U-{}^{14}C)$-GABA and $(3,4-{}^3H, U-{}^{14}C)$-glutamine were injected directly into the brain.

Time (min.)	GABA exp. $({}^3H)/({}^{14}C)$ in GABA	Glutamine exp. $({}^3H)/({}^{14}C)$ in glutamine
0	1.0	1.0
5	1.0(.005)	1.02
10	0.96(.019)	0.90
15	–	0.88
20	0.87(.005)	0.83
40	0.79(.06)	–

this is a closed circle, ie. we do not know whether the carbon-skeletons of a particular GABA pool do return to the same GABA pool. Such a proposition would be very difficult to prove, and may be very unlikely. Nevertheless, these data provide convincing evidence for the reutilization of degradation products of GABA for the resynthesis of GABA.

In most schemes of glutamate compartmentation, it is assumed that glutamine as the main degradation product moves from the astroglia cells to the GAD containing nerve-terminals. The evidence available comes partly from isotope kinetic studies and more recently from studies with isolated systems in which glutamine is indeed easily converted into GABA. But, direct prove that glutamine is moving is still not available. When one looks at the kinetics of $({}^3H, {}^{14}C)$ incorporation in amino acids, after the administration of labelled glutamine directly into the brain (Table 4), one can see that indeed GABA is rapidly labelled, but the time course of the $({}^3H, {}^{14}C)$ ratio's do not allow us to distinguish between glutamate or glutamine as the compound moving; they do however suggest that the glutamine is converted to glutamate at a site where this glutamate is directly related to α-oxoglutarate as a tricarboxylic acid cycle intermediate. This follows from the loss of tritium observed. As indeed most or all of the glutaminase in brain is mitochondrial, this proposition is in no way unexpected. But, we should realise that these data do not show that it is the glutaminase located in GAD containing nerve-terminals which is responsible for the formation of the glutamate precursor pool of GABA; it is still possible that the formation of glutamate from glutamine takes place elsewhere and that it is this glutamate which moves from those sites to the GAD containing nerve-terminals. A much more detailed kinetic analysis is required to settle this question.

Table 5.   Effect ammonia chloride administration on
           acetate and 3-hydroxybutyrate incorporation

dpm. 10^{-3}/100 mg protein/6 min.

		glutamate	glutamine	GABA
(3-^{14}C)-3-hydroxybutyrate				
Contr.	n=3	191+13	50+1	8.5+0.8
NH4Cl		180+12	61+6	8.3+1.3
(^{3}H)-acetate				
Contr.	n=6	34+10	56+16	5.0+0.7
NH4Cl		26+3	70+12	3.7+0.2 *

* $p < 0.05$

Table 6.   Ammonia and amino acid levels (μmol/gr. wet wt.)
           in mice brain. Averages $\pm$ SD (number of animals)

	Control	NH4Cl 7 mmol/kg, 5 min.	sign.
glutamate	11.41+1.73(49)	10.69+1.32(30)	–
aspartate	3.43+0.54(54)	3.05+0.51(42)	$p < 0.01$
glutamine	4.11+0.74(51)	5.17+1.01(43)	$p < 0.01$
GABA	1.61+0.26(74)	1.56+0.24(47)	–
Σ α-N	18.61+2.23(43)	19.08+2.13(40)	–

Concluding remarks

        Despite the enormous volume of data on the kinetics of amino
acid metabolism in the intact brain, or in isolated preparations,
there are still considerable problems in defining in very precise
terms the kinetics of the glutamate precursor pool of GABA; and
therefore exact estimates of the rate of GABA synthesis and of
changes in this rate due to experimental procedures cannot be made.
There is no doubt that the glutamate precursor pool of GABA has
some very unique properties; on one hand it is quickly labelled
from glucose, presumably with very little dilution and presumably
inside the GAD terminals (although this by no means proven), on
the other hand there is no doubt that compounds from structures
surrounding the GAD terminals move into those terminals to form
glutamate (see also Shank and Aprison, 1981).

But, are those compounds needed? Does ammonia exert its toxic action by an interruption of this source of glutamate? It may, but a definite proof has still to be given.

REFERENCES

Berl, S., Clarke, D. D., and Nicklas, W. J., 1970, Compartmentation of citric acid cycle metabolism in brain; effect of amino-oxyacetic acid, ouabain, and Ca^{++} on the labelling of glutamate, glutamine, aspartate, and GABA by (1-^{14}C)acetate, (U-^{14}C)-aspartate, J. Neurochem., 17: 999-1007.

Berl, S., Lajtha, A., and Waelsch, H., 1961, Amino acid and protein metabolism. VI Cerebral compartments of glutamic acid metabolism, J. Neurochem., 7: 186-197.

Berl, S., Takagaki, G., Clarke, D. D., and Waelsch, H., 1962, Carbon dioxide fixation in the brain, J. biol. Chem., 237: 2570-2573.

Bertilsson, L., and Costa, E., 1976, Mass fragmentographic quantitation of glutamic acid and γ-aminobutyric acid in cerebellar nuclei and sympathetic ganglion of rats, J. Chromatogr., 118: 395-402.

Bertilsson, L., Mao, C. C., and Costa, E., 1977, Application of principles of steady-state kinetics to the estimation of γ-aminobutyric acid turnover rate in nuclei of rat brain, J. Pharmacol. Exp. Ther., 200: 277-284.

Bradford, H. F., Ward, H. K., and Thomas, A. J., 1978, Glutamine - a major substrate for nerve endings, J. Neurochem., 30: 1453-1459.

Cremer, J. E., Sarna, G. S., Teal, H. M., and Cunningham, V. J., 1978, Amino acid precursors: their transport into brain and initial metabolism, in: "Amino Acids as Chemical Transmitters", F. Fonnum, ed., Plenum Press, New York, 669-689.

Gaitonde, M. K., Dahl, D. R., and Elliot, K. A. C., 1965, Entry of glucose carbon into amino acids of rat brain and liver in vivo after injection of uniformly ^{14}C-labelled glucose, Biochem. J., 94: 345-352.

Hyde, J. C., and Robinson, N., 1974, Appearance of γ-aminobutyrate transaminase activity in developing rat brain, J. Neurochem., 23: 365-367.

Hyde, J. C., and Robinson, N., 1976, Electron cytochemical localization of γ-aminobutyric acid catabolism in rat cerebellar cortex, Histochem., 49: 51-65.

Jung, M. J., Lippert, B., Metcalf, B. W., Schechter, P. J., Böhlen, P., and Sjoerdsma, A., 1977a, The effect of 4-amino hex-5-ynoic acid (γ-acetylenic GABA, γ-ethynyl GABA) a

Part of this investigation was supported by grants from FUNGO, Promeso and TNO-GO (Cleo).

catalytic inhibitor of GABA transaminase, on brain GABA
metabolism in vivo, J. Neurochem., 28: 717-723.

Jung, M. J., Lippert, B., Metcalf, B. W., Böhlen, P., and Schechter,
P. J., 1977b, γ-vinyl GABA (4-amino-hex-5-enoic acid), a
new selective irreversible inhibitor of GABA-T: Effects on
brain GABA metabolism in mice, J. Neurochem., 29: 797-802.

Kuriyama, K., Roberts, E., and Rubinstein, M. K., 1966, Elevation
of γ-aminobutyric acid in brain with aminooxyacetic acid and
susceptibility to convulsive seizures in mice: A quantitative
re-evaluation, Biochem. Pharmacol., 15: 221-236.

Löscher, W., and Frey, H. H., 1978, Aminooxyacetic acid: correlation
between biochemical effects, anticonvulsant action and toxicity
in mice, Biochem. Pharmacol., 27: 103-108.

Matheson, D. F., and Van den Berg, C. J., 1975, Ammonia and brain
glutamine: Inhibition of glutamine degradation by ammonia,
Biochem. Soc. Trans., 3: 525-528.

Matsui, Y., and Deguchi, T., Effects of GABAculine, a new
potent inhibitor of γ-aminobutyrate transaminase, on the brain
γ-aminobutyrate content and convulsion in mice, Life Sci.,
20: 1291-1296.

McLaughlin, B. J., Wood, J. G., Saito, K., Barber, R., Vaughn, J.
E., Roberts, E., and Wu, J. Y., 1974, The fine structural
localization of glutamate decarboxylase in synaptic terminals
of rodent cerebellum, Brain Res., 76: 377-391.

Norenberg, M. D., and Martinez-Hernandez, A., 1979, Fine structural
localization of glutamine synthetase in astrocytes of rat
brain, Brain Res., 161: 303-310.

Rando, R. R., and Bangerter, F. W., 1977, The in vivo inhibition
of GABA transaminase by GABAculine, Biochem. Biophys. Res.
Comm., 76: 1276-1281.

Reubi, J. C., Van den Berg, C. J., and Cuénod, M., 1978, Glutamine
as precursor for the GABA and glutamate transmitter pools,
Neuroscience Lett., 10: 171-174.

Salganicoff, L., and De Robertis, E., 1965, Subcellular distribution
of the enzymes of the glutamic acid, glutamine and γ-aminobutyric acid cycles in rat brain, J. Neurochem., 12: 287-309.

Salganicoff, L., and Koeppe, R. E., 1968, Subcellular distribution
of pyruvate carboxylase-diphosphopyridine nucleoticle and
triphosphopyridine nucleotode isocitrate dekydrogenase and
malate enzyme in rat brain, J. biol. Chem., 243: 3416-3420.

Shank, R. P., and Aprison, M. H., 1981, Present status and
significance of the glutamine cycle in neural tissue, Life
Sci., 28: 837-842.

Starr, M. S., 1975, Effects of metabolic inhibitors on amino acid
metabolism in rat retina: a comparison of aminooxyacetic
acid and ethanolamine-o-sulphate, J. Neurochem., 24: 122 -
1236.

Storm-Mathisen, J., 1976, Distribution of the components of the
GABA system in neuronal tissue: Cerebellum and Hippocampus -
Effects of Axotomy, in: "GABA in Nervous System Function",

E. Roberts, T. N. Chase and D. B. Tower, eds., Raven Press, New York, 149-168.

Tapia, R., and González, R. M., 1978, Glutamine and glutamate as precursors of the releasable pool of GABA in brain cortex slices, Neuroscience Lett., 10: 165-169.

Van den Berg, C. J., and Garfinkel, D., 1971, A simulation study of brain compartments: metabolism of glutamate and related substances in mouse brain, Biochem. J., 123: 211-218.

Van den Berg, C. J., Kržalic, Lj., Mela, P., and Waelsch, H., 1969, Compartmentation of glutamate metabolism in brain. Evidence for the existence of two different tricarboxylic acid cycles in brain, Biochem. J., 113: 281-290.

Van den Berg, C. J., Matheson, D. F., and Nijenmanting, W. C., 1978, Compartmentation of amino acids in brain: The GABA glutamine-glutamate cycle, in: "Amino Acids as Chemical Transmitters", F. Fonnum, ed., Plenum Press, New York, 709-723.

Van Gelder, N. M., 1966, The effect of aminooxyacetic acid on the metabolism of γ-aminobutyric acid in brain, Biochem. Pharmacol., 15: 533-539.

Van Kempen, G. M. J., Van den Berg, C. J., Van der Helm, H. J., and Veldstra, H., 1965, Intracellular localization of glutamate decarboxylase, γ-aminobutyrate transaminase and some other enzymes in brain tissue, J. Neurochem., 12: 581-588.

Wood, J. D., and Peesker, S. J., 1975, Anticonvulstant action of GABA-elevating agents: a re-evaluation, J. Neurochem., 28: 277-282.

Wood, J. D., Peesker, S. J., Gorechi, D. K., and Tsui, D., 1978, Effect of L-cycloserine on brain GABA metabolism, Can. J. Physiol. Pharmacol., 56: 62-68.

METABOLIC AND TRANSMITTER COMPARTMENTS FOR GLUTAMATE

A. Hamberger, I. Jacobsson, S.-O. Molin,
B. Nyström, M. Sandberg and U. Ungerstedt*

Institute of Neurobiology
U. of Göteborg, S-400 33 Göteborg, Sweden
*Karolinska Institutet
S-104 01 Stockholm, Sweden

Undoubtedly, the traditional concept of metabolic compartmentation as a means to understand certain aspects of amino acid-mediated
neurotransmission is excellently complemented by the results of
other approaches, as recent developments of agonists, antagonists
and analysis of membrane-binding sites have turned out to be promising and well suited to bridge gaps between neurochemistry and neuro-
physiology/neuropharmacology. The expanding mapping of an almost
daily increasing number of neuroactive substances is another factor
which adds to a more and more intricate pattern for neuronal communication in which the traditional putative amino acid transmitters
are to fit in. Although their role as "true" transmitters is still
debated, the formation of amino acids with excitatory and inhibitory
effects from basic respiratory fuels or from other amino acids seems
to be tightly regulated by fluxes of ions and other small molecules
between adjacent cells. The importance of neuron-glia interactions
at the perikaryal, axonal and nerve terminal level consequently can
not be stressed enough.

The theme of this chapter is to consider first one of the criteria for neurotransmission which is suitable for a biochemical
approach, the evoked release in vitro and in vivo. Secondly, to
describe the modulation of particularly glutamate secretion in vitro
by pathophysiological concentrations of ammonium ions and its possible relationship to neuron-glia interactions. Thirdly, to exemplify
neurochemical differences between normal and lesioned tissue, in
which the reduction of specific nerve terminals may provide information on transmitters, but where also glial cells play a role, as
neuronal degeneration induces glial proliferation which, in turn,
may provide signals for induction of neuronal plasticity.

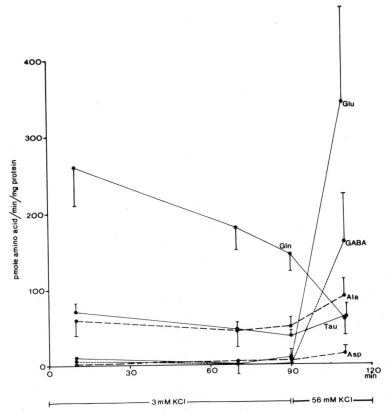

Fig. 1 "Spontaneous" and $|K^+|$-evoked efflux of endogenous amino acids from tissue slices prepared from the rat hippocampus. The slices (0.3 mg protein) were perfused in a closed perspex chamber at 0.2 ml/min and 37°. The tissue was equilibrating in the chamber for one hr before the beginning of the analyses. The medium was standard Krebs-Ringer bicarbonate, 10 mM glucose, 1.2 mM $CaCl_2$. The high $|K^+|$ medium contained 56 mM potassium chloride with a corresponding reduction in sodium chloride. Media were gassed with 95 % O_2 /5 % CO_2 and the pH kept at 7.4. The amino acid content in the perfusates was measured with high performance liquid chromatography after precolumn derivatization with O-phthaldialdehyde. Means of four experiments, the bars indicate S.E.

RELEASE OF NEUROTRANSMITTER AMINO ACIDS <u>IN VITRO</u> AND <u>IN VIVO</u>

     The release of substances with neurotransmitter or neuromodulator characteristics is generally investigated <u>in vitro</u> with tissue-slices or with more intact preparations as the isolated retina. Fractions, consisting mainly of nerve endings, Ca-dependency or tetrodotoxin sensitivity in the case of slices are employed to

ascertain that nerve terminals are the origins of the compounds released during depolarization evoked electrically or chemically, particularly with potassium or veratridine (cf. DeFeudis, 1975; Fonnum,
1978; Di Chiara and Gessa, 1981). Even the well oxygenated and
temperature-controlled tissue slice, maintained in isotonic conditions, is affected in many ways, so the final results of a release
experiment are dependent on the state of retention and uptake system
of cells.

The requirement of increasing sensitivity on the analytical side
has been met remarkably well, mainly due to the recent development
of high performance liquid chromatography techniques. Catecholamines
and amino acids are rapidly and conveniently measured at subpicomol
levels (Keller et al., 1976; Lindroth and Mopper, 1979; Mell,1979).

Fig. 1 shows the results of a typical tissue-slice experiment.
The rat hippocampus was chosen, because an extensive literature suggests that amino acids play important roles as neurotransmitters in
this region (Crawford and Connor, 1973; Storm-Mathisen, 1977;
Nadler et al., 1978). Following an equilibration period of tissue
perfusion with Krebs-Ringer bicarbonate medium, the slice was depolarized with a medium containing 56 mM potassium chloride. The evoked
release of particularly glutamate and GABA is largely Ca-dependent.
The more physiological, specific nerve tract stimulation is usually
less "effective" when the ratio stimulated/resting release is concerned (Bradford and Richards, 1976). The present system, in which
the bathing medium is continuously renewed, is often chosen because
the secretion from the tissue can be monitored with time, and reuptake phenomena are reduced. A disadvantage is the continuous loss
of substances from the tissue-slice, since resynthesis often occurs
to an insufficient extent. In order to overcome the problem, studies
on tissue-slices may be carried out with incubation in a constant
amount of medium, but then the time course of events are difficult
to assess. The more or less established transmitter amino acids,
glutamic acid, GABA and aspartic acid (Fig. 1) were secreted at very
low concentrations when the tissue is perfused with normal Krebs-
Ringer bicarbonate medium (the tissue content of glutamate and GABA
was higher than that of any other amino acid even in perfused slices
and was at 75 - 80 % of the preperfusion level). K^+-depolarization
had a dramatic effect on glutamic acid and GABA efflux. Other amino
acids, as glutamine, taurine and alanine, had a high "spontaneous"
efflux and little effect was seen during tissue depolarization. The
efflux of glutamine decreased somewhat during tissue depolarization
(Benjamin et al., 1980) while taurine secretion was slightly stimulated. The tissue contents of glutamine and taurine were, however,
greatly reduced during the perfusion period (down to 10 - 20 % of
preperfusion levels).

A further step towards evidence of true physiological activity
is to perform similar release experiments in vivo, using the freely

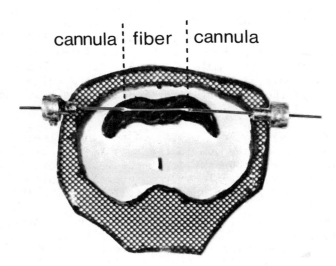

cannula | fiber | cannula

Fig.2 Frontal sec-
tion through the
skull and brain of
the rabbit approxi-
mately 4 mm behind
the intersection of
the sagittal and co-
ronal sutures. The
hippocampus is mar-
ked black. Holders
for cannulas are
fastened to the
skull with dental
cement. The hollow
fiber, to a length
of 10 mm, is glued
into cannulas and
inserted into the
hippocampal tissue.

moving, unanaesthetized animal. This is done by perfusion of brain,
either by application of cups to a specific surface area or by in-
serting push-pull cannulas into the desired region (Iversen et al.,
1971; Clark and Collins, 1976; van den Heyden et al., 1979;
Coutinho-Netto et al., 1980; Gauchy et al., 1980). In the present
work, the corresponding in vivo perfusion experiment employed the
method of Ungerstedt et al. (in press) which uses the principle of
brain dialysis.

     In order to withdraw only the few picomoles of amino acid which
are required for analysis, the hippocampus was perfused with a
closed system. A Diaflo hollow fiber (Amicon H 1 x 50, M.W. cut-off
50,000) was implanted. The fiber in the present study had a length
of 10 mm and an outer diameter of approximately 0.3 mm. It was connected to 0.7 mm steel cannulas which were attached to the skull
bone at a level 4 mm behind the intersection of the sagittal and
coronal sutures, as shown in Fig. 2. The hippocampus was then perfused at 2.5 µl/min with the Krebs-Ringer bicarbonate medium, and
5-10 min samples were collected for analysis of amino acids with
HPLC. Model experiments show that the fluid which has passed through
the dialysis tubing at this rate contains the amino acids at 15-20 %
of the concentration outside, with small difference between individual amino acids. Fig. 3 shows a histological section through the
hippocampus from a rabbit 8 days after the implantation of the fiber.
The fiber appears to take well to the tissue, it induced a certain
"endothelialization" and a moderate gliosis (Fig. 4). A few granular
cells are seen in the meshes of the fiber. Small bleedings can be
observed along the fiber. In addition to the advantage of a minimal

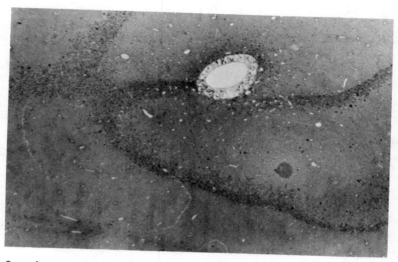

Fig. 3 Section of the hippocampus containing the hollow fiber (outer diameter 0.3 mm). Eight days after implantation, perfusion fixation with glutaraldehyde, plastic embedded, 1 µm section. Richardson's staining.

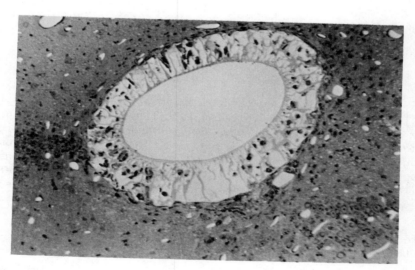

Fig. 4 Hollow fiber in the hippocampus at higher magnification (same section as Fig. 3). The fiber pores contain a few granular cells. The tissue shows a moderate gliosis and an "endothelialization" around the fiber.

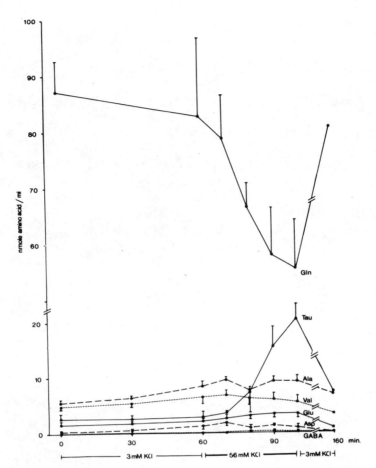

Fig. 5. Concentration of endogenous amino acids in perfusates from the hollow fiber implanted into the rabbit hippocampus 15 hr prior to the experiment. The fiber was perfused with Krebs-Ringer bicarbonate medium at a rate of 2.5 µl/min. The high |K⁺| medium which was introduced for 40 min contained 56 mM potassium chloride and had a corresponding reduction in sodium chloride. The amino acids were quantitated with high performance liquid chromatography as described.

interference with tissue fluids, the fiber appears to be less traumatic than push-pull cannulas and more versatile than surface cups.

The present perfusion experiments were performed when the animal was recovered for 15 hours after the fiber implantation. It was then unanaesthetized and freely moving. Fig. 5 shows the concentrations of endogenous amino acids when the rabbit hippocampus was perfused with normal Krebs-Ringer bicarbonate medium. The most striking observation in the steady state situation was the very high glutamine concentration. Alanine and valine were at intermediate concentration, followed by taurine and glutamate. Aspartate was very low and GABA hardly measurable. Small changes occurred with time over 3 - 4 hours, indicating that an actual steady state level was monitored in contrast to the situation in the in vitro experiment. The change to a 56 mM K^+ medium (Fig. 5) had an effect which differed quite strikingly from that of the in vitro experiment: A small increase in glutamate and GABA concentrations was seen while the increase in taurine release was 7 - 8 times. Although not easily observed in the figure, taurine levels started to increase one ten min fraction after the small increase in glutamic acid efflux. A similar delay in the evoked efflux of taurine has recently been reported in work with the rat retina where the release profiles of ^3H-taurine and ^3H-glycine were compared (Pycock and Smith, 1980). The effect by K^+ on the glutamine concentration was in principle similar to that seen in vitro, but the decrease in glutamine was here the quantitatively dominating change. All effects were rapidly (within 1 hour) reversible upon return to the normal medium.

An advantage of the dialysis fiber system is that the actual concentrations of amino acids in the extracellular space can be calculated from data in model experiments with known amino acid concentrations in the surrounding medium. The results from a series of experiments were thus calculated and compared with those for tissue amino acids and CSF amino acids (human, McGale et al., 1977). The calculated amino acid concentration in the extracellular space surrounding the fiber compared remarkably well with that for CSF (Fig. 6). The possibility that the similarity with the CSF profile could be due to the formation of a channel from the ventricles is contradicted by the morphological appearance of the fiber and the unlikeliness that a K^+ pulse would change the concentrations of amino acids in the CSF.

Consequently the concentration of glutamine appears to be in the range of 0.5 mM in the extracellular space, as assumed in a number of in vitro studies aiming at employing physiological glutamine concentrations in the incubation media (Bradford and Ward, 1976; Hamberger et al., 1979). The retention of glutamine brought about in vitro in the presence of high K^+ is not really comparable with the in vitro situation (Fig. 1) since decreasing glutamine concentrations in the in vitro perfusates there essentially reflect the depleted tissue pools, due to the questionable uptake affinity constants for glutamine (Weiler et al., 1979). A better parallel to the in vivo experiment are studies such as those of Benjamin et al. (1980) in which the tissue is incubated in a small and constant amount of medium with different K^+ concentrations. The ability of K^+ to retain glutamine in the tissue is apparently not present in nerve endings (Benjamin et al., 1980) and may represent a direct effect on astrocytic glial cells.

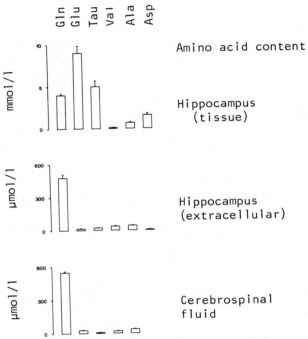

Fig. 6 Amino acid concentration of the freshly dissected rat hippocampus tissue (top), the extracellular space surrounding the hollow
fiber in the rabbit hippocampus (middle) and human cerebrospinal
fluid x) (bottom). x) Data from McGale et al. (1977).

        The strong decrease in glutamine secretion is in disagreement
with observations of an electrically or K^+ evoked increase in glutamine efflux (Clark and Collins, 1976; Abdul-Ghani et al., 1979).
Preliminary experiments in our laboratory have shown a biphasic
effect of veratridine on glutamine efflux, _i.e._ initial stimulation
followed by inhibition. This could be explained by an immediate
release of glutamine from the small pool in nerve terminals, followed
by a retention effect on the large glutamine pool in the glia. The
high glutamine content in the extracellular fluid appears to support
the proposed role of glutamine as a direct precursor of particularly
synaptically released GABA and glutamate (Bradford and Ward, 1976;
Cotman and Hamberger, 1978; Gauchy et al., 1980). The importance
of the extracellular glutamine pool is, however, still not well
established. It is easy to focus on the brain-glutamine relation and

forget that glutamine as such is regulated by similar mechanisms and is present in as high concentrations in most organs of the body, above all in skeletal muscle (cf. Mora and Palacios, 1980).

The direct application of KCl to the tissue surrounding the fiber is likely to stimulate most types of cells leading to the release of both excitatory and inhibitory amino acids. The placement of the fiber within the hippocampus may influence for example the relative recovery of the evoked release of glutamate and GABA in view of distinct distribution patterns demonstrated autoradiographically with the uptake of radiolabelled amino acids (Storm-Mathisen, 1977). Undoubtedly, several different areas of the hippocampus at a given level are perfused with a 10 mm long fiber. The K^+ stimulated release of glutamate and GABA in vivo appears negligible in Fig. 5, but represents a 2 - 3 fold increase above the resting level. The effect varied little between the present experiments or with experiments performed immediately after fiber implantation or with the fiber in the caudal part of the hippocampus. The ratio resting/stimulated release of endogenous glutamate and GABA efflux compares relatively well with results of in vivo studies employing surface cups or push-pull cannulas (Clark and Collins, 1976; Abdul-Ghani et al., 1979). The evoked efflux of exogenous transmitters is, however, often more impressive (Iversen et al., 1971; Gauchy et al., 1980).

Taurine has been placed beside GABA as an inhibitory transmitter, and occurs in high concentrations throughout the nervous system (cf. Rassin, 1981). It is released in vivo in response to K^+ stimulation (Clark and Collins, 1971; Davidson, 1979), but failure to release taurine with elevated K^+ has also been reported. Taurine has raised many questions, it is accumulated by both glia and neurons but its uptake systems display low capacities (Richelson and Thompson 1973; Schrier and Thompson, 1974). The present results tend to support the impression that the effect of taurine is a slowly appearing, long lasting inhibition or membrane stabilization when the tissue undergoes hyperexcitation (Gruener et al., 1975; Collins, 1977). An interdependence of taurine-glutamate-glutamine is indicated by a series of studies by Van Gelder (cf. Van Gelder, 1981): Hyperexcitation of the cerebral cortex may be a consequence of a release of glutamic acid in excess of what can be accumulated by glia and there transformed to glutamine. Cerebral taurine seems to influence such release of glutamate. This is the background to the successful treatment of certain types of epilepsy with taurine. It is therefore possible that a situation of tissue management of a K^+-induced hippocampal epilepsy is illustrated by Fig. 5.

TRANSMITTER GLUTAMATE DURING HYPERAMMONEMIA

The extensive literature on the pathogenesis of hepatic encephalopathy contains suggestions that a consequence of excess ammonia could be a depletion of the "transmitter pool" of glutamic acid (review: Conn and Lieberthal, 1979). The glutamic acid concentration is, however, not reduced when measured in total brain in different types of experimental hepatic coma (Williams et al., 1972). The apparently only resource for ammonia removal in the brain, the α-ketoglutarate-glutamate-glutamine pathway, results in one of the main characteristics of the patient with hepatic encephalopathy: the several - fold elevation of glutamine in the CSF (and the brain), the ammonia being recovered in the amide group of glutamine (Cooper et al., 1979). If glutamine, even at high concentrations, is harmless to brain membranes, the excess glutamine would correct for a low "transmitter glutamate" pool, as glutaminase is predominantly localized to nerve endings (Salganicoff and De Robertis, 1965; Bradford and Ward, 1975). An ammonia-induced depletion of glutamate due to accelerated glutamine formation would, on the other hand, affect mainly astrocytic glia, since glutamine synthetase appears exclusively localized in these cells (Norenberg and Martinez-Hernandez, 1979). The characteristic neuropathological feature in hyperammonemia is actually the hypertrophy of astrocytic glial cells (Cole et al., 1972).

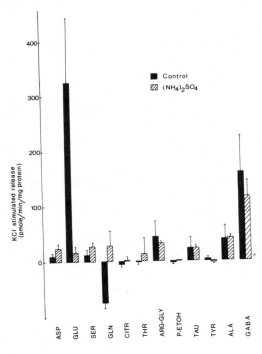

Fig. 7 Effect of 60 min perfusion with Krebs-Ringer bicarbonate medium containing 3 mM $(NH_4)_2 SO_4$ on the release of endogenous amino acids subsequently evoked with a 56 mM KCl medium. Slices from the rat hippocampus were perfused as described in legend to Fig. 1. The control tissue was perfused with normal medium and both control and ammonium perfused tissues were depolarized simultaneously with KCl.

The hyperammonemic state consequently appears ideal for the
purpose to gain insight into the effects of a competition between
nerve terminals and glia for the newly formed glutamate in a situation where the utilization of glutamine appears inhibited by several factors. Our aim was to correlate some biochemical data to the
clinical features of this type of hepatic failure which are hyperexcitation followed by coma. The best established physiological effect of ammonia so far is the inhibition of the chloride pump in
postsynaptic neuronal membranes which can increase neuronal excitability (Lux et al., 1970; Iles and Jack, 1978). The present results
are interpreted to indicate that the coma state which follows the
hyperexcitation is caused by a reduction of the pool of transmitter
glutamate, in agreement with previous suggestions by Bradford (1978).

The hippocampal tissue-slice preparation is, as discussed
above, ideal for in vitro studies on amino acid transmitter candidates. As shown (Fig. 1), the perfusion of tissue slices with a
medium containing 56 mM KCl causes a significant increase in the
release of particularly endogenous glutamate and GABA which is largely Ca-dependent and essentially in agreement with results obtained
with certain other regions, such as olfactory cortex (Collins et al.,
1981). The introduction of 3 mM $(NH_4)_2 SO_4$ into the standard Krebs-
Ringer bicarbonate medium had no effect on any amino acid but glutamate, the secretion of which increased slowly after a latency of 30
- 40 min which differs considerably from the prompt responses seen
with K^+-depolarization. The second observation, shown in Fig. 7, is
that K^+-depolarization, given after one hour of tissue perfusion
with 3 mM $(NH_4)_2 SO_4$, failed to evoke a release of glutamate while
the evoked release of GABA and the pattern of other amino acids
appeared unaffected. The tissue content of amino acids was not affected by perfusion with ammonia containing media, compared to with
control media. The glutamate/GABA balance in the extracellular space

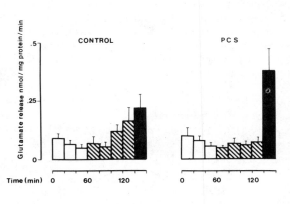

Fig. 8   Effects of per-
fusion of tissue slices
from the rat hippocampus
with ammonium chloride on
the subsequently evoked
release of glutamic acid
with 56 mM KCl. Compari-
son of tissue from con-
trol and porta-cava-
shunted (PCS) rats.

☐ = normal Krebs-Ringer
    bicarbonate medium.
▨ = + 3 mM NH_4Cl.
■ = + 3 mM NH_4Cl + 56
    mM KCl.

was thus pushed far in favor of GABA during tissue stimulation, which may offer an explanation to the coma state in vivo. A possible cause to the unaffected GABA release is that glutamic acid (a potent inhibitor of glutaminase), most likely is lower in GABAergic terminals than even in fairly "depleted" glutamatergic terminals.

It is thus apparent that the nerve terminal glutaminase is flooded with its substrate in hyperammonemia and hypothetically low in one of its inhibitors: glutamate. If the transmitter pool of glutamate is depleted or reduced, this must be caused by other factors, influencing either the transport of glutamine over the membrane of the nerve terminal, or inhibiting intraterminal glutaminase. The most obvious inhibitors of the enzyme is the ammonium ion (Bradford and Ward, 1975). The glutaminase in nerve endings appears to be exclusively of the phosphate-activated type (Svenneby, 1971). The phosphate-activated glutaminase is also stimulated by calcium ions (Benjamin, 1981), an effect which may be direct or via changing enzyme controlling factors. The close interdependence between phosphate and calcium homeostasis in the body may indicate that a role of calcium is to regulate phosphate availability to glutaminase. Calcium ions may also influence glutamate distribution in both tissue slices and homogenates since the depolarization-evoked glutamate release is Ca-dependent (White et al., 1977). Phosphate-depletion is another possibility to explain a decreased utilization of glutamine for glutamate formation. It may be a coincidence, but hypophosphatemia is noted frequently among alcoholic patients (Massry, 1977), a group most likely to be hyperammonemic. Almost all aspects of the daily life of a chronic alcoholic contribute to hypophosphatemia: poor food intake, use of antacids, alcohol ingestion per se via phosphaturia. Furthermore, the liver cirrhosis causes hyperventilation which leads to loss of phosphorous from the blood (Massry, 1977).

The porta-cava shunt (PCS) situation which is used to simulate chronic hepatic failure, was employed also in the present studies as a means to see whether hippocampal tissue could adapt to function properly with respect to glutamate release. Fig. 8 shows that tissue dissected from PCS rats operated 3 weeks earlier had acquired tolerance to ammonia perfusion in vitro (Hamberger et al., 1980). The tolerance may be partly attributed to effects on glutamine-metabolizing enzymes.

The contribution of neurons and glia to the formation of glutamate is frequently tested according to the present view of compartmentation of glutamate metabolism (Berl et al., 1962; Van den Berg and Garfinkel, 1971; Balasz and Cremer, 1973): the neuronal (large) pool is preferentially labelled by glucose while acetate is one of the substrates mainly labelling the glial (small) pool. The destruction of neurons by mechanical or chemical means leads to a

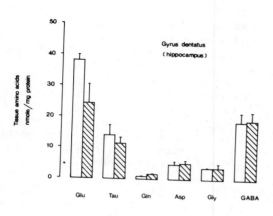

Fig. 9 a   Effect of lesion of the entorhinal cortex on content of amino acids in the molecular layer of the dentate gyrus of the rat hippocampus. (□ = contralateral side, ◩ = lesioned side).
The experiment was performed 7 days after the lesion. The tissue was chopped and incubated in a perfusion chamber for 60 - 90 min. The tissue slices were then homogenized in 70 % ethanol and the extracts analyzed for endogenous amino acids with the high performance liquid chromatography technique.

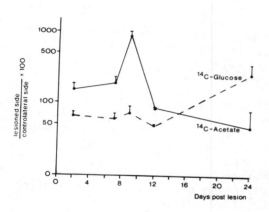

Fig. 9 b   Incorporation of ^{14}C-radioactivity from ^{14}C-glucose and ^{14}C-acetate into the amino acid fraction from tissue slices of the molecular layer of the dentate gyrus of the rat hippocampus. Time course of effects of unilateral lesion of the entorhinal cortex. The tissue was perfused for 30 min with radioactive precursors and then immediately homogenized in 70 % ethanol. The ethanol extracts were further analyzed as described in the legend to Fig. 10.

proliferation of astrocytes. The morphological change is then well correlated with a decreased glucose utilization and increased acetate utilization for glutamic acid and glutamine biosynthesis (Nicklas et al., 1979; Tursky et al., 1979). Fig. 9 (a and b) illustrates similar experiments with the rat hippocampus. The outer molecular layer of the dentate gyrus consists primarily of a single cell type (granule cell) which receives its major input from the entorhinal cortex. Ablation of the entorhinal cortex leads to a degeneration of approximately 60 % of the nerve terminals in the outer molecular layer of the dentate gyrus (Matthews et al., 1976). The input from the entorhinal cortex is excitatory and probably the best established glutamatergic tract (Nicoll and Iwamoto, 1978). The glutamate concentration in the outer molecular layer decreased

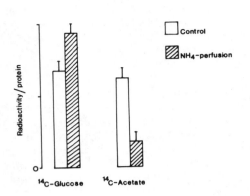

Fig. 10 Effect of 3 mM NH₄Cl on the incorporation of ^{14}C-radioactivity from ^{14}C-glucose and ^{14}C-acetate into the amino acid fraction extracted from rat hippocampal slices. The radioisotope was included for 30 min in the normal and ammonium containing Krebs-Ringer bicarbonate media, respectively. The glucose concentration was reduced to 2.5 mM in all experiments. The combined perfusates and tissue ethanol extracts were applied to an AG 50 (BioRad) column. The amino acid fractions were eluted from the columns with 1 M NH₄OH and analyzed for radioactivity.

significantly and specifically (Fig. 9 a) and the glucose-derived radioactivity in the amino acid pool decreased while that of acetate increased markedly, particularly one week after lesion (Fig. 9 b). The tissue contents of amino acids are shown in the tissue slice after a perfusion experiment (extensive loss of glutamine).

The possibility of a shift in the relative activity of the de novo synthesis of glutamate from nerve terminals towards glial cells during perfusion with ammonia was tested, and the results are shown in Fig. 10. They actually were opposite to what was expected, leading to the rapid conclusion that the glucose-acetate system is unsuitable in the presence of elevated ammonia. The main reason for this is that ammonia inhibits virtually all of the energy-requiring accumulation of acetate into the tissue-slice (data not shown). This appears to be analogous with the specific transport inhibition at the blood-brain-barrier level for acetate, but not for glucose in porta cava-shunted rats (Sarna et al., 1979). The uptake of acetate by the brain is also inhibited after removal of the liver (Tyce et al., 1981). The marked decrease in ^{14}C-acetate incorporation (Fig. 10) is consequently probably no definite proof of a decreased glutamate formation in the glia, since the two precursors are not strictly "compartmentated". On the other hand, if the present results are taken at face value, they could suggest that there is an inhibited glutamate formation in glia during hyperammonemia. Then glial cells might drain the neuronal compartment of glutamate for glutamine synthesis. It is, however, apparent that we have not arrived at an easily explained disturbance in the neuron/glia relationship.

Another metabolic correlate to neurotransmitter release which has been measured in brain slices are the changes in tissue NADH.

The method has been applied to evaluate the intermediary metabolism
in several organs (Chance et al., 1962). The fluctuations in redox
state are monitored "on line" with a spectrophotometric technique.
The cytoplasmic NAD/NADH potential is closely correlated with glucose
utilization and respiration in brain, so the metabolic reactions

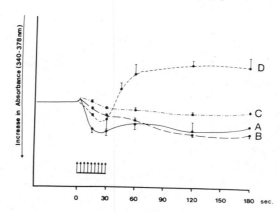

Fig. 11   Effects of 2.5 mM $(NH_4)_2$ SO_4 on directly measured NAD(P)H
levels in a cortex slice following electrical-field stimulation for
30 seconds (⬆⬆⬆⬆⬆). (A)Control perfusion, stimulation 15 - 20 min
after steady state was reached. (B) Control perfusion, stimulation after 60 min of steady state. (C) 2.5 mM $(NH_4)_2$ SO_4 in the
medium four min prior to stimulation, 15 - 20 min after steady-state
was reached. (D) 2.5 mM $(NH_4)_2$ SO_4 in the medium for 60 min prior
to stimulation。 Means ±SE of three experiments in each series.

that follow depolarization of brain cells, are likely to be reflected
in the level of NADH (Bull and O'Neill, 1975). Another coupling of
the NADH levels to the neurosecretory process is its Ca-dependency
(Cummins and Bull,(1971). Normally, high K^+-depolarization of the
hippocampal slice produces a long-lasting decrease in Nadh, while
electrical field stimulation of the slice evoked a transient increase
in NADH (Hamberger et al., 1978). A possible interpretation of
this difference is that potassium-depolarization involves larger
cell populations, including glia. Fig. 11 shows the effect of perfusion of tissue slices with ammonia-containing media. Ammonium ions
(3-5 mM) per se were without effect but inverted the NADH response
of the tissue during electrical stimulation (Cummins et al., 1981).
Thus, in the presence of ammonium ions both electrical and K^+-depola-
rization induced a decrease in NADH. Although the exact meaning of
these findings presently is unclear, they indicate that ammonium
ions influence certain regulatory mechanisms in cell populations in
the tissue slice which responds to depolarization with secretion of
neurotransmitters。

ACKNOWLEDGEMENT

This work was supported by grants from MRC (grant No. B80-12X-00164-16A) and Ax:son Johnsons Stiftelse. We are grateful to Dr. Hans-Arne Hansson for help with the histological work and to Miss Gull Grönstedt for secretarial aid.

REFERENCES

Abdul-Ghani, A.-S., Bradford, H.F., Cox, D.W.G., and Dodd, P.R., 1979, Peripheral sensory stimulation and the release of trans-mitter amino acids in vivo from specific regions of cerebral cortex, Brain Research, 171: 55.

Balasz, R. and Cremer, J.E., eds., 1973, "Metabolic Compartmentation in the Brain", MacMillan, London.

Benjamin, A.M., 1981, Control of glutaminase activity in rat brain cortex in vitro: influence of glutamate, phosphate, ammonium, calcium and hydrogen ions, Brain Research, 208: 363.

Benjamin, A.M., Verjee, Z.H., and Quastel, J.H., 1980, Effects of branched-chain L-amino acids, L-phenylalanine, and L-methionine on the transport of L-glutamine in rat brain cortex in vitro. Influence of cations, J. Neurochem., 35: 78.

Berl, S., Takagaki, G., Clarke, D.D., and Waelsch, H., 1962, Meta-bolic compartments in vivo: ammonia and glutamic acid metabolism in brain and liver, J. Biol. Chem., 237: 2562.

Bradford, H.F., 1978, Amino acid transmitters and their malfunction in disease, in: "Chemical Communication within the Nervous System and its Disturbance in Disease", Taylor and Jones, eds. Pergamon Press, Oxford and New York.

Bradford, H.F., and Ward, H.K., 1975, Glutamine as a metabolic sub-strate for isolated nerve-endings: Inhibition by ammonium ions, Biochem. Soc. Trans., 3 : 1223.

Bradford, H.F., and Ward, H.K., 1976, On glutaminase activity in mammalian synaptosomes, Brain Research, 110: 115.

Bradford, H.F., and Richards, C.D., 1976, Specific release of endo-genous glutamate from piriform cortex stimulated in vitro, Brain Research, 105: 168.

Bull, R.J., and O'Neill, 1975, Spectral changes in the respiratory chain of cerebral cortex slices. Correlation with the energy status of the tissue, Psychopharmacol. Commun., 1: 109.

Chance, B., Cohen, P., Jöbsis, F., and Schoener, B., 1962, Intracell-ular oxidation - Reduction states in vivo, Science, 137: 499.

Clark, R.M., and Collins, G.G.S., 1976, The release of endogenous amino acids from the rat visual cortex, J. Physiol., 262, 383.

Cole, M., Rutherford, R.B., and Smith, F.O., 1972, Experimental am-monia encephalopathy in the primate, Arch. Neurol., 26: 130.

Collins, G.G.S., 1977, On the role of taurine in the mammalian cen-
    tral nervous system, in:"Essays in Neurochemistry and Neuro-
    pharmacology",Vol. 1, M.B.H. Youdim, W.Lovenberg, D.F.Sharman,
    and J.R. Lagnado, eds., John Wiley, London.
Collins, G.G.S., Anson, J., and Probett, G.A., 1981, Patterns of
    endogenous amino acid release from slices of rat and guinea-pig
    olfactory cortex, Brain Research, 204, 103.
Conn, H.O., and Lieberthal, M.M., 1979,"The Hepatic Coma Syndromes
    and Lactulose", The Williams and Wilkins Company, Baltimore,USA.
Cooper, A.I.L., McDonald, I.M., Gelbard, A.S., Gledhill, R.F., and
    Duffy, T.E., 1979, The metabolic fate of ^{13}N-labeled ammonia
    in rat brain, J. Biol. Chem., 254 (No.12): 4982.
Cotman, C.W., and Hamberger, A., 1978, Glutamate as a CNS neurotrans-
    mitter: properties of release, inactivation and biosynthesis,
    in:"Amino Acids as Chemical Transmitters",F.Fonnum, ed., Plenum
    Press, New York and London.
Coutinho-Netto, J., Abdul-Ghani, A.S., and Bradford, H.F., 1980,
    Supression of evoked and spontaneous release of neurotransmit-
    ters in vivo by morphine, Biochem. Pharm., 29, 2777.
Crawford, I.L., and Connor, J.D., 1973, Localization and release of
    glutamic acid in relation to the hippocampal mossy fibre path-
    way, 1973, Nature, 244: 442.
Cummins, J.T., and Bull, R., 1971, Spectrophotometric measurement of
    metabolic response in isolated brain cortex, Biochem. Biophys.
    Acta, 253: 29.
Cummins, J.T., Hamberger, A., and Nyström, B., 1981, Effects of low
    ammonia levels on NAD(P)H levels and glutamate secretion during
    calcium-dependent depolarization of CNS slices, J.Neurosci.
    Res., 6: 217.
Davidson, N., 1979, High potassium, veratridine and electrically in-
    duced release of taurine from the cerebellar cortex, J.Physiol.
    (Paris), 75: 673.
De Feudis, F.V., 1975, Amino acids as central neurotransmitters, in:
    Annual Rev. of Pharmacol., Vol. 15, H.W.Elliot, R.George and
    R. Okun, eds.
Di Chiara, G., and Gessa, G.L., 1981, Glutamate as a neurotransmitter,
    Adv. Biochem. Psychopharmacol., 27.
Fonnum, F., ed., 1978,"Amino Acids as Chemical Transmitters",Plenum
    Press, New York and London.
Gauchy, C., Kemel, M.L., Glowinski, J., and Besson, M.J., 1981, In
    vivo release of endogenously synthesized (^{3}H) GABA from the
    cat substantia nigra and the pallido-entopedoneular nuclei,
    Brain Research, 193: 129.
Gruener, R., Markovitz, D., Huxtable, R., and Bressler, R., 1975,
    Excitability modulation by taurine: Transmembrane measurements
    of neuromuscular transmission, J. Neurol. Sci., 24: 351.
Hamberger, A., Cummins, J.T., Keller, E., and Cotman, C.W., 1978,
    Glutamate secretion and NAD(P)H levels during calcium-dependent
    depolarization of slices of the dentate gyrus, Brain Research,
    156: 253.

Hamberger, A., Hedquist, B., and Nyström, B., 1979, Ammonium ion in-
    hibition of evoked release of endogenous glutamate from hippo-
    campal slices, J. Neurochem., 33: 1295.
Hamberger, A., Hedquist, B., Lundborg, H., and Nyström, B., 1980,
    Hippocampal glutamate release after porta cava anastomosis:
    reduced sensitivity to ammonia inhibition, J. Neurosci.Res.,
    5: 313.
Iles, J.F., and Jack, J.J.B., 1978, Ammonia-mediated block of chlor-
    ide pumping in neurones, J. Physiol. (London), 280:20.
Iversen, L.L., Mitchell, J.F., and Srinivasan, V., 1971, The release
    of gamma-aminobutyric acid during inhibition in the cat visual
    cortex, J. Physiol. (London), 212: 519.
Keller, R., Oke, A., and Mefford, I., 1976, Liquid chromatographic
    analysis of catecholamines: routine assay for regional brain
    mapping, Life Sci., 19: 995.
Lindroth, P., and Mopper, K., 1979, High performance liquid chroma-
    tographic determination of subpicomole amounts of amino acids
    by precolumn fluorescence derivatization with o-phthaldialdehyde,
    Analyt. Chem., 51: 1667.
Lux, H.D., Loracher, C., and Neher, E., 1970, The action of ammonium
    on postsynaptic inhibition of cat spinal motoneurons, Exp.Brain
    Res., 11: 431.
Massry, S.G., 1978, The clinical syndrome of phosphate depletion,
    Adv. in Experim. Med. Biol., 103: 301.
Matthew, D.E., Cotman, C., and Lynch, G., 1976, An electron micro-
    scopic study of lesion-induced synaptogenesis in the dentate
    gyrus of the adult rat. 1 Magnitude and time course of degenera-
    tion, Brain Research, 115: 1.
McGale, E.H.F., Pye, I.F., Stonier, C., Hutchinson, E.C., and Aber,
    G.M., 1977, Studies on the inter-relationship between cerebro-
    spinal fluid and plasma amino acid concentrations in normal
    individuals, J. Neurochem., 29: 291.
Mell, L.D., 1979, Separation of biogenic amines by use of reversed-
    phase liquid chromatography and fluorescent detection, Clin.
    Chem., 25, 1187.
Mora, J., and Palacios, R., 1980,"Glutamine: Metabolism, Enzymology,
    and Regulation", Academic Press, N.Y.
Nadler, J.V., White, W.F., Vaca, K.W., Perry, B.W., and Cotman, C.W.,
    1978, Biochemical correlates of transmission mediated by gluta-
    mate and aspartate, J. Neurochem., 31: 147.
Nicklas, W.J., Nuñez, R., Berl, S., and Duvoisin, R., 1979, Neuronal-
    glial contributions to transmitter amino acid metabolism: stu-
    dies with kainic acid-induced lesions of rat striatum, J.Neuro-
    chem., 33: 839.
Nicoll, R.A., and Iwamoto, E.T., 1978, An evaluation of the proposed
    transmitter role of glutamate and taurine, in:"Neuronal Informa-
    tion Transfer", A.Karlin, V.M.Tennyson and H.J.Vogel,eds.
Norenberg, M.D., and Martinez-Hernandez, A., 1979, Fine structural
    localizations of glutamine synthetase in astrocytes of rat
    brain, Brain Research, 161: 303.

Pycock, C.J., and Smith, L.F.P., 1980, Effect of dopamine on the release of (^{3}H)-glycine and (^{3}H)-taurine from the rat isolated retina, Brit. J. Pharmacol., 70, 55.

Rassin, D.K., 1981, The function of taurine in the central nervous system, in:"Amino Acid Neurotransmitters", F.V. De Feudis and P. Mandel, eds., Raven Press, N.Y. Adv. Biochem. Psychopharmacol. Vol. 29.

Richelson, E., and Thompson, E.J., 1973, Transport of neurotransmitter precursors into cultured cells, Nature New Biol., 241: 201.

Salganicoff, L., and De Robertis, E., 1965, Subcellular distribution of the enzymes of the glutamic acid, glutamine and α-aminobutyric acid cycles in rat brain, J. Neurochem., 12: 287.

Sarna, G.S., Bradbury, N.W.B., Cremer, J.E., Lai, J.C.K., and Teal, H.M., 1979, Brain metabolism and specific transport of blood-brain barrier after portocaval anastomosis in the rat, Brain Research, 160: 69.

Schrier, B.K., and Thompson, E.J., 1974, On the role of glial cells in the mammalian nervous system, J. Biol. Chem., 249: 1769.

Storm-Mathisen, J., 1977, Localization of transmitter candidates in the brain: the hippocampal formation as a model, Prog. Neurobiol., 8: 119.

Svenneby, G., 1971, Activation of pig brain glutaminase, J. Neurochem., 18: 2201.

Tursky, T., Ruščák, M., Lassanová, M., and Ruscakova, D., 1979, (^{14}C) amino acid formation from labelled glucose and/or acetate in brain cortex slices with experimentally elicited proliferation of astroglia. Correlation of biochemical and morphological changes, J. Neurochem., 33: 1209.

Tyce, G.M., Ogg, J., and Owen Jr., C.A., 1981, Metabolism of acetate to amino acids in brains of rats after complete hepatectomy, J. Neurochem., 32: 640.

Ungerstedt, U., Zetterström, T., Tossman, U., and Jungnelius, U., in press, Brain dialysis - a new technique for the recovery of neurotransmitters in awake and asleep animals, Nature.

Van Den Berg, C.J., and Garfinkel, D.A., 1971, A simulation study of brain compartments: metabolism of glutamate and related substances in mouse brain, Biochem. J., 123: 211.

Van der Heiden, J.A.M., Venema, K., and Korf, J., 1979, In vivo release of endogenous GABA from rat substantia nigra measured by a novel method, J. Neurochem., 32: 469.

Van Gelder, N.M., 1981, Glutamic acid in nervous tissue and changes of the taurine content: its implication in the treatment of epilepsy, in:"Amino Acid Neurotransmitters", F.V. De Feudis and P. Mandel, eds., Raven Press, New York.

Weiler, C.T., Nyström, B., and Hamberger, A., 1979, Characteristics of glutamine vs. glutamate transport in isolated glia and synaptosomes, J. Neurochem., 32: 559.

White, W.F., Nadler, J.V., Hamberger, A., and Cotman, C.W., 1977, Glutamate as transmitter of hippocampal perforant path, Nature, 270: 356.

Williams, A.H., Mahta Kyu,   , Fenton, J.C.B., and Cavanagh, J.B.,
    1972, The glutamate and glutamine content of rat brain after
    portacaval anastomosis, J. Neurochem., 19: 1073.

GLUTAMATE AND GLUTAMINE TRANSPORT IN CULTURED NEURONAL AND GLIAL CELLS

Jacques Borg, Norbert Ramaharobandro and Jean Mark

Centre de Neurochimie du CNRS
5, rue Blaise Pascal
67084 Strasbourg Cedex, France

Glial cells are thought to be the main source of glutamine in the CNS, because of their high content in glutamine synthetase (Norenberg and Martinez-Hernandez, 1979). If glutamine is a precursor of GABA in Gabaergic neurons, one would expect a flow of glial glutamine towards the neurons. Neuronal and glial cells have been attributed different metabolic compartments which are in relation one with the other through the transfer of glutamate, GABA or glutamine in both directions (Benjamin and Quastel, 1972 ; Bradford et al., 1978 ; Hamberger et al., 1979).

The reports on L-glutamine uptake have given conflicting results, as several authors found a low affinity uptake (Km = 0.15 - 3.3 mM) (Balcar and Hauser, 1978 ; Cohen and Lajtha, 1972 ; Schousboe et al., 1979 ; Weiler et al., 1979), while others reported a high affinity uptake system (Km = 50 μM) (Balcar and Johnston, 1975 ; Roberts and Keen, 1974). In this study, we investigated the uptake of L-glutamine by neuronal and glial cultures of rat brain, in the conditions where the uptake of GABA is optimum (Borg et al., 1980). Further, in order to test the capacity of our cultures to transport L-glutamate we measured the kinetic parameters of the L-glutamate uptake mechanism.

Primary cultures of neuronal and glial cells as well as uptake experiments were performed as previously described (Borg et al., 1980). Glial and neuronal cultures originated from cerebral hemispheres of new born rats and twelve days old embryos respectively. Experiments were carried on neurons after 5 days of culture and in glial cells after 12 days. Glutamine synthetase and phosphate-dependent glutaminase activities were determined by previously described methods (Kulka et al., 1972 and Curthoys and Weiss, 1974 respectively). Both glutaminase and glutamine synthetase activities were shown to be present after the period of culture where the experiments were performed. Glutamine synthetase activity was about 10 times higher in the glial compared to the neuronal cells (24 versus 2.1 nmol/min/mg protein). Glutaminase activity was found to be 17 and 4.7 nmol/min/mg protein in the glial and neuronal cultures respectively.

L-glutamine and L-glutamate uptake were found to be linear for at least 10 min at 25°C in both cell types. The tissue to medium ratio at that time was found to be 13 and 18 in the neurons and glial cells respectively in the case of L-glutamine, while values of 25 in neurons and 300 in glial cells were found in the case of L-glutamate. The kinetic characteristics for L-glutamine uptake were those of a low affinity system with a rather high Vmax (Table 1). The Km values were much lower than the endogenous concentration of glutamine measured in both neuronal and glial cultures (50 mM). In the case of L-glutamate, the uptake was found to occur through a high affinity system and the glial cells exhibited a velocity 4 times higher than the neurons (Table 1). The Km values of glutamine uptake obtained with our glial cultures are identical to those found by Balcar and Hauser (1978) in similar cultures, but much lower than those reported by Schousboe et al. (1979) in cultures of mouse brain. It should be pointed out that no contribution of homoexchange could be measured in our experimental conditions.

The uptake of L-glutamine was found to be sodium dependent in the neuronal cells, while no such dependency could be detected in the glial cultures. When the concentration of potassium ions was increased in the incubation medium, glutamine uptake was significantly decreased in the glial but not in the neuronal cells. Concerning the inhibitors of L-glutamine uptake, only L-glutamate was efficient in neuronal cultures, while the uptake in glial cells was strongly inhibited by asparagine, N-methyl-glutamate, 4-fluoroglutamate and leucine and slightly by L-glutamate and L-aspartate. Thus neuronal carriers seem more specific for glutamine than glial ones.

When the efflux of radioactivity after incubating the cultures with ^{14}C glutamine was measured, glutamine and glutamate were shown to account for the major part (at least 60 %) of the released material in both cell types. Raising the potassium concentration to 50 mM in the superfusing medium increased the radioactivity released by neurons in a calcium-independent manner, but no effect could be measured in the case of glial cells.

Following neuronal depolarization, the level of potassium in the synaptic cleft increases, while that of calcium decreases. According to our results, it seems that these ionic variations tend

Table 1. Kinetic constants of the uptake of
L-/^{3}H/glutamine and L-/^{3}H/glutamate

	Km (µM)	Vmax (pmol.min^{-1} mg protein^{-1})
L-/^{3}H/GLUTAMINE		
Neuronal cells	116 ± 40 (28)	1034 ± 76 (28)
Glial cells	211 ± 48 (18)	2053 ± 119 (18)
L-/^{3}H/GLUTAMATE		
Neuronal cells	34 ± 18 (18)	588 ± 244 (18)
Glial cells	4 ± 1 (20)	2234 ± 157 (20)

L-/^{3}H/glutamine and L-/^{3}H/glutamate uptake were measured at nine
different concentrations after a 10 min incubation at 25°C. The
diffusion was determined at higher concentrations and the uptake
corrected for diffusion at each concentration. The values of Km
and Vmax and their standard deviations were computed using a
specially designed Fortran program with the number of experimental
values shown between brackets.

to inhibit the glial glutamine transport. Thus a larger amount of
glutamine will be available for neurons in the extracellular fluid,
allowing them to compensate the loss of aminoacids previously libe-
rated in the synaptic cleft. Moreover the release of sodium ion
from astrocytes following the repolarization, will stimulate the
neuronal glutamine uptake. A regulation mechanism triggered by the
astrocytes could be suggested, where astrocyte depolarization and
its repolarization would channel glutamine toward the neurons. It
seems that a flux of glutamate from neurons to glial cells is thus
closely related with a consecutive flux of glutamine in the
opposite direction.

Acknowledgement : This work was supported by a grant from the
INSERM (ATP 81.79.113).

REFERENCES

1. V. J. Balcar, and G. A. R. Johnston, High affinity uptake of L-
    glutamine in rat brain slices. J. Neurochem. 24:875 (1975).
2. V. J. Balcar, and K. L. Hauser, Transport of ^{3}H L-glutamate
    and ^{3}H L-glutamine by dissociated glial and neuronal cells in
    primary culture. Proc. Eur. Soc. Neurochem. 1:498 (1978).
3. A. M. Benjamin, and J. H. Quastel, Metabolism of aminoacids and
    ammonia in rat brain cortex slices _in vitro_ : a possible role
    of ammonia in brain function. J. Neurochem. 25:197 (1975).

4. J. Borg, N. Ramaharobandro, J. Mark, and P. Mandel, Changes in the uptake of GABA and taurine during neuronal and glial maturation. J. Neurochem. 34:1113 (1980).

5. H. F. Bradford, H. K. Ward, and A. J. Thomas, Glutamine, a major substrate for nerve endings. J. Neurochem. 30:1453 (1978).

6. S. R. Cohen, and A. Lajtha, Aminoacid transport, in "Handbook of Neurochemistry", A. Lajtha, ed., Plenum Press, New York, vol. 7, 543 (1972).

7. N. P. Curthoys, and R. F. Weiss, Regulation of renal ammoniagenesis subcellular localization of rat kidney glutaminase isoenzymes. J. Biol. Chem. 249:3261 (1974).

8. A. C. Hamberger, G. H. Chiang, E. S. Nylen, S. W. Scheff, and C. W. Cotman, Glutamate as a CNS transmitter. Brain Res. 168: 513 (1979).

9. R. G. Kulka, G. M. Tomkins, and R. B. Crook, Clonal differences in glutamine synthetase activity of hepatoma cells. J. Cell. Biol. 54:175 (1972).

10. M. D. Norenberg, and A. Martinez-Hernandez, Fine structure localization of glutamine synthetase in astrocytes of rat brain. Brain Res. 161:303 (1979).

11. P. J. Roberts, and P. Keen, High affinity uptake for glutamine in rat dorsal roots but not in nerve endings. Brain Res. 67: 352 (1974).

12. A. Schousboe, L. Hertz, G. Svenneby, and E. Kvamme, Phosphate activated glutaminase activity and glutamine uptake in astrocytes in primary cultures. J. Neurochem. 32:943 (1979).

13. C. T. Weiler, B. Nystrom, and A. Hamberger, Characteristics of glutamine vs glutamate transport in isolated glia and synaptosomes. J. Neurochem. 32:559 (1979).

STUDIES ON NEURONAL-GLIAL METABOLISM

OF GLUTAMATE IN CEREBELLAR SLICES

William J. Nicklas and Barbara Krespan

Departments of Neurology and Pharmacology
College of Medicine and Dentistry of
New Jersey-Rutgers Medical School
Piscataway, N.J. 08854, U.S.A.

Evidence has rapidly accumulated during the past few years that glia, as well as neurons, contribute to the metabolism and, therefore, the regulation of the transmitter function of the amino acids glutamate/aspartate and GABA (for recent reviews, Schoffeniels et al., 1978; Fonnum, 1978; Hertz, 1979). These conclusions are, for the most part, consistent with prior biochemical studies which demonstrated the compartmentation of glutamate metabolism in brain (Balazs and Cremer, 1973; Berl et al., 1975). Such studies have indicated that exogenously supplied glutamate, aspartate and GABA appear to be metabolized largely in a "small" compartment associated with glial cells. Since glial cells do have high affinity uptake systems for these amino acids, it may well be that one function of glial cells is to aid in the rapid inactivation of neuroactive amino acids released into the synaptic cleft (Schrier and Thomson, 1974; Nicklas and Browning, 1978). Central to this concept and consistent with the experimentally-observed rapid conversion of exogenous glutamate and ammonia to glutamine, is the demonstration by Norenberg and his colleagues (1979) of the astrocytic localization of glutamine synthetase. An understanding of the metabolism of glutamine in the various "compartments" of CNS tissue is probably pivotal to elaborating the regulation of the metabolism of transmitter glutamate/aspartate and GABA. Glutamine has been postulated to be a major precursor of neuronal, i.e. transmitter pools, of these neuroactive amino acids (Van den Berg, et al., 1975; Benjamin and Quastel, 1974), as well as being a deactivated form of the neuroexcitatory, and potentially neurotoxic, glutamate (Nicklas et al., 1980). Thus, glutamate (and GABA) levels within the nerve terminal can be maintained by glutamine derived from the

extracellular environment which, in turn, can be replenished by
synthesis in the glia via glutamine synthetase. This flow of
glutamate (and, perhaps, GABA) into glial cells with a return
flow of glutamine into nerve endings is consistent with a great
deal of available evidence. The latter point has been recently
questioned (Hertz, 1979). However, whether glutaminase is or is
not singularly localized in neurons, or whether glutamine is or
is not preferentially taken up by nerve endings may not be
overriding problems. Glutaminase activity can be regulated by a
number of factors, including the concentration of glutamate.
Release of glutamate during transmission will lower the intracellular concentration of glutamate and this event, in itself,
might trigger glutaminase activity (Bradford and Ward, 1976;
Benjamin, 1981). Therefore, the control of these systems may
depend not upon a differential distribution of glutaminase between neurons and glia but rather upon a delicate poising of
glutamate: glutamine ratios within these cells.

The in vivo complexity of the CNS makes a quantitative determination of the relative contribution of each compartment and
an elaboration of its specific function most difficult. The use
of intact tissue slices allows greater manipulation of the environment but the lack of specific agents to interact with amino
acid systems (as compared to, e.g., the monoamines) has hindered
a proper biochemical dissection of the systems. This report will
focus on the results of recent and ongoing studies with two substances which appear to interact with glutamate metabolism and/or
function in cerebellar slices. The first of these substances to
be discussed is kainic acid, a glutamate analog which is also a
potent neurotoxin (Olney, 1978). The second substance is 6-
diazo-5-oxo-norleucine (DON) which is a good inhibitor of phosphate-dependent glutaminase activity (Pinkus and Windmueller,
1977).

Studies with kainic acid

Kainic acid (KA) when injected into various brain areas, is
a potent excitotoxin (review, Olney, 1978). Specifically, KA
administered to cerebellum in vivo causes severe loss of neurons
with a relative sparing of the glutamergic granule cells
(Herndon and Coyle, 1977; Tran and Snyder, 1979). The mode of
action of this toxin is not clearly understood. The initial
event is believed to involve binding to a receptor-which is not
the "glutamate" receptor (Hall, et al., 1978; Davies, et al.,
1979)-followed by massive, irreversible neuronal depolarization
leading to cell death. A further constraint is put on any
interpretation by the demonstration that, e.g. for injections
of KA into rat neostriatum, the integrity of cortical, probably

glutamergic, afferents is necessary for the toxicity to occur
(McGeer, et al., 1978; Biziere and Coyle, 1978). This was also
observed by us in studies with corticostriatal tissue culture
(Whetsell et al., 1979). In attempting to understand the
mechanism(s) of toxicity we chose to look at what metabolic
changes occur acutely in cerebellar slices which contain an intrinsic glutamergic neuron-the granule cell (Tran and Snyder,
1979). In previous studies, it was found that KA consistently decreased ATP levels in the cerebellar slice and caused the
leakage of glutamate and aspartate (but not GABA) into the incubation medium (Nicklas et al., 1980). Most interestingly,
glutamine levels were severely depressed in the tissue slice with
no concomitant leakage into the medium (Table 1).

TABLE 1.   EFFECT OF INCUBATION WITH 1 mM KAINIC ACID ON AMINO
           ACID LEVELS IN CEREBELLAR SLICES AND INCUBATION MEDIUM

Tissue Amino Acid Levels (μmoles/100 mg protein)

	Control	1 mM Kainic Acid
Glutamic Acid	7.9 ± 0.7	7.1 ± 0.8
Aspartic Acid	1.7 ± 0.2	1.6 ± 0.2
Glutamine	2.3 ± 0.3	0.6 ± 0.2*
GABA	0.9 ± 0.2	0.9 ± 0.2

Medium Amino Acid Levels (μmoles/100 mg protein/2.5ml)

	Control	1 mM Kainic Acid
Glutamic Acid	0.26 ± 0.06	1.11 ± 0.08*
Aspartic Acid	0.11 ± 0.05	0.53 ± 0.07*
Glutamine	1.37 ± 0.42	1.60 ± 0.08

Cerebellar slices were preincubated for 30 minutes, then transferred to fresh Krebs-Ringer bicarbonate medium and 1 mM kainic
acid was added to some samples. The incubation continued for a
further 20 minutes. The tissue and medium were then separated
by centrifugation and amino acids in each analyzed. Values
are the mean ± S.D. (n=4). GABA in the medium of all samples
was below the level of detection (<.05 μmoles/100 mg protein/2.5
ml). * p. <0.001 when compared to control (from Krespan et al.,
1981).

To examine if this were a true decrease in glutamine synthesis, various labelled precursors were incubated with the slices in the presence or absence of KA. The relative specific activity (RSA) of glutamine to glutamate was decreased by 60% for ^{3}H-acetate, by 80% for ^{14}C-GABA, by 25% for ^{14}C-glucose and ^{14}C-glutamate as precursors (Table 2). All but the glucose data showed significant changes on statistical analysis. Thus, the data are consistent with a decrease in the glial synthesis of glutamine via glutamine synthetase. In other studies, it was found that KA does not directly inhibit the activity of this enzyme nor does it directly activate glutaminase activity.

TABLE 2. EFFECT OF 1 mM KAINIC ACID (KA) ON THE RELATIVE LABELLING OF GLUTAMINE FROM VARIOUS RADIOACTIVE PRECURSORS

PRECURSOR		GLUTAMINE RSA (glut=1)
^{3}H-Acetate	Control	7.93 ± 1.85
	1 mM KA	2.87 ± 0.28†
^{14}C-Glucose	Control	0.901 ± 0.189
	1 mM KA	0.679 ± 0.148
^{14}C-GABA	Control	1.74 ± 0.33
	1 mM KA	0.36 ± 0.13†
^{14}C-Glutamate	Control	4.43 ± 0.22
	1 mM KA	3.21 ± 0.92*

Different from control, *p <.05; †p <.005.

Cerebellar slices were preincubated for 15 minutes then transferred to fresh medium and 1 mM kainic acid was added to some samples. After a further 30 minute incubation various labelled precursors were added for an additional 10 min. Results are expressed as mean ± S.D. for 4 samples at each point and are ratio of the specific radioactivity (dpm/μmole) of glutamine compared to that of glutamic acid in the same tissue sample (from Krespan et al., 1981).

The problem that remains, then, is why glutamine formation from glutamate seems to be impaired. Our initial working hypothesis was that somehow a neuronal depolarization caused the metabolic changes in what appeared to be the glial compartment. This is consistent with the glial swelling often observed during the acute phases of KA toxicity in vivo (Olney and deGubareff, 1978) and the work of Hosli et al., (1979) who showed in culture that neuronal depolarization caused a K^+-mediated depolarization of adjacent glia. In this way, the ATP levels might be decreased in glial cells as well as neurones and this might cause the observed decrease in glutamine synthesis as well as the leakage of glutamate. That the mechanism of glutamate release into the medium is different from, e.g., veratridine-induced release is shown by the fact that tetrodotoxin (TTX) blocks veratridine-induced but not kainate-induced glutamate appearance in the medium (Table 3).

TABLE 3.   LEVELS OF GLUTAMATE IN MEDIUM OF CEREBELLAR TISSUE SLICES INCUBATED WITH KAINIC ACID OR VERATRIDINE IN THE PRESENCE AND ABSENCE OF TETRODOTOXIN

	GLUTAMATE
	μmoles/100 mg protein/2.5 ml
Control (4)	0.31 ± 0.08
1 mM Kainic Acid (3)	1.01 ± 0.12*
10 μM Veratridine (3)	0.72 ± 0.10*
1 mM Kainic Acid + 3 μM Tetrodotoxin (3)	1.04 ± 0.12†
10 μM Veratridine + 3 μM Tetrodotoxin (3)	0.35 ± 0.10ɣ

* Different from control, p. <.001
† Different from control, p <.001; not different from kainic acid treatment alone.
ɣ Different from veratridine alone, p. <005; not different from control.

Cerebellar slices were preincubated for 15 minutes, then transferred to fresh medium. Ten minutes later, 3 μM tetrodotoxin or vehicle (citrate buffer) was added. To some samples, 1 mM kainic acid or 10 μM veratridine was added 12 minutes later and the incubation continued for a further 15 minutes. Results are presented as mean ± S.D. for (N) preparations (from Krespan et al., 1981). TTX also blocks veratridine-induced decreases in ATP but not those seen with kainic acid.

Further information about the glutamate found in the medium after kainate treatment came from experiments in which the slices were prelabelled with ^{14}C-glucose and ^3H-acetate. Veratridine or kainate was then added and the glutamate in the tissue and medium isolated, measured and counted (Table 4). Consistent with findings using other preparations, (DeBelleroche and Bradford, 1972; Minchin, 1977; Bradford et al., 1978;

Hamberger et al., 1979) veratridine preferentially enhanced the
efflux of glucose-labelled glutamate over acetate-labelled
glutamate. On the other hand, kainate caused an increased release of glutamate labelled by either precursor. If one accepts
that acetate labels glial pools of glutamate, this is evidence
that there is a massive release of glial glutamate by kainate.

TABLE 4.   RELEASE OF LABELLED GLUTAMATE FROM CEREBELLAR SLICES
           PREVIOUSLY INCUBATED WITH D-($2-^{14}C$) GLUCOSE AND
           (^3H) ACETATE

Precursor	($2-^{14}C$) Glucose	Fraction Released [a] ^3H-Acetate
Control	0.017 ± 0.002	0.079 ± .007
1 mM KA (4)	0.126 ± 0.012*	0.475 ± .034*
Control (3)	0.014 ± 0.003	0.046 ±0.015
10 µM VER (3)	0.051 ± 0.007*	0.049 ±0.010

*$p < .005$ from corresponding control

[a] Fraction of   = glutamate in medium
    Tissue glutamate release   total glutamate

Values are the mean ± S.D. for (N) preparations (from Krespan
et al., 1981).

    These studies are an excellent illustration of the way in
which our knowledge of the compartmentation of glutamate
metabolism in CNS can aid in understanding the mechanism of
action of substances which interact with this system dele-
teriously such as kainic acid (Nicklas et al., 1979a,b). They
are also most supportive of suggestions that the glial metabolism of glutamate has a function in regulating the extracellular
content of this neuro-excitatory and, potentially, neurotoxic
amino acid.

Studies with 6-diazo-5-oxo-L-norleucine (DON)

    One of the principal problems in understanding glutamine
metabolism in the CNS is how to approach the hypothesis of a
functional flow of glutamine into neurones or nerve endings
where it can act as a source of transmitter amino acids. This
hypothesis suggests that acetate labels glutamine in glial cells
and this can form veratridine-releasable glutamate or GABA only
after transport into nerve endings. Therefore, inhibition of
glutaminase activity in the nerve ending should cause a decrease

in acetate-labelled, veratridine-releasable glutamate and/or GABA. The radioactive labelling and release of glucose-derived amino acids should be relatively unaffected. We have recently performed preliminary experiments with the diazoketone, DON, which irreversibly inhibits various glutaminases in vivo and in vitro by interacting with the glutamine binding site (Pinkus and Windmueller, 1977; Shapiro et al., 1979). It also inhibits glutamine-dependent activities of various amido-transferases (see Shapiro et al., 1979 for references). In our hands, pre-incubation of brain homogenates with 2 mM DON gives a 95% inhibition of the phosphate-activated glutaminase activity. To test whether DON could get into tissue slices and inhibit glutaminase, cerebellar slices were preincubated with various concentrations of DON, the DON removed by washing and residual glutaminase activity measured in tissue homogenates. The DON was able to penetrate the tissue and react with glutaminase as illustrated by a time dependent, dose dependent decrease in glutaminase activity (Table 5).

TABLE 5. GLUTAMINASE ACTIVITY IN HOMOGENATES OF CEREBELLAR SLICES PREINCUBATED WITH DON

Conc, DON mM	Activity μmoles/mg protein/0.5 hr.
0	2.76
2	1.70
4	1.22
6	0.89

Cerebellar slices were incubated for 30 min. at 37° in a Krebs-Ringer bicarbonate medium with above levels of DON. The incubation was stopped by dilution with ice-cold saline and centrifugation. After washing the tissue again with ice-cold saline, the tissue was homogenized in tris-phosphate, pH 8.0. Glutaminase activity was then measured as ^{14}C-glutamate formation from ^{14}C-glutamine in a medium containing 10 mM glutamine and 100 mM phosphate-tris, pH 8.0.

When cerebellar slices were labelled with a mixture of (2-^{14}C) glucose and ^{3}H-acetate after a 30 minute preincubation with DON, several interesting results were noted. In examining the relative specific activity of GABA to that of glutamate in the tissue, it was found that DON caused a 60% decrease in the RSA from acetate labelling with no change in that from glucose (Table 6).

TABLE 6.   EFFECT OF DON ON LABELLING OF GABA IN CEREBELLAR
           SLICES

	RSA TISSUE GABA	
	NO ADDITION	+ DON
	labelled from ^{14}C-glucose (glut=1)	
Control	0.96 ± 0.15	0.98 ± 0.13
+ Veratridine	1.14 ± 0.18	1.25 ± 0.06
	labelled from ^{3}H-acetate (glut=1)	
Control	0.41 ± .04	0.15 ± 0.01*
+ Veratridine	0.33 ± 0.06	0.15 ± 0.05*

*$p < 0.005$, N≈4

Cerebellar slices were treated as described in Table 7.
The data are expressed as average ± S.D. of the relative
specific activity of GABA to that of glutamate in the same slice.

This difference was also reflected in the labelling of the
GABA released by veratridine. Similarly DON caused a 35% decrease in the acetate-derived RSA of veratridine-released
glutamate to that in the tissue with no similar change in
glucose-derived, veratridine-releasable glutamate (Table 7).

TABLE 7.   EFFECT OF DON ON LABELLING OF GLUTAMATE RELEASED
           BY VERATRIDINE

	^{14}C-glucose	^{3}H-acetate
	RSA, medium/Tissue ± S.D.	
Control	1.06 ± 0.20	1.85 ± 0.18
+ DON	0.93 ± 0.19	1.23 ± 0.20*

*$p < .005$, N=4

Cerebellar slices were incubated in Krebs-Ringer bicarbonate
media with and without 5 mM neutralized DON for 30 min. at 37°.
After removing the DON medium by centrifugation and washing
with fresh medium, the slices were resuspended in medium con-

taining {2-^{14}C} glucose/^{3}H-acetate and incubated 15 min. After removing from this medium the slices were washed and resuspended again in fresh medium. 3 min. after addition of 10 μM veratridine (or carrier ethanol for control), medium and slices were separated and radioactive glutamate content in each found by ion-exchange chromatography. The results are expressed as the average of the ratio of the specific activity of the glutamate in the medium to that in its corresponding tissue.

These preliminary data are certainly consistent with the hypothesis that there is a functional connection between glutamine synthesis in the glia and maintenance of transmitter amino acid levels in the nerve endings. However, some caution must be exercised in these interpretations. This diazoketone reacts with other glutamine-dependent enzymes, such as γ-glutamyltranspeptidase, and effects on these systems being reflected in our observed changes in glutamate and GABA labelling must be taken into account before reaching any final conclusion.

ACKNOWLEDGEMENTS

This work was supported by U.S.P.H.S. grant NS 17360 as well as a GRS research grant from the College of Medicine and Dentistry of New Jersey.

REFERENCES

Balazs, R. and Cremer, J.E., eds., 1973. Metabolic Compartmentation in the Brain. MacMillan Press, London.

de Belleroche, J.S. & Bradford, H.F., 1972. Metabolism of beds of mammalian cortical synaptosomes: response to depolarizing influences. J. Neurochem. 19: 585-602.

Benjamin, A.M., 1981. Control of glutaminase activity in rat brain cortex in vitro: Influence of glutamate, phosphate, ammonium, calcium and hydrogen ions. Brain Res. 208: 363-377.

Benjamin, A.M. & Quastel, J.H., 1976. Cerebral uptakes and exchange diffusion in vitro of L- and D-glutamates. J. Neurochem. 26: 431-441.

Berl, S., Clarke, D.D. and Schneider, D., eds., 1975. Metabolic Compartmentation and Neurotransmission. Plenum Press, New York.

Biziere, K. & Coyle, J.T., 1978. Influence of corticostriatal afferents on striatal kainic acid neurotoxicity. Neuroscience Lett. 8: 303-310.

Nicklas, W.J., Nunez, R., Berl, S. & Duvoisin, R., 1979a.
Neuronal-glial contributions to transmitter amino acid metabolism:
studies with kainic acid-induced lesions of rat striatum.
J. Neurochem. 33: 839-844.

Nicklas, W.J., Duvoisin, R.C. & Berl, S., 1979b. Amino acids
in rat neostriatum: alteration by kainic acid lesion.
Brain Res. 167: 107-117.

Nicklas, W.J., Krespan, B. & Berl, S., 1980. Effect of kainate
on ATP levels and glutamate metabolism in cerebellar slices.
Eur. J. Pharmacol. 62: 209-213.

Norenberg, M.D. & Martinez-Hernandez, A., 1979. Fine structural
localization of glutamine synthetase in astrocytes of rat brain.
Brain Res. 161: 303-310.

Olney, J.W., 1978. Neurotoxicity of excitatory amino acids, in
Kainic Acid as a Tool in Neurobiology (E.G. McGeer, J.W. Olney
and P.L. McGeer, eds.) pp. 95-122, Raven Press, New York.

Olney, J.W. and de Gubareff, T., 1978. Extreme sensitivity of
olfactory cortical neurons to kainic acid toxicity, in
Kainic Acid as a Tool in Neurobiology (E.G. McGeer, J.W. Olney
and P.L. McGeer, eds.) pp. 201-218, Raven Press, New York.

Pinkus, L.M. & Windmueller, H.G., 1977. Phosphate-dependent
glutaminase of small intestine: Localization and role in
intestinal glutamine metabolism. Arch. Biochem. Biophys.
182: 506-517.

Schoffeniels, E., Franck, G., Hertz, L. and Tower, D.B., eds.,
1978. Dynamic Properties of Glial Cells. Pergamon Press,
Oxford.

Schrier, B.K. & Thompson, E.J., 1974. On the role of glial cells
in the mammalian nervous system. J. Biol. Chem. 249: 1769-1780.

Shapiro, R.A., Clarke, V.M. & Curthoy, N.P., 1979. Inactivation
of rat renal phosphate-dependent glutaminase with 6-diazo-5-oxo-
L-norleucine. J. Biol. Chem. 254: 2835-2838.

Tran, V.T. & Snyder, S.H., 1979. Amino acid neurotransmitter
candidates in rat cerebellum: selective effects of kainic acid
lesion. Brain Res. 167: 345-353.

Bradford, H. & Ward, H.K., 1976. On glutaminase activity in mammalian synaptosomes. Brain Res. 110: 115-125.

Bradford, H.F., de Belleroche, J.S. and Wark, H.K., 1978. On the metabolic and intrasynaptic origin of amino acid transmitters, in Amino Acids as Chemical Transmitters (F. Fonnum, ed.), pp. 367-377, Plenum Press, New York.

Davies, J., Evans, R.H., Francis, A.A. & Watkins, J.C., 1979. Excitatory amino acid receptors and synaptic excitation in the mammalian central nervous system. J. Physiol. (Paris) 75: 641-654.

Fonnum, F., ed., 1978. Amino Acids as Chemical Transmitters. Plenum Press, New York.

Hall, J.G., Hicks, T.P. & McLennan, H., 1978. Kainic acid and the glutamate receptor. Neuroscience Lett. 8: 171-175.

Hamberger, A.C., Chiang, G.H., Nylen, E.S., Scheff, S.W. & Cotman, C.W., 1979. Glutamate as a CNS transmitter. 1. Evaluation of glucose and glutamine as precursors for the synthesis of preferentially released glutamate. Brain Res. 168: 513-530.

Herndon, R.M. & Coyle, J.T., 1977. Selective destruction of neurons by a transmitter agonist. Science 198: 71-72.

Hertz, L., 1979. Functional interactions between neurons and astrocytes I. Turnover and metabolism of putative amino acid transmitters. Prog. in Neurobiology 13: 277-323.

Hosli, L., Andres, P.F. & Hosli, E., 1979. Action of amino acid transmitters on cultured glial cells of the mammalian peripheral and central nervous system. J. Physiol. (Paris) 75: 655-659.

Krespan, B., Berl, S. & Nicklas, W.J., 1981. Alteration in neuronal-glial metabolism of glutamate by the neurotoxin, kainic acid. J. Neurochem: in press.

McGeer, E.G., McGeer, P.L. & Singh, K., 1978. Kainic acid-induced degeneration of neostriatal neurons: dependency upon corticostriatal tract. Brain Res. 139: 381-383.

Minchin, M.C.W., 1977. The release of amino acids synthesized from various compartmented precursors in rat spinal cord slices. Exp. Brain Res. 29: 515-526.

Nicklas, W.J. & Browning, E.T., 1978. Amino acid metabolism in glial cells: homeostatic regulation of intra-and extra-cellular milieu by C-6 glioma cells. J. Neurochem. 30: 955-963.

Van Den Berg, C.J., Reijnierse, A., Blockhuis, G.G.D., Kroon, M.C., Ronda, G., Clarke, D.D. and Garfinkel, D., 1975. A model of glutamate metabolism in brain: a biochemical analysis of a heterogeneous structure, in Metabolic Compartmentation and Neurotransmission (S. Berl, D.D. Clarke and D. Schneider, eds.) pp. 515-543, Plenum Press, New York.

Whetsell Jr., W.O., Ecob-Johnston, M.S. and Nicklas, W.J., 1979. Studies of kainate-induced caudate lesions in organotypic tissue culture, in Advances in Neurology, Vol. 23 (T.N. Chase, N.S. Wexler and A. Barbeau, eds.) pp. 645-654, Raven Press, New York.

AMINO ACID COMPARTMENTS IN HIPPOCAMPUS:

AN AUTORADIOGRAPHIC APPROACH

Jon Storm-Mathisen

Anatomical Institute
University of Oslo
Oslo 1, Norway

INTRODUCTION

The purpose of the present communication is to show that certain amino acids when presented radiolabelled in the extracellular space, are taken up into distinct neuronal compartments. Thus, gammaaminobutyrate (GABA) was found to enter terminals of inhibitory neurons, whereas glutamate (Glu) and aspartate (Asp) entered excitatory terminals. By means of the metabolically inert acidic amino acid analogue D-Asp it was possible to show that a selective neuronal uptake occurs also in vivo. Once taken up, the amino acid, still in soluble form, enters a compartment which is subject to fast bidirectional axonal transport.

The studies were greatly facilitated by exploiting the unique anatomical organization of the hippocampal formation where various systems of nerve terminals are spatially segregated. The resulting zonal arrangement is suitable for microdissection and autoradiographic studies. More comprehensive treatments of the subject, including a survey of hippocampal pathways, are found elsewhere (Storm-Mathisen, 1981a, b).

GABA

Hippocampal slices incubated (10-30 min 25°) with μM concentrations of [^{3}H]GABA or [^{14}C]GABA in a physiological salt solution take up the labelled amino acid and retain

395

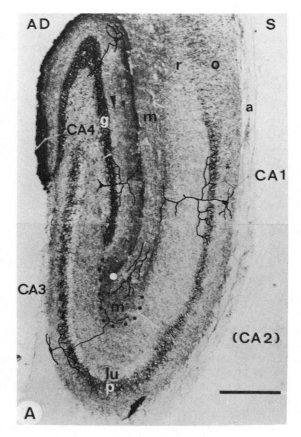

Fig. 1A.   Autoradiogram of hippocampal slice incubated
           with [^{3}H]GABA (1μM). Basket cells and other
           short axon neurons are indicated schematically.
           AD, area dentata; CA1-4, hippocampal subfields.
           Bottom of hippocampal fissure marked by circle.
           a, alveus; g, granular cell layer; lu, stratum
           lucidum (mossy fibre layer); m, molecular
           layer of hippocampus; p, pyramidal cell layer;
           o,r, strata oriens and radiatum (symbols mark
           limit CA1/subiculum); ▼▼, zone limits in
           molecular layer of AD. Bar 500 um. (Mofified
           from Taxt and Storm-Mathisen, 1979.)

about 2/3 of it when fixed in 5% glutaraldehyde. The
radioactivity in extracts of the tissue prior to fixation
is essentially pure GABA. To prepare autoradiograms of
the surface of the slice exposed to the incubating medium
the fixed slices are mounted on gelatinized slides,
covered with a protective polyvinylidene chloride film

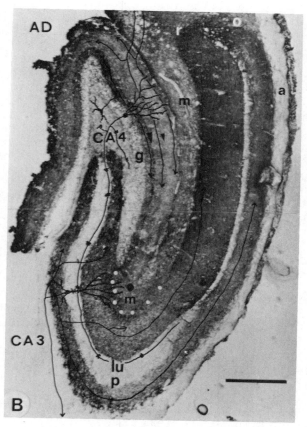

Fig. 1B. Autoradiogram of hippocampal slice incubated
with [^{3}H]-D-Asp (1μM). CA3 pyramidal cells
(terminals in strata oriens and radiatum of
CA1-3), CA4 pyramidal cells (terminals in inner
zone of molecular layer of area dentata), granular cells (terminating as mossy fibre boutons
in stratum lucidum of CA3 and in hilus, CA4)
and entorhinal afferents (perforant path, terminals in outer zones of the molecular layer of
area dentata) are indicated schematically in
india ink. Labelled as Fig. 1A. Note contrast
with distribution of [^{3}H]GABA. (Modified from
Taxt and Storm-Mathisen, 1979.)

and coated with Ilford L4 autoradiographic emulsion
(Storm-Mathisen, 1977; Taxt and Storm-Mathisen, 1977).
The resulting autoradiograms demonstrate a characteristic
zonal pattern (Fig. 1A), which is consistent with the
distribution of glutamate decarboxylase (GAD) as revealed

by microdissection (Storm-Mathisen and Fonnum, 1971;
Storm-Mathisen, 1972) and immunocytochemistry (Barber and
Saito, 1976). The highest concentrations are around the
pyramidal and granular cell bodies where the inhibitory
basket cell terminals are located. High concentrations
are also observed in the layers containing the most
superficial portions of the apical dendrites. GAD positive perikarya of local neurons (Ribak et al., 1978) and
a form of GABA mediated inhibition (Andersen et al.,
1980) occur in the superficial as well as in the cellular
layers. Clusters of autoradiographic grains appear
around perikarya even in CA4 ($\approx$ hilus fasciae dentatae)
and subiculum. Coarse, meandering axon-like structures
were seen in the less densely stained layers. Lesions of
afferent pathways do not change the GABA uptake pattern
or levels, nor those of GAD, as evidence of a localization in intrinsic structures. On the other hand, both
GABA uptake and GAD are reduced by injecting kainic acid,
which destroys local neurons and provokes glial proliferation (Fonnum and Walaas, 1978).

The pattern or intensity of labelling is not changed
by including 1 mM B-alanine in the incubation medium to
block the glial uptake system for GABA. When slices were
incubated with ^{3}H labelled glycine, taurine, B-alanine or
leucine under similar conditions only very weak uptake and
no distinct distribution pattern were observed autoradiographically.

These results suggest that exogenous radioactive
GABA can be used to label selectively likely GABAergic
nerve endings in the hippocampal formation. Others have
found that (^{3}H)GABA microinjected into the substantia
nigra labels striatal neurons by retrograde axonal
transport (Streit, 1980).

GLUTAMATE AND ASPARTATE

In vitro Studies

Unlike the situation for GABA, where theoretically
better methods (GAD immunohistochemistry) than GABA
uptake are available, the study of high affinity uptake
is so far the only way to visualize neurons that may use
Glu or Asp as their transmitter. When tissue is incubated in a physiological salt solution (high Na^+) at uM
concentration, essentially only the high affinity neuronal membrane transfer (uptake) is recorded. As for GABA,
there is very little metabolism. About 1/2 is fixed.

Autoradiograms of slices incubated with [^{3}H]Glu or
[^{3}H]Asp (Fig. 1B) showed maximum uptake in the hippocampal
zones containing the terminals of CA3 pyramidal cells,
and in the zone of area dentata containing the terminals
of CA4 cells. Lesion experiments confirmed that the
uptake was due to these fibre systems, since the uptake
in their target zones disappeared when the fibres degenerated. Further, biochemical assay in nerve terminal
containing homogenates of dissected samples showed that
CA3 afferents accounted for 80% of the high affinity
uptake of Glu and Asp in their target zones in CA1. The
Vmax was reduced on denervation, not the Km (about 1.5 μM
for D-Asp).

The mossy fibre layer, stratum lucidum, showed very
little uptake in surface autoradiograms. However, in
sections through the depth of incubated slices this layer
was clearly labelled and elctron microscopic autoradiograms showed the silver grains to be concentrated over
mossy fibre terminals, although the results suggested the
possible existence of populations with and without the
uptake (Storm-Mathisen and Iversen, 1979). Recent observations on surface autoradiograms dehydrated prior to
autoradiography (Bore and Storm-Mathisen, unpublished)
showed conspicuous labelling also of the mossy fibre
layer. The giant mossy fibre boutons are often larger in
diameter than the range of ^{3}H B-particles (2 μm, Rogers,
1979) and are likely to be damaged at the cut surface of
the slice. By drying the slice, or by cutting sections
through it, more deeply situated intact boutons would be
brought within the reach of the autoradiographic emulsion.

The target zones of the entorhinal afferents in the
molecular layer of area dentata have a moderate uptake of
Asp or Glu (Fig. 1B),the middle zone (target of the medial
perforant path) being slightly more labelled than the
outer zone (target of the lateral perforant path).
Measured biochemically the uptake of [^{3}H]Glu in these
zones is only 30% of that in oriens plus radiatum of CA1
based on protein (value for GAD 200%). The target of the
perforant path in the molecular layer of CA3 has a rather
high uptake of acidic amino acids.

After large lesions of the perforant path the uptake
of both Asp and Glu is reduced in all the target zones.
Biochemical assay in the outer two thirds of the dentate
molecular layer showed a reduction of 50% in Glu uptake
after such lesions. The lower normal uptake and the lower
reduction after axotomy suggest that the perforant path
axons have a lower density of Glu uptake sites in their

terminals than have the CA3 pyramidal cell axons. The
two pathways contribute similar, large proportions of the
total number of synapses in their target areas (Matthews
et al., 1976; Goldowitz et al., 1979). It is possible
that the perforant path contains fibres with and without
acidic amino acid uptake, and that the lateral and medial
perforant paths may differ in this respect.

To further investigate the subcellular sites of
[^{3}H]Glu uptake in the target of entorhinal afferents the
middle zone of the dentate molecular layer (target of
medial perforant path) was studied by electron microscopic autoradiography of incubated slices (Storm-Mathisen
and Iversen, 1979) applying the hypothetical grain analysis method of Blackett and Parry (1973; Parry 1976). By
this elegant method it is possible to tackle the cross-
firing problems in electron microscopic autoradiograms of
complex tissues, such as neuropil. A circle with radius
about equal to the "half radius" (i.e. a circle within
which there is a 50% probability of finding the source of
the B-particle that exposed the grain) is placed around
the centre of each autoradiographic grain, and the types
of structures within these "real grains" circles are
recorded. "Hypothetical grains" circles of the same size
are at random directions from "hypothetical sources", the
distances being governed by the range distribution function for the B-particles (Salpeter et al., 1969). Hypothetical grains and their hypothetical sources are placed
on the micrographs by means of a transparent overlay
screen, and the types of structures under each recorded.
A computer program is used to fit the distribution of
circle contents for hypothetical grains to that observed
for the real grains by testing various combinations of
radioactivity concentrations in the various hypothetical
sources. In this way it is possible to obtain likely
values for the concentrations of radioactivity in the
various tissue elements together with estimates of their
uncertainties. This method is clearly superior to
"conventional" grain counting (Fig. 2) and surprisingly
easy to apply. (A similar method has been published by
Salpeter et al., 1978.)

Results for the medial perforant path target zone
(Fig. 2, kindly computer-fitted by Dr. N. Blackett)
suggested that some 80% of the radioactivity in the
tissue could be accounted for by boutons and unmyelinated
axons, which had an activity 3-6 times the average for
the tissue. Glial elements accounted for about 13% of
the grains, but their radioactivity concentration was
about twice the average for the tissue. With the

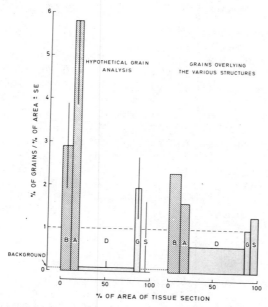

Fig. 2.   Hypothetical grain analysis of the middle zone
           of the dentate molecular layer (between arrow-
           heads in Fig. 1B), in electron microscopic auto-
           radiograms of a slice incubated with [³H]Glu.
           The analysis is based on 295 real grains and
           967 hypothetical grains. "Conventional" grain
           count data are given for comparison. (Data from
           Storm-Mathisen and Iversen, 1979; reproduced
           from Storm-Mathisen, 1981b.)

relatively small material the uncertainties are fairly
large. The results are consistent with the extent of
reduction of [³H]Glu uptake after degeneration of
entorhinal afferents.

Same or Different Uptake Carriers for Aspartate and Glutamate?

     According to the biochemical findings L-Glu, L-Asp
and D-Asp have very similar or identical high affinity
uptake carriers in cortical tissue (Balcar and Johnston,
1972). Similar uptake ratios for [³H]-D-Asp to [¹⁴C]-L-Glu
in hippocampus, septum and corpus mammillare, normally
and after denervation (Storm-Mathisen and Woxen Opsahl,
1978)   point in the same direction. Similarly the

autoradiographic patterns are very similar in hippocampal slices incubated with [3H]-L-Glu, [3H]-L-Asp and [3H]-D-Asp (Taxt and Storm-Mathisen, 1979). On the other hand there is some evidence that Asp and Glu uptake may not always be identical. The possibility should not be neglected that different neuronal sites might show some selectivity for one over the other. Thus Asp and Glu uptakes have different sensitivities to the presence of lithium ions (Davies and Johnston, 1976). In the cortico-pontine fibre system [3H]-D-Asp uptake is apparently more reduced by axotomy than [14C]-L-Glu uptake, measured in double labelling experiments (Thangnipon et al., 1980). Finally, Streit (1980) has reported that [3H]-D-Asp injected into the striatum labels a different set of cortical neurons (layer V) than does [3H]-D,L-Glu (layer VI).

Uptake in vivo

It is conceivable that some tissue compartments could be more vulnerable to the in vitro conditions than others. E.g. uptake in glial elements could be more suppressed than that in neuronal. Indeed, some reports from in vivo injections of [3H]-L-Glu in brain have suggested a diffuse or a glial localization of the label (Hökfelt and Ljungdahl, 1972; McLennan, 1976; Streit, 1980). Due to relatively rapid metabolism radiolabelled L-Glu or L-Asp are not easily handled in in vivo experiments on uptake. D-Asp appeared ideally suited for this purpose, being resistant to metabolic break-down and incorporation into proteins, and being a good substrate for the membrane carrier mediating high affinity uptake of L-Glu and L-Asp (Davies and Johnston, 1976).

We decided to infuse [3H]-D-Asp intracerebrally in anaesthetized rodents at concentrations close to the Km of the high affinity uptake carrier dissolved in artificial cerebrospinal fluid, in order to minimize participation of other uptake systems (Storm-Mathisen and Wold, 1981). After infusion the animals were perfusion fixed with 5% glutaraldehyde and processed for autoradiography. Indeed, a similar uptake pattern as in in vitro experiments was obtained in the hippocampal neuropil (Fig. 3), suggesting that the label was concentrated in the terminals of CA3 and CA4 pyramids also after uptake in vivo. Similarly, high uptake was seen in the juxtaventricular neuropil of septum and corpus striatum, other regions known to receive excitatory afferents capable of uptake of Asp and Glu in vitro (Fonnum et al., 1981). Small glial-like perikarya, ependymal cells and circumvascular

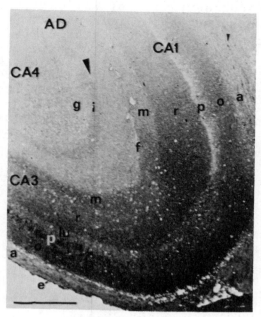

Fig. 3.   Uptake of [^{3}H]-D-Asp (5 uM) in vivo infused
           intraventricularly in Krebs' (1.1 ml) for 50
           min, followed by fresh Krebs' solution for 18
           min. Fixed by cardiac perfusion with 5% glu-
           taraldehyde. Horizontal kryostat section
           through dorsal hippocampus. e, ependymal
           cells; f, fissura hippocampi; i, inner part of
           dentate molecular layer; small arrow-head,
           possible glial cells. Other symbols: see
           Fig. 1. Scale bar, 500 μm. (Modified from
           Storm-Mathisen, 1981a.)

structures were also strongly labelled in vivo, although
the radioactivity in these structures apparently vanished
quickly if perfusion was continued without radioactivity
for some time before fixation.

Axonal Transport of D-Aspartate

    In the animals infused with [^{3}H]-D-Asp in vivo CA3
pyramidal cell bodies were conspicuously labelled (Fig. 3),
although this never was observed in vitro. This labelling could, in part, be due to uptake through the perikaryal membrane, but it seems more reasonable to assume

that this high concentration of radioactivity could
represent D-Asp retrogradely transported from the intensely labelled terminal fields of the cells. Indeed,
retrograde axonal transport has recently been demonstrated in several excitatory neuronal projections after
microinjection of higher concentrations (about 10^{-2}M) of
[^{3}H]-D-Asp (Streit, 1980; Baughman and Gilbert, 1980).
The present results suggest that such axonal transport
can occur even when the amino acid is administered in a
concentration and medium augmenting selective uptake by
the high affinity membrane carrier.

     Two hamsters were infused with D-Asp through a
cannula located in the hilus fasciae dentatae. The fluid
escaped to the subarachnoid space and the ventricles and
was drained through the cisterna magna. Intense labelling of the mossy fibre layer ensued (Fig. 4). The silver
grains were arranged in patterns suggesting labelling of
axons and large boutons. This was confirmed by electron
microscopic autoradiography (Fig. 5) which also demon-
stratred that the infusion did not result in oedema of the
mossy fibres or the interstices between them. The short
time scales involved (18 and 30 min) imply transport by
the fast axonal transport system. Fast anterograde axonal
transport of [^{3}H]-D-Asp was recently demonstrated in other
systems (Cuénod et al., 1981; Cuénod and Wiklund, personal
communication), and transported amino acid, still in
soluble form, was shown to be released Ca-dependently on
stimulation. These data would suggest that after uptake
the [^{3}H]-D-Asp enters a compartment, i.e. an organelle,
sequestering it from the cytosol to allow fast bidirectional axonal transport, and that this compartment is also
susceptible to Ca-dependent stimulation-induced release.
The synaptic vesicle would seem a likely candidate for such
a compartment.

     The giant mossy fibre boutons often show areas den-
sely packed with synaptic vesicles and other areas with
few vesicles (Fig. 5). The dimensions are such that it
would seem possible to determine by autoradiography
whether the radioactivity of axonally transported [^{3}H]-D-
Asp is situated mainly over vesicular or cytosol areas.
A survey of the preliminary material would suggest the
former possibility, but this can only be determined by
carefully applying the hypothetical grain analysis method
(see above).

     To study axonal transport further we have recently
made microinjections (100 µl) of [^{3}H]-D-Asp into the
hilus region through glass capillaries (Fischer and

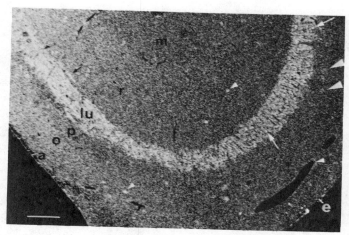

Fig. 4.   Anterograde transport of [³H]-D-Asp in the
           mossy fibres in hippocampus CA3 after infusion
           into the hilus fasciae dentatae (5.6 uM in
           Krebs 750 ul, 30 min). Dark field photograph
           of autoradiogram of Araldite section. There is
           also uptake in the neuropil in oriens (o) and
           radiatum (r) of CA3 and sign of retrograde
           axonal transport to CA3 pyramidal cells (▶).
           ✔, labelled axon- and bouton-like structures
           in mossy fibre layer;   ➤ , labelled glial-like
           perikarya and perivascular structures. Other
           labels as in Figs. 1 and 3. Scale bar 100 μm.
           (Modified from Storm-Mathisen, 1981a).

Storm-Mathisen, in preparation). As previous workers
(Streit, 1980) we used about 20 μM solutions in order to
have enough radioactivity in as small a volume as possible,
but dissolved the amino acid in 100 mM sodium phosphate
buffer pH 7.4 to insure enough Na⁺ for the high affinity
uptake system and a neutral pH. Preliminary results 12 h
after the injection showed labelling in oriens, radiatum
and the inner one third of the dentate molecular layer.
This was distinct contralateral to the injection site, as
evidence for anterograde axonal transport, and was very
intense ipsilaterally. By the same token, neuropil
labelling occurred also bilaterally in the dorsolateral
septum, which receives axons from CA3. CA3 and CA4 perikarya were heavily labelled on the side of the injection,
probably in part as a result of retrograde axonal
transport of [³H]-D-Asp from the intensely labelled ipsilateral terminals. In agreement, parikarya were labelled

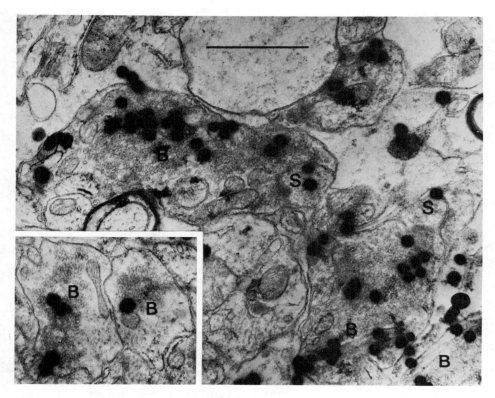

Fig. 5.   Electron microscopic autoradiograms of mossy
           fibre layer in a hamster infused with [^{3}H]-D-
           Asp into the hilus region as in Fig. 4 (18 min).
           Exposure three months, gold latensification
           (Bouteille, 1976) and phenidone development
           (Lettré and Paweletz, 1966). Mossy fibre boutons
           (B) are recognized by their large size, by con-
           taining heaps of synaptic vesicles and by
           making asymmetric synapses with dendritic
           spines (S) that often invaginate the boutons.
           Scale bar 1 μm.

also in the contralateral CA3/4 region. The relative
paucity of the contralateral labelling is consistent with
the relative paucity of the contralateral projections and
their relatively small contribution to the total uptake
activity for D-Asp (Storm-Mathisen, 1981b). On the
injected side granular cell perikarya were heavily
labelled close to the injection site, and the mossy fibre

layer was intensely radioactive along the trajectory from
the injection. It contained clusters of grains suggestive
of giant boutons. There was no conspicuous labelling of
glial perikarya. Thionine stained sections showed very
little sign of damage around the tip of the cannula.

CONCLUSIONS

Glutamate and aspartate are taken up in certain
excitatory neurons. If metabolic break-down is prevented
(D-Asp), neuronal uptake is clearly demonstrable in vivo,
and the acidic amino acid can remain for many hours in
the neurons and undergo axonal transport. Others have
observed synaptic release of axonally transported D-Asp
(Cuénod et al., 1981). These observations seem to provide
new insight into the storage, release and inactivation
mechanism of the alleged transmitter amino acids. The
anterograde and retrograde axonal transport of $[^3H]$-D-Asp
may become powerful tools for tracing neuronal connections
where Asp or Glu are likely to be transmitters. GABA is
taken up into some inhibitory neurones likely to use GABA
as transmitter. Axonal transport of $[^3H]$GABA or analogues,
may prove useful for tracing GABA pathways (Streit, 1980).
However, since different neurons may have different densities of membrane uptake sites for Asp/Glu or GABA
(Storm-Mathisen, 1981b), and possibly also different
capacities for storage and intracellular transport of the
amino acids, these methods may not be applicable to all
systems.

ACKNOWLEDGEMENTS

I would like to thank Mrs. Agnes Holter for typing
the manuscript. Supported by the Norwegian Research Council
for Science and the Humanities, Grant No. C 20.30-40.

REFERENCES

Andersen, P., Dingledine, R., Gjerstad,L., Langmoen,I.A.,
    and Mosfeldt Lausen, A., 1980, Two different responses
    of hippocampal pyramidal cells to application of
    gamma-amino butyric acid. J. Physiol. (Lond.),
    305:279-296.
Balcar, V.J., and Johnston, G.A.R.,1972, The structural
    specificity of the high affinity uptake of
    L-glutamate and L-aspartate by rat brain slices,
    J. Neurochem., 19:2657-2666.

Barber, R., and Saito, K., 1976, Light microscopic
    visualization of GAD and GABA-T in immunocytochemi-
    cal parations of rodent CNS, in: "GABA in Nervous
    System Function", E. Roberts, T.N. Chase, and D.B.
    Tower, eds., Kroc Foundation Series, Vol. 5, Raven
    Press, New York, pp.113-132.
Baughman, R.W., and Gilbert, C.D., 1980, Aspartate and
    glutamate as possible neurotransmitters of cells in
    layer 6 of the visual cortex, Nature (Lond.),
    287:848-850.
Blackett, N.M., and Parry, D.M., 1973, A method for ana-
    lyzing electron microscopic autoradiographs using
    hypothetical grain distributions, J. Cell Biol., 57:
    9-15.
Bouteille, M., 1976, The "LIGOP" meethod for routine ultra-
    structural autoradiography combination of single grid
    coating, gold latensification and Phenidon development,
    J. Microsc. Biol. cell., 27:124-128.
Cuénod, M., Beaudet, A., Canzek, V., Streit, P., and
    Reubi, J.C., 1981, Glutamatergic pathways in the
    pigeon and the rat brain, in: "Glutamate as a
    Neurotransmitter", Advances in Biochemical Psycho-
    pharmacology, Vol. 27, G. DiChiara and G.L. Gessa,
    eds., Raven Press, New York, pp.57-68.
Davies, L.P., and Johnston, G.A.R., 1976, Uptake and
    relase of D- and L-aspartate by rat brain slices,
    J. Neurochem., 26:1007-1014.
Fonnum, F., and Walaas, I., 1978, The effect of intrahip-
    pocampal kainic acid injections and surgical lesions
    on neurotransmitters in hippocampus and septum,
    J. Neurochem., 31:1173-1181.
Fonnum, F., Storm-Mathisen, J., and Divac, I.,1981, Bio-
    chemical evidence for glutamate as neurotransmitter
    in corticostriatal and corticothalamic fibres in rat
    brain, Neuroscience, 6:863-873.
Goldowitz, D., Scheff, S.W., and Cotman, C.W., 1979, The
    specificity of reactive synaptogenesis: a com-
    parative study in the adult rat hippocampal for-
    mation, Brain Res., 170:427-441.
Hökfelt, T., and Ljungdahl, Å., 1972, Application of cyto-
    chemical techniques to the study of suspected
    transmitter substances in the nervous system,
    Adv. biochem. Psychopharmacol., 6:1-36.
Lettré, H., und Paweletz, N., 1966, Probleme der elektron-
    mikroskopischen Autoradiographie, Naturwissenschaften,
    53: 268-271.

Malthe-Sørenssen, D., Skrede, K.K., and Fonnum, F., 1979, Calcium-dependent release of D-[^{3}H]aspartate evoked by selective electrical stimulation of excitatory afferent fibres to hippocampal pyramidal cells, Neuroscience, 4:1255-1263.

Matthews, D.A., Cotman, C., and Lynch, G., 1976, An electron microscopic study of lesion-induced synaptogenesis in the dentate gyrus of the adult rat - I. Magnitude and time course of degeneration, Brain Res., 115:1-21.

McLennan, H., 1976, The autoradiographic localization of L(^{3}H) glutamate in rat brain tissue, Brain Res., 115:139-144.

Parry, D.M., 1976, Practical approaches to the statistical analysis of electron microscope autoradiographs, J. Microsc. Biol. cell., 27: 185-190.

Ribak, C.E., Vaughn, J.E., and Saito, K., 1978, Immuno-cytochemical localization of glutamic acid decarboxylase in neuronal somata following colchicine inhibition of axonal transport, Brain Res., 140:315-332.

Rogers, A.W., 1979, "Techniques of Autoradiography", Third edition, Elsevier, Amsterdam, 429 pp.

Salpeter, M.M., Bachmann, L., and Salpeter, E.E., 1969, Resolution in electron microscope radioautography, J. Cell Biol., 41:1-20.

Salpeter, M.M., McHenry, F.A., and Salpeter, E.E., 1978, Resolution in electron microscope autoradiography. IV. Application to analysis of autoradiographs, J. Cell Biol., 76:127-145.

Storm-Mathisen, J., 1972, Glutamate decarboxylase in the rat hippocampal region after lesions of the afferent fibre systems. Evidence that the enzyme is localized in intrinsic neurones, Brain Res., 40:215-235.

Storm-Mathisen, J., 1977, Glutamic acid and excitatory nerve endings: reduction of glutamic acid uptake after axotomy, Brain Res., 120:379-386.

Storm-Mathisen, J., 1981a, Glutamate in hippocampal pathways, in: "Glutamate as a Neurotransmitter", Advances in Biochemical Psychopharmacology, Vol. 27, G. DiChiara and G.L. Gessa, eds., Raven Press, New York, pp.43-55.

Storm-Mathisen, J., 1981b, Autoradiographic and microchemical localization of high affinity glutamate uptake, in: "Glutamate: Transmitter in the Central Nervous System", P.J. Roberts, J. Storm-Mathisen and G.A.R. Johnston, eds., Wiley, Chichester, pp.89-115.

Storm-Mathisen, J., and Fonnum, F., 1971, Quantitative histochemistry of glutamate decarboxylase in the rat hippocampal region, J. Neurochem., 18:1105-1111.

Storm-Mathisen, J., and Iversen, L.L., 1979, Uptake of [^{3}H]glutamic acid in excitatory nerve endings: Light and electronmicroscopic observations in the hippocampal formation of the rat, Neuroscience, 4:1237-1253.

Storm-Mathisen, J., and Woxen Opsahl, M., 1978, Aspartate and/or glutamate may be transmitters in hippocampal efferents to septum and hypothalamus, Neurosci. Lett., 9:65-70.

Streit, P., 1980, Selective retrograde labelling indicating the transmitter of neuronal pathways, J. comp. Neurol., 191:429-463.

Taxt, T., and Storm-Mathisen, J., 1979, Tentative localization of glutamergic and aspartergic nerve endings in brain, J. Physiol. (Paris), 75:677-684.

Thangnipon, W., Taxt,T., Brodal, P., and Storm-Mathisen, J., 1980, Glutamate (Glu) and aspartate (Asp): transmitters in the corticopontine pathway? Neurosci. Lett., Suppl.5: S79.

THE DISTRIBUTION AND REGULATION IN NERVE CELLS AND ASTROCYTES OF
CERTAIN ENZYMES ASSOCIATED WITH THE METABOLIC COMPARTMENTATION OF
GLUTAMATE

Ambrish J. Patel

MRC Developmental Neurobiology Unit
Institute of Neurology, 33 John's Mews
London   WC1N 2NS

INTRODUCTION

Kinetic studies on the fate of labelled substances oxidized in
the brain, carried out initially in the laboratory of the late
Professor Waelsch and his colleagues (for references see Balazs and
Cremer, 1973), have indicated that the metabolism of glutamate and
the associated tricarboxylic acid cycle intermediates are compartmented in the brain. The first model considering the structural
correlates on metabolic compartments was put forward by Garfinkel
(1966) and this has been further modified in the light of new
information (cf. Balazs et al., 1970). In 1973, on the basis of
these studies of the metabolism of labelled GABA and glucose in vitro
(Balazs et al., 1970; Machiyama et al., 1970) and of the fate of
other labelled substrates in vivo (Berl and Clarke, 1969; Van den Berg,
1970; Patel and Balazs, 1970), and, in particular, of our studies on
the influence of metabolic factors on the development of metabolic
compartmentation of glutamate (Patel and Balazs, 1971; 1975),
Dr. Balazs and myself postulated that the 'small' glutamate
compartment, where most of the labelled glutamine is formed, was
located in glial cells and the 'large' compartment in neuronal
structures (Balazs et al.,1973). It must be emphasized, however,
that each "compartment" probably results from the summation of a
number of different units with more or less similar metabolic
patterns; moreover, the compartments are not static but depend on
the experimental conditions under which they are observed (Patel
et al., 1970; Balazs et al., 1973; Patel et al., 1974; Mohler et al.,
1974; 1976; Van den Berg et al., 1975).

A simplified scheme based on two-compartment models, where
compartments assigned to neuronal structures by Balazs et al (1973)

411

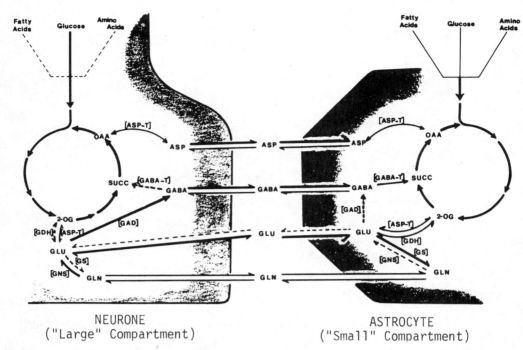

Fig. 1.   Simplified scheme of metabolic compartmentation of glutamate
          and associated Krebs cycle intermediates. In this scheme,
          based on two-compartment models, the compartments assigned
          to neuronal structures (II and III) in Balazs et al (1973)
          are combined. Abbreviations used, for intermediates: OAA-
          oxaloacetate, SUCC-succinate, 2-OG - 2-oxoglutarate, ASP-
          aspartate, GABA-γ-aminobutyrate, GLU-glutamate and GLN-
          glutamine; and for enzymes: [ASP-T]-aspartate aminotrans-
          ferase, [GABA-T]-GABA aminotransferase, [GAD] -glutamate
          decarboxylase, [GS] -glutamine synthetase, [GNS]-glutaminase
          and [GDH]-glutamate dehydrogenase.

are combined, is given in Fig. 1. Briefly, it shows that when the
transmitter amino acids (glutamate, GABA and aspartate) are released
from nerve terminals, a large part is taken up by the glial cells
and there converted into glutamine. Glutamine diffuses out continuously into the extracellular space, from which it is taken up by
neurones and hydrolysed to glutamate, thus balancing the loss of
carbon units in the tricarboxylic acid cycle that occurs as a result
of release of amino acid transmitters. During the last few years a
number of studies have corroborated certain aspects of our hypothesis

(cf. Patel, 1981). The most important new observations have been: (a) the course of metabolism of neuronal glutamate differs from that of glial glutamate (Benjamin and Quastel, 1974); (b) after incubation of rat dorsal root ganglia with [^{14}C]acetate followed by autoradiography silver grains appeared mainly on satellite glial cells, while they were seen on nerve cell bodies when the ganglia were incubated with [^{14}C]glucose (Minchin and Beart, 1974); (c) as shown independently both in the laboratories of Bradford (Bradford et al., 1978) and of Cotman (Hamberger et al., 1979), glutamine is a better precursor than exogenous glutamate of the 'transmitter' glutamate in vitro, and (d) glutamine synthetase, the enzyme responsible for glutamine formation, is present predominantly in glial structures (Martinez-Hernandez et al., 1977). With the recent availability of relatively pure cell types in our Unit (Balazs et al., 1980) we are now able to estimate some of the enzymes directly involved in these processes, and if our model is correct they should have a selective distribution between neurones and glia (Patel et al., 1981a). The present report also describes other results supporting the involvement of glutamine synthetase in processes associated with amino acid neurotransmission and discusses the regulation of this enzyme in developing brain in vivo.

THE ACTIVITIES OF ENZYMES RELATED TO GLUTAMATE METABOLISM IN NEURONES AND ASTROCYTES

Previously, the distribution of enzymes associated with glutamate metabolism has been studied in preparations of isolated perikarya and in subcellular fractions from brain (e.g. Salganicoff and de Robertis, 1965; Balazs et al., 1966; Rose, 1968; Neidle et al., 1969; Van den Berg et al., 1975; Dennis et al., 1977; Hamberger et al., 1978; Weiler et al., 1979a). Such studies of subcellular distribution provides evidence about morphological correlates of metabolic compartments but it is circumstantial. Moreover, much of the information previously obtained from studies on separated cell types must be questioned because the structural preservation of the cells, and thus presumably their metabolic competence was inadequate (Wilkin et al., 1976; Bálazs et al., 1980).

In the present studies ultrastructurally preserved and metabolically competent cell bodies were isolated by mild trypsinization of cerebellum from 8-day old rats and were separated into various relatively pure cell types (Purkinje cells, granule cells and astrocytes), by unit-gravity sedimentation as described previously by my colleagues (Cohen et al., 1978, 1979; Woodhams et al., 1980). Alternatively, a selection for neuronal and glial cell types was achieved by tissue culture techniques (Messer, 1977; Balazs et al., 1980; Patel et al., 1981a).

Marked differences were observed in the distribution of the enzymes studied in the various classes of cells (Fig. 2). In

general, the profile of 'glutamate' enzymes in the nerve cells
differed from that in astrocytes (Gordon et al., 1981; Patel et al.,
1981a).

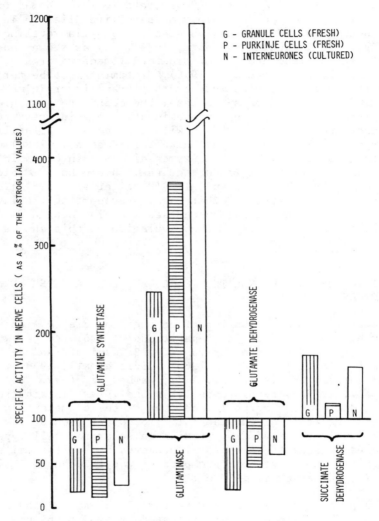

Fig. 2.   The cellular distribution of certain enzymes associated with
          the metabolic compartmentation of glutamate has been estim-
          ated in ultrastructurally preserved and metabolically
          competent perikarya fractions that were enriched in astro-
          cytes, granule cells and Purkinje cells and derived from 8
          day old rat cerebellum, and in monolayer cultures (14 DIV)
          composed principally of interneurones or astrocytes. The
          specific activity (µmol/h/mg protein) in neuronal cells are
          expressed as a percentage of the respective astrocyte values
          (From Patel et al., 1981a).

Glutamine Synthetase

In the freshly isolated perikarya preparations the activity of glutamine synthetase was respectively 5 and 8 times higher in the astrocytes than in the granule and Purkinje cells. This difference between the cell classes was also maintained in the cultured cells, as the enzyme activity of the isolated granule cells or astrocytes was similar to that in the respective cultures. The activity in the cultured interneurones, which consisted mainly of granule cells, was one quarter of that in astrocyte cultures (Fig. 2). The first systematic attempt to determine the cellular distribution of this enzyme has been made by Rose (1968), who reported that the activity of glutamine synthetase in neurones is nearly double that in glia, a finding radically different from our observations (Table 1). Similarly, a relative enrichment of glutamine synthetase in neurones and in subcellular fractions derived from neurones, such as synaptosomes, has also been reported by Hamberger and co-workers (Hamberger et al., 1978; Weiler et al., 1979a), but not by others (Salganicoff and De Robertis, 1965; Ward and Bradford, 1979). However, Schousboe et al (1977) observed that the glutamine synthetase activity in primary astrocyte cultures is similar to that in the whole brain (Table 2). Our results are also in good agreement with the immunocytochemical demonstration of the localization of glutamine synthetase in rat brain (Martinez-Hernandez et al., 1977).

Table 1. The Distribution of Certain Enzymes Associated With the Metabolic Compartmentation of Glutamate in Relatively Enriched Neuronal and Glial Cell Fractions

	Specific activity ratio of neuronal/glial cells		
	Rose, 1968	Hamberger et al., 1978	Patel et al., 1981a
Glutamine synthetase	1.77	0.82	0.12 - 0.19
Glutaminase	-	0.37	2.46 - 3.71
Glutamate dehydrogenase	2.61	-	0.19 - 0.45
Succinate dehydrogenase	-	-	1.18 - 1.72

Table 2. The Distribution of Certain Enzymes Associated With the
          Metabolic Compartmentation of Glutamate in Relatively
          Pure Neuronal and Glial Cell Primary Cultures

	Specific activity (μmol/h per mg protein)		
	Schousboe et al., 1977;1979	Patel et al., 1981a		22-Day old cerebellum
	Astroglial	Astroglial	Neuronal	
Glutamine synthetase	1.55	1.33	0.34	1.32
Glutaminase*	0.23	0.11	1.31	0.41
Glutamate dehydrogenase	0.74	6.08	3.65	11.19
Succinate dehydrogenase	–	0.60	0.96	2.24

* The initial rate obtained at optimal substrate concentration (8 mM
  glutamine) or at suboptimal substrate concentration (0.5 mM)
  multiplied by 10 (see, Patel et al., 1981a).

Glutaminase

       In contrast to glutamine synthetase, the glutaminase activity
was about 3 times higher in the isolated perikarya of granule and
Purkinje cells than in astrocytes (Fig. 2). The differences between
these two neural cell types in monolayer cultures were much greater,
about 12 fold. This was due to the fact that in comparison with the
isolated cell bodies the activity in cultured astroglia was half
while in interneurone cultures it was double (Patel et al., 1981a).
These results are in good agreement with the values previously
reported for synaptosomes, in which the enzyme activity is found to
be enriched by about 2-4 fold on a protein basis (Salganicoff and
De Robertis, 1965; Bradford and Ward, 1976; Ward and Bradford, 1979).
However, Hamberger and his co-workers (Hamberger et al., 1978;
Weiler et al., 1979a) have reported that in bulk prepared neural cell
types the activity of this enzyme is about 2 - 3 fold higher in
glial cells than in neurones (Table 1). Schousboe et al (1979) have

also reported that the activity of glutaminase in astrocyte cultures
is relatively high as it is similar to that in adult brain. On the
other hand, in our study, the activity in astrocyte cultures was less
than 10% or 14% respectively of that in the interneurone cultures or
in adult cerebellum (Patel et al., 1981a). Schousboe and Divac (1979)
have suggested that the properties of astrocytes derived from various
regions of the brain differ and this may contribute to the discrepant
results (astrocyte cultures were prepared from mouse forebrain by
Schousboe et al., 1979 and from the rat cerebellum in our studies,
Patel et al., 1981a). In addition the differences may also relate
in part to the culture conditions (see below).

Glutamate Dehydrogenase

On the basis of $^{15}NH_3$-infusion experiments, Berl et al (1962)
have proposed that glutamate dehydrogenase is associated with the
'small' compartment of glutamate, which in our model is related to
glial structures. This was supported by the present results showing
respectively 2.2 and 5.3 fold higher enzyme activity in the astrocytes than in the Purkinje and granule cells (Fig. 2). Similar
enrichment of glutamate dehydrogenase activity has been reported in
C_6 glioma compared to neuroblastoma cells (Passonneau et al., 1977).
In contrast, Rose (1968) has claimed that the activity of glutamate
dehydrogenase is higher in neurones than in glia (Table 1). A
histochemical electron microscopic study on the localization of
glutamate dehydrogenase in the cerebellum has also failed to reveal
a clear-cut distinction between neurones and glial cells, both cell
classes showing random variation in the activity in different
cellular regions (Toledano et al., 1979). It is possible that the
differences in the enzyme activity between neuronal and glial cells
is too small for detection by the histochemical method. Furthermore,
in comparison with our astrocyte cultures, the cultures of Schousboe
et al (1977) show very low glutamate dehydrogenase activity (Table 2).
One of the major differences between our culture conditions (Patel
et al., 1981a) and that of Schousboe et al (1977) is that during
the last week they withdrew serum and added cyclic AMP in their
culture medium to induce the differentiation of astrocytes (i.e.
rapid growth of cell processes), and these may relate in part to
these differences. However, in cultured cells the activities of
enzymes reported in Table 2 in general and mitochondrial enzymes in
particular were lower than in the cerebellum at a comparable age.

Succinate Dehydrogenase

Glutamate dehydrogenase and glutaminase are both mitochondrial
enzymes; therefore, in order to correct for the possible effect of
differences in mitochondrial concentration in the different cell
types, the activity of succinate dehydrogenase was also measured

(Fig. 2). The enzyme activity was more uniformly distributed in the
different cells than were the other mitochondrial enzymes assayed,
and the differences in the activity of glutamate dehydrogenase and
glutaminase between neuronal and glial cells persisted even after
the correction for the activity of succinate dehydrogenase (Patel
et al., 1981a).

CORRELATION BETWEEN REGIONAL DISTRIBUTION OF GLUTAMINE SYNTHETASE
AND GLUTAMATE DECARBOXYLASE

In previous studies on glutamine synthetase the most commonly
used method has been the colorimetric assay of γ-glutamylhydroxamate
formed from an activated glutamine residue and hydroxylamine
(Levintow, 1954; Pamiljans et al., 1962). A number of studies
have shown that the ratio of synthetase to transferase activity
exhibited by the enzyme depended upon the conditions employed for
the activity determination (see, Herzfeld, 1973). It is possible
that when unpurified tissue preparations have been studied, the
estimation of glutamine synthetase was vitiated by the action of
other enzymes such as glutaminases and glutamine amidotransferases
that can also catalyse formation of γ-glutamylhydroxamate from
glutamate and hydroxylamine (Meister, 1980). Therefore, it seems
that the more appropriate method for the estimation of glutamine
synthetase is by measurement of labelled glutamine formed from the
precursor $[1-^{14}C]$glutamate (Patel and Hunt, 1981a), and the assay
system should contain both a Na^+-K^+ ATPase inhibitor and an ATP
regenerating system (Ward and Bradford, 1979).

Using this optimised method we have measured the developmental
increase in the specific activity of glutamine synthetase in three
brain regions (Fig. 3). The results showed that at the ages when
the rate of cell acquisition is at a maximum the increase in
glutamine synthetase is low. The major increase in enzyme activity
in all the three brain regions is after cell acquisition has more
or less ceased, suggesting that the increase in glutamine synthetase
mainly reflects the differentiation of astrocytes. When the daily
increase in glutamine synthetase was compared with that of the S-100
protein (Herschman et al., 1971; Ghandour et al., 1981) which is
also believed to be localized in astrocytes, it became evident that
the maximum acquisition of both these astrocytic proteins occurs at
a comparable age. However, glutamine synthetase, particularly in
the cerebellum, continues to increase at an appreciably higher rate
and for a much longer time than S-100 protein.

Marked differences were observed in different brain regions in
the distribution of glutamine synthetase (Fig. 4) and the range,
between the lowest value in the spinal cord (not given in the Figure)
and the highest value in the olfactory bulbs, is about 3 - 4 fold
(Patel and Hunt, 1981b). In any given brain region the activity of

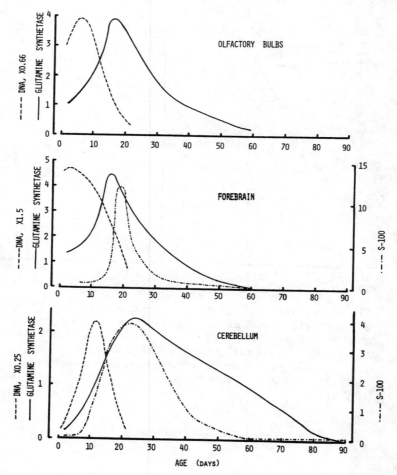

Fig. 3.   The daily increase in the amount of glutamine synthetase,
           cell number and S-100 protein in the olfactory bulbs, fore-
           brain and cerebellum of the rat during development. The
           results for glutamine synthetase (from Patel and Hunt,
           1981a), DNA (from Patel and Balazs, 1980) and S-100 (from
           Herschman et al., 1971; Ghandour et al., 1981) are given
           as a percentage of the adult amount deposited each day.

glutamine synthetase was at least 8-10 fold higher than that of
glutamate decarboxylase. Furthermore, in different regions of the
brain the activity of glutamine synthetase was significantly (P<0.001)

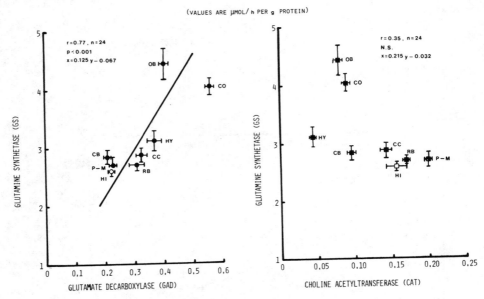

Fig. 4. The correlation of glutamine synthetase with glutamate
         decarboxylase and choline acetyltransferase in different
         regions of the rat brain. Abbreviations used: OB- olfactory
         bulbs, CO- colliculi, HY- hypothalamus, CC- cerebral cortex,
         CB- cerebellum, P-M- pons-medulla, HI- hippocampus and RB-
         residual brain. (From Patel et al., 1978; Patel and Hunt,
         1981b).

correlated with that of glutamate decarboxylase (a marker of GABA-
ergic systems), but not with that of choline acetyltransferase
(a marker of cholinergic systems). This indicates that the high
concentration of glutamine synthetase in certain regions may suggest
an equally high proportion of nerve cells in that brain part
functioning with amino acids as neurotransmitter. These observations
provide further evidence for the involvement of glutamine synthetase
in processes associated with amino acid neurotransmission.

NEURONAL-ASTROCYTIC INTERACTIONS IN THE METABOLISM OF NEUROTRANS-
MITTER AMINO ACIDS

    The cell type specific distribution of enzymes related to
glutamate metabolism and a selective correlation of glutamine
synthetase with glutamate decarboxylase and not with choline

acetyltransferase in different brain regions, are consistent with the view that the inactivation of neurotransmitter amino acids and the loss of carbon units resulting from transmitter release involve intercellular metabolic co-operation between neurones and astrocytes. In particular, the enrichment of glutamine synthetase in astrocytes and glutaminase in neurones are key factors for these enzymes catalyse the conversion of glutamate to glutamine and of glutamine to glutamate, respectively. Furthermore, the rate of glutamate transport (Vmax) is very high in glial cells relative to neuronal structures (for cerebellar cells, see chapter by R. Balazs; Gordon et al., 1980; Hertz, 1979). Therefore, it would appear that a considerable fraction of the glutamate which is released from neurones is likely to be taken up by astrocytes. Thus a 'large' compartment comprising neurones is losing tricarboxylic acid constituents to a 'small' compartment associated with astroglia, and this loss should be balanced by a flow of glutamine in the opposite direction. The situation regarding the uptake of glutamine into neuronal structures is not at present very clear. Some workers have reported a high affinity uptake (K_m about 50 μM) of glutamine into chopped brain slices (Balcar and Johnson, 1975) and synaptosomes (Roberts and Keen, 1974), while others observed a low affinity uptake that had a K_m of about 250 μM in synaptosomes (Baldessarini and Yorke, 1974; Weiler et al., 1979b) and about 680 μM in slices (Benjamin et al., 1980). However, all preparations showed a Vmax of 0.2 to 1 μmol/min per g wet weight. Glutamine concentration in cerebrospinal fluid is relatively high (about 0.5 mM; Gjessing et al.,1972), and if this reflects the extracellular concentration in the brain, then the above uptake process can supply neurones with sufficient exogenous glutamine. Furthermore, an increase in extracellular K^+ concentration during neurotransmission will facilitate the uptake of glutamine (Machiyama et al., 1970), and this will probably be more in nerve cells than in glial cells because of the expected lower intracellular glutamine concentration in the former than in latter, due to selective localisation of glutamine catabolizing and synthesizing enzymes in these cell types. The activity of glutaminase was high in nerve cells, and it is possible that the transported glutamine could be converted in these cells to glutamate, which would serve as a compensating source of carbon and nitrogen. Therefore, the present findings strongly support our model assigning metabolic compartments to particular morphological structures, underlying the importance of metabolic interaction between neuronal and glial cells in the brain.

REGULATION OF IN VIVO GLUTAMINE SYNTHETASE ACTIVITY BY GLUCOCORTICOIDS

In prokaryotic systems the regulation of glutamine synthetase is subject to a variety of control mechanisms including covalent modification of the enzyme by the reversible adenylylation of a specific tyrosyl residue on each subunit and feedback regulation by

several metabolites (see review, Tyler, 1978). However in eukaryotic
systems the regulation of the enzyme is far less well understood.
The liver enzyme can be activated by α-oxoglutarate and inhibited by
glycine, alanine and carbamylphosphate, but these compounds have
relatively little effect on brain glutamine synthetase (Tate et al.,
1972). Glutamine-mediated regulation of glutamine synthetase has
been observed in cultured HeLa cells (DeMars, 1958), mouse L cells
(Barnes et al., 1971) and Chinese hamster cells (Tiemeimer and
Milman, 1972).

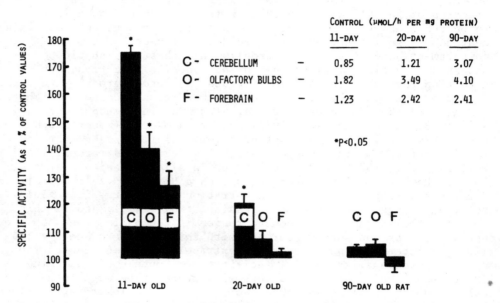

Fig. 5.   Induction by glucocorticoids of glutamine synthetase in
          developing rat brain in vivo. Three groups of rats aged
          8, 17, and 87 days were given daily subcutaneous injections
          of corticosterone-21-acetate (40 mg/kg) for 3 days and
          killed 24h after the last injection. The specific activities
          of glutamine synthetase in the cerebellum, olfactory bulbs
          and forebrain of experimental rats are given as a percentage
          of the respective control values. The mean control values
          based on 3 - 5 observations are given in inset. (From
          Patel et al., 1981b).

     Glutocorticoids have been shown to regulate the activity of
glutamine synthetase in a variety of mammalian cells, including chick
embryonic retina (Moscona et al., 1980), cultured hepatoma cells

(Kulka and Cohen, 1973; Crook et al., 1978), mouse fibroblasts
(Miller et al., 1978), and cultured cells of neural origin, such as
primary cultures enriched in astrocytes (Vaccaro et al., 1979;
Juurlink et al., 1981; Hallermayer et al., 1981) and established
glioma cell lines (Pishak and Phillips, 1980; Hallermayer et al.,
1981). In agreement with these in vitro findings, we have now
observed that glucocorticoids can induce the activity of glutamine
synthetase in developing rat brain in vivo (Patel et al., 1981b).
As mentioned before (see Fig. 3 and inset in Fig. 5), the specific
activity of glutamine synthetase increased linearly up to day 50
in the cerebellum before reaching the adult level, while in the
forebrain the activity at birth (0.28 µmol/h per mg protein) was a
little higher than in cerebellum (0.24 µmol/h per mg protein) and
increased at a much faster rate reaching the adult value by day 20.
On the other hand, in the olfactory bulbs the activity at birth
(0.59 µmol/h per mg protein) was about twice as much as in forebrain,
increased much more rapidly until the first 20 days after birth and
then at a lower rate up to day 60 (Patel and Hunt, 1981a). Corticosterone treatment resulted in increases in glutamine synthetase
activity of magnitude depending on age (Fig. 5). In 8 day old rats
the increase was about 70% in the cerebellum, 40% in the olfactory
bulbs and 30% in the forebrain. The effect was markedly diminished
during development and at day 20 a marked increase was detectable
only in the cerebellum. The induction of glutamine synthetase also
depended on the dose of corticosterone and the duration of the
hormonal treatment. The large induction was also observed after
treatment with dexamethasone, but not with other steroid hormones
(testosterone, estradiol or progesterone).

SUMMARY

     The cellular distribution of certain enzymes associated with the
metabolic compartmentation of glutamate was estimated in ultrastructurally preserved and metabolically competent perikarya fractions
that were enriched in astrocytes, granule cells and Purkinje cells
and derived from 8 day old rat cerebellum, and in monolayer cultures
(14 DIV) composed principally of interneurones or astrocytes. The
activities of glutamine synthetase and glutamate dehydrogenase in
astrocytes were respectively about 4 - 8 fold and 2 - 5 fold higher
than in neurones, depending upon the class of neurone and the type
of preparation used for comparison. By contrast, glutaminase
activity was about 3.- 12 fold higher in neuronal than in astrocyte
preparations. The specific activity of succinate dehydrogenase was
more even in the different cell types, indicating that the differences
in the distribution of mitochondrial enzymes are not simply related
to variations in the concentration of mitochondria in the two classes
of cells. The possible involvement of glutamine synthetase in

processes associated with amino acid neurotransmission was also suggested by the two findings: the activity of this enzyme was unevenly distributed throughout the central nervous system, and in the different regions of the brain its activity was significantly correlated with that of glutamate decarboxylase but not with that of choline acetyltransferase. The findings presented provide direct evidence in support of our model assigning the 'small' glutamate compartment, where most of the labelled glutamine is synthesized, to glial cells, and the 'large' compartment to neurones, and also underline the metabolic interaction between these two cell types in the brain.

In agreement with previous studies on glutamine synthetase in chick retina and various avian and mammalian cells in vitro, we observed that the activity of this enzyme in the mammalian brain in vivo was increased by glucocorticoids. The increase was more marked in young than in adult rats and comparison of the effect in various brain areas suggested that elevation of glutamine synthetase was dependent on the maturational state of the region at the time of the hormone treatment. Glutamine synthetase induction was also observed after treatment with dexamethasone, but not with testosterone, estradiol or progesterone.

ACKNOWLEDGMENTS

The author is indebted to Dr. R. Balazs for his advice, encouragement and active collaboration over many years, and gratefully acknowledges the collaboration of Mr. R.D. Gordon, Mr. A. Hunt and Dr. C.S.M. Tahourdin in these studies. The author also thanks Dr. B.W.L. Brooksbank for critically reading this manuscript.

REFERENCES

Balazs, R., and Cremer, J.E., Eds., 1973, "Metabolic Compartmentation in the Brain", Macmillan, London.
Balazs, R., Dahl, D., and Harwood, J.R., 1966, Subcellular distribution of enzymes of glutamate metabolism in rat brain, J. Neurochem., 13: 897-905.
Balazs, R., Machiyama, Y., Hammond, B.J., Julian, T., and Richter, D., 1970, The operation of the γ-aminobutyrate bypath of the tricarboxylic acid cycle in brain tissue in vitro, Biochem. J., 116: 445-467.
Balazs, R., Patel, A.J., and Richter, D., 1973, Metabolic compartments in the brain: their properties and relation to morphological structures, in: "Metabolic Compartmentation in the Brain" (R. Balazs and J.E. Cremer, eds.) pp. 167-184, Macmillan, London.

Balazs, R., Regan, C., Meier, E., Woodhams, P.L., Wilkin, G.P., Patel, N.J. and Gordon, R.D., 1980, Biochemical properties of neural cell types from rat cerebellum, in: "Tissue Culture in Neurobiology" (E. Giacobini, A. Vernadakis and A. Shahar, eds.), pp. 155-168, Raven Press, New York.

Balcar, V.J. and Johnston, G.A.R., 1975, High affinity uptake of L-glutamine in rat brain slices, J. Neurochem., 24: 875-879.

Baldessarini, R.J., and Yorke, C., 1974, Uptake and release of possible false transmitter amino acids by rat brain tissue, J. Neurochem., 23: 839-848.

Barnes, P.R., Youngberg, D., and Kitos, P.A., 1971, Factors affecting production of glutamine in cultured mouse cells, J. Cell Physiol., 77: 135-144.

Benjamin, A.M., and Quastel, J.H., 1974, Fate of L-glutamate in the brain, J. Neurochem., 23: 457-464.

Benjamin, A.M., Verjee, Z.H., and Quastel, J.H., 1980, Kinetics of cerebral uptake processes in vitro of L-glutamine, branched-chain L-amino acids, and L-phenylalanine: effect of ouabain, J. Neurochem., 35: 67-77.

Berl, S., and Clarke, D.D., 1969, Compartmentation of amino acid metabolism, in: "Handbook of Neurochemistry", Vol. 2 (A. Lahtha, ed.), pp. 447-472, Plenum Press, New York.

Berl, S., Takagaki, G., Clarke, D.D., and Waelsch, H., 1962, Metabolic compartments in vivo. Ammonia and glutamic acid metabolism in brain and liver, J. Biol. Chem., 237: 2562- 2573.

Bradford, H.F., and Ward, H.K., 1976, On glutaminase activity in mammalian synaptosomes, Brain Res., 110: 115-125.

Bradford, H.F., Ward, H.K., and Thomas, A.J., 1978, Glutamine - a major substrate for nerve-endings, J. Neurochem., 30: 1453-1459.

Cohen, J., Balazs, R., Hajos, F., Currie, D.N., and Dutton, G.R., 1978, Separation of cell types from the developing cerebellum, Brain Res., 148: 313-331.

Cohen, J., Woodhams, P.L., and Balazs, R., 1979, Preparation of viable astrocytes from the developing cerebellum, Brain Res., 161: 503-514.

Crook, R.B., Louie, M., Deuel, T.F., and Tomkins, G.M., 1978, Regulation of glutamine synthetase by dexamethasone in hepatoma tissue culture cells, J. Biol. Chem., 253: 6125-6131.

DeMars, R., 1958, The inhibition by glutamine of glutamyl transferase formation in cultures of human cells, Biochem. Biophys. Acta, 27: 435-436.

Dennis, S.C., Lai, J.C.K., and Clark, J.B., 1977, Comparative studies on glutamate metabolism in synaptic and non-synaptic rat brain mitochondria, Biochem. J., 164: 727-736.

Garfinkel, D., 1966, A simulation study of the metabolism and compartmentation in brain of glutamate, aspartate, the Krebs cycle and related metabolites, J. Biol. Chem., 241: 3918-3929.

Ghandour, M.S., Labourdette, G., Vincendon, G., and Gombos, G., 1981, A biochemical and immunohistological study of S100 protein in developing rat cerebellum, Dev. Neurosci., 4: 98-109.

Gjessing, L.R., Gjesdahl, P., and Sjaastad, O., 1972, The free amino acids in human cerebrospinal fluid, J. Neurochem., 19: 1807-1808.

Gordon, R.D., Wilkin, G.P., Gallo, V., Levi, G., and Balazs, R., 1980, High affinity transport of L-glutamate and D-aspartate into cell types of the cerebellum, Neurosci. Lett., Suppl. 5: 78.

Gordon, R.D., Hunt, A. and Patel, A.J., 1981, The cellular distribution of certain enzymes associated with the metabolic compartmentation of glutamate, Biochem. Soc. Trans., 9: 115-116.

Hallermayer, K., Harmening, C., and Hamprecht, B., 1981, Cellular localization and regulation of glutamine synthetase in primary cultures of brain cells from newborn mice, J. Neurochem., 37: 43-52.

Hamberger, A., Cotman, C.W., Sellstrom, A., and Weiler, C.T., 1978, Glutamine, glial cells and their relationship to transmitter glutamate, in: "Dynamic Properties of Glial Cells" (E. Schoffeniels, G. Franck, L. Hertz and D.B. Tower, eds.), pp. 163-172, Pergamon Press, New York.

Hamberger, A., Chiang, G.H., Hylen, E.S., Schiff, S.W., and Cotman, C.W., 1979, Glutamate as a CNS transmitter, I. Evaluation of glucose and glutamine as precursors for the synthesis of preferentially released glutamate, Brain Res., 168: 513-530.

Herschman, H.R., Levine, L., and De Vellis, J., 1971, Appearance of a brain-specific antigen (S-100 protein) in the developing rat brain. J. Neurochem., 18: 629-633.

Hertz, L., 1979, Functional interactions between neurons and astrocytes. I. Turnover and metabolism of putative amino acid transmitters, Prog. Neurobiol., 13: 277-323.

Herzfeld, A., 1973, The distribution between γ-glutamylhydroxamate synthetase and L-glutamine-hydroxylamine glutamyltransferase activities in rat tissues studies in vitro, Biochem. J., 133: 49-57.

Juurlink, B.H.J., Schousboe, A., Jorgensen, O.S. and Hertz, L., 1981, Induction by hydrocortisone of glutamine synthetase in mouse primary astrocyte cultures, J. Neurochem., 36: 136-142.

Kulka, R.G., and Cohen, H., 1973, Regulation of glutamine synthetase activity of hepatoma tissue culture cells by glutamine and dexamethasone, J. Biol. Chem., 248: 6738-6743.

Levintow, L., 1954, The glutamyltransferase activity of normal and neoplastic tissues, J. Natl. Cancer Inst., 15: 347-352.

Machiyama, Y., Balazs, R., Hammond, B.J., Julian, T., and Richter, D., 1970, The metabolism of γ-aminobutyrate and glucose in potassium ion-stimulated brain tissue in vitro, Biochem. J., 116: 469-481.

Martinez-Hernandez, A., Bell, K.P., and Norenberg, M.D., 1977, Glutamine synthetase: glial localization in brain, Science, 195: 1356-1358.

Meister, A., 1980, Catalytic mechanism of glutamine synthetase; overview of glutamine metabolism, in: "Glutamine: Metabolism, Enzymology and Regulation" (J. Mora and R. Palacios, eds.), pp. 1-40, Academic Press, New York.

Messer, A., 1977, The maintenance and identification of mouse cerebellar granule cells in monolayer culture, Brain Res., 130: 1-12.

Miller, R.E., Hackenberg, R., and Gershman, H., 1978, Regulation of glutamine synthetase in cultured 3T3-LI cells by insulin hydrocortisone, and dibutyryl cylic AMP, Proc. Natl. Acad. Sci. USA, 75: 1418-1422.

Minchin, M.C.W., and Beart, P.M., 1974, Compartmentation of amino acid metabolism in the rat dorsal root ganglion. A metabolic and autoradiographic study, Brain Res., 83: 437-449.

Mohler, H., Patel, A.J., and Balazs, R., 1974, Metabolic compartmentation in the brain: metabolism of a tricarboxylic acid cycle intermediate, $[1,4-^{14}C]$- succinate, after intracerebral administration, J. Neurochem., 23: 1281-1289.

Mohler, H., Patel, A.J., and Balazs, R., 1976, Gamma-hydroxybutyrate degradation in the brain in vivo: negligible direct conversion to GABA, J. Neurochem., 27: 253-258.

Moscona, A.A., Linser, P., Mayerson, P., and Moscona, M., 1980, Regulatory aspects of the induction of glutamine synthetase in embryonic neural retina, in: "Glutamine: Metabolism, Enzymology and Regulation" (J. Mora and R. Palacios, eds.), pp. 299-313, Academic Press, New York.

Neidle, A., Van den Berg, C.J., and Grynbaum, A., 1969, The heterogeneity of rat brain mitochondria isolated on continuous sucrose gradients, J. Neurochem., 16: 225-234.

Pamiljans, V., Krishnaswamy, P.R., Dunnville, G., and Meister, A., 1962, Studies on the mechanism of glutamine synthetase: isolation and properties of the enzyme from sheep brain, Biochemistry, 1: 153-158.

Passonneau, J.V., Lust, W.D., and Crites, S.K., 1977, Studies on the GABAergic system in astrocytoma and neuroblastoma cells in culture, Neurochem. Res., 2: 605-617.

Patel, A.J., 1981, Amino acids and the nervous system, in: "Amino acid Analysis" (J.M. Rattenbury, ed.), pp. 237-256, Ellis Horwood, Chichester.

Patel, A.J., and Balazs, R., 1970, Manifestation of metabolic compartmentation during the maturation of the rat brain, J. Neurochem., 17: 955-971.

Patel, A.J., and Balazs, R., 1971, Effect of thyroid hormone on metabolic compartmentation in the developing rat brain, Biochem. J., 121: 469-481.

Patel, A.J., and Balazs, R., 1975, Factors affecting the development of metabolic compartmentation in the brain, in: "Metabolic Compartmentation and Neurotransmission. Relation to Brain Structure and Function" (S. Berl, D.D. Clarke and D. Schneider, eds.), pp. 363-383, Plenum Press, New York.

Patel, A.J., and Balazs, R., 1980, Hormones and cell proliferation in the rat brain, in: "Progress in Psychoneuroendocrinology" (F. Brambilla, G. Racagni and D. de Wied, eds.), pp. 621-632, Elsevier/North-Holland Biomedical Press, Amsterdam.

Patel, A.J., and Hunt, A., 1981a, Maturation of astrocytes followed by changes in the activity of glutamine synthetase in three brain areas of the rat during development, in preparation.

Patel, A.J., and Hunt, A., 1981b, The regional distribution of glutamine synthetase and its correlation with glutamate decarboxylase in the rat brain, in preparation.

Patel, A.J., Balazs, R., and Richter, D., 1970, Contribution of the GABA bypath to glucose oxidation, and the development of compartmentation in the brain, Nature, 226: 1160-1161.

Patel, A.J., Johnson, A.L., and Balazs, R., 1974, Metabolic compartmentation of glutamate associated with the formation of γ-aminobutyrate, J. Neurochem., 23: 1271-1279.

Patel, A.J., del Vecchio, M., and Atkinson, D.J., 1978, Effect of undernutrition on the regional development of transmitter enzymes: glutamate decarboxylase and choline acetyltransferase, Dev. Neurosci., 1: 41-53.

Patel, A.J., Hunt,A., Gordon, R.D., and Balazs, R., 1981a, The activities in different neural cell types of certain enzymes associated with the metabolic compartmentation of glutamate, Brain Res., in press.

Patel, A.J., Hunt, A. and Tahourdin, C.S.M., 1981b, Induction by glucocorticoids of glutamine synthetase in developing rat brain in vivo, 8th Meet. Int. Soc. Neurochem., Nottingham, (Abstr.), p. 174.

Pishak, M.R., and Phillips, A.T., 1980, Glucocorticoid stimulation of glutamine synthetase production in cultured rat glioma cells, J. Neurochem., 34: 866-872.

Roberts, P.J., and Keen, P., 1974, High affinity uptake for glutamine in rat dorsal roots but not in nerve endings, Brain Res., 67: 352-357.

Rose, S.P.R., 1968, Glucose and amino acid metabolism in isolated neuronal and glial cell fractions in vitro, J. Neurochem., 15: 1415-1429.

Salganicoff, L., and De Robertis, E., 1965, Subcellular distribution of the enzymes of the glutamic acid, glutamine and gamma-aminobutyric acid cycles in rat brain, J. Neurochem., 12: 287-309.

Schousboe, A., and Divac, I., 1979, Differences in glutamate uptake in astrocytes cultured from different brain regions, Brain Res., 177: 407-409.

Schousboe, A., Svenneby, G., and Hertz, L., 1977, Uptake and meta-
    bolism of glutamate in astrocytes cultured from dissociated
    mouse brain hemispheres, J. Neurochem., 29: 999-1005.
Schousboe, A., Hertz, L., Svenneby, G., and Kvamme, E., 1979, Phos-
    phate activated glutaminase activity and glutamate uptake in
    primary cultures of astrocytes, J. Neurochem., 32: 943-950.
Tate, S.S., Leu, F., and Meister, A., 1972, Rat liver glutamine
    synthetase, J. Biol. Chem., 247: 5312-5321.
Tiemeier, D.C., and Milman, G., 1972, Regulation of glutamine
    synthetase in cultured Chinese hamster cells, J. Biol. Chem.,
    247: 5722-5727.
Toledano, A., Barca, M.A., Perez, C., and Martinez-Rodriguez, R.,
    1979, Histochemical electron microscope study of the enzyme
    glutamate dehydrogenase in cerebellum, Cell. Mol. Biol., 24:
    113-125.
Tyler, B., 1978, Regulation of the assimilation of nitrogen compounds,
    Ann. Rev. Biochem., 47: 1127-1162.
Vaccaro, D.E., Leeman, S.E., and Reif-Lehrer, L., 1979, Glutamine
    synthetase activity in vivo and in primary cell cultures of
    rat hypothalamus, J. Neurochem., 33: 953-957.
Van den Berg, C.J., 1970, Glutamate and glutamine, in: "Handbook of
    Neurochemistry", Vol. 3 (A. Lajtha, ed.), pp. 355-379,
    Plenum Press, New York.
Van den Berg, C.J., Matheson, D.F., Ronda, G., Reijnierse, G.L.A.,
    Blokhuis, G.G.D., Kroon, M.G., Clarke, D.D., and Garfinkel, D.,
    1975, A model of glutamate metabolism in brain: a biochemical
    analysis of a heterogeneous structure, in: "Metabolic
    Compartmentation and Neurotransmission. Relation to Brain
    Structure and Function" (S. Berl, D.D. Clarke and D. Schneider,
    eds), pp. 515-543, Plenum Press, New York.
Ward, H.K. and Bradford, H.F., 1979, Relative activities of glutamine
    synthetase and glutaminase in mammalian synaptosomes,
    J. Neurochem., 33: 339-342.
Weiler, C.T., Nystrom, B., and Hamberger, A., 1979a, Glutaminase and
    glutamine synthetase activity in synaptosomes, bulk-isolated
    glia and neurons, Brain Res., 160: 539-543.
Weiler, C.T., Nystrom, B., and Hamberger, A., 1979b, Characteristics
    of glutamine vs glutamate transport in isolated glia and
    synaptosomes, J. Neurochem., 32: 559-565.
Wilkin, G.P., Balazs, R., Wilson, J.E., Cohen, J., and Dutton, G.R.,
    1976, Preparation of cell bodies from the developing cerebellum.
    Structural and metabolic integrity of the isolated 'cells',
    Brain Res., 115: 181-199.
Woodhams, P.L., Cohen, J., Mallet, J., and Balazs, R., 1980, A
    preparation enriched in Purkinje cells identified by morpho-
    logical and immunocytochemical criteria, Brain Res., 199:
    435-442.

COMPARTMENTATION OF THE SUPPLY OF THE ACETYL MOIETY FOR ACETYLCHOLINE SYNTHESIS

J. B. Clark, R.F.G. Booth[+], S.A.K. Harvey,
S.F. Leong and T.B. Patel*
Biochemistry Department
St. Bartholomew's Hospital Medical College
University of London
Charterhouse Square, London, EC1M 6BQ

In mammalian brain, acetylcholine is synthesised by the enzyme choline acetyl transferase from the precursors choline and acetyl CoA. Since the brain 'in situ' appears to be unable to synthesise choline de novo (see Tucek, 1978), much interest has centred around the supply of acetyl CoA for acetylcholine synthesis. Although early work suggested that choline acetyl transferase might be bound to a particulate fraction in brain, Fonnum (1968) established that this was an artefact of isolation and the bulk of the enzyme is now generally accepted as being cytosolic, with approximately half of its activity located at the nerve ending (see Tucek, 1978). The work of Gibson and Blass (1976) and Jope and Jenden (1977) has demonstrated that conditions which reduce the availability of acetyl CoA in general bring about proportional reductions in acetyl choline synthesis although the flux into the acetyl group of acetyl choline is less than 1% of the total carbon throughput in whole brain. Two immediate questions which arise from this are: a) Is choline supply the principal control point in acetylcholine syntheis (Simon & Kuhar, 1976) b) What is the nature of the carbon pool which supplies the acetyl CoA for acetyl-

---

+Biochemistry Dept., Chelsea College, U. of London
Manresa Road, London SW3 6LK

*Biochemistry Dept., U. of Texas, Health Science Center
San Antonio, Texas 78284

choline synthesis.   Observations by Lefresne et al. (1973) and
other groups (Browning & Schulman, 1968; Grewaal & Quastel,
1973) that radioactive pyruvate is incorporated into acetyl choline
with little or no dilution implies that the endogenous pool is extremely small with a rapid turnover rate.

   The adult brain of many species utilizes glucose as the principal
substrate both for respiration and acetylcholine synthesis. Current
dogma, would by analogy to other tissues such as the liver
(Lowenstein, 1968) suggest that the supply of acetyl CoA for acetylcholine synthesis would be a compartmented process involving
both the mitochondrion and the cytosol of the nerve ending. This
would involve the movement of carbon from glucose across the
inner mitochondrial membrane in the form of pyruvate into the
matrical compartment and subsequently the passage of carbon out
of the mitochondria to generate acetyl CoA in the cytosol (see
Scheme). The general acceptance that the mitochondrial membrane is impermeable to acetyl CoA as such, means that a carrier
molecule must be involved that is synthesised from acetyl CoA in

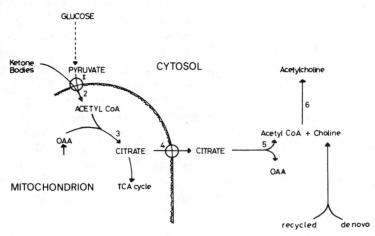

SUBCELLULAR SYNTHESIS OF ACETYLCHOLINE

Scheme
1) Monocarboxylate translocase. 2) Pyruvate dehydrogenase.
3) Citrate synthase.   4) Tricarboxylate translocase.
5) ATP-Citrate lyase.   6) Choline acetyl transferase

the mitochondrial matrix, transported across the membrane and which subsequently generates acetyl CoA in the cytosol. This problem is of course not unique to neurotransmitter synthesis but also includes lipid synthesis in, for example, the developing brain which involves intercompartmental acetyl group transfer. The problem lies as to the identity of the carrier molecule. By analogy to other tissues the most favoured candidate is probably citrate which is formed intramitochondrially by citrate synthase (E.C.4. 1.3.7) may be transported out on the tricarboxylate translocase (Patel & Clark, 1981) and may regenerate acetyl CoA in the cytosol under the influence of the ATP-citrate lyase (E.C.4.1.3.8). However, evidence to support this proposed mechanism has not been forthcoming. Although radioactive citrate is taken up and metabolised in whole brain (Tucek & Cheng, 1974) and synaptosomes (Lefresne et al., 1977) this does not result in significant labelling of acetylcholine. As a consequence a number of other potential acetyl group carriers have been proposed, e.g. N-acetyl aspartate (D'Adamo et al., 1968), acetate (Tucek, 1978), acetylcarnitine (Tucek et al. 1981), acetoacetate (Rous, 1976) and 2-oxoglutarate (D'Adamo and D'Adamo, 1968). However, no potential acetyl transfer group so far tested, when added exogenously in a radioactive form, results in significant labelling of acetylcholine (Tucek & Cheng, 1974; Lefresne, et al. 1977; Tucek, et al. 1981).

This situation has in fact lead to the suggestion that the supply of acetyl CoA from glucose for acetylcholine synthesis is not a two-compartment process but resides solely in the cytosol of the nerve ending. This suggestion derives from the work of Lefresne et al. (1977; 1978) using rat striatal synaptosomes in which they studied incorporation of labelled glucose into $^{14}CO_2$ and acetylcholine in the presence of an inhibitor of pyruvate transport- - cyanocinnamate and an 'irreversible' inhibitor of pyruvate dehydrogenase-bromopyruvate. They concluded from their results that there were two functional pools of pyruvate dehydrogenase one of which did not appear to be within the mitochondria, hence suggesting the possibility of acetyl CoA production for acetylcholine synthesis within a single intracellular compartment - the cytosol. The main objection to this model is that pyruvate dehydrogenase activity has yet to be found outside the mitochondria in any other mammalian tissue and that direct attempts to detect pyruvate dehydrogenase in the cytosol of synaptosomes from regions of the brain both high and low in cholinergic activity have not been successful (Jope & Jenden, 1980).

Although much work on the brain is still carried out using whole brain slices the use of the nerve ending preparation or synaptosome for certain investigations is becoming more common. Indeed, over the last 10 or so years it has been demonstrated that synaptosomes may be used as reasonable models of the nerve ending and that in many respects they show analogous properties to cortical slices (see review, Barondes, 1974). They do, however, have as far as neurotransmitter synthesis is concerned, distinct advantages over the slice. This derives from the localisation of the bulk of the neurotransmitter synthetic enzymes at the nerve ending (Coyle & Axelrod, 1972) which means that they have an effective increase in specific activity of neurotransmitter synthesis over the slice together with a reduction in the number of metabolic pools which are not directly related to this function of the nerve ending. If the problem of acetylcholine synthesis specifically is considered, then the synaptosome has a further advantage over the slice with respect to studies on the incorporation of labelled precursors. This relates to the relative simplicity of the membrane/barrier system of the nerve ending as compared to the slice which permits not only more clearly defined access of substrates to the system under study but also a better controlled external environment. A problem intrinsic to the use of the synaptosome, however, lies in its purity and artefacts which are derived from its preparative procedure. The original methods of synaptosome preparation (see Whittaker, 1969) involved high speed centrifugation on discontinuous sucrose gradients of a hyperosmolar nature. Continued exposure to such conditions gave rise to some concern about the metabolic capabilities of these preparations and with the advent of the sucrose polymer Ficoll a number of laboratories - ourselves included (Kurokawa et al., 1965; Abdel-Latif, 1966; Autilio, et al., 1968; Cotman & Matthews, 1971; Booth & Clark, 1978a) sought to develop preparative procedures for metabolically improved preparations of synaptosomes which had not been subjected to long periods of exposure to hyperosmotic gradients. The method that we have developed takes less than two hours, less than half the time of the original method of Gray & Whittaker (1962) and the preparation is both metabolically active and minimally (3-4%) contaminated with 'free' (non-synaptosomal) mitochondria (see Booth & Clark, 1978a), thus providing a suitable model preparation of the nerve ending to investigate the compartmentation of the acetylcholine synthesis. The first few figures are introduced by way of justification of the use of this preparation for these studies. Fig. 1 shows the ability of a forebrain synaptosomal preparation to oxidise $U-^{14}C$ — glucose to $^{14}CO_2$.

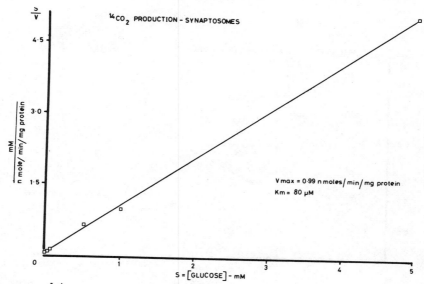

Fig. 1. $^{14}CO_2$ production from U-^{14}C glucose by rat brain synaptosomes

Synaptosomes were prepared by the method of Booth and Clark (1978a). They were resuspended in a medium comprising 136 mM NaCl, 5.6 mM KCl, 16.2 mM $NaHCO_3$, 1.2 mM $MgCl_2$, 1.2 mM NaH_2PO_4, 2.2 mM $CaCl_2$, 0.2 mM choline chloride and 0.1 mM physostigmine. Aliquots were incubated in the presence of U-^{14}C -D-glucose [1.36 µC /µmole] at $37°C$ with shaking, in an atmosphere of 95% O_2, 5% CO_2 and $^{14}CO_2$ collected. Incubations were stopped by injection of 1 ml of 20% w/v trichloroacetic acid containing 15-50 nCi of ^3H-acetyl -choline (used for expts. in Fig. 2). For each point 20 > n > 5. S.E.M. bars for these data are shown in Fig. 3. $^{14}CO_2$ output estimated given that it will have one-sixth the specific radioactivity of the original glucose.

There is a linear relationship with a Vmax of 0.99 nmols. $^{14}CO_2$ produced min.$^{-1}$mg protein together with an apparent Km for glucose of 80 µM. In Fig. 2 the relationship between glucose concentration and the rate of ^{14}C acetylcholine synthesis has been plotted. The Vmax is 12.5 pmoles ^{14}C- acetylcholine formed min.$^{-1}$mg protein, i.e. more than 80-fold less than for $^{14}CO_2$, whereas the Km at 150 µM is approx. twice as high. If the relative incorporation of radioactivity from U-^{14}C D-glucose into

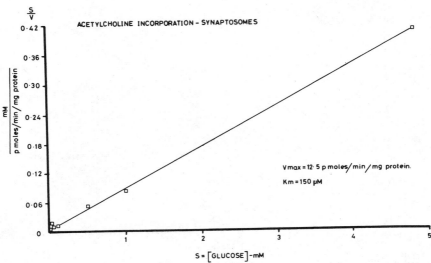

Fig. 2. ^{14}C acetylcholine synthesis from U-^{14}C glucose by
rat brain.

Incubation conditions as in Fig. 1 legend.   The acidified
aqueous extracts were neutralised by extensive washing with water-
saturated ether followed by addition of sodium phosphate buffer
(pH 7.2, final concentration 10 mM).   Preliminary extraction of
acetylcholine was by the method of Fonnum (1969) using tetra-
phenylboron in 3-heptanone.   Characterisation of acetylcholine
after back-extraction into aqueous phase was by high voltage
electrophoresis after Potter and Murphy (1967) or by hydrolysis
using purified acetylcholinesterase followed by organic re-extrac-
tion.   Recovery of acetylcholine was assessed by recovery of the
^{3}H-acetylcholine   tracer added, after ^{3}H and ^{14}C content of the
characterised acetylcholine had been determined by scintillation
counting.
     Both ^{14}CO$_2$ and ^{14}C-acetyl choline synthesis were linear with
time up to the maximum incubation period used for any given glucose concentration.   For each point $20 > n > 5$.   S.E.M. bars for
these data are shown in Fig. 3.   Synthesis of ^{14}C-acetyl choline
was estimated given that the acetyl moiety will have one-third the
specific radioactivity of original glucose (Grewaal and Quastel,
1973).

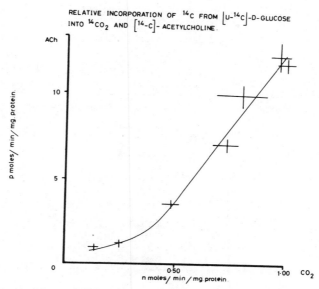

Fig. 3. Data as determined for Figs. 1 and 2. ^{14}C-acetylcholine
synthesis is plotted as a function of $^{14}CO_2$ output.

both $^{14}CO_2$ and ^{14}C acetylcholine is compared, Figure 3 results.
This indicates that above a glucose concentration of about 50-100µM
there exists a directly proportional relationship between ^{14}C
incorporation into acetylcholine and $^{14}CO_2$ output, the latter being
representative of the overall activity of the citric acid cycle. As
the glucose concentration falls, however, whilst the rate of glucose oxidation as represented by $^{14}CO_2$ output is maintained, the
level of ^{14}C incorporation into acetylcholine decreases (Fig. 3).
This suggests that at low glucose concentrations when the energetic
status of the synaptosome may be at risk by a decreased rate of
ATP synthesis with a possible disturbance in the maintenance of
normal mitochondrial potentials, that acetylcholine synthesis is
impaired. This further suggests, of course, that directly or
indirectly acetylcholine synthesis is a compartmented system
involving the mitochondria (see later).

     Further support for the synaptosome as a model for the study
of acetylcholine synthesis is depicted in Table I. This shows the

TABLE I.   INCORPORATION OF ^{14}C FROM 1 mM U-^{14}C-D-
GLUCOSE INTO ^{14}CO$_2$ AND ^{14}C-ACETYLCHOLINE
BY SYNAPTOSOMES FROM DIFFERENT REGIONS.

Region	^{14}CO$_2$ nmole/min /mg protein	^{14}C-ACh pmole/min /mg protein
Whole forebrain	1.00 ± 0.04	11.8 ± 0.39
	n = 20	n = 20
Cortex	1.05 ± 0.01	10.9 ± 0.61
	n = 11	n = 9
Striatum	0.95 ± 0.04	18.7 ± 0.31
	n = 11	n = 9

Table 1. Synaptosomes were prepared from material dissected
by the method of Glowinski and Iversen (1966). ^{14}CO$_2$ output and
^{14}C-acetyl choline synthesis were determined as described for
Figs. 1 and 2 using 1 mM glucose as substrate. Results are expressed as means $\pm$ S.D.

rates of ^{14}CO$_2$ output and ^{14}C-acetylcholine synthesis from
U-^{14}C -D-glucose in synaptosomal preparations from different
regions of rat brain. Whilst it is apparent that the rate of activity
of the energy metabolising pathways as judged by ^{14}CO$_2$ production
is reasonably constant in the 3 areas, the rate of ^{14}C-acetyl-
choline synthesis is almost twice as high in the striatal region as
compared with the cortex and whole forebrain preparations. These
results are of course in agreement with neurophysiological studies
which suggest that the striatum is densely innervated with systems
using acetylcholine as the neurotransmitter. Table II has been
compiled to provide some data on the kinetic parameters of various
metabolic activities involving glucose measured in synaptosomes
or in certain cases slices or purified enzyme systems, by which
the status of our synaptosomal preparation may be compared. The
whole spectrum of apparent Km s for glucose fall in the range
50-250 µM, and relate to a wide variety of metabolic activities.
In particular, the apparent Km for glucose for incorporation into
acetylcholine between our system and that of Lefresne et al.

TABLE II   GLUCOSE CONCENTRATION REQUIRED FOR
HALF-MAXIMAL VELOCITY OF SYNAPTOSOMAL
FUNCTIONS

Function	Glucose uM	
Glucose uptake	200[a]	Heaton & Bachelard, 1973
	240	Diamond & Fishman, 1973
Oxygen uptake	50	Bradford, 1969
Hexokinase	40-100[b]	Thompson & Bachelard, 1970
Acetylcholine synthesis	200[c]	Lefresne et al., 1973
	440[d]	Lefresne et al., 1978
	150	This lab.
$^{14}CO_2$ output	80	This lab.

Rat brain synaptosomes except : [a]guinea pig; [b]enzyme from
whole brain; [c]striatal slices; [d]approx. Vmax.
Table II.   Summary of Km values from the literature values are
as published except for those attributed to Bradford (1969) and
Lefresne et al. (1973) which have been calculated from published
data.

(1973, 1978) is very comparable as is the Km for oxygen consumption (Bradford, 1969) and $^{14}CO_2$ output (this paper) both of
which may be taken as representative of the activity of the energy
metabolising systems in the synaptosomes.

Further support for the hypothesis that acetylcholine synthesis
is a compartmented system comes from studies on the effects of
anoxia and veratridine on synaptosomal acetylcholine synthesis.
In the present studies we have investigated the relationship between
the bioenergetics of the nerve ending and acetylcholine synthesis.
The synaptosome has clear advantages in this context as a model
system since the extramitochondrial ATP demand may be varied
by altering the rate of ion cycling at the plasma membrane by the
addition of the alkaloid veratridine.   This alkaloid acts by stabilization of the high conductance conformation of the potential-
dependent Na$^+$ channel in the plasma membrane (Ohta et al., 1973)

hence inducing a prolonged depolarisation of the plasma membrane (Blaustein & Golding, 1975). Therefore if the Na^+ permeability of the membrane is normally limited, the addition of veratridine will lead to an increased rate of ion cycling across the plasma membrane and as a consequence an increased Na^+-K^+-ATPase activity, ATP turnover and rate of synaptosomal respiration. Hence veratridine causes a 260% increase in synaptosomal respiration coupled with a fall in the plasma membrane potential from 45 to 35 mV and of the mitochondrial membrane potential from 150 to 125mV (Scott & Nicholls, 1980) (see Table III). In contrast to veratridine, rotenone, an inhibitor of mitochondrial electron transport at the NADH-CoQ reductase segment of the respiratory chain, inhibits synaptosomal respiration, causes a similar decrease in the mitochondrial membrane potential but has no effect on the plasma membrane potential. It is suggested that under these circumstances despite the inhibition of oxidation a relatively high mitochondrial membrane potential is maintained by glycolytically produced ATP (Scott & Nicholls, 1980). When both veratridine and rotenone were added together cytosolic ATP was severely depleted (Scott & Nicholls, 1980) and both the plasma membrane and mitochondrial membrane potentials fell indicating that anaerobic glycolysis was unable to generate sufficient ATP to meet the

TABLE III   EFFECTS OF INHIBITORS ON SYNAPTOSOMAL MEMBRANE POTENTIALS

Inhibitor	Respiration	Membrane Potentials (mV)	
		Plasma	Mitochondrial
Rotenone (4 µM) ($\equiv$ Anoxia)	Inhibited	45 —— 45	150 —— 125
Veratridine (100 µM)	+ 260%	45 —— 35	150 —— 125
Rotenone + Veratridine	Inhibited	45 —— 20	150 —— 75

Data derived from paper by I.R. Scott and D.G. Nicholls, 1980.

demands of both the Na^+-K^+-ATPase and the mitochondrial ATP-ase and hence maintain membrane potentials (Scott & Nicholls, 1980). These effects are summarized in Table III and serve to show how synaptosomal energy metabolism may be artificially regulated with a view to studying its relationship with acetylcholine synthesis. Subjecting synaptosomes to an 'anoxic' episode may be likened to the situation in which rotenone is present. Fig. 4

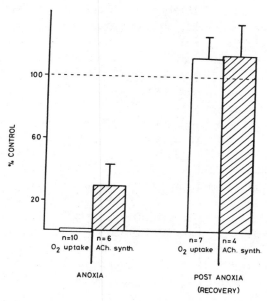

Fig. 4.   Synaptosomal oxygen uptake and ^{14}C-acetyl choline synthesis were measured before, during and after a 10 minute period of anoxia. Synaptosomes in saline medium were incubated at 37°C with stirring. Oxygen uptake was measured using a Clark-type electrode, with 1 mM unlabelled glucose as substrate. After 10 minutes anoxia, the oxygen content of the medium was raised by the addition of aliquots of catalase and H_2O_2.
    ^{14}C-acetyl choline synthesis during any given period was measured by adding high specific activity U-^{14}C -D-glucose at the beginning of the period, and stopping the reaction with trichloro-acetic acid containing ^{3}H-acetyl choline at the end. Determination of ^{14}C-acetyl choline synthesis was as described in legend to Fig. 2.   Number of determinations and standard deviation bars are shown: '100%' or initial aerobic characteristics are 3.42 $\pm$ 0.98 nmoles O_2/mg protein/min. (S.D. n = 20) and 11.0 $\pm$ 2.2 pmoles ACh/mg protein/min (S.D. n = 12).

indicates the changes occurring in the rate of oxygen uptake and acetylcholine synthesis in the synaptosome during and after a period of anoxia. It is clear from Fig. 4 that during the anoxic period ^{14}C – acetylcholine synthesis from U-^{14}C - glucose falls by about 75% and on reoxygenation a full recovery in both the rate of oxygen consumption and acetylcholine synthesis occurs. It may be suggested that the effects of anoxia on acetylcholine synthesis may be localised at the level of the mitochondrial membrane potential which falls and leads to a decreased activity of the acetyl group transfer mechanism. In addition, the increased conversion of pyruvate to lactate in anaerobic conditions will make less carbon available to the mitochondrial compartment for transfer for acetyl-choline synthesis. Tables IV and V extend these studies in assessing the effects of anoxia and veratridine both individually and together on synaptosomal metabolic activity as measured by $^{14}CO_2$ output from U-^{14}C -D-glucose, ^{14}C – acetyl choline synthesis and bioenergetic states as measured by ATP, ADP and creatine phosphate concentrations. Thus Table IV indicates that the synaptosomal $^{14}CO_2$ production and ^{14}C acetylcholine synthesis is fully capable of recovering from an anoxic period in the absence of veratridine. This is reflected in Table V which shows that the energetic status of the synaptosome has also virtually returned to the aerobic levels. The inclusion of veratridine in the synaptosomal incubation is observed to result in a large stimulation (almost 4-fold) in the rate of $^{14}CO_2$ production from U-^{14}C glucose whilst ^{14}C-acetylcholine synthesis decreases by 50% (Table IV). The increased rate of $^{14}CO_2$ production is presumably due to the increased energy demand made on the synaptosome in order to maintain its ion homeostasis in the presence of veratridine. This is reflected in the lowered creatine phosphate concentrations and ATP/ADP ratio shown for similar conditions in Table V. The fact that ^{14}C-acetylcholine synthesis is also decreased suggests that this process is either directly sensitive to the bioenergetic status of the synaptosome or being a compartmented system involving the mitochondria is indirectly linked to it via the mito-chondrial membrane potential. If synaptosomes are subjected to anoxic insult and then incubated in the presence of veratridine whilst the $^{14}CO_2^-$ production from U-^{14}C glucose is only stimulated twofold (Table IV - cf. aerobic incubation) ^{14}C-acetylcholine synthesis is decreased even more drastically to approx. 30% of the rate seen with the control (aerobic) incubations. These marked changes are reflected in the severely decreased energy status of the synaptosome after an anoxic episode and subsequently in the presence of veratridine as indicated by the marked decrease in

TABLE IV.   INCORPORATION OF ^{14}C FROM U-^{14}C -D-GLUCOSE INTO ACETYLCHOLINE AND CO_2 IN SYNAPTOSOMES SUBJECTED TO DIFFERENT TREATMENTS

Incubation	$^{14}CO_2$ output nmoles/min/mg	^{14}C-ACh synthesis pmoles/min/mg
Aerobic	0.91 ± 0.03 n = 19	11 ± 0.65 n = 12
Post anoxic	1.07 ± 0.07 n = 9 *	9.6 ± 1.2 n = 8 ns
Aerobic + Veratridine	3.53 ± 0.04 n = 9 **	5.5 ± 0.3 n = 9 **
Post anoxic + Veratridine (100 μM)	2.17 ± 0.14 n = 9 **	3.5 ± 0.45 n = 11 **

* $p < 0.05$ ** $p < 0.005$

Table IV. Synaptosomes were incubated with unlabelled 1mM glucose as described in the legend to Fig. 4, except that following 10 minutes anoxia reoxygenation was by dilution into a 10-fold excess of fresh saline containing U-^{14}C -D-glucose (1 mM final concentration). The metabolic characteristics ($^{14}CO_2$ output and ^{14}C-acetyl choline synthesis) of the synaptosomes were then determined as in the legends to Figs. 1 and 2.

Synaptosomes were resuspended without being exposed to anoxia (aerobic) as well as after exposure ('post-anoxic'). In some experiments, veratridine was present in both primary and secondary incubations at 100 μM final concentration. Veratridine increased the oxygen uptake in the primary incubation to 6.84 ± 1.08 nmoles/mg/protein/min (S.D. n = 29). Results are expressed as means $\pm$ S.D.

TABLE V.   ENERGY METABOLITES IN SYNAPTOSOMES FROM
            NORMOXIC RATS SUBJECTED TO DIFFERENT
            TREATMENTS

| Incubation | nmoles/mg. protein | | | |
	ATP	ADP	CP	ATP/ADP
aerobic	1.46±0.10	1.09±0.15	2.18±0.28	1.45±0.17
	n = 13	n = 12	n = 12	n = 11
post anoxia	1.04±0.11	1.11±0.15	1.74±0.26	1.01±0.15
	n = 9	n = 9	n = 3	n = 9
	*	ns	ns	ns
aerobic + 100µM veratridine	1.40±0.16	2.05±0.30	1.44±0.13	0.77±0.09
	n = 7	n = 6	n = 6	n = 6
	ns	**	ns	*
post anoxia + 100µM veratridine	0.64±0.16	2.00±0.37	0.73±0.35	0.41±0.18
	n = 4	n = 4	n = 4	n = 4
	**	**	*	*

* $p < 0.05$ ** $p < 0.005$

Table V. Synaptosomes were incubated as in legend to Table IV,
except that reoxygenation was by stirring with exposure to air for
2 minutes. Neutralised acid-extracts of synaptosomes were
assayed for ATP and CP by the method of Lamprecht (1974) and
for ADP by the method of Jaworek et al. (1974) or by the HPLC
method described by Booth and Clark (1979). Results are expressed as means ± S.D. CP = creatine phosphate.

creatine phosphate and ATP/ADP ratio (approx. 30% of the control). These data clearly indicate that the rate of synaptosomal
[14]C-acetylcholine synthesis is sensitive to the energy states in
both the mitochondrial and cytosolic compartments of the synaptosome since it is observed that a fall in either the mitochondrial

membrane potential (anoxia, Fig. 4) or in the cytosolic ATP/ADP ratio (veratridine, Tables IV and V) leads to a decreased acetylcholine synthesis. It may therefore be concluded that acetylcholine is either a compartmented system involving the mitochondrial and cytosolic compartments of the synaptosome or if not, it is indirectly sensitive to the energy status of these compartments of the nerve ending.

If it is accepted that acetylcholine synthesis is a compartmented system then there are a number of questions which should be asked: a) do the compartments involved, viz. the synaptic mitochondria and cytosol possess the necessary enzyme complements for the synthesis of candidate carriers and regeneration of acetyl CoA ? b) are isolated synaptic mitochondria capable of synthesising and exporting candidate carriers ? c) can the use of particular carrier be detected either directly or indirectly, in vivo or in vitro ? Although the last question would be the most informative, technically it presents considerable difficulties. However, the answers to the first two questions do provide some useful pointers. There have been a number of proposals as to the chemical nature of the carriers involved - citrate (including 2-oxoglutarate), acetate (Tucek, 1978), acetyl carnitine (Sterri & Fonnum, 1980, Dolezal & Tucek, 1981), N-acetyl aspartate (D'Adamo et al., 1968) and acetoacetate (Buckley & Williamson 1973). Some of these proposed carriers seem less likely than others; acetoacetate for example would require an acetoacetyl CoA synthetase activity in the cytosol in excess of that reported (Buckley & Williamson, 1973) to maintain acetylcholine concentrations; n-acetyl aspartate on the basis of present information would appear to be hydrolysed to acetate and aspartate in the cytosol rather than producing acetyl CoA (D'Adamo et al., 1968; Patel & Clark, 1979); acetylcarnitine does not dilute the radioactivity in labelled acetylcholine synthesised from labelled glucose and whilst carnitine acetyl transferase activity has been measured in brain mitochondria (McCaman et al., 1966; Tucek, 1967) and cholinergic terminals (Sterri & Fonnum, 1980) it is not clear whether it is appropriately located in the mitochondrial membrane to provide cytosolic acetyl CoA.

With respect to the first of our questions, the brain and the nerve ending in particular certainly exhibit the appropriate enzymatic activities for the involvement of citrate as the carrier, viz. citrate synthase, ATP citrate-lyase (see Scheme). In our hands the citrate synthase activity of synaptic mitochondria from cortex, striatum or medulla is high ($\sim 0.4 - 0.6$ umole min.$^{-1}$ mg. mitochondrial protein - S.F. Leong and J.B. Clark, unpublished observations), and taken together with the low apparent Kms of the brain enzyme for its substrates (Clark & Land, 1974) this must mean that the bulk of the intramitochondrial acetyl CoA at the synapse is metabolised to citrate as the equilibrium constant of this reaction is of the order of 10^6. The activity of the ATP-citrate lyase enzyme, which undertakes energy dependent reversal of the citrate synthase step in the cytosol of nerve endings is shown in Table VI. Whilst the maximal activity of this enzyme is lower than that of choline acetyl transferase in synaptosomes

TABLE VI.   SYNAPTOSOMAL ACTIVITIES OF ATP-CITRATE LYASE AND CHOLINE ACETYL TRANSFERASE (CAT)

Region	Enzyme activity - nmol mg prot.min.$^{-1}$		Acetylcholine turnover pmol/min/mg protein
	Choline acetyl transferase	ATP citrate-lyase	
Medulla oblongata and pons	1.22±0.05 (n = 7)	0.49±0.02 (n = 4)	ND
Cortex	1.1±0.11 (n = 8)	0.46, 0.45	10.9±0.61 (n = 9)
Striatum	2.52±0.10 (n = 6)	0.41±0.02 (n = 3)	18.7±0.31 (n = 9)

Table VI.   Synaptosomes for enzyme assays were prepared from dissected regions essentially by the method of Glowinski and Iversen (1966). ATP-citrate lyase activity was measured essentially as described by Hoffman et al (1978), except that p-(p-aminophenylazo)benzene sulphonic acid (AABS) was used instead of p-nitroaniline. Choline acetyltransferase (ChAT) activity was measured by the method of Fonnum (1969) as described by Burgess et al (1978).

Acetylcholine synthesis figures are from Table 1 and enzyme activities are expressed as means ± S.D.

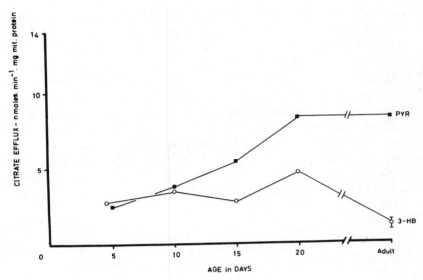

Fig. 5.   Rat brain mitochondria were prepared from animals of
different ages by the method of Clark and Nicklas (1970).   The
mitochondria were incubated in a medium containing 100 mM K$^+$
containing 5 mM pyruvate + 2.5 mM malate or 10 mM DL-3-
hydroxybutyrate + 2.5 mM malate in the presence of ADP and a
hexokinase trap, i.e. state 3 - (for details see Patel and Clark,
1981).   The data are expressed as a rate of efflux in nmoles min^{-1}
mg protein and each value is a mean of at least 2 distinct experiments in each of which the citrate concentrations were measured
at minimum of 3 points.

made from regions of the brain of differing cholinergic innervation,
it is clear that it is much higher than the estimated rate of acetylcholine synthesis (Table VI). Data is also available to show that in
the appropriate conditions brain mitochondria are capable of exporting considerable quantities of citrate. Fig. 5 shows the capa-
bility of brain mitochondria during development to efflux citrate
utilising either 3-hydroxybutyrate + malate or pyruvate + malate
as substrates.   In the young animal (5 days) 3-hydroxybutyrate is
a marginally better substrate for citrate efflux than pyruvate.
However, as the brain develops pyruvate becomes a progressively
better precursor for citrate, whereas the 3-hydroxybutyrate

remains fairly constant during suckling but decreases in the adult.
This is interesting in that it has been suggested that in the young
suckling rat brain ketone bodies may be more effective precursors
of lipid than glucose (Patel & Owen, 1977; Patel & Clark, 1980;
Patel & Clark, 1981) whereas the opposite is true in the adult.
Furthermore, similar observations have been made in the case
of incorporation of carbon into acetylcholine (Gibson & Blass,
1979). Thus the marked increase in citrate efflux from brain
mitochondria develops at a time after the major period of structural lipid synthesis in the brain (7 - 10 days after birth -
Dhopeshwarker et al, 1969; Patel & Owen, 1977) and is associated
with the period of onset of neurological activity ($\sim$ 15 days, Land
et al, 1977).

Table VII shows the rates of citrate efflux from 'synaptic'
and 'free' mitochondria from adult rat brain utilising either

TABLE VII.   CITRATE EFFLUX FROM 'FREE' AND
             'SYNAPTIC MITOCHONDRIA

Substrate	State	Free mitochondria	Synaptic mitochondria
		nmoles min^{-1} mg protein	
Pyruvate + malate	3	8.6 ± 0.7	3.4 ± 0.3
	4	8.7 ± 0.8	7.6 ± 0.5
3-hydroxybutyrate + malate	3	1.1 ± 0.1	2.1 ± 0.2
	4	3.5 ± 0.2	2.9 ± 0.2

Mean $\pm$ S.D. - measured at 3 time points in 3 separate experiments

Table VII.   Free brain mitochondria were prepared by the method
of Clark and Nicklas (1970), synaptic mitochondria by the method
of Lai and Clark (1979). Incubations were carried out as outlined
in the legend to Fig. 5 either in the presence of 1 mM ADP and
a hexokinase trap (state 3) or in the absence of ADP (state 4).

pyruvate + malate or 3-hydroxybutyrate + malate as substrates.
The characteristics of citrate efflux from 'syaptic' mitochondria
are different to those of 'free mitochondria. Whilst the maximal

rate of citrate efflux with either substrate is similar in both mitochondrial populations, citrate-efflux from pyruvate as substrate
in synaptic mitochondria is sensitive to the energy status of the
mitochondria, whereas that in free mitochondria is not. This
distinction is not artifactual since in the case of 3-hydroxybutyrate
as substrate the opposite is the case; however, this latter effect
is unlikely to be of physiological significance since ketone bodies
are not normally an important substrate in the fed adult.

     The direct incorporation of exogenously added radioactive
citrate into acetylcholine by brain slices (Cheng, Nakamura &
Waelsch, 1967) or synaptosomes (Lefresne et al, 1977) has proved
difficult to demonstrate satisfactorily. Such results may be explained if a) synaptic mitochondria differentiate metabolically
between exogenously added and endogenously generated citrate,
b) ATP-citrate lyase in the synapse was compartmented in some
fashion which meant it effectively only used mitochondrially produced and effluxed citrate. Some evidence to support the first of
these possibilities has been demonstrated by Rafalowska &
Ksiezak (1979) who have reported that synaptic mitochondrial uptake and oxidation of added citrate is only 24% and 6% respectively
of the rates exhibited by free mitochondria. Taking into account
the data already presented (Fig. 5, Table 7) this means that
synaptic mitochondria will tend to export endogenous citrate rather
than import exogenous citrate. Evidence of ATP-citrate lyase
compartmentation is less good although there have been reports of
'cytosolic' ATP-citrate lyase being associated with particulate
fractions in brain (Szutowicz & Lysiak, 1980) and liver (Janski &
Cornell, 1980). The loose association of 'cytosolic' enzymes with
brain mitochondria permitting preferential use of effluxed sub-
states has precedents in the case of hexokinase (Land et al. 1977)
and creatine kinase (Booth & Clark, 1978b). In an attempt to
obtain more evidence for the direct involvement of citrate in acetylcholine synthesis we carried out experiments following the incorporation of doubly labelled glucose $6-^3H$, ^{14}C into acetylcholine
with synaptosomes prepared from whole forebrain, along the lines
of similar experiments using brain slices reported by Sollenberg
& Sorbo (1970) and Sterling & O'Neill (1978). The principles underlying these experiments are shown in Fig. 6 and much of the
support for this has come from the elegant studies of Walter &
Soling (1976) on liver. Attachment of the acetyl group from acetyl
CoA to oxaloacetate at the citrate synthase step results in the loss
of proton from the methyl carbon which, if $6-^3H$, ^{14}C-glucose
or $3-^3H$, ^{14}C-lactate are substrates, may be detected as a re-

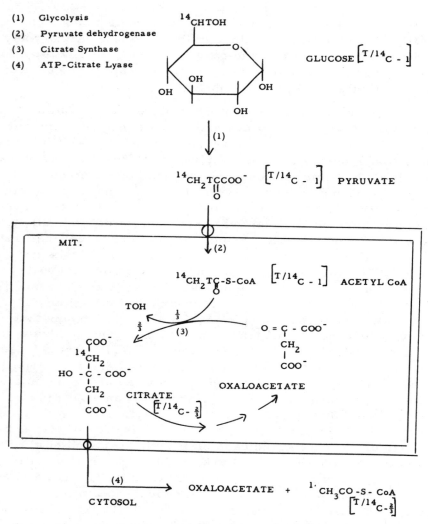

(1) Glycolysis
(2) Pyruvate dehydrogenase
(3) Citrate Synthase
(4) ATP-Citrate Lyase

Fig. 6.   Outline of passage of tritium (^3H) label (T) and ^{14}C
label from 6-^3H, ^{14}C glucose into acetyl CoA in the cytosol via
the citrate mechanism (see scheme). If glucose is assigned
T/^{14}C ratio of 1, then intramitochondrial acetyl CoA has T/^{14}C
ratio = 1, but intramitochondrial citrate and cytosolic acetyl CoA
have T/^{14}C ratio = 0.67.

duction in the ^{3}H/^{14}C ratio at citrate and subsequent metabolites.
The loss may not be as great as one third (i.e. citrate ^{3}H/^{14}C
ratio $>$ 0.67) as the synthase discriminates slightly against tritium,
(Walter & Soling, 1976). There are other possibilities for an
apparent loss of ^{3}H in metabolites apart from the citrate synthase
step. These are mainly exchange reactions in glycolysis, at the
citrate synthase step without net formation of citrate and at the
citrate lyase step. From various control experiments carried
out by Walter & Soling these do not contribute significantly,
However, significant modification of the ^{3}H/^{14}C ratio of citrate
may occur by labelling of the oxaloacetate/malate pool by a
previous turn of the citric acid cycle. Given a ^{3}H/^{14}C ratio of
AcCoA of 1, then the ratios in malate/oxaloacetate and total
citrate pool after n turns of the TCA cycle will be:

No. of turns.	Malate	OAA	Citrate
0	-	-	0.67
1	0.32	0.16	0.42
2	0.16	0.08	0.28
∞	0.08	0.04	0.21

This assumes no anaplerotic influx into the TCA cycle which
would increase the ^{3}H/^{14}C ratio of oxaloacetate. This would
seem reasonable as pyruvate carboxylase activity in the adult
brain is extremely low (Land & Clark, 1975). Some of the data
we have obtained from these experiments is shown in Table VIII
and compared to those of Sollenberg & Sorbo (1970) and Sterling
& O'Neill (1978). Some important differences between our experiments and the others should be noted. Sollenberg & Sorbo (1970)
and Sterling & O'Neill (1978) used cortex slices and incubated them
for periods of an hour or more using 10 mM glucose as substrate.
In our experiments synaptosomes from whole forebrain were incubated for 6-10 mins with 1 mM glucose. The advantages of the
latter are:- the need for only low (1 mM) glucose concentrations
with synaptosomes permits a high specific radioactivity to be
attained; the use of synaptosomes excludes the glial and perikary-
onal compartments, although the synaptosomes themselves are
metabolically heterogenous; the short incubation period reduces
recycling which will occur and obscure isotope ratio changes.
In fact, the isotope ratios in the case of the slice work (see Table
VIII) for the total citrate are considerably lower than those in the
synaptosomal experiments. This probably results from the extended incubation times, which result in more cycling of the TCA
cycle. The 'total' citrate value for our data is closer to that re-

TABLE VIII. ^{3}H/^{14}C RATIO OF METABOLITES GIVEN ^{3}H/^{14}C
-D-GLUCOSE SUBSTRATE AS UNITY

Metabolite	Slices[1]	Slices[2]	Synaptosomes[3]
Lactate/Pyruvate	0.95 ± 0.02 n = 4 (L)	0.91 ± 0.01 n = 5 (L)	0.96 (P)
Citrate (Total	0.56 ± 0.03 n = 2	0.39 ± 0.01 n = 5	0.72 ± 0.01 n = 3
Citrate (4, 5-)	0.65 ± 0.01 n = 2	0.62 ± 0.02 n = 4	ND
Acetylcholine	0.67 ± 0.00 n = 4	0.67 ± 0.02 n = 5	0.81 ± 0.03 n = 4

All systems unstimulated (High Na$^+$ medium)
[1]Sollenberg & Sorbo (1970);   [2]Sterling & O'Neill (1978);
[3]This paper.
Table VIII.   Synaptosomes were incubated as described for Figs.
1 and 2 except that protein concentration was higher (20 mg/ml),
incubation time shorter (6-15 min.) and glucose substrate was
6-^{3}H, ^{14}C labelled.   No ^{3}H-acetylcholine was added when the
reaction was terminated   After neutralisation, the incorporation
of ^{3}H and ^{14}C into acetylcholine was determined as for Fig. 2.
Incorporation of isotopes into pyruvate was determined as described by Lindsay and Bachelard (1966), and into citrate by an
HPLC method.   The latter involves utilisation of a nucleotide-type
HPLC column (see legend to Table V).

ported for citrate in the 4, 5 positions for the slice work, which
suggests that there has not been any extensive anaplerotic function
from pyruvate.   The main difference between our work with synaptosomes and the other data with slices is that whilst our citrate
^{3}H/^{14}C ratio is very close to what would theoretically be predicted
(0.67), the acetylcholine ratio is considerably higher at 0.81. This
contrasts with the slice data both of which show a citrate ratio of
0.45 and an acetylcholine ratio of approximately 2/3, which is as
theory predicts.   Our data may be interpreted as suggesting that
citrate cannot be the only contributor of acetyl groups to acetylcholine;   in fact on the basis of the observed isotope ratios, one
would expect it to contribute just over one half of the carbon

required. However, further work will be necessary to exclude the possibility of a kinetic isotope effect contributing to this higher ratio in cholinergic nerve endings.

When hydroxycitrate, an inhibitor of ATP-citrate lyase is used to interfere with either lipid synthesis or acetylcholine synthesis in whole brain preparations (Sterling & O'Neill, 1978; Tucek et al, 1981) production of these metabolites is reduced but not completely inhibited which suggests that some acetyl group transfer not involving citrate does occur. Our results also suggest when compared with the slice data that acetyl groups for acetylcholine synthesis at the nerve ending tend to be derived less from citrate than those from the whole brain. Indirect support for this comes from the work of Sterling & O'Neill (1978) who showed that when cortical slices were stimulated, the only metabolite $^3H/^{14}C$ ratio that changed significantly was that of acetylcholine which increased. Such stimulation would be expected to specifically increase synthesis of acetylcholine in the nerve ending pool. If this pool had a greater contribution of 'acetate' level acetylcholine such an increase could be explained. Indeed, preliminary data from experiments in which synaptosomes have been incubated and subsequently split into cytosol and mitochondrial compartments (see method of Booth & Clark, 1979) has shown that the mitochondrial acetyl CoA has a $^3H/^{14}C$ isotope ratio close to 0.95. It is also of interest in this context that the citrate output of 'synaptic' mitochondria is energy sensitive - Table 7, since depolarisation of the plasma membrane will increase energy demands on the mitochondria (i.e. put them into State 3) and hence reduce citrate efflux.

The question still remains as to the likely identity of the second acetyl group carrier. Two recent papers have both suggested that the possibility of acetyl carnitine being involved should be reassessed. Sterri & Fonnum (1980) have shown that lesions leading to degeneration of specific cholinergic tracts cause a much greater decrease in pyruvate dehydrogenase and carnitine acetyl transferase (total) than in citrate synthase and ATP citrate-lyase. Tucek et al. (1981) on the basis of radioactively labelled acetyl carnitine studies with brain slices have also indicated that acetyl carnitine may be a possible candidate. Whilst our data are compatible with this suggestion, further experimental data on the mitochondrial/cytosolic acetyl CoA isotope ratios after incubation with labelled acetylcarnitine and carnitine acetyl transferase distribution would be necessary to give firm support to this hypothesis.

This work has been supported by the MRC, SRC and NIH.

REFERENCES

Abdel-Latif, A.A., 1966. A simple method for isolation of nerve ending particles from rat brain. Biochim. Biophys. Acta 121: 403-406.

Autilio, L.A., Appel, S.M., Pettis, P. and Gambetti, P.L., 1968. Biochemical Studies of synapses in vitro. I. Protein synthesis. Biochemistry 7: 2615-2622.

Barondes, S.H. 1974. Synaptic macromolecules: Identification and metabolism. Ann. Rev. Biochem. 43: 147-168.

Blaustein, M.P. and Goldring, J.M., 1975. Membrane potentials in pinched-off presynaptic nerve terminals monitored with a fluorescent probe: evidence that synaptosomes have potassium diffusion potentials. J. Physiol. (Lond.) 247: 589-615.

Booth, R.F.G. and Clark, J.B. , 1978a. A rapid method for the preparation of relatively pure metabolically competent synapto-somes from rat brain. Biochem. J. 176: 365-370.

Booth, R.F.G. and Clark, J.B., 1978b. Studies on the mitochon-drially bound form of rat brain creatine kinase. Biochem. J. 170: 145-151.

Booth, R.F.G. and Clark, J.B., 1979. Method for the rapid separation of soluble and particulate components of rat brain syn-aptosomes. Febs. Letts. 107: 387-392.

Bradford, H.F., 1969. Respiration in vitro of synaptosomes from mammalian cortex. J. Neurochem. 16: 675-684.

Browning, E.T., Schulman, M.P. , 1968. C^{14}acetylcholine syn-thesis by cortex slices of rat brain. J. Neurochem. 15: 1391-1405.

Buckley, B. and Williamson, P.H., 1973. Acetoacetate and brain lipogenesis: Developmental pattern of acetyacetyl CoA synthetase in the soluble fraction of rat brain. Biochem. J. 132: 653-656.

Burgess, E.J., Atterwill, C.K. and Prince, A.K., 1978. Choline acetyltransferase and the high affinity uptake of choline in corpus striatum of reserpinized rats. J. Neurochem., 31: 1027-1033.

Cheng, S-C., Nakamura, R. and Waelsch, H., 1967. Krebs cycle and acetylcholine synthesis in nervous tissue. Biochem. J. 104: 52P

Clark, J.B. and Nicklas, W.J., 1970. The metabolism of rat brain mitochondria. J. biol. Chem. 245: 4724-4731.

Clark, J.B. and Land, J.M., 1974. Differential effects of 2-oxo-acids on pyruvate utilisation and fatty acid synthesis in rat brain. Biochem. J. 140: 25-29.

Cotman, C.W. and Matthews, D.A., 1971. Synaptic plasma membranes from rat brain synaptosomes. Isolation and partial characterization. Biochim. Biophys. Acta 249: 380-394.

Coyle, J.T. and Axelrod, J., 1971. Dopamine β-hydroxylase in the rat brain. Developmental characteristics. J. Neurochem. 19: 449-459.

D'Adamo, A.F., Gidez, L.I. and Yatsu, F.M., 1968. Acetyl transport mechanisms. Involvement of N-acetyl aspartate in de novo fatty acid biosynthesis in developing rat brain. Expt. Brain Res. 5: 267-273.

D'Adamo, A.F. and D'Adamo, A.P., 1968. Acetyl transport mechanisms in the nervous system. The oxoglutarate shunt and fatty acid synthesis in developing rat brain. J. Neurochem. 15: 315-323.

Dhopeshwarker, G.A., Maier, R. and Mead, J.F., 1969. Incorporation of $1-^{14}C$ acetate into the fatty acids of the developing rat brain. Biochim. Biophys Acta 187: 6-12.

Diamond, I. and Fishman, R.A., 1973. High affinity transport and phosphorylation of 2-deoxy-D-glucose in synaptosomes. J. Neurochem. 20: 1533-1542.

Dolezal, V. and Tucek, S., 1981. Utilization of citrate, acetyl-carnitine, acetate, pyruvate and glucose for synthesis of acetyl-choline in rat brain slices. J. Neurochem. 36: 1323-1330.

Fonnum, F., 1968. Choline acetyltransferase binding to and release from membranes. Biochem. J. 109: 389-398.

Fonnum, F., 1969. Radiochemical microassays for the determination of choline acetyltransferase and acetylcholinesterase activities. Biochem. J. 115: 465-472.

Gibson, G.E. and Blass, J.P., 1976. Impaired synthesis of acetylcholine in brain accompanying mild hypoxia and hypoglycaemia. J. Neurochem. 26: 1073-1078.

Gibson, G. E. and Blass, J.P., 1979. Proportional inhibition of acetylcholine synthesis accompanying impairment of 3-hydroxy-butyrate oxidation in rat brain slices. Biochem. Pharm. 28: 133-139.

Glowinski, J. and Iversen, L.I., 1966. Regional studies of catecholamines in rat brain. I. The disposition of [3H]-norepi-nephrine, [3H]-dopamine and [3H] in various regions of the brain. J. Neurochem. 13: 655-559.

Gray, E.G. and Whittaker, V.P., 1962. The isolation of nerve endings from brain: An E.M. study of cell fragments derived by homogenisation and centrifugation. J. Anatomy (Lond.) 96: 79-87.

Grewaal, D.S. and Quastel, J.H., 1973. Control of synthesis and release of radioactive acetylcholine in brain slices from the rat. Biochem. J. 132: 1-14.

Heaton, G.M. and Bachelard, H.S., 1973. The kinetic properties of hexose transport into synaptosomes from guinea pig cerebral cortex. J. Neurochem. 21: 1099-1108.

Hoffman, G., Weiss, L. and Wieland, O.H., 1978. Measurement of ATP citrate-lyase and acetyl-CoA synthetase activity using arylamine acetyltransferase. Analytical Biochem. 84: 441-448.

Janski, A.M. and Cornell, N.W., 1980. Subcellular distribution of enzymes determined by rapid digitonin fractionation of isolated hepatocytes. Biochem. J. 186: 423-429.

Jaworek, D., Gruber, J. and Bergmeyer, H.U. , 1974. in 'Methods of Enzymatic Analysis' (H.U. Bergmeyer, ed.) 4: pp.2127-2131 3nd edition, Verlag Chemie.

Jope, R.S. and Jenden, D.J., 1977. Synaptosomal transport and acetylation of choline. Life Sciences 20: 1389-1392.

Jope, R.S. and Jenden, D.J., 1980. The utilization of choline and acetyl CoA for the synthesis of acetylcholine. J. Neurochem. 35: 318-325.

Kurokawa, M., Sakamoto, T. and Kato, M., 1965. Distribution of Na^+ and K^+ stimulated ATPase activity in isolated nerve ending particles. Biochem. J. 97: 833-844.

Lai, J.C.K. and Clark, J.B., 1979. Preparation of synaptic and non-synaptic mitochondria from mammalian brain. in 'Methods in Enzymology', 55: 51-60.

Lamprecht, W., Stein, P., Heinz, F. and Weisser, H., 1974. In 'Methods of Enzymatic Analysis' (H.U. Bergmeyer, ed.) 4: 1777-179. Verlag-Chemie - Academic Press, New York & London.

Land, J.M. and Clark, J.B., 1973. Effect of phenylpyruvate on enzymes involved in fatty acid synthesis in rat brain. Biochem. J. 134: 545-555.

Land, J.M. and Clark, J.B., 1975. in 'Normal and Pathological Development of Energy Metabolism.' (Hommes, F.A. and Van den Berg, C.J. eds.) pp.155-167.

Land, J.M, Booth, R.F.G., Berger, R. and Clark, J.B., 1977. Development of mitochondrial energy metabolism in rat brain. Biochem. J. 164: 339-348.

Lefresne, P., Guyenet, P. and Glowinski, J., 1973. Acetyl-choline synthesis from $2-^{14}C$ pyruvate in rat striatal slices. J. Neurochem. 20: 1083-1097.

Lefresne, P., Harman, M., Beaujouan, J.C. and Glowinski, J., 1977. Origin of the acetyl moiety of acetylcholine synthesised in rat striatal synaptosomes. Biochimie 59: 197-215.

Lefresne, P., Beaujouan, J.C. and Glowinski, J., 1978. Evidence for extra-mitochondrial pyruvate dehydrogenase involved in acetylcholine synthesis in nerve endings. Nature, 274: 497-500.

Lindsay, J.R. and Bachelard, H.S., 1966. Incorporation of ^{14}C from glucose into α-ketoacids and amino acids in rat brain and liver in vivo. Biochem. Pharmacol. 15: 1045-1052.

Lowenstein, J.M., 1968. Citrate and conversion of carbohydrate into fat. In 'The Metabolic Roles of Citrate' (Goodwin, T.W. ed.) pp. 61-86. Academic Press.

McCaman, R.E., McCaman, M.W. & Stratford, M.L., 1966. Carnitine acetyltransferase in nervous tissue. J. biol. Chem. 241: 930-934.

Ohta, M., Narahashi, T. and Keeler, R.F., 1973. Effects of veratrum alkaloids on membrane potential and conductance of squid and crayfish giant axons. J. Pharmacol. Exp. Therap. 184: 143-154.

Patel, M.S. and Owen, O.E., 1977. Development and regulation of lipid synthesis from ketone bodies by rat brain. J. Neurochem. 28: 109-114.

Patel, T.B. and Clark, J.B., 1979. Synthesis of N-acetyl aspartate by rat brain mitochondria and its involvement in mitochondrial/cytosolic carbon transport. Biochem. J. 184: 539-546.

Patel, T.B. and Clark, J.B., 1980. Lipogenesis in the brain of suckling rats. Studies on the mechanism of mitochondrial-cytosolic carbon transfer. Biochem. J. 188: 163-168.

Patel, T.B. and Clark, J.B., 1981. Mitochondrial/cytosolic carbon transfer in developing rat brain. Biochim. Biophys. Acta. in press.

Potter, L. T. and Murphy, W., 1967. Electrophoreis of acetyl-choline, choline and related compounds. Biochem. Pharmacol. 16: 1386-1388.

Rafalowska, U. and Ksiezak, H., 1979. Uptake of citrate by synaptosomes and synaptosomal mitochondria from rat brain. IRCS Med. Sci. 7: 1979

Rous, S., 1976. On the occurrence of enzymes of ketone body metabolism in human adipose tissue. Biochem. Biophys. Res. Comm. 69: 74-78.

Scott, I.D., Nicholls, D.G., 1980. Energy transduction in intact synaptosomes. Influence of plasma-membrane depolarisation on the respiration and membrane potential of internal mitochondria determined in situ. Biochem. J. 186: 21-33.

Simon, J.R. and Kuhar, M.J., 1976. High affinity choline up-take: ionic and energy requirements. J. Neurochem. 27: 93-99.

Sollenberg, J. and Sörbo, B., 1970. On the origin of the acetyl moiety of acetylcholine in brain studied with a differential labelling technique using ^{3}H-^{14}C-mixed labelled glucose and acetate. J. Neurochem. 17: 201-207.

Sterling, G.H. and O'Neill, J.J., 1978. Citrate as the precursor of the acetyl moiety of acetylcholine. J. Neurochem. 31: 525-530.

Sterri, S.H. and Fonnum, F., 1980. Acetyl-CoA synthesizing enzymes in cholinergic nerve terminals. J. Neurochem. 35: 249-253.

Szutowicz, A. and Lysiak, W., 1980. Regional and subcellular distribution of ATP-citrate lyase and other enzymes of acetyl-CoA metabolism in rat brain. J. Neurochem. 35: 775-785.

Thompson, M.F. and Bachelard, H.S., 1970. Cerebral cortex hexokinase. Comparison of properties of solubilized mitochondrial and cytoplasmic activities. Biochem. J. 118: 25-34.

Tucek, S., 1967. The use of choline acetyl transferase for meas-uring the synthesis of acetyl CoA and its release from brain mito-chondria. Biochem. J. 104: 749-756.

Tucek, S., 1978. in 'Acetylcholine Synthesis in Neurons.'
Chapman & Hall.

Tucek, S. and Cheng, S.C., 1974. Provenance of the acetyl
group of acetylcholine and compartmentation of acetyl CoA and
Krebs cycle intermediates in the brain in vivo.   J. Neurochem.
22: 893-914.

Tucek, S., Dolezal, V. and Sullivan, A.C., 1981. Inhibition of
synthesis of acetylcholine in rat brain slices by (-) HO citrate
and citrate.   J. Neurochem.   36: 1331-1337.

Walter, U. and Soling, H.D., 1976. Transfer of acetyl-units
through the mitochondrial membrane: Evidence for a pathway
different from the citrate pathway. Febs. Letts. 63: 260-266.

Whittaker, V.P., 1969. The Synaptosome.   in 'Handbook of
Neurochemistry' (Lajtha, A. ed.) 2: 327-364.   Plenum Press,
New York.

INTER—CELL REGULATION OF METABOLISM AND FUNCTION

Jill E. Cremer

MRC Toxicology Unit
Medical Research Council Laboratories
Woodmansterne Road, Carshalton
Surrey SM5 4EF, U.K.

The application of techniques that give conceptual images of dynamic events in the brain have made us aware more than ever before, of the fine control constantly exerted over metabolism and function from moment to moment and region to region. The mechanisms by which such synchrony is achieved are only beginning to be understood and most current studies are still of phenomenological nature. The work here falls into this category and perhaps its main purpose will be to ensure that any mechanistic interpretation will encompass the various observations.

Synaptic mitochondrial phosphoprotein

There has been considerable interest in proteins, enriched in synaptosomal preparations, that undergo rapid phosphorylation and dephosphorylation. Of two such proteins which appear to have particularly high rates of phosphate turnover both _in vivo_ and _in vitro_ one is associated with mitochondria and the other with the synaptic plasma membrane (Mitrius _et al_., 1981). The mitochondrial phosphoprotein is almost undoubtedly the α subunit of pyruvate dehydrogenase (Morgan & Routtenberg, 1980; Browning _et al_., 1981 a & b; Magilen _et al_., 1981). Its apparent molecular weight is 41,000 and the phosphorylation of this protein band _in vitro_ has been shown to be sensitive to two known inhibitors of pyruvate dehydrogenase kinase namely dichloroacetate and pyruvate (Morgan & Routtenberg, 1980; Browning _et al_., 1981 b). Cyclic AMP appears not to influence the phosphorylation which distinguishes it from most other phosphoproteins of synaptic membranes (Browning _et al_., 1979 a; Berman _et al_., 1980).

461

From their evidence of a rapid phosphate turnover in vivo Mitrius et al. (1981) have suggested that the phosphorylation state could change in response to rapid changes in neuronal activity.   Indeed, such changes have been observed following repetitive electrical stimulation of hippocampal slices (Browning et al., 1979 a & b).   If this protein represents the activity of pyruvate dehydrogenase in vivo as appears to be the case, then a link between neurotransmitter events and oxidative metabolism comes closer.

In a study on 'whole brain' Cremer & Teal (1974) showed that in the conscious adult rat about two-thirds of the pyruvate dehydrogenase was in its active (non-phosphorylated) form.   Furthermore the rate at which the active portion of the enzyme decarboxylated pyruvate in vitro was comparable to the activity expected in vivo if most of the glucose used by brain is metabolised via pyruvate.   The authors commented that these findings implied that the enzyme could be finely controlled in vivo by the extent to which it was phosphory- lated.   The recent evidence showing high rates of phosphate turnover of this enzyme protein would seem to endorse this view.

The role of calcium

A connection between the regulation of the activity of pyruvate dehydrogenase and synaptic neurotransmission could involve calcium.   This has been postulated by Browning et al. (1981 a) based on the known influences of calcium ions on neuronal function and the ability of mitochondria to sequester calcium.   When the activity of pyruvate dehydrogenase increases, i.e. when less of the enzyme is in the phospho- rylated form, there is also an increase in the intramito- chondrial Ca^{2+} concentration.   Browning et al. (1981 a) have suggested that the change in pyruvate dehydrogenase activity might be the major mechanism for the control of cytoplasmic calcium ion concentration.   Unravelling cause and effect is difficult however, since the phosphatase that dephosphorylates pyruvate dehydrogenase is activated by Ca^{2+} so that it could be argued that Ca^{2+} movement into mitochondria drives oxida- tive metabolism (Denton & McCormack, 1981).   What is not in doubt is that there are specific mechanisms for cycling Ca^{2+} in and out of mitochondria, including those in brain (Nicholls & Crompton, 1980).   It therefore follows that mitochondria do have the ability to buffer cytoplasmic calcium ion concentra- tion which would be so important in nerve terminals.   An interesting description of morphological relationships between mitochondria and other structures within nerve terminals is given by E.G. Gray, in this book.

Compartmentation of pyruvate

Although the implication that pyruvate dehydrogenase might play a general regulatory role in the release and uptake of neurotransmitters in synaptic terminals is only speculation the enzyme's close association with the synthesis of one neurotransmitter, acetylcholine, is not in question.

A radioactive tracer study by Gibson et al. (1978) on acetylcholine synthesis is particularly pertinent. These authors showed that in mouse brain in vivo acetylcholine was formed from a specific pool of pyruvate. This pyruvate compartment was on a direct route from glucose because although the specific radioactivity of acetylcholine was several-fold greater than that of total brain pyruvate it showed a classical product relationship to brain glucose. Assuming that acetylcholine synthesis is predominantly within synaptic terminals this evidence of metabolic compartmentation implies a tight coupling between the following sequence of events. The entry of glucose into terminals, its phosphorylation by hexokinase and further metabolism via the glycolytic pathway to pyruvate which is acted upon by pyruvate dehydrogenase to form acetyl-CoA which becomes incorporated into acetylcholine.

A similar compartmentation effect has been found for glutamate in relation to brain glucose and lactate labelling in the adult rat brain (Fig.1). Because of the high activity of lactate dehydrogenase it can be assumed that lactate and pyruvate will have the same specific radioactivity so that glutamate must have been formed from a small pool of more highly labelled pyruvate (+ lactate) which was on a direct route from glucose.

This type of compartmentation is not seen in the brains of young animals (Fig.2) and probably reflects an increase in synaptic density and function with maturation. It is interesting that in autoradiographs of localised glucose utilization it can be seen that neuropil regions rich in synaptic terminals, as opposed to neuron cell bodies, have high rates of glucose utilization. One region in which this can be clearly seen is the hippocampus, as pointed out by Schwartz & Sharp (1978). Thus when measurements are made of the amount of glucose utilized in a particular brain region it may be presumed that a substantial proportion will represent that occurring in synaptic terminals. It may be worth noting in this context that Wilson (1972) found that mitochondria located in synaptic terminals had an enrichment of hexokinase activity.

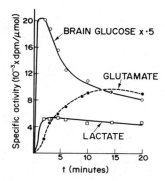

Fig.1. Evidence that in adult rats ^{14}C from glucose becomes
       incorporated into glutamate faster than it equilibrates
       with the total pools of brain pyruvate and lactate.

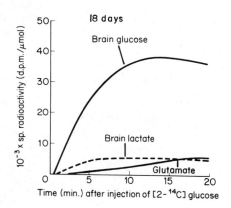

Fig.2. Evidence that in young rats the incorporation of ^{14}C
       from glucose into glutamate occurs after equilibration
       with total brain pyruvate and lactate.

Supply and utilization of glucose in relation to neuronal function

An association between the rate of glucose utilization and the functional state of the brain has been known for some time. For example, pentobarbital anaesthesia in adult rats was shown to reduce the rate to about half (Hawkins et al., 1974).

It is only more recently that it has been possible to show that alterations in glucose utilization can be confined to very specific regions. Such changes can be visualised by the application of the autoradiographic technique of Sokoloff et al. (1979). Studies of this type have shown that administration of the glutamate analogue, kainic acid systemically to rats brings about an early selective increase in glucose utilization in the hippocampus (Collins et al., 1980; Ben-Ari, 1981). Outwardly the animals at this stage showed only mild symptoms. Later convulsions developed and changes in glucose utilization became more widespread, some areas showing a decrease and others an increase. Differences between regions in the rate at which glucose is utilized makes it of interest to consider whether the supply of glucose to the tissue from blood is also regulated regionally.

It is known that the rate at which glucose can pass into brain tissue from blood by simple diffusion is too slow to meet the metabolic requirements. Faster rates are achieved by a facilitated transport mechanism (Crone, 1965; Oldendorf, 1971). This process is probably mediated by protein carriers located in the plasma membranes of capillary endothelial cells. The properties of the process show characteristics similar to those of an enzyme and its substrate particularly in saturability and selectivity (Oldendorf, 1971; Betz et al., 1973; Cremer & Cunningham, 1979). Although these characteristics have been well established there have been few studies attempting to determine the activity of the transporter in localized regions of the brain either in normal situations or in response to altered neuronal activity.

We have recently described a method which allows the simultaneous estimation of regional rates of glucose transport and of glucose utilization in the brain of individual animals (Cunningham & Cremer, 1981). It has been applied to several situations in which motor disturbances were induced chemically (Cremer et al., 1981). Some of the results will be mentioned here, together with some previously unpublished observations.

The method is based on carefully timed sequential intravenous injection of $[^{14}C]-$ and $[^{3}H]2$-deoxyglucose and subsequent inactivation of brain enzymes by focussed microwave irradiation to the head.   The experiment lasts between 4 to 5 minutes and arterial blood samples are obtained throughout this time.   The brain is sliced and punched to give selected regions of between 5 to 20 mg.   Each region is analysed for glucose, and the label separated by ion exchange resin into 2-deoxyglucose and 2-deoxyglucosephosphate.   The data for plasma and brain are analysed to give simultaneous estimates of R_1 and R_3 based on the following simple model:

$$\boxed{\begin{array}{c}\text{Plasma} \\ \text{glucose}\end{array}} \xrightarrow[\text{Efflux } (R_1-R_3)]{\overset{\text{Influx } (R_1)}{\mu\text{mol}\cdot\text{g}^{-1}\cdot\text{min}^{-1}}} \boxed{\begin{array}{c}\text{Brain} \\ \text{glucose}\end{array}} \xrightarrow[\mu\text{mol}\cdot\text{g}^{-1}\cdot\text{min}^{-1}]{\text{Phosphorylation } (R_3)}$$

Since the isotopic tracer used is 2-deoxyglucose two conversion factors are required to correct for the differences between this analogue and glucose in the relative rates of transport across the blood brain barrier and relative rates of phosphorylation by hexokinase.   Full details are given by Cunningham & Cremer (1981).

        In adult rats the rate of simple diffusion of glucose between plasma and brain is low, about 0.008 $\text{ml}\cdot\text{g}^{-1}\cdot\text{min}^{-1}$ (Cremer et al., 1979) so that R_1, the rate of influx of glucose from plasma to a given brain region represents almost entirely the functioning of the specific hexose transporter.   The rate of phosphorylation, R_3, as determined is equivalent to the net rate of glucose utilization.

Table 1.   Estimates of Glucose Transport and Utilization in Brain Regions of Normal Awake Rats

		Influx (R_1) $\mu\text{mol}\cdot\text{g}^{-1}\cdot\text{min}$	Phosphorylation (R_3) $\mu\text{mol}\cdot\text{g}^{-1}\cdot\text{min}$
Sensory cortex	(7)	$2.02 \pm .08$	$1.11 \pm .07$
Inferior Colliculus	(4)	$2.13 \pm .08$	$1.03 \pm .06$
Thalamus	(4)	$1.56 \pm .13$	$0.85 \pm .07$
Caudate Putamen	(7)	$1.46 \pm .07$	$0.95 \pm .05$
Hippocampus	(6)	$1.21 \pm .05$	$0.71 \pm .03$
Cerebellum	(7)	$1.72 \pm .08$	$0.82 \pm .03$

Data are taken from Cremer et al. (1981).

        Estimated values for several brain regions in normal, lightly restrained awake rats are given in Table 1.   It can be seen that for each region the rate of influx of glucose is close to twice the net rate of glucose utilization.   Since the

animals were in a steady-state the difference between the rate
of influx and the rate of phosphorylation gives the rate of
efflux of glucose from brain to blood.   Efflux and phosphorylation in normal awake rats are about equal.

The average plasma glucose concentration in these animals
was 10 mM.   This is very close to the estimated K_m value for
the transporter (Daniel et al., 1978; Cremer et al., 1979)
therefore the rates of influx would be expected to be half the
estimated V_{max} value.   In fact for each region the rate of
influx was considerably higher.   The explanation almost certainly lies in the fact that the kinetic properties of the
transport carrier have been determined from experiments carried
out in pentobarbital anaesthetized animals (Daniel et al., 1978;
Cremer et al., 1979).   In such animals the net rate of glucose
utilization is only half that of awake animals (Hawkins et al.
1974; Sokoloff et al., 1977) so that influx is also likely to
be less.   This raises the possibility that not only is the
rate of glucose utilization directly linked to neuronal
activity and metabolic demand but that the activity of the
glucose transporter in capillary endothelial cells is also
coupled.

This has been tested further by carrying out experiments
in animals with stimulated motor activity.   Continuous, strong
body tremors were induced in rats by intravenous injection of
cismethrin.   [This chemical is one of a series of synthetic
pyrethroids known to interact with the Na^+ channel of nerve
membranes inducing a prolongation of the transient increase in
sodium permeability during the action potential.   These compounds act synergistically with veratridine and their effects
are blocked by tetrodotoxin;   see Jaques et al., 1980].

In rats dosed with cismethrin the cerebellum, cerebellar
nuclei and inferior colliculi always showed a significant
increase in the net rate of glucose utilization.   Concomitantly
there was a regional increase in the rate of glucose transport.   Furthermore, this increase was sustained even at a
lower concentration of plasma glucose (Table 2).   In the
latter situation there is clear evidence that the kinetics of
glucose entry from plasma into brain tissue had changed.
This has been expressed as the PS product in Table 2.   There
could have been localised recruitment of more carriers and/or
a change in the rate at which the carriers in these regions
transported glucose.   A distinction between the various
possible mechanisms cannot be made from present data.   Since
the supply of glucose is so essential for the maintenance of
neuronal function a better understanding of the regulatory
factors involved seem worthy of further study.

Table 2.   Altered Rates of Glucose Influx and Phosphorylation
in Brain Regions of Rats with Continuous Body Tremors

Animal	Plasma glucose (mM)	Brain region	Brain glucose $\mu mol.g^{-1}$	Glucose influx $\mu mol.g^{-1}.min^{-1}$	Glucose utilization $\mu mol.g^{-1}.min$	PS product $ml.g^{-1}.min^{-1}$
Control	10.7	Cerebellum	3.4	1.74	0.85	0.16
	10.7	Inferior colliculus	3.0	2.29	1.03	0.21
Cismethrin induced tremors	12.2	Cerebellum	2.4	2.72	1.58	0.22
	6.0	Cerebellum	1.4	5.31	1.98	0.89
	12.2	Inf.collic.	2.6	2.94	1.57	0.23
	6.0	Inf.collic.	1.5	3.65	1.47	0.61

Summarizing comments

     The theme of this chapter has been to outline various
regulatory links between nerve terminal activity and glucose
metabolism including its localized transport through capillary
endothelial cells.   Examples have been taken mostly from
excitatory situations but recent studies on the striate cortex
of Macaca monkeys have shown a correlation between high rates
of glucose utilization and inhibitory GABAergic terminals
(Hendrickson et al., 1981).   The interplay between capillary
permeability and neuronal function is just beginning to be
studied and may not only involve glucose.   One interesting
example is the marked influence of tricyclic antidepressants
on cerebral capillary permeability (Preskorn et al., 1980).

REFERENCES

Ben-Ari, Y., 1981 in 'Glutamate as a neurotransmitter'
(DiChiava G and Gessa G.L. eds). Advances in Biochemical
Psychopharmacology 27: 385-394.

Berman, R.F., Hullihan, J.P., Kinnier, W.J. and Wilson, J.E.,
1980. Phosphorylation of synaptic membranes. J.Neurochem.
34 (2): 431-437.

Betz, A.L., Gilboe, D.D., Yudilevich, D.L. and Drewes, L.R.,
1973. Kinetics of unidirectional glucose transport into the
isolated dog brain. Am.J.Physiol. 225: 586-592.

Browning, M., Dunwiddie, T., Bennett, W., Gispen, W. and
Lynch, G., 1979 a.   Synaptic phosphoproteins: specific
changes after repetitive stimulation of the hippocampal slice.
Science 203: 60-62.

Browning, M., Bennett, W. and Lynch, G., 1979 b.   Phsophorylase
kinase phosphorylates a brain protein which is influenced by
repetitive synaptic activation. Nature 278: 273-275.

Browning, M., Baudry, M., Bennett, W.F. and Lynch, G., 1981 a.
Phosphorylation-mediated changes in pyruvate dehydrogenase
activity influence pyruvate-supported calcium accumulation by
brain mitochondria. J.Neurochem. 36 (6): 1932-1940.

Browning, M., Bennett, W.F., Kelley, P. and Lynch, G., 1981 b.
Evidence that the 40,000 Mr phosphoprotein influenced by high
frequency synaptic stimulation is the alpha subunit of pyruvate dehydrogenase. Brain Research 218: 255-266.

Collins, R.C., McLean, M. and Olney, J., 1980. Cerebral metabolic response to systemic kainic acid: 14-C-deoxyglucose studies. Life Sciences 27: 855-862.

Cremer, J.E. and Cunningham, V.J. 1979. Effects of some chlorinated sugar derivatives on the hexose transport system of the blood/brain barrier. Biochem.J. 180: 677-679.

Cremer, J.E., Cunningham, V.J., Pardridge, W.M. Braun, L.D. and Oldendorf, W.H., 1979. Kinetics of blood-brain barrier transport of pyruvate, lactate and glucose in suckling, weanling and adult rats. J.Neurochem. 33: 439-445.

Cremer, J.E., Ray, D.E., Sarna, G.S. and Cunningham, V.J., 1981. A study of the kinetic behaviour of glucose based on simultaneous estimates of influx and phosphorylation in brain regions of rats in different physiological states. Brain Research 221:331-342.

Cremer, J.E. and Teal, H.M., 1974. The activity of pyruvate dehydrogenase in rat brain during postnatal development. FEBS Letters 39: 17-20.

Crone, C., 1965. Facilitated transfer of glucose from blood into brain tissue. J.Physiol.Lond. 181: 103-113.

Cunningham, V.J. and Cremer, J.E., 1981. A method for the simultaneous estimation of regional rates of glucose influx and phosphorylation in rat brain using radiolabelled 2-deoxyglucose. Brain Research 221: 319-330.

Daniel, P.M., Love, E.R. and Pratt, O.E., 1978. The effect of age upon the influx of glucose into the brain. J.Physiol. Lond. 274: 141-148.

Denton, R.M. and McCormack, J.G., 1981. Calcium ions, hormones and mitochondrial metabolism. Clinical Science 61: 135-140.

Gibson, G.E., Blass, J.P. and Jenden, D.J., 1978. Measurement of acetylcholine turnover with glucose used as precursor: evidence for compartmentation of glucose metabolism in brain. J.Neurochem. 30: 71-76.

Hawkins, R.A., Miller, A.L., Cremer, J.E. and Veech, R.L., 1974. Measurement of the rate of glucose utilization by rat brain in vivo. J.Neurochem. 23: 917-923.

Hendrickson, A.E., Hunt, S.P. and Wu J.-Y., 1981. Immunocytochemical localization of glutamic acid decarboxylase in
monkey striate cortex. Nature Lond. 292: 605-607.

Jaques, Y., Romey, G., Cavey, M.T., Kartalovski, B. and
Lazdunski, M., 1980. Interaction of pyrethroids with the
Na$^+$ channels in mammalian neuronal cells in culture. Biochim.
Biophys.Acta. 600: 882-897.

Magilen, G., Gordon, A., Au, A. and Diamond, I., 1981.
Identification of a mitochondrial phosphoprotein in brain
synaptic membrane preparations. J.Neurochem. 36 (5):1861-1864.

Mitrius, J. C., Morgan, D. G. and Routtenberg, A., 1981. In
vivo phosphorylation following [^{32}P]orthophosphate injection
into neostriatum or hippocampus: selective and rapid labeling
of electrophoretically separated brain proteins. Brain
Research 212: 67-81.

Morgan, D.G. and Routtenberg, A., 1980. Evidence that a
41,000 dalton brain phosphoprotein is pyruvate dehydrogenase.
Biochem.Biophys.Res.Comm. 95: 569-576.

Nicholls, D.G. and Crompton, M., 1980. Mitochondrial calcium
transport. FEBS Letters 111: 261-268.

Oldendorf, W.H., 1971. Brain uptake of radiolabelled amino
acids, amines and hexoses after arterial injection. Am.J.
Physiol. 221: 1629-1639.

Preskorn, S.H., Hartman, B.K., Raichle, M.E. and Clark, H.B.,
1980. The effect of dibenzazepines (tricyclic antidepressants)
on cerebral capillary permeability in the rat in vivo.
J.Pharmacol.Exp.Ther. 213: 313-320.

Schwartz, W.J. and Sharp, F.R., 1978. Autoradiographic maps
of regional brain glucose consumption in resting, awake rats
using [^{14}C]2-deoxyglucose. J.Comparative Neurol.177: 335-359.

Sokoloff, L., Reivich, M., Kennedy, C., Des Rosiers, M.H.,
Patlak, C.S., Pettigrew, K.D., Sakurada, O. and Shinohara, M.
1977. The [^{14}C]-deoxyglucose method for the measurement of
local cerebral glucose utilization: theory, procedure and
normal values in the conscious and anesthetized albino rats.
J.Neurochem. 28: 897-916.

Wilson, J.E., 1972. The localization of latent brain hexokinase on synaptosomal mitochondria. Arch.Biochem.Biophys.
150: 96-104.

MACROMOLECULAR INTERACTIONS BETWEEN NEURONS AND PERIPHERAL GLIA IN

CELL CULTURE

S. Varon and M. Manthorpe

Department of Biology, School of Medicine
University California, San Diego, La Jolla, CA 92093 USA

It has become increasingly evident that development, maintenance, functional performance and repair.of neurons are extensively
influenced by humoral and surface interactions with glial cells
(Varon & Somjen, 1979; Varon & Manthorpe, 1981). In the past, neuroglia was viewed as providing physical scaffolding, insulation
(myelin), and monitoring of chemical exchanges between blood and
neurons. It has also been suggested that glial cells may remove
excess K^+ from the vicinity of firing neurons and dissipate it via
intraglial and interglial (gap junctions) redistribution--thereby
contributing to slow electrical activities of the brain and, possibly, the onset of epileptic foci. More recently, considerable
evidence has been gathered both in vivo and in vitro that glial
cells can take up and release neurotransmitters and other neuroactive molecules, suggesting another possible way for glial cells
to regulate neuronal function or intervene in neuronal pathology.
Conversely, K^+ and transmitters may be viewed as <u>microsignals</u> from
neurons to glia, causing the glial cells to change their own performance. It is only in the last decade, however, that serious
attention has been given to <u>macrosignals</u> between neurons and glia,
that is two-way communications mediated by macromolecular agents
presented by one cell type to regulate behaviors of the other
(Varon & Adler, 1981).

NEURONAL AND GLIAL CELL CULTURES

Glia-neuron interactions, like many other neurobiological problems, can be analyzed in considerable detail by use of in vitro
cultures (Varon 1975b; Varon & Saier 1975; Fedoroff & Hertz 1978;
Giacobini <u>et al</u>., 1980). Of particular importance for such investigation is the availability of purified and viable populations of
individual classes of glial and neuronal cells to be studied in

isolation so as to define their own properties, or after recombin-
ation so as to investigate heterotypic cell interactions. Several
methods are now available to obtain purified neuronal and glial
cultures from both central and peripheral neural tissues (cf. Varon
1977), and further improvements in methodology are likely to derive
in the near future from the use of monoclonal antibodies against
cell-specific surface antigens (cf. Varon & Manthorpe 1980).

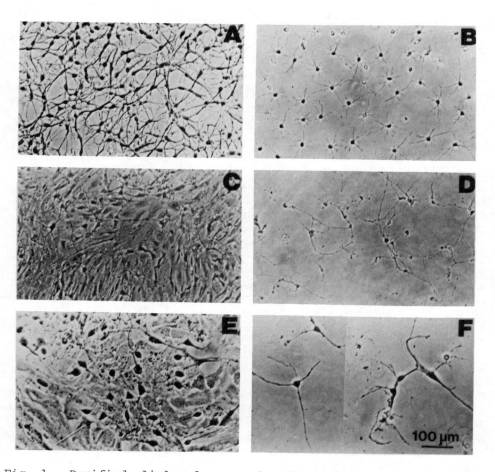

Fig. 1. Purified glial and neuronal cultures from central neural
tissues. A,B: selective seeding densities and in vitro ages can
produce nearly pure astrocytic (A) or oligodendrocytic (B) populations from neonatal rat cerebrum. C,D: fetal calf serum (C) but
not horse serum (D) promotes glial proliferation in embryonic
chick spinal cord cell cultures. E,F: glial proliferation from
rodent central tissues (neonatal cerebrum, here) is supported by
horse serum (E): use of the serum-free, N1 supplement prevents
glial growth while fully supporting neuronal survival (F).

Purification of glial cells is theoretically easier than that
of neurons, since glial cells can proliferate and rapidly outnumber
the neuronal elements: the main problem, here, is to segregate
different classes of nonneuronal elements.   In contrast, neuronal
purification is limited by the number of viable neurons obtained in
the original cell dissociate, and requires culture conditions that
are both suitable for neuronal survival and restrictive on nonneuronal growth.   Figure 1 illustrates how selective manipulations of
the culture conditions can yield purified glial and neuronal populations from central neural tissues.

When neonatal rat (or mouse) cerebrum is dissociated, the en-
suing cultures consist almost exclusively of nonneuronal, "flat"
cells which rapidly proliferate to a confluent cell monolayer (e.g.
Varon & Raiborn 1969; Sensenbrenner 1977; Hertz 1977).   Many of
these "flat" cells assume a more typical astrocytic morphology
when deprived of serum and treated with cyclic AMP-elevating
agents (e.g. Lim et al., 1973; Moonen et al., 1976; Sensenbrenner
1977). A detailed study (Manthorpe et al., 1979) has revealed the
importance of seeding densities and in vitro ages for the selection of astroglial and oligodendroglial cells. With the appropriate conditions, one can thus obtain glial cell cultures, more than
90% of which are astroglial by their content of the astroglial-
specific glial fibrillary acidic protein (GFA) and their ability
to assume the astrocytic morphology (Fig. 1 A). With high seeding
densities and increasing age in culture, a second population appears, which spontaneously displays several fine processes and is
more loosely attached to the culture substratum or, more often,
the astroglial flat cell layer. It is possible to dislodge these
cells from their attachment surfaces, collect them off the mixed
culture, and re-seed them as a nearly homogenous population
(Manthorpe et al., 1979; McCarthy & DeVellis 1980). Their distinct
behavior and morphology (Fig. 1 B) proposes an oligodendroglial
identity, further confirmed by the absence of GFA and the presence of several oligodendroglial biochemical markers.

Until recently, both neurons and glial cells have required
serum supplementation of the medium for their survival in culture.
Differential serum effects, however, may determine whether the
glial cells will or will not grow. For example, nonneuronal cells
from embryonic chick, but not rodent, central neural tissues require fetal calf serum for in vitro proliferation, as shown with
cell cultures from spinal cord (Popiela et al., 1978), optic lobe
(Adler et al., 1979) or neural retina (Hyndman & Adler 1981). Fig.
1, C and D show the dramatic contrast between cultures of 8 day
chick embryo spinal cord that were supplemented with fetal calf
serum (C) and those that were supplemented with horse serum (D).
Horse serum provides adequate support for the neurons but not the
nonneuronal elements, thereby yielding nearly pure neuronal populations.   Nonneuronal growth might be controlled even in rodent

cultures, if one could omit serum altogether while still supporting neuronal survival. Nearly purified neuronal cultures can now
be obtained in serum-free media, with additional advantages offered
for biochemical investigations. These results were obtained by re-
placing serum with chemically defined supplements, designated as N1
or N2 and consisting of insulin, transferrin, putrescine, progesterone and selenite (N1 only differs from N2 by its lower content
of transferrin). We demonstrated this competence of the N1 supplement with neuronal cultures from a variety of avian and rodent central neural tissues (Skaper et al., 1979). Fig. 1, E and F illustrate the contrasting effects of using horse serum (E) or N1 supplement (F) on cerebral cells from neonatal mouse.

The serum-free, N1-supplemented medium supports neuronal survival but not nonneuronal growth also in cultures from peripheral
neural tissues, such as dorsal root ganglia (DRG) (Bottenstein et
al., 1980) or sympathetic ganglia (Varon & Skaper 1981) from embryonic chick--provided Nerve Growth Factor (NGF), the classical
neuronotrophic factor for these neurons, is also present.

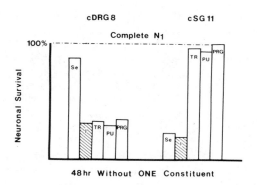

Fig. 2. Differential requirements of N1 constituents by different
neurons. Cells from 8 day DRG (cDRG8) or 11 day sympathetic ganglia (cSG11) were cultured 2 days on collagen in serum-free medium
containing NGF and the N1 supplement, from which a single constituent (symbols in histograms) was omitted at a time. Se = selenite
$(3.10^{-8}M)$; I = insulin (5 µg/ml); TR = transferrin (5 µg/ml); PU =
putrescine (100 µM): PRG = progesterone $(2.10^{-8}M)$.

Figure 2 shows that the individual Nl constituents which are critical for neuronal survival in vitro need not be the same for different neuronal populations. With 8 day chick embryo DRG neurons, the
single omission of selenite had little effect on survival, while
any one of the other four Nl constituents could not be omitted
without a drastic reduction (Bottenstein et al., 1980). In contrast, neurons from 11 day chick embryo sympathetic ganglia toler-
ated the single omission of transferrin, or putrescine, or progesterone, but suffered greatly from the omission of either selenite
or insulin (Varon & Skaper 1981). Such analyses are now being
extended to other neuronal cultures from both central and peripheral sources, and may reveal yet another approach to the selective
elimination of distinct subsets of neurons from heterogenous, albeit nonneuron-free neuronal cultures. One should note that, at
present, no information is available on i) what role the relevant
Nl constituents play in neuronal survival, or ii) how their actions
relate to that of the traditional neuronotrophic factors (such as
the equally required NGF in the ganglionic cultures of Fig. 2).

    A different way to segregate neurons and nonneurons from a
mixed neural cell suspension, which has the advantage of yielding

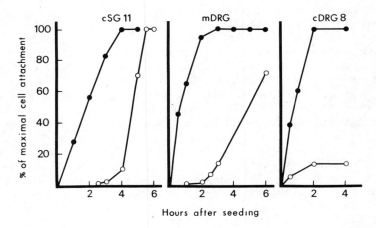

Fig. 3.   Fractionation of neurons and nonneuronal cells by differential attachment. Dissociates from chick embryo sympathetic ganglia (cSG11), neonatal mouse DRG (mDRG), or chick DRG (cDRG8) are
seeded on collagen in serum-containing medium. Most nonneurons (●)
are attached by 2-3 hr, while nearly no neurons (O) are.

both subpopulations, is to take advantage of differential cell
attachment. Upon seeding a neural dissociate on a substratum of
appropriate adhesiveness, nonneuronal cells will attach more
promptly than neurons. At the correct time, therefore, one can
collect the still unattached cells as a "neuron-enriched" cell suspension, and leave behind a "neuron-free" nonneuronal cell culture
(which can then be grown under the appropriate mitogenic conditions). Such a differential attachment approach was first described
for chick embryo cerebral cells (Varon & Raiborn 1969) and has been
successfully applied to dissociates from chick sympathetic ganglia
(Varon & Raiborn 1972), mouse DRG (Varon et al., 1973), and chick
DRG (Fishel, Skaper, Varon, unpublished). Figure 3 illustrates the
different attachment curves of neurons and nonneurons in the three
cases. Similar approaches are now routinely used for ganglionic
cells in several laboratories (e.g. McCarthy & Partlow 1976; Barde
et al., 1980; Edgar et al., 1981).

SCHWANN CELL CULTURES

     Glial cells in the peripheral nervous system are usually cate-
gorized as "satellite" cells surrounding the ganglionic cell bodies
and "Schwann" cells associated with peripheral axons.   There are
reasons to believe that both categories represent the same cell
type in different topographic and functional situations (cf. Bunge
1970; Webster 1974; Aguayo et al., 1976 a,b, 1979; Varon & Bunge
1978; Varon & Manthorpe 1981; Pannese 1980). The close physical
association between peripheral glial cells (to which we shall refer here collectively as Schwann cells) and various parts of the
peripheral neurons (as well as central neurons projecting outside
the central nervous system) has long inspired the view that equally
close biochemical and functional interactions must occur between
the two partners. Myelin formation, maintenance, breakdown and
restoration--the most conspicuous Schwann-neuron interaction--have
been extensively investigated in vivo and, more recently, in vitro
(e.g. Salzer & Bunge 1980; Bunge & Bunge 1978; Bunge et al., 1980),
and will not be discussed in this chapter (for reviews, see Varon
& Bunge 1976; Varon & Manthorpe 1981). Rather, we shall be concerned with macromolecular signals from neurons to Schwann cells
other than the myelinogenic ones, and with converse signals from
Schwann cells to neurons. Once again, these problems have become
more directly accessible with the advent of purified Schwann cell
cultures from rat DRG, rat sciatic nerve and mouse DRG. Each of
these three preparations and the methodology by which they are obtained have brought to light interesting--and different--features
of Schwann cell regulation.

Rat DRG Schwann cells (Wood 1976). Late fetal DRG (16-20 day) are
dissected free of their capsule (a major source of fibroblasts)
and explanted on collagen in a heavily supplemented medium (human
placental serum, chick embryo extract, Nerve Growth Factor). The

outgrowth from the explant displays neurites, Schwann cells and relatively fewer fibroblasts. Alternate-day treatments with antimitotic drugs suppress preferentially the proliferation of fibroblasts. After several weeks, the body of the explant (containing
the ganglionic neuronal somata) is excised and re-explanted in another dish, to generate a second outgrowth of neurites and Schwann
cells practically devoid of fibroblastic contaminants. The operation can be repeated several times until no cells are left inside
the ganglionic mass, thereby yielding a pure "neuronal" ganglion
which can be cultured as an explant or after dissociation. The
outgrowth zones remaining after transfer of the ganglionic mass
contain only Schwann cells and amputated neurites, which rapidly
degenerate yielding a pure Schwann cell bed. Two main features
have emerged from this approach (Wood & Bunge 1975; Wood 1976;
Salzer & Bunge 1980). In the neurite-free Schwann cell bed (or in
dissociated cell cultures derived from it), the Schwann cells behave as postmitotic elements: less than 1% of the population will
display labeled nuclei after ^{3}H-thymidine exposure, despite the
medium supplementation with placental or fetal calf serum and embryo extract. In contrast, the presence or subsequent presentation
of neurites acts as a potent mitogen for the Schwann cells (but not
the fibroblasts): the mitogenic effects of neurites in the mixed
culture decrease with increasing time of Schwann-neurite association. One should also note the manner by which the fibroblastic
component of a ganglionic population is removed, first by excising
its main source, i.e. the ganglionic capsule, and then by differentially suppressing its proliferation with the antimitotic
treatment.

Rat sciatic Schwann cells (Brockes et al., 1977, 1979). Cell dissociates from neonatal sciatic nerve, containing Schwann cells and
relatively few fibroblasts (no neurons), are cultured in medium
supplemented with 10% fetal calf serum (FCS). These rat sciatic
Schwann cells, unlike the rat DRG ones, display some proliferative
response to the FCS (up to 20% of them label with ^{3}H-thymidine)
which is still, however, much more modest than that of the fibroblasts. Antimitotic treatments, therefore, preferentially destroy
the fibroblastic population, the remnants of which are eliminated
by immunocytolytic treatment with complement and anti-Thy-1.1 antibodies (Thy-1.1 is a surface antigen present on the rat fibroblasts but not the rat sciatic Schwann cells). The resulting, highly purified sciatic Schwann cell population is re-seeded and prop-
agated in medium containing, in addition to the 10% FCS, a potent
and selective mitogen for these Schwann cells obtained from extracts of bovine pituitary gland or brain. Rat sciatic and DRG
Schwann cells, unlike their partner fibroblasts or neurons, carry
on their surface the Ran-1 antigen, which permits their immunochemical identification (Fields et al., 1978). Thus: (1) rat
sciatic Schwann cells do respond, although modestly, to FCS mitogens, (2) they are strongly and selectively stimulated by a

pituitary mitogen, and (3) immunochemical methods could be used to
further the Schwann cell purification (antibody to Thy-1.1), as
well as to characterize the resulting cells (Ran-1 antigen).

Mouse DRG Schwann cells (Skaper et al., 1980; Manthorpe et al.,
1980a). Neonatal mouse DRG cell cultures, in a study comparing the
effects of N1 and FCS-supplemented media, have revealed that: (1)
N1 supported survival not only of these neurons (provided NGF was
also present), but also of their partner Schwann and fibroblast
cells; (2) in the presence of neurons, the N1-supported Schwann
cells assumed the typical spindle morphology, aligned themselves
along the neuritic processes and underwent considerable proliferation; and (3) FCS-supported Schwann cells assumed a "flat" morphology, abandoned their association with neurites (if present), and
displayed vigorous proliferation as did the fibroblastic elements.
These observations have led to a procedure for the purification and
propagation of mouse DRG cells. The three main steps are illustrated in Figure 4.

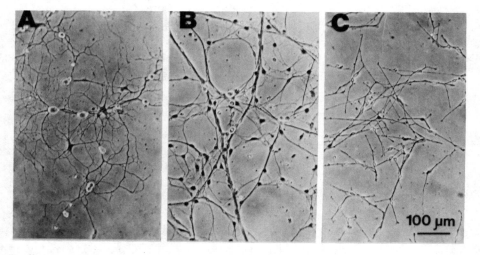

Fig. 4. Different stages of mouse Schwann cell purification and
expansion. A = neuronal fraction obtained by differential attachment, 24 hr in culture. B = primary culture, after 9 days of expansion in N1 medium (+NGF). C = secondary culture, expanded in
serum for 6 days, then treated 24 hr with serum-free, N1 medium:
98% of the cells resume the typical Schwann morphology.

     The DRG dissociate is first subjected to a differential
attachment step, to remove most of the fibroblasts and free
Schwann cells. The unattached cell population, containing the
neurons, their satellite cells and a few remaining free nonneuronal elements, is then cultured in serum-free N1 medium with NGF, so

that the neurons grow neurites and the Schwann cells associate
with them and respond to the neuritic mitogen with a 20-fold expansion. The primary culture is harvested and cultured further in
NGF-free, FCS-supplemented medium, where the neurons fail to survive: the serum mitogens cause another 20-fold expansion of the
Schwann cells, accompanied by a similar proliferation of the residual fibroblasts (no more than 2% of the total population).

Schwann cell identification criteria. The problem of cell identification is a recurrent one in neural cell cultures and, even more
so, in neural cell purification work. As has been extensively
discussed elsewhere (e.g. Varon & Somjen 1979; Varon & Manthorpe
1980, 1981), cell behavior is modulated by developmental age, by
cell-cell interactions and by the extrinsic influences imposed by
both medium and substratum of the culture. Thus, morphological,
biochemical or immunochemical markers for Schwann cells need not
be expressed under all conditions and cannot be viewed as absolute
criteria for cell identification, however specific they may appear
for a given cell type in a particular set of circumstances. Furthermore, some criteria (e.g. electron microscopy, myelination)
are excellent ones to document the occurrence of Schwann cells,
but are impractical or inadequate tools to quantitate their presence. The three groups of Schwann cell studies just reviewed
have used several kinds of criteria, which it is instructive to
compare:
i) Most cell markers have to be initially correlated with morphological criteria. In culture, as in vivo, the typical Schwann
cell displays a "spindle" morphology (two narrow and tapering processes, 50-100 µm, extended in opposite directions from a small
oval body), and the tendency to join with other Schwann cells into
linear or branching chains. Both the spindle morphology and the
chain-like associations are especially conspicuous when neurites
are available for Schwann cell alignment with them. On the other
hand, in most circumstances one also sees small, roughly triangu-
lar flat cells that by other criteria can still be classified as
Schwann cells (Varon & Manthorpe 1981; Krikorian et al., 1981).
The mouse DRG Schwann cell studies make it particularly obvious
that flat and spindle morphologies, as well as Schwann-neurite
association, can be drastically influenced by the culture conditions, e.g. the presence of FCS. Thus, the morphological criterion, while sufficient in practice when expressed, is not a necessary concomitant of the Schwann cell identity: conversely, the
use of serum-free N1 medium may help the morphological identification.
ii) A physical association with neurites appears to be a unique
attribute of Schwann cells--again when culture circumstances permit it (cf. Varon & Bunge 1978). Both rat DRG and mouse DRG
Schwann cell preparations exhibit it, as do chick DRG cells (e.g.
Peterson & Murray 1955; Varon 1977). The physical association is
likely to have important functional counterparts, such as the
presentation of mitogenic and myelinogenic signals from neurite to

Schwann cell or elongation and guidance signals from Schwann cell
surface to neurite.
iii) <u>Biochemical markers</u> can be important supplementary tools for
cell identification if they can be readily visualized at the individual cell level. While such markers are now available for central glial cells (cf. Varon & Somjen 1979), this is not yet the
case for Schwann cells. Unlike oligodendrocytes, Schwann cells do
not retain the ability to make myelin-related glycolipids and proteins once dissociated from their source tissue (cf. Brockes <u>et al</u>.,
1980a). Uptake of certain neurotransmitters, reported for ganglionic satellite cells in vivo (e.g. Schon & Kelly 1974; Bowery
<u>et al</u>., 1979), has not yet been examined in vitro.
iv) A most promising category is that of <u>immunochemical markers</u>
(particularly surface antigens), the investigation of which has
only just begun. Two Schwann surface antigens have been described.
One is the already mentioned Ran-1, which has been detected on rat
Schwann cells of advanced fetal age (Fields <u>et al</u>., 1978) but not
on mouse or avian ones, thus far. The other is an antigen detected
on both Schwann cells and oligodendrocytes of the rat by an antiserum raised against bovine oligodendrocytes (Lisak <u>et al</u>., 1980):
no information is yet available about its presence in other animal
species. Clearly, such markers cannot yet be generalized to all
Schwann cell preparations regardless of source, age or conditions.

SCHWANN CELL MITOGENS

Proliferation of Schwann cells <u>in vivo</u> appears to be subject
to different regulations during development, in the mature organ-
ism, or after nerve injury (cf. Webster 1974; Romine <u>et al</u>., 1975,
1976; Asbury & Johnson 1978; Varon & Manthorpe 1981; among others).
During development, Schwann cells migrate down already growing
neurites, proliferate on them until the neuritic domain is fully
occupied, and then stop replicating whether or not myelin formation
is undertaken. Local injury of a mature nerve will trigger renewed proliferation, both in the proximal segment where axons are
regenerating and in the distal segment where the amputated axons
are degenerating. No definitive information is available on the
nature and the number of mitogenic signals that operate in each of
these situations. The recent <u>in vitro</u> studies reviewed here have
provided evidence for at least two classes of Schwann cell mitogens.

<u>Neuritic mitogens</u>. We have already noted that neurites supply a
strong, and selective, mitogenic signal for DRG Schwann cells from
both the rat (Wood & Bunge 1975; Wood 1976) and the mouse (Skaper
<u>et al</u>., 1980; Manthorpe <u>et al</u>., 1980a). The mitogenic competence
of the neurites appears to decline with the age of the cultures,
being progressively restricted to the growing portion of the neurite until all Schwann cells become quiescent (Salzer & Bunge 1980).
The neuritic mitogen resides in the neuritic membrane, being absent
in nerve extracts or nerve-conditioned media and retained (at least

for a time) by axolemmal particulate preparations, and is likely to
involve glycoprotein constituents on the surface of the neurite
(Salzer et al., 1980 a,b). Mitogenic competence for Schwann cells
has been observed with several peripheral neurites (Wood & Bunge
1975), as well as with axolemmal preparations from adult rat brain
(DeVries et al., 1980), but not with membranes from fibroblasts or
neuroblastoma clonal cultures (Salzer et al., 1980 a,b). An important point, brought out by the mouse Schwann cell studies, is that
serum is not required for the Schwann cell response to the neuritic
mitogen (Manthorpe et al., 1980a). It is not yet known, however,
whether the N1 supplement used in those studies is needed to support Schwann cell proliferation (as it is for neuroblastoma pro-
liferation--Bottenstein & Sato 1979), or only to maintain neuronal
survival and thus neuritic growth.

Soluble mitogens. Raff et al. (1978 a,b) have reported that proliferation of rat sciatic Schwann cells is stimulated by several
agents that elevate their cyclic AMP content, such as choleratoxin.
These mitogenic effects (though not the cyclic AMP elevation) were
potentiated by several tissue extracts, themselves without mitogenic competence, and required the concurrent presence of fetal calf
serum. Choleratoxin, however, may have little or no mitogenic
effects on rat DRG Schwann cells (Salzer et al., 1980a). Neither
rat sciatic nor rat DRG Schwann cells responded to several other
agents presumed to be mitogenic for different cell systems, such as
lectins, neurotransmitter, hormones, prostaglandins, proteases,
epidermal growth factor (EGF) or fibroblast growth factor (FGF)
(Raff et al., 1978 a,b; Salzer & Bunge 1980). In contrast, FGF
(but not EGF) preparations displayed mitogenic effects on mouse
Schwann cells even in the presence of very low serum levels
(Krikorian et al., 1981). Of the several tissue extracts tested on
rat sciatic Schwann cells (Raff et al., 1978b), only bovine pitui-
tary--and to a much lesser extent brain--extract displayed mitogenic activity, provided again that fetal calf serum (though not
other sera) be also present. Partial purification of the pituitary
mitogen (Brockes et al., 1980b) suggests that it resides with a
dimeric, 60,000 dalton acidic protein, which is different from FGF
and is also effective on astrocytes (but not oligodendroglia or
microglia cells). Finally, mouse DRG Schwann cells are highly
responsive to fetal calf and other sera (Manthorpe et al., 1980a;
Krikorian et al., 1981), in contrast with rat DRG cells which are
not affected (Wood & Bunge 1975; Salzer & Bunge 1980) and rat
sciatic cells which respond only moderately (Brockes et al., 1979).
Serum plays an important role in the attachment and maintenance of
Schwann (as well as other) cells, and with mouse cells it is important to distinguish between these and the mitogenic effects
(Krikorian et al., 1981). No information is yet available on i)
the nature of the serum mitogens involved in the mouse Schwann cell
response, or ii) the basis for the different responsiveness to
serum mitogens by the three preparations of rodent Schwann cells.

NEURONOTROPHIC FACTORS OF SCHWANN CELL ORIGIN

Just as neurons can regulate proliferation and other behaviors of their Schwann cells, Schwann cells can influence survival and growth of their neuronal partners. It has long been known that DRG and sympathetic ganglionic neurons require for their maintenance, growth and expression of differentiated functions the availability of Nerve Growth Factor (NGF). This soluble protein factor is found in many sources but is most abundant in the adult mouse submaxillary gland, from which is has been isolated and characterized (cf. Levi-Montalcini & Angeletti 1968; Varon 1975a; Greene & Shooter 1980; Varon & Skaper 1982; among others). NGF has been viewed as the model for other neuronotrophic factors (NTFs), that is, macromolecular agents responsible for survival and general growth of their target neurons. Neuronotrophic factors may be supplied to the neurons by either their innervation territories or their partner glial cells (cf. Varon & Adler 1980). Recent work in several laboratories has now recognized the occurrence of several such NTFs (reviewed in Varon & Adler 1981).

Ganglionic neuronotrophic factors (GNTFs). The first demonstration that ganglionic nonneuronal cells could serve as sources of trophic factors for their partner neurons came from studies of neonatal mouse DRG cultures (Burnham et al., 1972). In these studies (reviewed in Varon 1975a; Varon & Manthorpe 1981), neurons could be made to survive equally well with NGF in the medium, or by the presence of adequate numbers of ganglionic nonneurons with an NGF-free medium. The specific trophic competence of these cells (which comprised both Schwann and fibroblastic elements) was abolished by treatment with antiserum against mouse NGF, demonstrating the NGF-like nature of their contribution. Neuronotrophic activities for various chick embryo ganglionic neurons have been subsequently reported in conditioned media (CMs) from several cell cultures. CMs from C6 clonal cell cultures (derived from a central glioma of the rat) contain NGF-like activity recognizable by anti-NGF antibodies (Schwartz et al., 1977; Perez-Polo et al., 1977), but also trophic activities for DRG and sympathetic ganglionic neurons which are not blocked by those antibodies (Barde et al., 1980; Edgar et al., 1981). Heart conditioned medium displays NTF activities for the same ganglia as well as for ciliary ganglion cells (Helfand et al., 1976, 1978; Varon et al., 1979, 1981), which are also not sensitive to anti-NGF antibody. Thus, these studies reveal the occurrence of ganglionic neuronotrophic factors (GNTFs), which differ at least by some immunochemical features from the classical mouse NGF.

A quantitative comparison of GNTF activities has been carried out among conditioned media from mouse purified Schwann cells, rat Schwannoma RN22 clonal cultures and the already mentioned chick heart cell cultures, using test neurons from neonatal mouse DRG, 8 day chick embryo DRG and 11 day chick embryo sympathetic ganglia

(Varon et al., 1981). All three CMs supported survival of the mouse DRG and chick sympathetic neurons, but not those from the 8 day chick DRG. Essentially the same number of neurons were supported by the CMs alone, NGF alone or a combination of both treatments (each at its optimal dose), indicating that the CMs address the same neurons as does NGF. Inclusion of antibodies against mouse NGF blocked the NGF activity, but not that of the CMs. Since the Schwann-CM was also derived from mouse cells, there can be no question that at least this CM contains NTFs which are different from the traditional mouse submaxillary NGF. The presence of NGF-unlike NTFs in all three CMs was, of course, also suggested by their failure to support 8 day chick DRG neurons. More recent work (Fishel, Skaper & Varon, unpublished) has shown that chick DRG neurons do respond to these CMs but only at older embryonic ages. Barde et al. (1980) have already pointed out, in an elegant developmental study, that their C6-CM becomes increasingly effective on chick DRG neurons as their age increases, while conversely the trophic support of NGF for the survival of the same neurons declines. Taken together, these studies suggest that i) DRG neurons carry two sets of receptors (one for NGF, one for GNTFs), the relative number of which varies with development, and ii) survival may require a minimal number of "occupied" receptors, regardless of the set and the factor involved (cf. Varon & Skaper 1982).

The top and central panels of Figure 5 illustrate the similar appearance of neurons from mouse DRG or chick sympathetic ganglia, respectively, when cultured with their traditional NGF (left) or with GNTFs produced by Schwann cells (right). We have recently detected GNTF activity, with the same neuronal target spectrum as these CMs, in fluid collected in vivo from chambers surrounding a regenerating sciatic nerve in the rat (Lundborg et al., 1981; Longo et al., 1982). It remains to be determined what is the actual cell source of the GNTFs in this fluid and whether GNTFs from different provenances (in vivo fluid, in vitro conditioned media, or tissue extracts--cf. Manthorpe et al., 1981b) represent the same molecular agents.

Trophic factors for spinal cord neurons. Spinal cord motor neurons have their somata located in the central nervous system and could, therefore, derive trophic influences from central glial cells and other central neurons. On the other hand, their axons project outside the central nervous system and associate with Schwann cells as do those from ganglionic neurons. Like ganglionic neurons, too, spinal motor neurons innervate peripheral territories (skeletal muscle) and are likely to be subject to "target-derived" neuronotrophic factors (Varon & Adler 1981; Varon et al., 1982). Indeed, conditioned medium from skeletal muscle cells has been reported by various investigators to support in vitro survival of spinal cord neurons (reviewed in Varon et al., 1982).

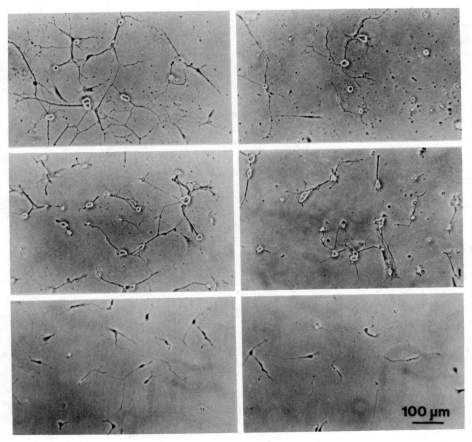

Fig. 5. Trophic effects of conditioned media from Schwann cells for ganglionic and spinal cord neurons. Top to bottom: 24 hr cultures from neonatal mouse DRG, 11 day chick embryo sympathetic ganglia, and 4 day chick embryo lumbar cord. Left panels: medium was supplemented with NGF (ganglia) or with skeletal muscle conditioned medium (cord). Right panels: medium supplemented with conditioned medium from RN22 schwannoma cells.

We have recently demonstrated that NTFs for such neurons are also present in CMs from normal mouse and clonal rat Schwann cell cultures (Longo et al., 1981). Figure 5 (bottom panels) shows the similar effects of schwannoma CM (right) and skeletal muscle CM (left) on cultures from 4 day chick embryo lumbar cord which, by virtue of the age and location of their source, are expected to be greatly enriched in motor neurons (cf. Varon et al., 1982). A similar survival of spinal neurons has been obtained with the fluid collected in vivo from the nerve-regeneration model chambers mentioned above (Longo et al., 1982). Work is now in progress to define molecular properties of the spinal cord NTFs from both the in vitro and the in vivo sources.

NEURITE-PROMOTING FACTORS OF SCHWANN CELL ORIGIN

In the course of investigating heart conditioned medium effects on ciliary ganglionic cells, it has been found that this CM contains an agent which selectively binds to polyornithine (or other polycationic substrata) and elicits extensive neuritic growth from such neurons (Collins 1978; Varon et al., 1979). This poly-ornithine-binding neurite promoting factor (PNPF) is clearly different from the neuronotrophic factors present in the CM in that i) it has no trophic activity by itself (neuronal survival still requires the additional presence of NTF) and ii) it operates from its bound condition rather than in solution (and thus readily segregates on the polyornithine surface from the NTFs which remain in the medium) (Adler & Varon 1980). Ciliary ganglia explanted on untreated polyornithine release their own PNPF, which coats the surrounding substratum to make it conducive to neurite elongation and imposes on the neuritic outgrowth from the ganglion a distinctive "circular"pattern (Adler & Varon 1981a). This ganglionic PNPF is likely to originate from the ganglionic nonneurons, since neuritic outgrowth from the same ganglia explanted on collagen (to which PNPF does not bind) remains restricted to the surface of the nonneurons migrating out of the explant (Adler & Varon 1981b). A survey of a large number of CMs indicated that PNPFs are released by a great variety of peripheral cells (Adler et al., 1981a).

PNPF sources include Schwann cell cultures from both normal (mouse DRG) and clonal (rat RN22) origin (Adler et al., 1981) Thus, Schwann cells not only release into their media neuronotrophic factors (see preceding section), they also release neurite promoting agents. The RN22 schwannoma-conditioned medium (RCM) is relatively rich in PNPF even when prepared free of serum. Fractionation studies have indicated that its PNPF resides with an acidic, high molecular weight glycoprotein (Manthorpe et al., 1981a; Adler et al., 1981b).

A comparison of neuritic behaviors on untreated polyornithine and PNPF-treated polyornithine has been carried out in several neural cell cultures, beside those from ciliary ganglia (Adler et al., 1981a). Representative results are illustrated in Figure 6. Ciliary ganglionic neurons from 8 day chick embryos, cultured in media containing serum as well as their appropriate trophic factor (e.g. Manthorpe et al., 1980b), will grow no neurites on polyornithine unless it has been treated with PNPF. DRG neurons from either mouse or chick and chick sympathetic neurons, supported by NGF or GNTF in the medium, grow some neurites even on untreated

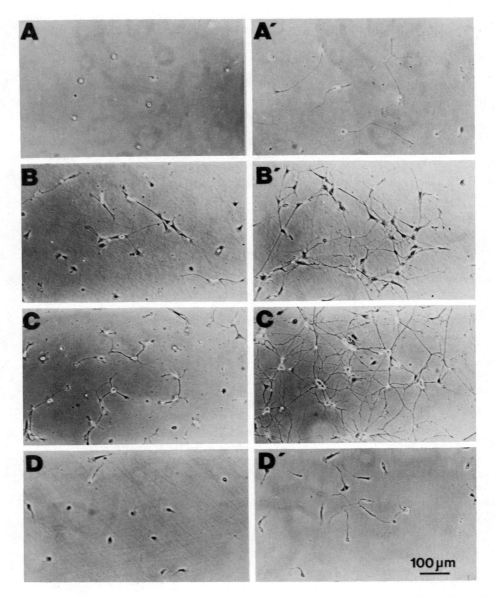

Fig. 6.   Effects of polyornithine-binding neurite promoting factors
(PNPFs) on neuritic growth.   Left panels = untreated polyornithine.
Right panels = polyornithine with PNPF from schwannoma conditioned
medium.   A,A' = 8 day chick embryo ciliary ganglion.   B,B' = neonatal mouse DRG.   C,C' = 11 day chick embryo sympathetic ganglia.
D,D' = 4 day chick embryo lumbar cord.   Cultures (24 hr) in serum-
supplemented medium containing the appropriate neuronotrophic
factors.

PORN, but both the number of neurite-bearing cells and the length of neuritic outgrowth are dramatically enhanced by PNPF. It is yet to be determined whether the modest neuritic growth in the absence of exogenously supplied PNPF may not be due to some PNPF contributed directly by these ganglionic dissociates. Finally, all cell cultures examined from central neural tissues (both avian and rodent), with one exception, displayed similar neuritic growth in the absence or presence of PNPF. Such a lack of sensitivity to, as well as dependence from, exogenous PNPF may signify truly different properties of central neurites or, more likely, also reflect the indigenous availability of PNPF (or a "central" PNPF) from within the culture themselves. The one exception observed in those studies was the culture of spinal cells from 8 day chick embryos, where some 6% of the neurons displayed very long neurites only if the polyornithine had been pretreated with PNPF. When spinal cultures were prepared from embryos only 4 day old (Longo et al., 1981), the proportion of neurons displaying neurites exclusively on PNPF-treated polyornithine rose to 60% (see Fig. 6, bottom panels). These cultures are presumably much enriched in motor neurons.

Altogether, the available information on PNPFs has encouraged the following speculations (Adler & Varon 1981 a,b; Varon & Adler 1980, 1981): (1) PNPFs are surface constituents of cells (including glial ones) normally encountered by neurites growing outside the central nervous system, regardless of the location of the neuronal somata; (2) these constituents, or fragments thereof, are released by the cells in culture and can re-anchor to polycationic surfaces so as to keep their active sites exposed; (3) neuritic growth cones recognize, in vivo or in vitro, the PNPF active sites as promoting or permitting neuritic growth; (4) the same surface materials may play a role in neuritic guidance, if they are temporally or spacially restricted to particular domains--in accordance with the guidance role often attributed to Schwann cells during nerve regeneration (cf. Varon & Manthorpe 1982).

ACKNOWLEDGEMENTS

This work has been supported by NINCDS grant NS-16349 and by a grant from the Muscular Dystrophy Association. We are especially grateful to Ms. Marilee Bateman whose patience and skill are responsible for the existence of this typescript.

REFERENCES

Adler, R. & Varon, S., 1980. Cholinergic neuronotrophic factors:
V. Segregation of survival- and neurite-promoting activities in
heart conditioned media. Brain Res. 188: 437-448.

Adler, R. & Varon, S., 1981a. Neuritic guidance by polyornithine-
attached materials of ganglionic origin. Dev. Biol. 81: 1-11.

Adler, R. & Varon, S., 1981b. Neuritic guidance by nonneuronal
cells of ganglionic origin. Dev. Biol. 85: in press.

Adler, R., Manthorpe, M. and Varon,S.,1979. Separation of neuronal
and nonneuronal cells in monolayer cultures from chick embryo optic
lobe. Dev. Biol. 69: 424-435.

Adler, R., Manthorpe, M., Skaper, S.D. and Varon, S., 1981a. Poly-
ornithine-attached neurite-promoting factors (PNPFs): Culture
sources and responsive neurons. Brain Res. 206: 129-144.

Adler, R., Manthorpe, M. and Varon, S., 1981b. Lectin affinities of
PNPF, a polyornithine-binding neurite promoting factor. Soc.
Neurosci. Abstr. 7: in press.

Aguayo, A., Charron, L. and Bray, G., 1976a. Potential of Schwann
cells from unmyelinated nerves to produce myelin: a quantitative
ultrastructural and radiographic study. J. Neurocytol. 5: 565-573.

Aguayo, A., Epps, J., Charron, L. and Bray, G., 1976b. Multipoten-
tiality of Schwann cells in cross-anastomosed and grafted myelinated and unmyelinated nerves: quantitative microscopy and radioautography. Brain Res. 104: 1-20.

Aguayo, A., Bray, G. and Perkins, S., 1979. Axon-Schwann cell
relationships in neuropathies of mutant mice. Ann. New York Acad.
Sci. 317: 512-531.

Asbury, A.K. & Johnson, P.C., 1978. 'Pathology of Peripheral Nerve'
W.B. Sanders Co., Philadelphia.

Barde, Y.-H., Edgar, D. and Thoenen, H., 1980. Sensory neurons in
culture: Changing requirements for survival factors during embryonic development. Proc. Natl. Acad. Sci. USA 77: 1199-1203.

Bottenstein, J.E. & Sato, G., 1979. Growth of a rat neuroblastoma
cell line in serum-free supplemented medium. Proc. Natl. Acad.
Sci. USA 76: 514-517.

Bottenstein, J.E., Skaper, S.D., Varon, S. and Sato, G., 1980.
Selective survival of neurons from chick embryo sensory ganglionic

dissociates by use of a defined, serum-free medium. Exp. Cell. Res. 125: 183-190.

Bowery, N.G., Brown, D.A., White, R.D. and Yamini, G., 1979. [^{3}H]-γ Aminobutyric acid uptake into neuroglial cells of rat superior cervical sympathetic ganglia. J. Physiol. 293: 51-74.

Brockes, J.P., Fields, K.L. and Raff, M.C., 1977. A surface anti-genic marker for rat Schwann cells. Nature 266: 364-366.

Brockes, J.P., Fields, K.L. and Raff, M.C., 1979. Studies on cul-tured rat Schwann cells. I. Establishment of purified populations from cultures of peripheral nerve. Brain Res. 165: 105-118.

Brockes, J.P., Raff, M.C., Nishiguchi, D.J. and Winter, J., 1980a. Studies on cultured rat Schwann cells. III. Assays for peripheral myelin proteins. J. Neurocytol. 9: 67-78.

Brockes, J.P., Lemke, G.E. and Balzer, D.R., 1980b. Purification and preliminary characterization of a glial growth factor from the bovine pituitary. J. Biol. Chem. 255: 8374-8377.

Bunge, R.P., 1970, in 'The Neurosciences: Second Study Program' (F.O. Schmitt, ed.) pp. 782-797, Rockefeller University Press, New York.

Bunge, R.P. & Bunge, M.B., 1978. Evidence that contact with con-nective tissue matrix is required for normal interaction between Schwann cells and nerve fibers. J. Cell Biol. 78: 943-950.

Bunge, M.B., Williams, A.K., Wood, P.M., Uitto, J. and Jeffrey, J.J., 1980. Comparison of nerve cell and nerve plus Schwann cell cultures, with particular emphasis on basal lamina and collagen formation. J. Cell Biol. 84: 184-202.

Burnham, P., Raiborn, C. and Varon, S., 1972. Replacement of Nerve Growth Factor by ganglionic non-neuronal cells for the survival in vitro of dissociated ganglionic neurons. Proc. Natl. Acad. Sci. USA 69: 3556-3560.

Collins, F., 1978. Induction of neurite outgrowth by a conditioned medium factor bound to culture substratum. Proc. Natl. Acad. Sci. USA 75: 5210-5213.

DeVries, G.H., Salzer, J.L. and Bunge, R.P., 1980. Stimulation of Schwann cell proliferation by axolemma-enriched fractions. Trans. Am. Soc. Neurochem. 11: 111.

Edgar, D., Barde, Y.-A. and Thoenen, H., 1981. in 'Development of the Autonomic Nervous System' (R.D.G. Milner and G. Burnstock, eds.)

CIBA Found. Symp. #83, in press.

Fedoroff, S. & Hertz, L. (eds.), 1977. 'Cell, Tissue, and Organ Cultures in Neurobiology', Academic Press, New York.

Fields, K.L., Brockes, J.P., Mirsky, R. and Wendon, L.M.B., 1978. Cell surface markers for distinguishing different types of rat dorsal root ganglion cells in culture. Cell 14: 43-51.

Giacobini, E., Vernadakis, A. and Shahar, A. (eds.), 1980. 'Tissue Culture in Neurobiology', Raven Press, New York.

Greene, L.A. & Shooter, E.M., 1980. The Nerve Growth Factor: Biochemistry, synthesis and mechanism of action. Ann. Rev. Neurosci. 3: 352-402.

Helfand, S.L., Smith, G. and Wessells, N., 1976. Survival and development in culture of dissociated parasympathetic neurons from ciliary ganglia. Dev. Biol. 50: 541-547.

Helfand, S.L., Riopelle, R.J. and Wessells, N.K., 1978. Non-equivalence of conditioned medium and Nerve Growth Factor for sympathetic, parasympathetic, and sensory neurons. Exp. Cell. Res. 113: 39-45.

Hertz, L., 1977. in 'Cell, Tissue and Organ Cultures in Neurobiology' (S. Fedoroff and L. Hertz, eds.), pp. 39-71, Academic Press, New York.

Hyndman, A.G. & Adler, R., 1981. Neural retina development in vitro: Effects of tissue extracts on cell survival and neuritic development in purified neuronal cultures. Dev. Neurosci.: in press.

Krikorian, D., Manthorpe, M. and Varon, S., 1981. Purified mouse Schwann cells: Mitogenic effects of fetal calf serum and fibroblast growth factor. Dev. Neurosci.: in press.

Levi-Montalcini, R. & Angeletti, P., 1968. Nerve Growth Factor. Physiol. Rev. 48: 534-569.

Lim, R., Mitsunobo, K. and Li, W. K-P., 1973. Maturation-stimulating effect of brain extract and dibutyryl cyclic AMP on dissociated embryonic brain cells in culture. Exp. Cell Res. 79: 243-246.

Lisak, R.P., Pruss, R.M., Kennedy, P.G.E., Abramsky, O., Pleasure, D.E. and Silberberg, D.H., 1980. Antisera to bovine oligodendroglia raised in guinea pigs bind to surface of rat oligodendroglia and Schwann cells. Neurosci. Lett. 17: 119-124.

Longo, F.M., Manthorpe, M. and Varon, S., 1981. Spinal cord neuron-otrophic factors (SCNTFs): I. Bioassay of Schwannoma and other conditioned media. Dev. Brain Res.: in press.

Longo, F.M., Lundborg, G., Manthorpe, M., Skaper, S.D. and Varon, S., 1982. Neuronotrophic activities in fluid collected in vivo from nerve regeneration model chambers. Submitted.

Lundborg, G., Longo, F.M. and Varon, S., 1981. Nerve regeneration and the production of neuronotrophic factors in vivo. Submitted.

Manthorpe, M., Adler, R. and Varon, S., 1979. Development, re-activity and GFA immunofluorescence of astroglia-containing mono-layer cultures from rat cerebrum. J. Neurocytol. 8: 605-621.

Manthorpe, M., Skaper, S.D. and Varon, S., 1980a. Purification of mouse Schwann cells using neurite-induced proliferation in serum-free monolayer cultures. Brain Res. 196: 467-482.

Manthorpe, M., Skaper, S.D., Adler, R., Landa, K.B. and Varon, S., 1980b. Cholinergic neuronotrophic factors: IV. Fractionation properties of an extract from selected chick embryonic eye tissues. J. Neurochem. 34: 69-75.

Manthorpe, M., Varon, S. and Adler, R., 1981a. Neurite-promoting factor (NPF) in conditioned medium from RN22 schwannoma cultures: bioassay, fractionation and other properties. J. Neurochem. 37: in press.

Manthorpe, M., Skaper, S.D., Barbin, G. and Varon, S., 1981b. Ciliary neuronotrophic factors (CNTFs): Concurrent activities on certain nerve growth factor-responsive neurons. J. Neurochem.: in press.

McCarthy, K. & Partlow, L., 1976. Preparation of pure neuronal and non-neuronal cultures from embryonic chick sympathetic ganglia: a new method based on both differential cell adhesiveness and the formation of homotypic neuronal aggregates. Brain Res. 114: 391-414.

McCarthy, K. & DeVellis, J., 1980. Preparation of separate astro-glial and oligodendroglial cell cultures from rat cerebral tissues. J. Cell Biol. 85: 890-902.

Moonen, G., Heinen, E. and Goessens, G., 1976. Comparative ultra-structural study of the effects of serum-free medium and dibutyryl cyclic AMP on newborn rat astroblasts. Cell and Tissue Res. 167: 221-227.

Pannese, E., 1980. Satellite cells of the sensory ganglia. Adv. Anat. Embryol. and Cell Biol. 65: 1-100.

Perez-Polo, J.R., Hall, K., Livingston, K. and Westlund, K., 1977. Steroid induction of Nerve Growth Factor synthesis in cell culture. Life Sci. 21: 1535-1544.

Peterson, E.R. & Murray, M.F., 1955. Myelin sheath formation in cultures of avian spinal ganglia. Am. J. Anat. 96: 319-346.

Popiela, H., Manthorpe, M., Adler, R. and Varon, S., 1978. Choline acetyltransferase-promoting activity of medium exposed to skeletal muscle cell culture from chick embryo. Trans. Am. Soc. Neurochem. 9: 49.

Raff, M.C., Hornby-Smith, A. and Brockes, J.P., 1978a. Cyclic AMP as a mitogenic signal for cultured rat Schwann cells. Nature 273: 672-673.

Raff, M.C., Abney, E., Brockes, J.P. and Hornby-Smith, A., 1978b. Schwann cell growth factors. Cell 15: 813-822.

Romine, J.S., Aguayo, A.J. and Bray, G., 1975. Absence of Schwann cell migration along regenerating unmyelinated nerves. Brain Res. 98: 601-606.

Romine, J.S., Bray, G.M. and Aguayo, A.J., 1976. Schwann cell multiplication after crush injury of unmyelinated fibers. Arch. Neurol. 33: 49-54.

Salzer, J.L. & Bunge, R.P., 1980. Studies of Schwann cell proliferation during development, wallerian degeneration and direct injury. J. Cell Biol. 84: 739-752.

Salzer, J.L., Williams, A.K., Glaser, L. and Bunge, R.P., 1980a. Studies of Schwann cell proliferation. II. Characterization of the stimulation and specificity of the response to a neurite membrane fraction. J. Cell Biol. 84: 753-766.

Salzer, J.L., Bunge, R.P. and Glaser, L., 1980b. Studies of Schwann cell proliferation. III. Evidence for the surface localization of the neurite mitogen. J. Cell Biol. 84: 767-778.

Schon, F. & Kelly, J.S., 1974. Autoradiographic localization of [^{3}H]GABA and [^{3}H]glutamate over satellite glial cells. Brain Res. 66: 275-288.

Schwartz, J.P., Chuang, D.N. and Costa, E., 1977. Increase in Nerve Growth Factor content of C6 glioma cells by the addition of a beta-adrenergic receptor. Brain Res. 137: 369-375.

Sensenbrenner, M., 1977, in 'Cell, Tissue and Organ Cultures in Neurobiology' (S. Fedoroff and L. Hertz, eds.), pp. 191-213, Academic Press, New York.

Skaper, S.D., Adler, R. and Varon, S., 1979. A procedure for purifying neuron-like cells in cultures from central nervous tissues with a defined medium. Dev. Neurosci. 2: 233-237.

Skaper, S.D., Manthorpe, M., Adler, R. and Varon, S., 1980. Survival, proliferation and morphological specialization of mouse Schwann cells in a serum-free, fully defined medium. J. Neurocytol. 9: 683-697.

Varon, S., 1975a. Nerve Growth Factor and its mode of action. Exp. Neurol. 48(#3, part 2): 75-92.

Varon, S., 1975b. Neurons and glia in neural cultures. Exp. Neurol. 48(#3, part 2): 93-134.

Varon, S., 1977, in 'Cell, Tissue and Organ Cultures in Neurobiology' (S. Fedoroff and L. Hertz, eds.), pp. 237-261, Academic Press, New York.

Varon, S. & Adler, R., 1980. Nerve growth factors and control of nerve growth. Curr. Topics Dev. Biol. 16: 207-252.

Varon, S. & Adler, R., 1981. Trophic and specifying factors directed to neuronal cells. Adv. Cell Neurobiol. 2: 115-163.

Varon, S. & Bunge, R.P., 1978. Trophic mechanisms in the peripheral nervous system. Ann. Rev. Neurosci. 1: 327-361.

Varon, S. & Manthorpe, M., 1980. Separation of neurons and glial cells by affinity methods. Adv. Cell Neurobiol. 1: 405-442.

Varon, S. & Manthorpe, M., 1981. Schwann cells: An in vitro perspective. Adv. Cell Neurobiol. 3: in press.

Varon, S. & Raiborn, C.W., 1969. Dissociation, fractionation and culture of embryonic brain cells. Brain Res. 12: 180-199.

Varon, S. & Raiborn, C.W., 1972. Dissociation, fractionation and culture of chick embryo sympathetic ganglionic cells. J. Neurocytol. 1: 211-221.

Varon, S. & Saier, M., 1975. Culture techniques and glial-neuronal interrelationships in vitro. Exp. Neurol. 48(#3, part 2): 135-162.

Varon, S. & Skaper, S.D., 1981, in 'Development of the autonomic nervous system' (R.D.G. Milner and G. Burnstock, eds.) CIBA Found.

Symp. #83: in press.

Varon, S. & Skaper, S.D., 1982, in 'Somatic and Autonomic Nerve-Muscle Interactions' (G. Burnstock, G. Urbova and R. O'Brien, eds.) Elsevier-North Holland, Amsterdam: in press.

Varon, S. & Somjen, G., 1979. Neuron-glia interactions. Neurosci. Res. Prog. Bull. 17: 1-239.

Varon, S., Raiborn, C.W. and Tyszka, E., 1973. In vitro studies of dissociated cells from newborn mouse dorsal root ganglia. Brain Res. 54: 51-63.

Varon, S., Manthorpe, M. and Adler, R., 1979. Cholinergic neurono-trophic factors: I. Survival, neurite outgrowth and choline acetyl-transferase activity in monolayer cultures from chick embryo ciliary ganglia. Brain Res. 173: 29-45.

Varon, S., Skaper, S.D. and Manthorpe, M., 1981. Trophic activities for dorsal root and sympathetic ganglionic neurons in media condi-tioned by Schwann and other peripheral cells. Dev. Brain Res. 1: 73-87.

Varon, S., Manthorpe, M. and Longo, F.M., 1982, in 'International Conference on Human Motor Neuron Diseases' (L.P. Rowland, ed.), Raven Press, New York: in press.

Webster, deF., 1974, in 'The Peripheral Nervous System' (J.I. Hubbard, ed.), pp. 3-26, Plenum Press, New York.

Wood, P.M., 1976. Separation of functional Schwann cells and neu-rons from normal peripheral nerve tissue. Brain Res. 115: 361-375.

Wood, P.M. & Bunge, R.P., 1975. Evidence that sensory axons are mitogenic for Schwann cells. Nature 256: 662-664.

PROLIFERATION AND MATURATION OF NEURONAL CELLS FROM THE CENTRAL

NERVOUS SYSTEM IN CULTURE

Monique Sensenbrenner, Ibtissam Barakat and Gérard
Labourdette

Centre de Neurochimie du C.N.R.S.
5, rue Blaise Pascal
67084 Strasbourg Cedex

INTRODUCTION

During embryogenesis the behaviour and the development of nerve
cells in its successive steps of neuronal and glial evolution are
influenced by the surrounding environment, cell contacts as well as
trophic factors (Sherbet and Lakshmi, 1974 ; Le Douarin et al., 1975 ;
England and Cowper, 1976 ; Toivonen et al., 1976 ; Noden, 1978 ;
Cochard et al., 1979). The use of dissociated nerve cells in culture
has facilitated investigations of the influence of growth factors on
the development of these cells (Varon et al., 1973 ; De Vellis et al.,
1977 ; Greene, 1977a, 1977b ; Lim et al., 1977 ; Sensenbrenner,
1977 ; Hanson and Partlow, 1978 ; Patterson, 1978 ; Prochiantz et al.,
1979 ; Sensenbrenner et al., 1980a ; Thoenen and Barde, 1980).

In our laboratory studies have been undertaken to detect and
identify stimulatory factors present in brain extracts. It has been
found that several brain extracts can stimulate the maturation of
nerve cells in culture (Sensenbrenner et al., 1972 ; Athias et al.,
1974 ; Sensenbrenner, 1977 ; Pettmann et al., 1980a, 1980b ;
Sensenbrenner et al., 1980a ; Pettmann et al., 1981). Until now
neurotrophic factors, endogenous to the nervous system and which may
control neuronal cell proliferation in the early embryonic central
nervous system, are not known. Therefore, a research was started with
the view to determine factors, present in brain extracts, which might
be involved in controlling the proliferation of neuroblasts (morphologically undifferentiated neuronal cells). Such a study could be
achieved by stimulating mitoses when neuronal cells are still capable

497

of dividing. We have previously shown that neuroblasts from dissociated cerebral hemispheres of young chick embryo (3 to 7 day-old)
can undergo division when put in culture (Sensenbrenner et al.,
1980b ; Barakat et al., in press). Therefore, such cultures can be
considered as an adequate system to investigate the influence of
factors on the proliferation of neuroblasts and the effects of brain
extracts on the proliferative activity as well as on the maturation
of neuronal cells in culture will be herein reviewed.

PROLIFERATION OF NERVE CELLS FROM CEREBRAL HEMISPHERES OF CHICK
EMBRYOS CULTURED IN STANDARD NUTRIENT MEDIUM

     Incorporation of radioactive thymidine combined with autoradio-
graphic methods was used to analyse the proliferative activity of
cultured nerve cells. Cerebral hemispheres from 5, 6 and 7-day old
chick embryos were dissected and mechanically dissociated. The
dissociated cells were collected in nutrient medium (Eagle's minimum
essential medium with 20 % fetal calf serum) and grown in Falcon
plastic petri dishes on a collagen substrate. The cultures were incubated for 24 h with [^{14}C]thymidine (0.1 µCi/ml ; sp. activ. 33 mCi/
mole) or [^{3}H]thymidine (0.5-1 µCi/ml ; sp. activ. 26 Ci/mmole),
washed and supplied with fresh medium without labeled thymidine.
Radioactive thymidine have been given at different time intervals
from 0 to 7 days and the cultures were fixed after 4, 7 or 14 days,
then submitted to the autoradiographic method (Sensenbrenner et al.,
1980b). The neuronal cells were visualized by toluidine blue staining.

     Many neuronal cells were labeled in cultures from 5 to 6 day-
old embryos treated with [^{3}H]thymidine during the first 3 days of
culture (Fig. 1). In contrast, very few flat polygonal astroblasts
had incorporated [^{3}H]thymidine. Conversely in the cultures treated
with radioactive thymidine after 4 days fewer neurons were labeled,
while many astroblasts presented a labeling. In the cultures derived
from 7 day-old embryos and incubated with radioactive thymidine
during the first 48 h many neuronal cells and all astroglial cells
were labeled. When the radioactive precursor was added to the culture
medium between 2 and 4 days or between 7 and 8 days only few or no
neurons respectively incorporated thymidine.

     These observations indicated that in nerve cell cultures from
5 and 6 day-old chick embryos many neuronal precursors (neuroblasts)
were capable of proliferation until the 4th day. Later neuronal proliferating activity slowed down, while astroblasts started to multiply
after the third day. In the 7 day-old embryo cultures, the astroblasts
divided actively as soon as the cells were in the culture medium,
while most neuroblasts had stopped dividing after 2 days. From these
findings it appears that the culture of dissociated brain cells from
5-6 day-old chick embryos is a good model system to study neuronal
proliferation.

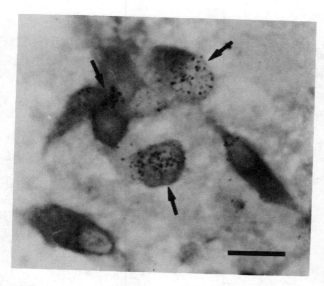

Fig. 1. Autoradiograph of dissociated brain cells from 6 day-old chick embryo in culture (14 days) after [^{3}H]thymidine incorporation (label was given between 24 and 48 h of culture). Toluidine blue stain. Bar = 20 μm. Note the presence of labeled neuronal cells (arrows).

INFLUENCE OF BRAIN EXTRACTS ON THE PROLIFERATION OF NEUROBLASTS FROM CHICK EMBRYO

The effects of brain extracts from chick embryos, chicken as well as from fish, rat and beef on the proliferative activity of neuroblasts from cerebral hemispheres of 6 day-old chick embryo have been studied. The dissociated nerve cells were cultured on a collagen substrate in standard nutrient medium either in absence or in presence of brain extracts. The extracts were prepared by hand homogenizing the whole brain in Tyrode solution (200 mg fresh weight/ml). After centrifugation of the homogenate at 105,000 g for 1 h, the supernatant was sterilized by filtration and added to the nutrient medium in a proportion of 1 ml/10 ml (Barakat and Sensenbrenner, 1981).

Morphological observations have shown the formation of small and medium sized clumps of young neuroblasts when cultured in standard nutrient medium (Fig. 2a) or in the presence of brain extracts from 12 and 15 day-old chick embryos. In the presence of brain extract from fish no cellular clusters were formed and the cells quickly degenerated. After addition of brain extracts from 8 day-old chick embryo, chicken, rat and beef, the number of clusters remained constant if compared to control cultures and moreover predominantly large cellular aggregates were observed (Fig. 2b). The cells forming the aggregates were identified as neurons by thionine

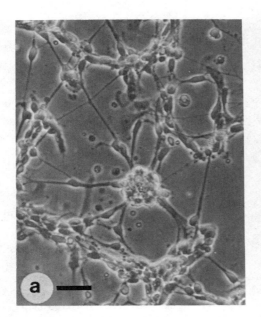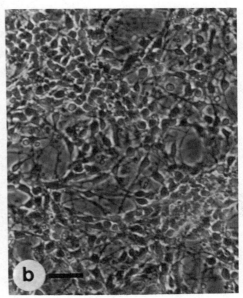

Fig. 2. Phase contrast micrographs of dissociated brain cells from
6 day-old chick embryo after 3 days in culture. 2a : Control
culture in standard nutrient medium ; 2b : Culture treated
with brain extract from 8 day-old chick embryo. Bar = 50 µm.

staining, by histochemical demonstration of acetylcholinesterase
(AChE) activity according to the method of Karnovsky and Roots (1964)
(Fig. 3) and by immunohistochemical presence of the neuronal specific
membrane protein D2 (Bock et al., 1980) (Fig. 4).

The proliferation of the neuroblasts was characterized by determination of DNA content, quantitative evaluation of the neuronal
cells, measurement of [^{3}H]thymidine incorporation into DNA and autoradiographic analysis. For these studies the cultures were used over
a short time period of 6 days, when they were mainly constituted of
neuronal cells, before the occurence of extensive growth of non-
neuronal elements.

Under standard culture conditions the amount of DNA per culture
dish increased regularly for 6 days from a value of 16.1 ± 2.0 to
a value of 29.9 ± 2.7 µg DNA. In the presence of brain extract from
8 day-old chick embryo the DNA level increased throughout the entire
culture period studied from a value of 18.12 ± 1.2 to a value of
33.3 ± 3.2 µg DNA per dish with a rapid phase between 2 and 3 days.
In treated cultures the DNA content was significantly higher between
2 and 5 days compared to those of control cultures.

Quantitative evaluation of the neuronal cells was made on

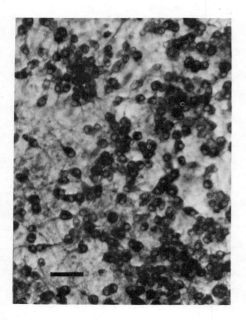

Fig. 3. Dissociated brain cells
from 6 day-old chick embryo
after 5 days in culture in
presence of brain extract
from 8 day-old chick embryo
and stained for AChE activity. Bar = 50 μm.

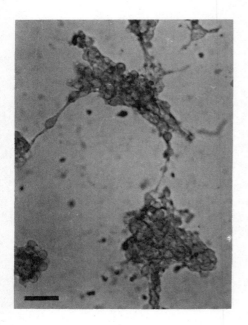

Fig. 4. Dissociated brain cells
from 6 day-old chick
embryo after 2 days in
culture in presence of
brain extract from 8 day-
old chick embryo. Immuno-
peroxidase technique using
an anti-D2 serum. Note the
presence of many stained
cells. The antiserum is
bound to the neuronal cell
bodies as well as on the
fibers. Bar = 50 μm.

preparations stained for AChE activity after 5 days of culture. It
has been demonstrated that in cultures from cerebral hemispheres of
chick embryos, all neurons contain an AChE activity, while glial cells
lack this enzyme activity (Sensenbrenner et al., 1972, 1973). In
the presence of brain extract from 8 day-old chick embryo more neuronal cells (257.7 ± 5.6 cells per sq. mm of the culture dish) were
present compared to control cultures (141.3 ± 4.0 cells).

Incorporation of [^{3}H]thymidine in dissociated brain cells was
measured after various periods of culture either in the absence or
in the presence of brain extracts from chick embryos, chicken, rat
(Fig. 5) or beef. Analysis of the labeled macromolecules was carried
out using a filter disc technique and scintillation counting
(Barakat and Sensenbrenner, 1981). In control cultures the incorporation of [^{3}H]thymidine was shown to decrease between 2 and 3 days,
i.e. when the cultures were mainly constituted of neuronal cells and
therefore indicating a decrease of proliferative activity of neuroblasts. Afterwards, when cellular aggregates had increased in size
and glial elements had appeared the thymidine incorporation increased.
In cultures treated by brain extracts from 8 day chick embryos incorporation of the thymidine was, at all times, significantly higher
than in the control cultures. Brain extracts from 12 and 15 day

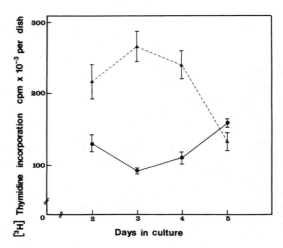

Fig. 5. [^{3}H]Thymidine incorporation by cultured brain cells from 6
         day-old chick embryo. Cultures in standard nutrient medium
         (●——●) and in presence of brain extract from adult rat
         (▲---▲). [^{3}H]Thymidine (0.5 μCi/ml) was added to each culture
         at different culture time after plating and cultures were
         harvested 24 h later. Results are expressed as the mean of
         4 determinations ± S.D.

chick embryos had a stimulatory effect on young cultures (1 to 3 days) and no effect on older cultures. This stimulatory effect was lower than that obtained with brain extract from 8 day-old embryo (Barakat and Sensenbrenner, 1981). On the other hand, brain extracts from chicken, rat (Fig. 5) and beef produced a very strong stimulatory effect, which was more effective between the 2nd and 4th day. This period correspond to intense neuroblast proliferation. Afterwards, when glial cells had appeared the thymidine incorporation declined.

Finally autoradiographic analysis after [^{3}H]thymidine incorporation were performed to evaluate the proportion of proliferating cells. The pulses (2 h exposure) of thymidine (2 µCi/ml) were given at different time intervals from 1 to 6 days. The cultures were fixed immediately after the exposure time and the autoradiographic preparations were stained with toluidine blue. The labeled and unlabeled cells were counted. Table 1 shows that in the presence of brain extracts more cells had incorporated the radioactive label.

However, from the autoradiographic data alone it was difficult to state that synthesis of DNA was always followed by cell division since some of the cultured cells might become polyploid. Therefore, cytophotometric measurements of DNA content of cells grown for 4 days in standard nutrient medium and in the presence of brain extract from 8 day-old chick embryo were undertaken. The results indicated that cultured neuronal cells from cerebral hemispheres are diploid and are capable of synthesizing DNA before undergoing mitotic division (Barakat and Sensenbrenner, 1981).

These observations indicate that the proliferative activity of neuroblasts from young chick embryos is stimulated by some components present in embryonic and adult brain extracts. Moreover it is possible to suggest that soluble factors present in the brain may contribute to the control of neuronal growth.

Several authors have found mitogenic activity in extracts of central nervous tissues for a number of cultured cell types (fibroblasts, endothelial cells, myoblasts and glial cells) (Gospodarowicz et al., 1975 ; Lim et al., 1977 ; Jabaily and Singer, 1978 ; Jennings et al., 1979 ; Maciag et al., 1979). Our study demonstrates the presence in brain of factors which are mitogenic for neuroblasts.

PURIFICATION OF THE ACTIVE FACTORS AFFECTING THE PROLIFERATION OF NEUROBLASTS IN CULTURE

Soluble beef brain extracts enhance the proliferation of chick embryo neuroblasts in culture. Since large quantities of beef brain are easily available we decided to purify the mitogenic factors from this material.

Table 1. Total numbers of neural cells in cultures from 5 day-old chick embryo and numbers incorporating [3H]thymidine

Culture	Age days	Neural cells (neuroblasts and glioblasts)		
		Total	Labeled	% Labeled
C	1	2905	365	12.5
E		3406	424	12.4
C	2	2351	206	8.7
E		1284	120	9.3
C	4	1849	144	7.7
E		2122	171	8.0
C	5	2547	202	7.9
E		1517	146	9.6
C	6	1922	175	9.1
E		2263	258	11.4

The neural cells were grown either in standard medium alone (C = control culture) or supplemented with brain extract from 8 day-old chick embryo 24 h after plating (E = experimental culture). [3H]Thymidine (2 μCi/ml) was added at different time of culture ; cultures were exposed to label for 2 h, fixed and processed for autoradiography.

The first step of the purification was the homogenization of the beef brains in chloroform-methanol, filtration and acetone-drying of the crude brain extract. The powder was then extracted several times with Tris-buffer. The supernatant obtained after centrifugation was submitted to DEAE-cellulose column chromatography. The mitogenic activity was retained. A first active fraction was eluted at about 0.12 M NaCl (Fig. 6). A second active fraction was eluted from a concentration of 0.3 M NaCl.

The activity of the crude extract and of the different fractions was determined by incorporation of [^{3}H]thymidine in 2 and 3 day-old cultures of neuroblasts. In these experiments the Eagle's minimum essential medium was supplemented by 5 % fetal calf serum. This

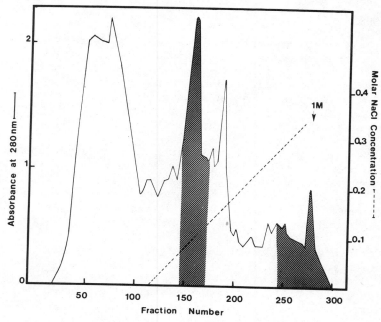

Fig. 6. DEAE cellulose chromatography of soluble brain extract. One hundred g of chloroform-methanol powder from 1 kg of beef brain were extracted 3 times for 12 h with 50 mM Tris-HCl, pH 8.0. About 1 liter of extract was applied onto the column (4.3 x 40 cm). This was washed with 800 ml of buffer and retained material was eluted with 2.6 liters of a linear gradient of NaCl from 0 to 0.35 M in the buffer. Subsequently the column was washed with 1 M NaCl, the last peak was thus eluted. Fractions were analyzed for their activity to stimulate neuroblasts proliferation in culture. The hatched areas represent the active fractions.

particular concentration of serum was chosen to provide optimal cell
proliferation in the neural cell cultures.

Our results showed that beef brain extract contains at least
two stimulatory fractions which enhance the proliferation of chick
embryo neuronal cells.

EFFECTS OF BRAIN EXTRACTS ON THE MATURATION OF NEURONAL CELLS IN
CULTURE

The data presented above show that proliferation of neuroblasts
from cerebral hemispheres of 6 day-old chick embryo was stimulated
during the first week of culture under the influence of various
embryonic and adult brain extracts. The behavioral aspects of these
neuronal cells over a period of 3 to 4 weeks were then investigated
and the effects of brain extracts on the maturation of these cells
were extended.

Morphological observations have shown that after 7 days of
culture in standard nutrient conditions many spindle-shaped neurons
developed and formed interconnections. Between the first and the
second week many nerve fibers were organized in bundles, forming an
interlacing network between isolated cells and cell clusters. After
14 days mature bipolar and multipolar neuronal cells were observed
upon a layer of flat polygonal glial cells (Fig. 7a).

In the presence of a brain extract from 8 day-old chick embryo
at 2 weeks the cell bodies of neuronal cells were larger, the nerve
fibers appeared to be thicker and more ramified than in control
cultures (Fig. 7b). Between 2 and 3 weeks large bipolar and multipolar neurons differentiated. Brain extracts from older chick embryos,
chicken, rat and beef produced similar effects.

After one week in culture some neuronal cells were already
degenerating in control as well as in treated cultures. Between the
second and the third week there was a significant cell decrease in
these dissociated cell cultures. However, in the presence of the
brain extract there were always more neuronal cells present, even
after 3 weeks, when compared to untreated cultures.

These observations lead to the conclusion that brain extracts
enhance the morphological maturation of neuronal cells and also have
an influence on the survival of differentiated neurons during longer
periods of culture. We have previously reported similar observations
on cultured nerve cells from 5 and 7 day-old chick embryos using
brain extracts from chick embryos as well as from new-born rats
(Sensenbrenner et al., 1972 ; Athias et al., 1974).

In 6 day-old chick embryo cultures brain extracts were shown
to stimulate the proliferation of neuroblasts (see section on
neuroblast proliferation). During their subsequent stages of

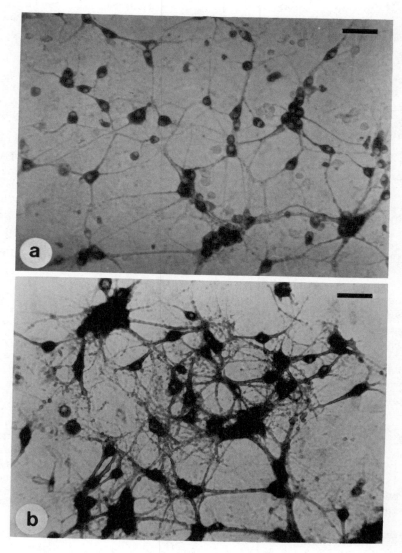

Fig. 7. Dissociated brain cells from 6 day-old chick embryo after 14 days in culture and stained for AChE activity. 7a : Control culture in standard nutrient medium ; 7b : Culture treated with brain extract from 8 day-old chick embryo. Bar = 50 μm.

development the biochemical maturation of these cells might be
influenced by the surrounding environment and, in particular, the
presence of (a) brain extracts might direct the neuroblasts to
develop into specific neuronal types. In order to follow the development of neurons measurement of transmitter-synthesizing enzyme activities in neuronal cell cultures might provide useful information.

In this study choline acetyltransferase (CAT ; EC 2.3.1.6) and
acetylcholinesterase (AChE ; EC 3.1.1.7) activities were measured in
neural cell cultures in the presence and in the absence of brain
extracts over a period of 3 weeks. A measurable AChE activity was
already detected after 2 days of culture, while CAT activity became
measurable after 4 days.

It is generally admitted that CAT is a specific marker for
cholinergic neurons and any change in the activity of this enzyme
during the evolution of the culture might give information about the
growth and maturation of cholinergic neurons. In contrast, AChE
activity can be considered in our culture system as a general neuronal marker. Histochemical staining of AChE activity have indeed
demonstrated the localization of this enzyme in all cultured neuronal cells from cerebral hemispheres of chick embryos (Sensenbrenner
et al., 1972, 1973).

The results (Table 2) showed in control cultures a progressive
increase of AChE activities per culture during the first 10 days
and then a continuing decline. The increase of AChE activity can be
explained as due to proliferation of the neuroblasts as well as to
neuronal maturation. The subsequent gradual decrease in AChE activity
can be ascribed to the partial degeneration and death of neuronal
cells which occured after 10 days in culture.

In the presence of a brain extract from 8 day-old chick embryo
the enzymatic activities were higher throughout the entire culture
period compared to the controls indicating the presence of more
neuronal cells and/or of more differentiated cells under these
conditions. A rapid increase in enzyme activities observed between
3 and 4 days may reflect the sharp rise in the number of neuroblasts
which occured during this period as pointed out in the section on
neuroblast proliferation.

The activity of CAT per culture remained low and relatively
constant in control cultures during the period under study (Table 2).
This may indicate that in dissociated cell cultures from 6 day-old
chick embryo cerebral hemispheres only few neurons acquire the
enzymatic equipment to synthesize acetylcholine.

In previous investigations (Werner et al., 1971) and in our
laboratory (Ebel et al., 1974 ; Pettmann, 1979) it was shown that

Table 2. Acetylcholinesterase and choline acetyltransferase activities in brain cell cultures

Ages (days)	AChE μmoles ACh hydrol./h/culture		CAT nmoles ACh synth./h/culture	
	Control culture	Culture treated with brain extract	Control culture	Culture treated with brain extract
2	0.59 ± 0.12	0.78 ± 0.08		
3	0.91 ± 0.16	1.25 ± 0.08		
4	1.59 ± 0.45	2.85 ± 0.14	1.43 ± 0.16	1.34 ± 0.08
5	1.54 ± 0.33	2.32 ± 0.63		
6	1.82 ± 0.48	2.46 ± 0.56		
7	1.72 ± 0.23	2.35 ± 0.28	1.36 ± 0.22	1.79 ± 0.16
10	1.94 ± 0.40	2.66 ± 0.13	1.56 ± 0.1	3.0 ± 0.06
14	1.45 ± 0.19	2.26 ± 0.04	1.37 ± 0.05	2.19 ± 0.13
18	1.06 ± 0.09	1.7 ± 0.24	1.51 ± 0.33	2.23 ± 0.06
21	1.15 ± 0.06	1.39 ± 0.15	1.43 ± 0.32	1.77 ± 0.14

Cells dissociated from cerebral hemispheres from 6 day-old chick embryo were cultured in absence or in presence of brain extract from 8 day-old chick embryo in 60 mm diameter Falcon petri dishes. The data are means of 3 or 6 cultures ± S.D.

neuronal cells from older chick embryos (7 and 12 day embryos) developed cholinergic properties when cultured under conditions similar
to those described in the present study and suitable for glial cell
proliferation. However, in cell cultures from 7 day or older chick
embryos the glial cells divided actively as soon as the cells were
in the culture medium, while in the cultures from 5 and 6 day embryos
the glial cells started to multiply only after the third day
(Sensenbrenner et al., 1980b). That the presence of glial cells
might stimulate neuronal chick embryo cells to develop CAT activity
has already been suggested (Werner et al., 1971 ; Pettmann, 1979 ;
Louis et al., 1981).

    The importance of interactions between neurons and glial or
other non-neuronal cells as well as of the influence of conditioned
media to induce transmitter-synthesizing enzymes in neurons has been
recently reported (Le Douarin et al., 1978 ; Patterson, 1978 ;
Heumann et al., 1979 ; Bird, 1980). In the present study, the values
of CAT activity were always higher after incubation with brain extract
for 7 days than in controls. The low activity at 4 days, increased
rapidly to reach a peak at 10 days and then declined until 21 days
(Table 2). The sharp increase of CAT activity from 4 to 10 days immediately followed a period of massive proliferation of neuroblasts
(see section above) and may indicate the development and maturation
of cholinergic neurons under this culture condition. A stimulation of
CAT activity by brain extracts in cultured neural cells has already
been briefly described (Pettmann, 1979 ; Cam et al., 1980). The
marked decrease of CAT activity from day 10 to 21 may reflect a
degeneration of cholinergic neurons in this culture system.

    In order to define the presence of other specialized neurons in
the dissociated neural cell cultures from cerebral hemispheres of
6 day-old chick embryo, catecholaminergic neurons were visualized
by the histofluorescence technique of Lindvall and Björklund (1974).
After 2 and 3 weeks in culture most of the cells exhibited very bright
fluorescence. Furthermore, using electron microscopy, most cells
were found to contain dense-cored vesicles. These granule-containing
cells were considered as electron microscopic equivalent of the
brightly fluorescent cells. Similar observations have been previously
reported in our laboratory for mixed cultures of neuronal and glial
cells from 7 and 12 day-old chick embryos (Bastien-Miehe, 1977).
These data actually showed that the majority of the neurons from
chick embryo cerebral hemispheres grown in dissociated cultures and
which survive in long-term culture were aminergic-containing neurons.
Recently, Louis et al. (1981) have reported that neurons cultured in
the absence of glial cells acquired essentially dopaminergic properties during their development.

    At this stage of our investigations further quantitative evalua-
tions of neurotransmitter-synthesizing enzyme activities are required
to provide evidence of development of specific neurons under the

influence of brain extract in dissociated neural cell cultures.

CONCLUSION

We have demonstrated that neuroblasts from cerebral hemispheres of 6 day-old chick embryos undergo multiplication in standard nutrient medium during the first week in culture. Under the influence of various brain extracts the proliferation of these nueroblasts was enhanced. Two active fractions with itogenic activity were isolated from a beef brain extract. Furthermore, brain extracts were shown to stimulate the morphological maturation of the neuronal elements over a period of 3 to 4 weeks. The biochemical maturation of these neurons was also enhanced by brain extracts and a substantial elevation of CAT activity occured between 4 and 10 days in culture. This phenomenon might be due to the rise in the number of differentiating cholinergic cells. After 10 days CAT activity started to decline and became very low at 21 days, at which time most neuronal cells present contained dense-cored vesicles. These observations may indicate that cholinergic neurons degenerate in long term culture, while catecholaminergic neurons are able to survive. From the findings discussed in this paper it is possible to suggest that soluble factors present in the brain may contribute to the control of neuronal growth and maturation.

ACKNOWLEDGEMENTS

This research was supported by DGRST Grant n° 80.7.0349 and by a Grant from the Fondation pour la Recherche Médicale Française. The authors thank Dr. E. Bock for the gift of antisera-D_2 and Mrs. M.F. Knoetgen for her technical assistance. The authors are also grateful to Drs. R. Massarelli, B. Pettmann, R.V. Rechenmann and E. Wittendorp-Rechenmann for their collaboration.

REFERENCES

Athias, P., Sensenbrenner, M. and Mandel, P., 1974, The behaviour of dissociated chick embryo brain cells in long-term cultures in presence and absence of brain extracts, Differentiation, 2:99.

Barakat, I. and Sensenbrenner, M., 1981, Brain extracts that promote the proliferation of neuroblasts from chick embryo in culture, Dev. Brain Res., 1:355.

Barakat, I., Wittendorp-Rechenmann, E., Rechenmann, R.V. and Sensenbrenner, M., Influence of meningeal cells on the proliferation of neuroblasts in culture, Dev. Neurosci., in press.

Bastien-Miehe, M., 1977, Comportement in vitro de cellules dissociées provenant d'hémisphères cérébraux d'embryons de poulets, Thèse de Doctorat 3ème Cycle, Strasbourg.

Bird, M.M., 1980, The development and ultrastructure of previously dissociated embryonic chick corpus striatum cultured on feeder layers of liver cells, Anat. Embryol., 159:115.

Bock, E., Yavin, Z., Jørgensen, O.S. and Yavin, E., 1980, Nervous
    system-specific proteins in developing rat cerebral cells
    in culture, J. Neurochem., 35:1297.
Cam, Y., Ledig, M., Ebel, A., Sensenbrenner, M. and Mandel, P.,
    1980, Study of some enzyme activities in cultured chick
    embryo brain nerve cells treated by chick embryo brain
    extract, Neurochem. Res., 5:831.
Cochard, P., Goldstein, M. and Black, I.B., 1979, Initial develop-
    ment of the noradrenergic phenotype in autonomic neuroblasts
    of the rat embryo in vivo, Dev. Biol., 71:100.
De Vellis, J., Mc Ginnis, J.F., Breen, G.A.M., Leveille, P., Bennet,
    K. and Mc Carthy, K., 1977, Hormonal effects on differen-
    tiation in neural cultures, in "Cell, Tissue and Organ Cultu-
    res in Neurobiology", S. Fedoroff and L. Hertz, eds.,
    Academic Press, New York.
Ebel, A., Massarelli, R., Sensenbrenner, M. and Mandel, P., 1974,
    Choline acetyltransferase and acetylcholinesterase activities
    in chicken brain hemispheres in vivo and in cell culture,
    Brain Res., 76:461.
England, M.A. and Cowper, S.V., 1976, A transmission and scanning
    electron microscope study of primary neural induction,
    Experientia, 32:1578.
Gospodarowicz, D., Weseman, J. and Moran, J., 1975, Presence in brain
    of a mitogenic agent promoting proliferation of myoblasts in
    low density culture, Nature, 256:216.
Greene, L.A., 1977a, Quantitative in vitro studies on the Nerve
    Growth Factor (NGF) requirement of neurons. I. Sympathetic
    neurons, Dev. Biol., 58:96.
Greene, L.A., 1977b, Quantitative in vitro studies on the Nerve
    Growth Factor (NGF) requirement of neurons. II. Sensory
    neurons, Dev. Biol., 58:106.
Hanson, G.R. and Partlow, L.M., 1978, Stimulation of non-neuronal
    cell proliferation in vitro by mitogenic factors present in
    highly purified sympathetic neurons, Brain Res., 159:195.
Heumann, R., Öcalan, M. and Hamprecht, B., 1979, Factors from glial
    cells regulate choline acetyltransferase and tyrosine hydro-
    xylase activities in a hybrid-hybrid cell line, FEBS Letters,
    107:37.
Jabaily, J. and Singer, M., 1978, Neurotrophic and hepatotrophic
    stimulation of proliferation of embryonic chick muscle cells
    in vitro : assay and partial characterization of mitogenic
    activity in chick embryonic organ and tissue extracts,
    Dev. Biol., 64:189.
Jennings, T., Jones, D. and Lipton, A., 1979, A growth factor from
    spinal cord, J. Cell Physiol., 100:273.
Karnovsky, M.J. and Roots, L., 1964, A "direct-coloring" thiocholine
    method for cholinesterases, J. Histochem. Cytochem. 12:219.

Le Douarin, N.M., Renaud, D., Teillet, M.A. and Le Douarin, G.H., 1975, Cholinergic differentiation of presumptive adrenergic neuroblasts in interspecific chimeras after heterotopic transplantations, Proc. Natl. Acad. Sci. U.S.A., 72:728.

Le Douarin, N.M., Teillet, M.A., Ziller, C. and Smith, J., 1978, Adrenergic differentiation of cells of the cholinergic ciliary and Remak ganglia in avian embryo after in vivo transplantation, Proc. Natl. Acad. Sci. U.S.A., 75:2030.

Lim, R., Turriff, D.E., Troy, S.S. and Kato, T., 1977, Differentiation of glioblasts under the influence of glia maturation factor, in : "Cell, Tissue and Organ Cultures in Neurobiology", S. Fedoroff and L. Hertz, eds., Academic Press, New York.

Lindvall, O. and Björklund, A., 1974, The glyoxylic acid fluorescence histochemical method : a detailed account of methodology for the vizualization of central catecholamine neurons, Histochem., 39:97.

Louis, J.C., Pettmann, B., Courageot, J., Rumigny, J.F., Mandel, P. and Sensenbrenner, M., 1981, Developmental changes in cultured neurons from chick embryo cerebral hemispheres, Exp. Brain Res., 42:63.

Maciag, T., Cerundolo, J., Ilsley, S., Kelley, P.R. and Forand, R., 1979, An endothelial cell growth factor from bovine hypothalamus : Identification and partial characterization, Proc. Natl. Acad. Sci. U.S.A., 76:5674.

Noden, D.M., 1978, The control of avian cephalic neural crest cytodifferentiation. II. Neural tissues, Dev. Biol., 67:313.

Patterson, P.H., 1978, Environmental determination of autonomic neurotransmitter functions, Ann. Rev. Neurosci., 1:1.

Pettmann, B., 1979, Recherches sur la maturation de cellules nerveuses en culture, Thèse de Doctorat 3ème Cycle, Strasbourg.

Pettmann, B., Delaunoy, J.P., Courageot, J., Devilliers, G. and Sensenbrenner, M., 1980a, Rat brain glial cells in culture : effects of brain extracts on the development of oligodendroglia-like cells, Dev. Biol., 75:278.

Pettmann, B., Labourdette, G., Devilliers, G. and Sensenbrenner, M., 1981, Effects of brain extracts from chick embryo on the development of astroblasts in culture, Dev. Neurosci., 4:37.

Pettmann, B., Sensenbrenner, M. and Labourdette, G., 1980b, Isolation of a glial maturation factor from beef brain, FEBS Letters, 118:195.

Prochiantz, A., Diporzio, U., Kato, A., Berger, B. and Glowinski, J., 1979, In vitro maturation of mesencephalic dopaminergic neurons from mouse embryos is enhanced in presence of their striatal target cells, Proc. Natl. Acad. Sci. U.S.A., 76:5387.

Sensenbrenner, M., 1977, Dissociated brain cells in primary cultures, in : "Cell, Tissue and Organ Cultures in Neurobiology", S. Fedoroff and L. Hertz, eds., Academic Press, New York.

Sensenbrenner, M., Booher, J. and Mandel, P., 1973, Histochemical study of dissociated nerve cells from embryonic chick cerebral hemispheres in flask cultures, Experientia, 29:699.

Sensenbrenner, M., Labourdette, G., Delaunoy, J.P., Pettmann, B., Devilliers, G., Moonen, G. and Bock, E., 1980a, Morphological and biochemical differentiation of glial cells in primary culture, in : "Tissue Culture in Neurobiology", E. Giacobini, A. Vernadakis and A. Shahar, eds., Raven Press, New York.

Sensenbrenner, M., Springer, N., Booher, J. and Mandel, P., 1972, Histochemical studies during the differentiation of dissociated nerve cells cultivated in the presence of brain extracts, Neurobiology, 2:49.

Sensenbrenner, M., Wittendorp, E., Barakat, I. and Rechenmann, R.V., 1980b, Autoradiographic study of proliferating brain cells in culture, Dev. Biol., 75:268.

Sherbet, G.V. and Lakshmi, M.S., 1974, Follicle stimulating hormone and the differentiation of neural tissue, Differentiation, 2:51.

Thoenen, H. and Barde, Y.A., 1980, Physiology of Nerve Growth Factor, Physiol. Rev., 60:1284.

Toivonen, S., Tarin, D. and Saxen, L., 1976, The transmission of morphogenetic signals from amphibian mesoderm to ectoderm in primary induction, Differentiation, 5:49.

Varon, S., Raiborn, Ch. and Tyszka, E., 1973, In vitro studies of dissociated cells from newborn mouse dorsal root ganglia, Brain Res., 54:51.

Werner, I., Peterson, G.R. and Shuster, L., 1971, Choline acetyltransferase and acetylcholinesterase in cultured brain cells from chick embryos, J. Neurochem., 18:141.

CERTAIN SURFACE PROPERTIES OF ISOLATED

AND CULTURED CEREBELLAR CELLS

R. Balázs, C.M. Regan, R.D. Gordon, P. Annunziata*
Ann E. Kingsbury and E. Meier**

Developmental Neurobiology Unit
Medical Research Council
33 John's Mews
London WC1N 2NS

INTRODUCTION

In order to further the understanding of the biochemical properties of the different neural cell types we have been engaged over the last few years in studies aimed at the separation and characterization of perikarya of various classes of cells from the rodent cerebellum (for review cf Garthwaite and Balázs, 1981). The investigations have recently been extended employing tissue culture techniques for selection of cell type enriched preparations. This approach has the advantage that information can be obtained on the development of cells in vitro and also facilitates the examination of interactions of the different cell types underlying the functional organization of the nervous system. The preparations we have mainly used in these studies are primary cultures greatly enriched respectively in cerebellar internuerones and astrocytes (cf Balázs et al., 1980; Woodhams et al., 1981). The former contain principally two neuronal classes, predominantly excitatory granule cells and inhibitory interneurones (stellate/ basket cells) constituting about 80% and 7 - 16% of the neurones respectively, while astrocytes are the most numerous non-neuronal cells (about 7-15%). (Lasher, 1974, Currie and Dutton, 1980, and unpublished observations from our Unit). The glial cultures consist of about 80% glial fibrillary acidic protein (GFA) positive astrocytes, and endothelial cells are the most abundant contaminants (Woodhams et al., 1981).

---

*Department of Neurology, University of Siena, Italy
**Department of Biochemistry, The Panum Institute, Copenhagen

In this chapter we will describe current investigations especially on the neuronal cultures concerning cell surface constituents which are thought to have important roles in cell-cell interaction and the recognition of molecular signals. Firstly certain properties related to neurotransmission will be considered and these will be compared with the characteristics of cultured astrocytes and of the perikarya of different classes of separated cells.

Secondly we will describe the developmental changes in the profile of surface exposed proteins in the neuronal cultures, including attempts to identify one of the major constituents and the demonstration that the masking of these molecules with antibodies under certain conditions interferes with the long-term survival of the nerve cells.

NEUROTRANSMISSION RELATED PROPERTIES

The trypsinization procedure employed in the dissociation of the tissue resulted not only in the amputation of the neuronal processes but also in a marked loss of certain surface constituents including transmitter receptors. Thus it was of interest to investigate whether the development of the nerve cells in vitro is accompanied by the expression of transmission associated functions. The following considerations prompted the study of the muscarinic choninergic and the GABA receptors: it is believed that the rat cerebellum has no intrinsic cholinergic cells and that cholinergic afferents with associated postsynaptic muscarinic receptors are confined to a relatively small part of the tissue, the archicerebellum (Kása and Silver, 1969, Rotter et al, 1979). Thus the investigations may reveal whether transmitter receptors can develop on the interneurones, which are derived randomly from all parts of the cerebellum, in the absence of cholinergic innervation. On the other hand, there is evidence (eg Kingsbury et al, 1980, Palacios et al, 1980) indicating that GABA receptor binding is very high on the most abundant cells in these cultures, the granule cells which are presumably innervated here by the inhibitory interneurones.

The culture conditions adopted from previous studies (Lasher and Zagon, 1972, Messer, 1977, Currie and Dutton, 1980) selected for the survival of the cerebellar interneurones. These included the seeding of the mixed cells suspension obtained usually from 8 day old rat cerebella on polylysine coated dishes (Yavin and Yavin, 1974), preventing the replication of non-neuronal cells (eg using fluorodeoxyuridine, FDU, or preferably cytosine arabinoside, ARA-C), and the inclusion of relatively high concentrations of K^+ ions (25 mM) in the medium (Dulbecco's modified Eagle medium, DMEM or preferably Eagle's (modified) basal medium, BMEM, supplemented with 10% foetal calf serum).

Soon after seeding (2 5x10^6 cells per 35 mm diameter dish) the small nerve cells attached to the plastic, started to grow fibres and assembled into rows comprising less than ten cells. Progressive fibre growth was accompanied by migration of cells along the fibres, and clumps were formed by the end of the first day in vitro (DIV). The further development of the cultures was characterized by the growth of the aggregates, formation of thick interconnecting fibre bundles and the disappearance of many of the non-neuronal cells. Large neurones were very rarely encountered under these conditions. The appearance of the interneurone cultures using phase contrast microscopy is shown in Fig. 2 and 5.   In further electromicroscopic studies synapse formation was also detectable in these cultures (unpublished observations by P. Woodhams in the Unit; see also Burry and Lasher, 1978).

Transmitter Receptors

Previous studies (Patel et al.,1980) showed that muscarinic receptor binding is maximal, in terms of unit protein, in the cerebellum during the first 6 - 10 days after birth when cells have been prepared for cultivation.   Although a great proportion of the receptors were lost during the trypsinization step, they were rapidly reconstituted in culture and after 3 days their level was even somewhat higher than in the whole cerebellum at the corresponding age (Table 1).   Muscarinic receptor binding per unit protein decreases during the development of the cerebellum in vivo (Patel et al.,1980).   In contrast, it was found that the concentration of muscarinic receptors progressively increased in vitro, and by 14 DIV it was about three times higher than it was in the tissue from which the cultured cells were derived. Furthermore, at that time the values were about four-fold greater than at the comparable age in vivo. We have proposed previously that the decrease in the concentration of muscarinic receptors during ontogenesis is due to the dilution of the archicerebellum with the later developing principally non-cholinoceptive parts of the cerebellum, that constitutes ultimately a much greater proportion of the whole organ (Patel et al., 1980.   This is consistent with the observation that total receptor binding per cerebellum increases approximately nine-fold during the period 6 - 21 days, since the germinal matrix, the external granular layer is still present in the archicerebellum, and thus here both the newly formed and the existing cholinoceptic cells may acquire new receptors. In contrast, under the present culture conditions, nerve cell replication was precluded, thus the three-fold increase in the concentration of muscarinic receptors compared reasonably with in vivo development. However, the most important conclusion from these results was that the formation of the cholinergic receptors does not depend on the cells receiving cholinergic innervation, but is an intrinsic property of this population of nerve cells. As a matter of fact, the absence of

Table 1. Development of Transmitter Receptors in the Cerebellar Interneurone Cultures[a]

	8	11	12	15	21	22	35
Age in vivo (days)[b]	8	11	12	15	21	22	35
Age in vitro (DIV)[c]		3		7		14	
Muscarinic receptor binding[d]							
in vitro		0.33±0.07		0.5±0.13		0.87±0.07	
in vivo	(0.27)[e]		0.26		0.22		0.16
GABA receptor binding[d]							
in vitro		0.81±0.48		2.31±0.76		3.59±1.21	
in vivo	(0.48)[e]		0.85		1.22		3.0

[a]Surface cultures enriched in nerve cells were obtained from 8-day old dissociated cerebella, and receptor binding in crude membrane preparations was estimated as described by Patel et al.(1980).

[b]The in vivo estimates are from Patel et al (1980). In order to compare the development of receptor binding in vitro and in vivo the 'age' of the cultured cells is also expressed as the time in culture plus the age of the animals (8-day old) from which the cells were derived.

[c]DIV - days in vitro

[d]Specific binding was estimated as the difference between triplicate samples containing 3nM L-[3H]QNB or 12nM[3H]-muscimiol in the presence or absence of the displacing agent (100µM oxotremorine or 200µM GABA). Receptor binding is expressed as pmol/mg membrane protein and is the mean ±SE of 3-4 separate experiments. (QNB=quinuclidinylbenzilate).

[e]Extrapolated values from the in vivo age-curves of Patel et al (1980).

cholinergic innervation may have contributed to the relatively high
QNB binding, since it has been shown previously that muscarinic
receptor stimulation, even at the physiological level, results in
a decrease in receptor binding (Siman and Klein, 1979; Burgoyne
and Pearce, 1981).

Transport of Putative Amino Acid Transmitters

It is generally considered that nerve cells operating with a
particular transmitter also have a high affinity transport system
for that substance. Autoradiographic studies have indeed shown
that [^{3}H]GABA is taken up only by a small population of nerve cells
in the cerebellar neuronal cultures (see also Lasher, 1974; Currie
and Dutton, 1980). These results were consistent with biochemical
findings on separated cell types (Table 2; Cohen et al.,1980;
East et al., 1980) and with autoradiographic observations on structurally preserved cerebellar slices (Wilkin et al., 1981a). These
studies showed that in contrast with the Purkinje cells and inhibitory
interneurones high affinity GABA uptake is not detectable in the
most abundant cerebellar neurones, the excitatory granule cells.

It was also found that both the separated and cultured astrocytes are endowed with high affinity GABA transport systems (Shousboe
et al., 1977; Cohen et al., 1980). Compared with a GABA-ergic
neurone, the Purkinje cell, the separated astrocytes showed lower
maximal velocity (V_{max} about one sixth) but higher affinity (about
double) (Table 2). Furthermore, differences could be detected in
the properties of the GABA carrier using structural analogues,
β-alanine being a good uptake inhibitor in the astrocytes, while
cis - 1, 3 - aminocyclohexane carboxylic acid (Bowery et al., 1976)
in the Purkinje cells (Cohen et al., 1980). We have now observed
that when astrocytes are grown in vitro certain changes occur in
the properties of the GABA transport system. Thus, in comparison
with the freshly separated astrocytes, the affinity was about eight-
fold lower and β-alanine was no longer a potent inhibitor. Furthermore, autoradiographic studies showed that [^{3}H]GABA uptake was
different in the two types of GFA-positive astroglial cells detectable
in culture, the process-bearing astrocytes displaying a very much
higher grain density than the polygonal astroblast-like cells (Wilkin, Gordon and Bourne, in preparation).

It is generally believed that glutamate is the transmitter of
the granule cells (Young et al., 1974; McBride et al., 1976; Sandoval and Cotman, 1978; however, cf Patel and Balazs, 1975). We
investigated, therefore, [^{3}H]glutamate uptake in the neuronal cultures. Autoradiographic studies showed that in the cerebellar cultures the nerve cells and their processes were conspicuously unlabelled, in contrast to the astrocytes which were heavily labelled.
In contrast with the report of Le Campbell and Shank (1978) similar

Table 2. Kinetics of High Affinity Uptake in Separated and Cultured Cerebellar Cells[a]

Preparations	[3H]Glutamate		[3H]GABA	
	K_t (µM)	V_{max}[b]	K_t (µM)	V_{max}[b]
Separated cell types				
Granule cells	2.3±0.3	52±12	-	-
Replicating cells	3.1±0.4	432±155	-	-
Astrocytes	2.9±0.1	1331±210 (18.13±2.86)[c]	1.05±0.19[d]	51±17[d] (0.695±0.1.77)[c]
Purkinje cells	3.8±0.2	547±105	2.15±0.21[d]	310±33[d]
Astrocyte-cultures				
6 DIV	19.3±3.9	22.3±4.0	8.32±1.036	0.342±0.0697
14 DIV	27.5±5.5	20.8±6.98	-	-

[a]Uptake was estimated as described by Cohen et al. (1980). The results are the mean ±S.E. of 3-4 experiments, except for [3H]GABA uptake into separated cells (n=5).

[b]V_{max} for the separated cells is expressed in pmol/10^6 cells per min. and for the cultured cells in nmol/mg protein per min.

[c]In brackets the V_{max} for separated astrocytes is also expressed in nmol/mg protein per min.

[d]These results are taken from Cohen et al (1980). This study has also shown that [3H]GABA uptake into granule cells is negligible.

results were obtained using separated cell types (see also East et al., 1980). Table 2 shows that the rate of [^{3}H]glutamate uptake into granule cell perikarya is very low, and if corrections were made for astrocyte contamination in this fraction, it is negligible. On the other hand, astrocytes transport [^{3}H]glutamate with a high rate, which exceeds by a factor of 8 the rate found in cerebellar synaptosomal preparations (Rohde et al., 1979) and by a factor of 3 the highest levels reported in the review of Hertz (1979) for brain synaptosomes.

These results are at variance with those of Weiler et al (1979) whose values for bulk separated glia are only a fraction of the estimates (about 3%) given in Table 2. There are certain important differences in these two studies. The cells in our work were isolated from 8-day old rat cerebella, whereas Weiler et al., (1979) used 1.5 - 2 kg rabbits. However, it seems unlikely that these factors could account fully for the observed differences, especially as the rate of high affinity glutamate uptake, measured simultaneously by Weiler et al. (1979) in rabbit synaptosomes, is similar to the values reported for the rat preparations. Rather the discrepancy may relate to the differences in the structural preservation of the isolated glial perikarya.

It was also observed in these studies that the rate of high affinity [^{3}H]glutamate uptake is comparable in the cultured and isolated astrocytes (Table 2), and is similar to the estimates reported by Hertz et al.(1978) and Schousboe and Divac (1979) for cultured astrocytes derived from the mouse brain. Furthermore, autoradiographic studies using both adult and 8-day old cerebellar slices showed a preferential uptake of the glutamate analogue, D-[^{3}H]aspartate, into astrocytes (Wilkin et al., 1981b). These electron microscopic autoradiographic studies also demonstrated that the perikarya, dendrites and axons of the granule cells exhibit negligible acidic amino acid uptake which, however, may take place in the synaptic terminals of these cells. The resolution of the technique did not permit a definitive conclusion, as the parallel fibre terminals are too small and are ensheathed by glial processes. Evidently these observations do not exclude the possibility that granule cells function with acidic amino acids as their transmitter. However, they introduce a note of caution concerning the uncritical application of putative transmitter substance uptake for the identification of transmitter-specific neuronal structures. The high glutamate uptake in astrocytes relative to neurones also has implications concerning metabolic interactions between different cell types in the CNS and this is discussed in detail in the Chapter by Patel.

PROTEINS EXPOSED ON THE CELL SURFACE

In these experiments developmental changes in the neuronal
cell surface were studied during the period 1 - 8 DIV, when mature
looking cultures, comprising clumps of cells with interconnecting
fibre tracts, are established from the initially plated rounded
perikarya.

Lactoperoxidase-Catalysed Iodination of Cell Surface Constituents

The amount of ^{125}I combined in proteins exposed on the cell
surface was relatively high in the first few days in vitro, reaching a peak at 4 DIV (Annunziata et al., 1981). This was followed
by a sharp fall, the degree of ^{125}I-iodination at 8 DIV being only
about 30% of that at the maximum. Autoradiography of the iodinated
constituents after separation by sodium dodecyl sulphate-polyacryla-

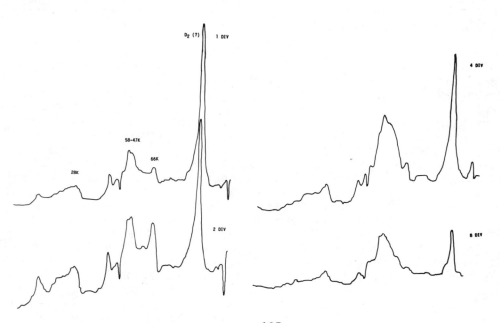

Fig. 1. Scan of autoradiograms of ^{125}I-labelled surface constituents
of cerebellar interneurone cultures separated by SDS-PAGE(10% gels).
Lactoperoxidase mediated iodination as described by Hubbard and Cohn
(1976). The apparent molecular weight of the iodinated bands and the
length of the cultivation time are indicated; the component marked
D2(?) has a molecular weight 140K dalton.

mide gel electrophosesis (SDS-PAGE) showed that the profile was different and very much simpler than that seen either after making the cells permeable to the reagents or following metabolic label- ling with [^{35}S]methionine. The scan of autoradiograms of the surface-^{125}I-iodinated proteins revealed that changes also took place during the development of the cultures in the relative pro- portion of ^{125}I which was combined in the intensively labelled bands (Fig. 1). The band which initially showed the most pronounced labelling had an approximate molecular weight of 140K (P140).

A major surface iodinated protein comprises the D2 antigen. In order to attempt the identification of the surface labelled proteins we have used a brain specific antiserum previously obtained in our Unit (Balázs et al., 1980; Meier et al., 1981). The anti- serum was raised in rabbits against plasma membrane preparations from immature rat cerebella (anti-BPM serum), and recognised pre- dominantly one brain specific antigen, as indicated by crossed immunoelectrophoresis using Triton-X100 solubilized extracts of brain and other tissues. In immunofluorescence studies the anti- serum labelled specifically the entire surface, both perikarya and processes of cultured nerve cells (Fig. 2). A light background staining of astrocytes occasionally encountered with some antiserum batches could be virtually eliminated by absorption of the serum with cells from an astroglial culture. Other cell types which are usually present in the cerebellar cultures, such as endothelial cells and fibroblasts, were not stained by the antiserum.

The nerve cell specific antigen(s) recognised by the anti- BPM serum were identified (Balázs et al.,1980; Meier et al., 1981) using an antiserum raised against synaptosomal membrane preparations (we are indebted to Dr. O. S. Jørgensen for the gen- erous gift of this antiserum). It was demonstrated, using Triton- X-100 solubilized adult brain tissue as an antigen source that the anti-BPM serum incorporated into the intermediate gel retarded markedly the mobility of one antigen only, the D2 protein (Jørgen- sen and Bock, 1974) while another, the D3, was slightly affected. It should be noted here that in independent immunofluorescence studies using an anti-D2 serum Bock et al (1980) reported a similar selective staining of the surface of nerve cells in primary brain cultures as observed by us after the application of the anti-BPM serum .

The anti-BPM serum was used for the isolation of the nerve cell specific antigen(s) from the protein mixture of surface ^{125}I-iodinated cultures by extracting the Coomassie-blue stained precipitation arc after crossed immunoelectrophoresis. This ex- tract was subjected to SDS-PAGE and it was found that the major ^{125}I-iodinated component was located in the same position as the P140 after the separation of the surface labelled proteins in the adjacent lane (Fig. 3). The apparent molecular weight of the D2

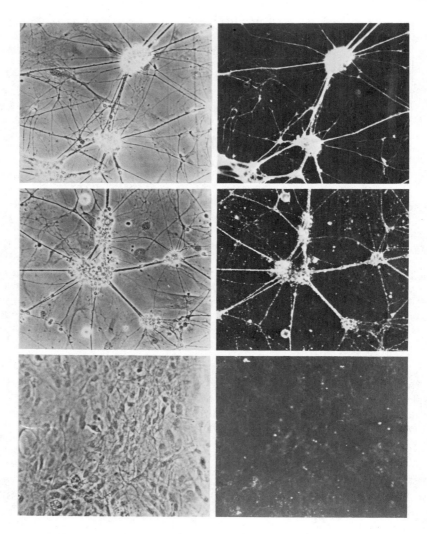

Fig. 2. Immunofluorescence (on the right) and phase contrast (on the left) views of cultures enriched in cerebellar interneurones (top and center) or astrocytes (bottom) using anti-BPM serum (top and bottom) and tetanus toxin/anti-tetanus serum (centre). The indirect sandwich technique was used (Steinberger, 1974); anti-BPM serum (1:20) followed by fluorescein isothiocyanate (FITC) conjugated anti-rabbit IgG or tetanus toxin (10µg/ml), horse anti-tetanus toxoid serum (1:50) followed by rabbit anti-horse IgG-FITC. Note that anti-BPM serum and tetanus stained comparable structures, the cell bodies and fibres of the nerve cells, while non-neuronal cells evident in the phase contrast micrographs were unlabelled. This was further corroborated by the absence of staining by anti-BPM serum of cells in the astrocyte cultures (bottom).

protein is about 140K, while D3 comprises three smaller polypeptides (14K, 23.5K and 34.4K; Jørgensen, 1979). The results showed, therefore, that one of the major surface ^{125}I-iodinated proteins in the cerebellar neuronal cultures comprises the D2 protein.

It seems appropriate to make now a few comments concerning the apparent similarities between the anti-BPM serum and the anti-NS-4 serum, which recognizes surface components on mouse brain cells

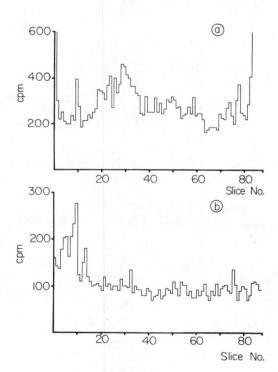

Fig. 3. The surface ^{125}I-iodinated k40K M.W. constituent (P140) comprises the D2 protein. ^{125}I-labelled proteins obtained after lactoperoxidase mediated iodination of 4 DIV cultures were subjected to crossed immunoelectrophoresis (Bjerrum and Bøg-Hansen, 1976). The D2 precipitate in the anti-BPM serum containing gel was cut out, extracted and separated by SDS-PAGE (10% gels) as described by Jørgensen (1980) (b). The ^{125}I content was measured after slicing the gel and this showed a peak coinciding in mobility with the P140 obtained by separating the solubilized proteins of the iodinated cultures in an adjacent lane (a).

(Schachner et al., 1975). Goridis et al (1978) and Rohrer and
Schachner (1980) have found that the anti-NS-4 serum precipitates
from extracts of surface iodine labelled primary cultures of mouse
cerebellum a limited number of antigens principally including
proteins with apparent molecular weights of 200K and 145K. Although Goridis et al. (1978) questioned whether P145 carries the
NS-4 antigenic determinants the available information cannot yet
provide a definitive answer (Rohrer and Schachner, 1980). However,
the P145 and the D2 protein have some common properties, such as
similar molecular weight, surface localization and greater concentration in the immature than the adult brain (see below and Jacque
et al., 1976; Schachner et al., 1975). Certain differences have
also been noted, for example the anti-NS-4 serum reacts with mouse
sperm, whereas the D2 protein has not been detected in the rat
testis (Jørgensen, 1980).

Developmental Changes Affecting the D2 Protein

These were studied and the development in vitro was compared
with that in vivo. It was observed that the amount of D2 per
unit protein was maximal during the period 6 - 12 days in vivo.
After this time the values declined progressively to about 50%
of the maximum by day 30 when the adult levels were approached.
Cells dissociated from 8-day old cerebella contained much less D2
protein than found in the whole tissue. This may be due to either
the trypsin treatment or the exclusion of neuronal processes from
the cell suspension. During the first 2 h in vitro a further decline occurred, but this was followed by a rapid increase to a peak
at 8 DIV, when the levels were similar to that at the corresponding
age in vivo. Beyond that time there was a moderate decline in the
amount of D2 protein.

The observation showing a progressive increase of D2 concentration during the first 8 DIV were not consistent with the results
demonstrating a decrease in the amount of ^{125}I combined in P140
after 2 DIV (Fig. 4). A lead to the understanding of these apparently discrepant findings was provided by further studies on the D2
protein during development.

It was observed that the D2 protein is subject not only to
quantitative changes (described above) but also to qualitative
alterations during development. Two molecular forms of D2 could
be distinguished, an 'anodic' form (aD2) dominant during the first
2 weeks after birth and a 'cathodic' form (cD2) later (constituting
all the D2 by about day 30 (see Jørgensen and Møller, 1980). These
maturational changes were also reproduced in vitro: initially
aD2 was expressed on the cultured cells, but by 2 DIV the concen-

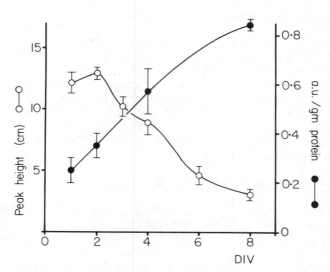

Fig. 4.   The concentration of the D2 protein (●) progressively
increases during 8-day period in vitro, while the amount of ^{125}I
combined in P140(D2) decreases after 2DIV (0).

tration of the two forms was similar, while cD2 became dominant
later accounting for all the D2 by 8 DIV.   The accelerated
maturation observed in vitro was probably related to the culture
conditions, which precludes cell replication, thus the differentiation of the interneurones occurs during a period when in vivo
cell proliferation is still extensive.

   The developmental change in the molecular forms of D2 could
be reproduced by treating plasma membrane preparations containing
both D2 forms with neuraminidase.   It was found that under these
conditions aD2 was converted into cD2 (see also Jørgensen and
Møller, 1980).   The hypothesis was therefore tested that the
decrease during cultivation in the degree of ^{125}I-iodination of
P140 ,in spite of the progressive increase of the concentration of
D2,is related to the developmental change involving desialidition
of this protein.   2DIV neuronal cultures, in which the iodination
of P140 is maximal and the concentration of aD2 still exceeds

somewhat that of the cD2, were therefore treated with neuraminidase. It was indeed observed that the amount of ^{125}I combined in P140 was markedly reduced when compared with untreated cultures.

These results are therefore consistent with the view that the developmental changes in the accessibility to the extracellular reagents of the tyrosine residues of the D2 polypeptide chain on the cell surface are due to alterations of the conformation of the protein consecutive to desialidation. Furthermore, the changes detected in the amount of ^{125}I combined not only in the D2, but also in other surface exposed polypeptides (Fig. 1) indicate that active reorganization of the plasma membrane takes place during the development of the nerve cells in vitro.

Release and Phosphorylation of the D2 Protein

Some of the surface ^{125}I-iodinated proteins including P140 were found to be released from the cultivated cells into the medium (see also Røhrer and Schachner, 1980). These findings were corroborated by labelling the cultures metabolically with [35S]methionine. The proteins released into a fresh, unlabelled medium were immunoprecipitated using anti-BPM-serum followed by anti-rabbit IgG. Analysis using SDS-PAGE showed that labelled P140 was present in the medium and it was completely removed from the released mixture of proteins by the immunoprecipitation. The structural requirements for antibody recognition were therefore retained in the protein which is shed from the cells.

The next series of experiments showed that the D2 protein is phosphorylated in the plasma membrane. Interneurone cultures were incubated in inorganic ^{32}P-phosphate containing media. After 4.5 h. the medium was removed and the proteins were precipitated with trichloroacetic acid, while a crude membrane preparation was obtained from the thoroughly washed cultures. The Triton-extracted membrane proteins were analysed by crossed immunoelectrophoresis using anti-BPM-serum. Autoradiography showed that the D2 precipitation arc was heavily labelled. On the other hand, ^{32}P incorporation into the medium proteins could not be detected.

These results, in conjunction with observations on the surface ^{125}I-iodination of the neuronal cultures, indicated that a significant part of the polypeptide chain of D2, which is an integral neuronal membrane constituent, is exposed on the cell surface, though with an anchorage within the membrane that can be phosphoylated but is apparently not released when D2 is shed into the medium.

Effect of the Neuronal Surface Specific Antiserum (Anti-BPM Serum) on the Survival of Neural Cells in Culture

Finally we have attempted to understand the physiological role of the cell surface constituent(s) recognised by the anti-BPM serum by masking the antigen(s) with the antibodies and following the effect of this perturbation on the development of the nerve cells in vitro (Regan et al., 1981). When added 4h after plating the anti-BPM serum did not interfere with the attachment of the cells. Furthermore the neurones emitted processes and migrated to produce beads of cells and small clumps (Fig. 5). However, during a period of a few days after this apparently unaffected initial phase of development, the survival of the nerve cells was compromised and by 3-5 DIV most of the neurones were apparently dead. The results were similar, when the antiserum was added at 8 DIV, i.e. no immediate cytotoxic effect was evident, but the nerve cells died usually 2 - 4 days later, although the variation in the length of survival was greater. The same results were obtained using the IgG fraction or the $F(ab')_2$ fragments derived from the anti-BPM serum, including the consistent finding that the non-neuronal cells were unaffected by the treatment. However, in contrast to the effects of $F(ab')_2$ fragments, the Fab' fragments failed to interfere with the survival of the nerve cells in culture, although in immunofluorescence studies they stained the nerve cells as well as the $F(ab')_2$ fragments. The different effects of the $F(ab')_2$ and Fab' fragments may relate to the higher dissociation rate of Fab' fragments at physiological temperature (Mason and Williams, 1980) or are the consequences of crosslinking the antigen, and these alternatives are currently under investigation.

It is of interest to note here that the Fab' fragments of D2 antibodies inhibit the fasciculation of neurites in rat sympathetic ganglia in culture (Jørgensen et al., 1980). Furthermore similarities have been noted in the properties of D2 and the cell adhesion molecule (CAM) isolated from chick embryo neural tissue (Rutishauser et al., 1979) including molecular weights, membrane distribution and immunological crossreactivity and it has been proposed that D2 and CAM may be evolutionarily and functionally related proteins (Jørgensen et al., 1980). CAM has been implicated in the chick in adhesion among cells and neurites in the developing nervous tissue and seems to be involved in histogenesis in the retina (Buskirk et al., 1980). The present observations suggest a further role for the D2 protein by demonstrating that divalent antibodies primarily directed against this protein interfere with the long-term survival of cerebellar neurones in culture.

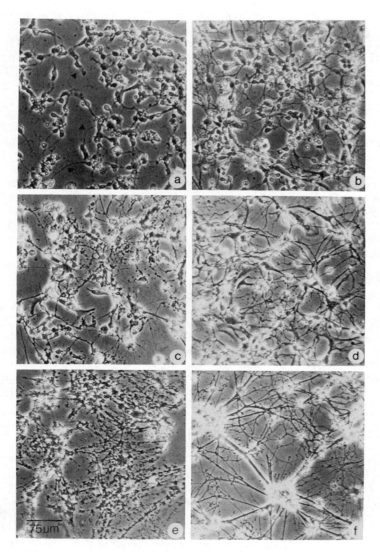

Fig. 5.   Phase-contrast views of cerebellar nerve cells cultured
in DMED containing 10% heat inactivated FCS in the presence of
anti-BPM serum derived IgG fraction (2 mg/ml). a and c, -cells cultured for 2 and 5 days respectively after the addition of rabbit
anti-BPM IgG-s 4h after seeding. Cells attached and grew fibres
(arrowheads) by 2DIV, but the nerve cells died by 5 DIV. e,-cells
cultures for 4 days after the addition of the anti-BPM IgG-s at 8
DIV.   On the right (b,d,f) the corresponding controls cultured
in the presence of anti-BPM IgG-s absorbed with cerebellar plasma
membrane preparations.

REFERENCES

Annunziata, P., Regan, C. M., Meier, E. and Balázs, R., 1981, Surface
properties of cerebellar interneurones in culture.   Proc. 8th
Meet. ISN, p.215.

Balázs, R., Regan, C., Meier, E., Woodhams, P.L., Wilkin, G.P., Patel,
A.J. and Gordon, R.D., 1980, Biochemical properties of neural
cell types from rat cerebellum, in: "Tissue Culture in Neurobiology", E. Giacobini, A. Vernadakis and A. Shahar, eds.,
Raven Press, New York, pp. 155-168.

Bjerrum, O.S. and Bøg-Hansen, T.C., 1976, Immunochemical gel precipitation techniques in membrane studies, in "Biochemical Analysis
of Membranes", A. H. Maddy, ed., Chapman and Hill, London, pp.
378-427.

Bock, E., Yavin, Z., Jørgensen, O.S. and Yavin, E., 1980, Nervous system specific proteins in developing rat cerebral cells in culture, J. Neurochem., 35: 1297-1302.

Bowery, N.G., Jones, G.P. and Neal, M., 1976, Selective inhibition of
neuronal GABA uptake by cis-1,3-aminocyclohexane carboxylic
acid, Nature, 264, 281-284.

Burgoyne, R.D. and Pearce, B., 1981, Muscarinic acetylcholine receptor
regulation and protein phosphorylation in primary cultures of
rat cerebellum, Dev. Brain Res., 2:55-63.

Burry, R.W. and Lasher, R.S., 1978, Electron microscopic autoradiography of the uptake of [³H]GABA in dispersed cell cultures of
rat cerebellum.   II.   The development of the GABA-ergic
synapses. Brain Res., 151:19-29.

Buskirk, D.R., Thiery, J.-P., Rutishauser, V. and Edelman, G.M., 1980,
Antibodies to a neural cell adhesion molecule disrupt histogenesis in cultured chick retinae, Nature, 285: 488-489.

Cohen, J., Balazs, R. and Woodhams, P.L., 1980, Characterization of
separated cell types from developing rat cerebellum. Transport of [³H]GABA by preparations enriched in Purkinje cells
and astrocytes. Neurochem. Res., 5, 963-981.

Currie, D.N. and Dutton, G.R., 1980, [³H]GABA uptake as a marker for
cell type in primary cultures of cerebellum and olfactory bulb,
Brain Res., 199: 473-481.

East, J.M., Dutton, G.R. and Currie, D.N., 1980, Transport of GABA,
β-alanine and glutamate into perikarya of postnatal rat cerebellum, J. Neurochem., 34, 523-530.

Garthwaite, J. and Balázs, R., 1981, Separation of cell types from
the cerebellum and their properties, in: "Adv. Cell. Neurobiol", Vol. 2, S. Fedoroff and L. Hertz, eds., Academic Press,
New York, pp. 461-489.

Goridis, C., Joher, M.A., Hirsch, M. and Schachner, M., 1978, Cell
surface proteins of cultured brain cells and their recognition by anti-cerebellum (anti-NS4) antiserum, J. Neurochem.,
31: 531-539.

Hertz, L., 1979, Functional interactions between neurones and astrocytes.   I.   Turnover and metabolism of putative amino acid
transmitters. Progr. Neurobiol., 13:277-323.

Hertz, L., Schousboe, A., Boechler, N., Mukerji, S. and Fedoroff, S., 1978, Kinetic characteristics of glutamate uptake into normal astrocytes in culture. Neurochem. Res., 3, 1-14.

Hubbard, A.L. and Cohn, Z.A., 1976, Specific labels for cell surfaces, in "Biochemical Analysis of Membranes", A.H. Maddy, ed., Chapman and Hall, London, pp. 427-501.

Jacque, C.M., Jørgensen, O.S., Baumann, N.A. and Bock, E., 1976, Brain-specific antigens in the quaking mouse during ontogeny, J. Neurochem., 27: 905-909.

Jørgensen, O.S., 1979, Polypeptides of the synaptic membrane antigens D1, D2 and D3, Biochim. Biophys. Acta, 581: 153-162.

Jørgensen, O.S. and Bock, E., 1974, Brain specific synaptosomal membrane proteins demonstrated by crossed immunoelectrophoresis, J. Neurochem., 23: 879-880.

Jørgensen, O.S. and Møller, M., 1980, Immunocytochemical demonstration of the D2 protein in the presynaptic complex, Brain Res., 194: 412-429.

Jørgensen, O.S.,Delouvee, A., Thiery, J.-P. and Edelman, G.M., 1980, The nervous system specific protein D2 is involved in adhesion among neurites from cultured rat ganglia, FEBS.Lett.111:39-42.

Kasa, P. and Silver, A., The correlation between choline acetyltransferase and acetylcholinesterase in different areas of the cerebellum of rat and guinea pig, J. Neurochem., 16: 389-397.

Kingsbury, A.E., Wilkin, G.P., Patel, A.J. and Balazs, R., 1980, Distribution of GABA receptors in the rat cerebellum, J. Neurochem., 35: 739-742.

Lasher, R.S., 1974, The uptake of [^{3}H]GABA and differentiation of stellate neurons in cultures of dissociated newborn rat cerebella, Brain Res., 69, 235-254.

Lasher, R.S. and Zagon, I.S., 1972, The effect of K$^+$ on neuronal differentiation in cultures of dissociated newborn rat cerebella, Brain Res., 41, 482-488.

Le Campbell, M.G. and Shank, R.P., 1978, Glutamate and GABA uptake by cerebellar granule and glial cell enriched populations. Brain Res., 153: 618-622.

McBride, W.J., Nadi, N.S., Altman J. and Aprison, M.H., 1976, Effects of selective doses of X-irradiation on the levels of several amino acids in the cerebellum of the rat. Neurochem. Res., 1:141-152.

Mason, D.W. and Williams, A.F., 1980, The kinetics of antibody binding to membrane antigens in solution and at the cell surface, Biochem. J., 187: 1-20.

Meier, E., Regan, C., Balazs, R. and Wilkin, G.P., 1981, Nerve-specific marker obtained by immunization with plasma membranes from immature cerebellum (submitted for publication).

Messer, A., 1977, The maintenance and identification of mouse cerebellar granule cells in monolayer culture. Brain Res., 130: 1-12.

Palacios, J.M., Niehoff, D.L. and Kuhar, M.J., 1980, Autoradiographic localization of γ-aminobutyric acid (GABA) receptors in the rat cerebellum, Proc. Natl. Acad. Sci., 77: 670-674.

Patel, A.J. and Balázs, R., 1975, Effect of x-irradiation on the bio-chemical maturation of rat cerebellum: metabolism of

^{14}C-glucose and ^{14}C-acetate, Radiat. Res., 62: 456-469.

Patel, A.J., Smith, R.M., Kingsbury, A.E., Hunt, A. and Balazs, R., 1980, Effects of thyroid state on brain development: muscarinic cholinergic and GABA receptors. Brain Res., 198: 389-402.

Regan, C.M., Meier, E. and Balázs, R., 1981, Effect of a neuron-specific antiserum on the survival and maturation of neural cells in culture, Biochem. Soc. Trans, 9: 315-316.

Rohrer, H. and Schachner, M., 1980, Surface proteins of cultured mouse cerebellar cells, J. Neurochem., 35: 792-803.

Rohde, B. H., Rea, M.A., Simon, J.R. and McBride, W.J., 1979, Effects of x-irradiation-induced loss of cerebellar granule cells in the synaptosomal levels and high affinity uptake of amino acids. J. Neurochem. 32: 1431-1435.

Rotter, A., Field, P.M. and Raisman, G., 1979, Muscarinic receptors in the central nervous system of the rat. III. Postnatal development of binding of [^{3}H] propylbenzylcholine mustard, Brain Res. Rev. 1: 185-205.

Rutishauser, V., Brackenbury, R., Thiery, J.-P. and Edelman, G.M., 1979, Surface molecules involved in interactions among nerve cells during development, in "Recent Advances in Developmental Biology and CNS Malformations" N.C. Myrianthopoulous and D. Bergsma, eds., Alan Liss, New York, pp. 79-92.

Sandoval, M.E. and Cotman, C.W., 1978, Evaluation of glutamate as a neurotransmitter of cerebellar parallel fibres, Neuroscience 3: 199-206.

Schachner, M., Wortham, K.A., Carter, L.D. and Chaffee, J.K., 1975, NS-4 (Nervous system antigen-4) a cell surface antigen of developing and adult mouse brain and sperm. Develop. Biol., 44: 313-325.

Schousboe, A. and Divac, I., 1979, Differences in glutamate uptake in astrocytes cultured from different brain regions. Brain Res. 177: 407-409.

Schousboe, A., Hertz, L. and Svenneby, G., 1977, Uptake and metabolism of GABA in astrocytes cultured from dissociated mouse brain hemispheres. Neurochem. Res., 2: 217-229.

Siman, R.G. and Klein, W.L., 1979, Cholinergic activity regulates muscarinic receptors in central nervous system cultures, Proc. Natl. Acad. Sci., USA, 76: 4141-4145.

Steinberger, C.A. (1974). "Immunocytochemistry." Prentice Hall, New Jersey.

Weiler, C.J., Nystrom, B. and Hamberger, A., 1979, Characteristics of glutamine and glutamate transport in isolated glia and synaptosomes. J. Neurochem., 32: 559-565.

Wilkin, G.P., Csillag, A., Balázs, R., Kingsbury, A.E. Wilson, J.E. and Johnson, A.L., 1981a, Localization of high affinity [^{3}H]glycine transport sites in the cerebellar cortex, Brain Res., 216: 11-13.

Wilkin, G.P., Garthwaite, J. and Balázs, R., 1981b, Putative acidic amino acid transmitters in the cerebellum. II. Electron microscopic localization of transport sites, Brain Res.(submitted).

Woodhams, P.L., Wilkin, G.P. and Balázs, R., 1981, Rat cerebellar
    cells in tissue culture.   II. Immunocytochemical identifi-
    cation of replicating cells in astrocyte-enriched cultures.
    Dev. Neurosci., 4: 307-321.
Yavin, E. and Yavin, Z., 1974, Attachment and culture of dissociated
    cells from rat embryo cerebral hemispheres on polylysine
    coated surface, J. Cell Biol., 62: 540-546.
Young, A.B., Oster-Granite, M.L., Herndon, R.M. and Snyder, S.H.,
    1974, Glutamic acid: selective depletion by viral-induced
    granule cell loss in hamster cerebellum.   Brain Res. 73: 1-13.

IMMUNOCYTOCHEMICAL LOCALIZATION OF GLUTAMIC ACID DECARBOXYLASE,

GAMMA-AMINOBUTYRIC ACID TRANSAMINASE IN THE CEREBELLUM

Victoria Chan-Palay

Department of Neurobiology
Harvard Medical School, Boston, Massachusetts, USA

GAMMA-AMINOBUTYRIC ACID PATHWAYS IN THE CEREBELLUM STUDIED BY
RETROGRADE AND ANTEROGRADE TRANSPORT OF GLUTAMIC ACID
DECARBOXYLASE (GAD) ANTIBODY AFTER IN VIVO INJECTIONS

Gamma-aminobutyric acid (GABA) is a major inhibitory neurotransmitter in the mammalian central nervous system, and deficits
of GABA have been implicated in certain neurological and psychia-
tric disorders, such as Huntington's chorea, Parkinson's disease,
and schizophrenia. Considerable interest attaches to the identification of GABA-containing neurons and receptor sites for GABA,
and cells and processes with GABA-synthesizing enzymes and with
GABA uptake systems have been identified morphologically (Chan-
Palay, 1977, Hokfelt and Ljungdahl, 1970, McLaughlin et al, 1974,
Ribak et al, 1976). The present investigations extend the applications of a new technique for the retrograde and anterograde
tracing of chemically specific pathways by the injection of specific, characterized antibodies directly into the central or
peripheral nervous system (Chan-Palay, 1979a; b; see Figure 1C).
A specific antibody can be used to localize and to identify neurons known to contain the antigen in the live animal by in vivo
injections directly into nervous tissue. The method allows localization of a putative transmitter molecule in the central and
peripheral nervous system without the use of agents such as
colchicine, which are necessary in most experiments that apply
the primary antibody onto fixed tissue. The antigen-antibody
complex is largely associated with lysosomal or prelysosomal
particles in the somatic cytoplasm, and such complexes mark the
dendritic and axonal processes of Substance P (SP) immunoreactive
cells. Further, the antigen-antibody complexes are carried by

axoplasmic flow in retrograde or anterograde directions and
therefore the method can be adapted for use in tracing chemically
specific pathways.

      Glutamic acid decarboxylase (GAD) is the enzyme that converts
glutamic acid to γ-aminobutyric acid (GABA). GAD has been isolated and purified from mouse brain and its properties extensively characterized (Matsuda et al, 1973; Wu, 1976; Wu and Roberts,
1974; Wu et al, 1973). Antibodies specific to GAD have been
obtained for immunocytochemical studies (Saito, 1976; Wong et al,
;074; Wu, 1976). These antibodies have been applied to fixed
tissue sections in order to detect GAD in the brain. In the mammalian cerebellum, GAD immunoreactivity has already been localized
to stellate, basket, and Golgi cells and their porcesses (Barber
and Saito, 1976; McLaughlin et al, 1974; Wood et al, 1976) and to
Purkinje cell somata after treatment with colchicine (Ribak et al,
1976). Other histochemical studies with ^{3}H-GABA uptake (Ljungdahl
et al, 1973), GABA-transaminase immunoreactivity (Barber and
Saito, 1976; Chan-Palay et al, and ^{3}H-muscimol detection of
the muscimol-GABA receptors (Chan-Palay 1978a; Chan-Palay and
Palay, 1978) in the cerebellum have strengthened the evidence
for GABA as a major transmitter in most of the intracortical
cerebellar neurons (except for granule cells and Lugaro cells)
and some neurons of the deep cerebellar nuclei (Barber and Saito,
1976; Chan-Palay, 1977; 1978a and b; Chan-Palay et al, 1979).

      Up to the present time GAD immunoreactivity has been found
to be confined to neuronal sites and is not apparently found in
neuroglia. In a series of recent experiments, a characterized
antibody against GAD was used to study the reciprocal pathways in
the cerebellum (Chan-Palay et al, 1979). These studies validated
the known corticonuclear projections from Purkinje cells to the
deep cerebellar nuclei and vestibular nuclei, by utilizing chemically specific transport of GAD antigen-antibody complexes in
the anterograde and retrograde directions, and investigated the
chemical nature of the nucleocortical pathways recently demonstrated to run between the deep cerebellar nuclei and the cortex
(Chan-Palay, 1977; Gould, 1977; Tolbert et al, 1976).

      Experiments were designed to label GAD-containing neurons,
particularly the Purkinje cells, and to study the transport of
GAD antigen-antibody complexes in anterograde transport from
cerebellar cortex to the corresponding underlying deep cerebellar
nucleus, as well as retrograde transport of the tracer from
cerebellar cortical terminals to the deep nuclei. Multiple doses
of 0.025 µl of undiluted antibody were ejected by pressure from a
glass micropipette (Chan-Palay, 1977, 1978a, 1979b) into the
cerebellar cortical surface less than 0.1 mm to 0.5 mm deep into
the brain of rats. Single amounts of 0.01 µl were injected into

the dentate nucleus and care was taken to avoid leakage of the label into overlying cortex and to secure as small an injection site as possible, confined within the boundaries of the dentate nucleus. A dorsal posterior approach through occipital cortex was used to avoid damaging cerebellar cortex as much as possible. These injections were intended to label dentate neurons by means of immunoreactivity to GAD and to examine the transport of GAD antigen-antibody complexes from dentate nucleus to Purkinje cells in the cortex.

Controls were carried out by injecting undiluted preimmune sera in equal volumes (0.025 µl) unilaterally into the vermis, simple lobule, and lateral hemispheres of the cerebellar cortex. In other control animals, colchicine, a drug that inhibits fast axonal transport (Dahlstrom, 1968), was given as a single intra-isternal injection into the fourth ventricle (3 µg/µl; 10 µl/100 g body weight) 24 h prior to injections of GAD antibody into the cerebellum. These controls were intended a. to alter the rate of retrograde and anterograde transport of GAD antigen-antibody complexes, and b. to enhance the visualization of GAD immunoreactivity.

GAD was isolated and purified from mouse brain. The purity of GAD preparations was established according to previously published procedures (Saito, 1976; Wong et al, 1974; Wood et al, 1976). Preimmune and/or normal rabbit sera served as controls. Antibody against GAD was used undiluted throughout these studies. Three separate batches of antibody against GAD were tested; each produced equivalent results. Pilot studies with sera diluted at 1:10, 1:50, and 1:100 showed less intense and less reliable results. On the basis of previous experiences with in vivo injections of SP antibodies into the rat medulla, the technique for tissue preparation was standardized and used as described previously (Chan-Palay, 1979 a, b).

After survival times of 1, 2, 4, 24 and 48 h, tissues from the separate groups of animals were examined in order to evaluate a. the initial size of the injection, b. the rate of regression of the injection site, and c. the GAD immunoreactivity obtained in cells and terminals at various times after injection. Optimal results as judged by the number and intensity of cells and terminals labeled at the injection site, after anterograde and retrograde transport of GAD, were obtained from animals with postinjection survivals of 2 to 4 hours.

The animals were fixed by perfusion through the heart (Chan-Palay, 1977, Palay and Chan-Palay, 1974). The animals were anesthetized with ether for the perfusion and maintained under artificial respiration through a tracheotomy tube with a mixture of 95% oxygen and 5% carbon dioxide. The blood was washed out

with cold Ca++-free Tyrode's buffer (50 ml at 4°C) followed immediately with cold 4% formaldehyde in 0.2 M phosphate buffer, pH 7.4
(500 ml at 4°C) for 20 min. Throughout, the animal was immersed
in ice. Following perfusion the brain was dissected from the
skull and soaked in fresh fixative. The optimum duration of this
postperfusion fixation was 2 h. Then the entire cerebellum was
sectioned on a freezing microtome or in a cryostat. Through the
region of the injection site and the deep cerebellar nuclei and
vestibular nuclei, all sections were saved and mounted in series.

       Two light microscopic immunocytochemical techniques were
performed; the indirect immunofluorescence method of Coons (1958)
and the peroxidase-antiperoxidase (PAP) method of Sternberger
(1979). Immunofluorescence studies were conducted on coronal
serial sections through the cerebellum and brainstem on a cryostat
(Dittes, -20° C), 10 μm thick, or on a freezing microtome, 30 μm
thick. The sections were mounted on chrome alum-gelatin-coated
slides, treated directly with goat anti-rabbit immunoglobulin
(IgG) conjugated to fluorescein isothiocyanate (FITC) and coverslipped in buffer-glycerol (3:1 v/v). No other application of
primary antibody was used (Chan-Palay, 1979a and b). Sections
were examined with a Zeiss fluorescence microscope fitted with
epi-illumination.

       More permanent preparations were obtained by using the PAP
technique. Coronal sections through the injection sites in the
cerebellar cortex and the deep cerebellar nuclei were cut serially
20-25 μm thick, on a Vibratome. The sections were treated with
goat anti-rabbit IgG (1:10 in 0.05 M Tris buffer, Triton X 100
0.5%, room temperature, 30 min.), then with rabbit PAP followed
by a reaction with 0.022% diaminobenzidine (DAB) in the presence
of 0.3% H_2O_2. No further application of primary antibody was
introduced (Chan-Palay, 1979a, b). The sections were mounted on
chrome alum-gelatin-coated slides, counterstained lightly with
0.5% cresyl violet and coverslipped in Permount for examination
by light or darkfield microscopy.

       The injection sites of GAD antibody were readily located in
the cerebellum by either immunofluorescence or the PAP method.
In cerebellar cortical folia injected discretely with 0.025 μl of
undiluted GAD antibody, only neuronal elements were found to be
immunoreactive. The neurons most intensely reactive were Purkinje
cells (Fig. 1a, b) with intense label in their perikarya and less
label in their dendrites. Sections parallel to the Purkinje
cell layer (Fig. 1a) showed that even within the injection site
all Purkinje cells did not exhibit the same level of immunoreactivity for GAD antibody. Some cells were intensely labeled
(arrows) and others were less (crossed arrows), and still others
in between these were not GAD immunoreactive at all. This observation brings up several questions: a. Does this patchy labeling

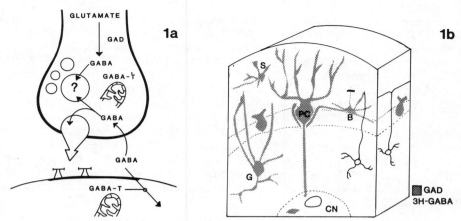

Fig. la: Schematic diagram to show the synthesis and metabolism
     of GABA.

Fig. lb: The cerebellar cortical and nuclear neurons with GAD im-
     munoreactivity and uptake capacities for 3H-GABA are indicated
     by stippling. These are the stellate (S), basket (B), Purkin-
     je cells (PC), Golgi cells (G) of the cortex and some small
     neurons in the deep cerebellar nuclei (CN).

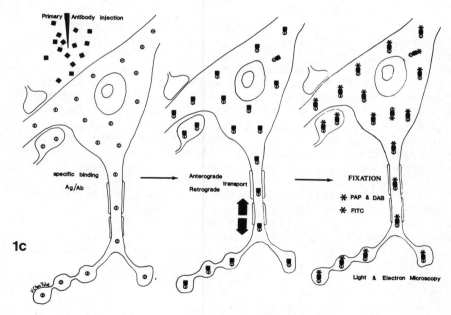

Fig. lc: Schematic diagram to summarize the steps involved in
    chemically specific labeling by in vivo injection of the prim-
    ary antibody. Primary antibody molecules are indicated by
    black squares; antigen molecules (or precursor molecules) are
    indicated by circles; subsequent immunocytochemical labels
    are indicated by asterisks.

of Purkinje cells reflect deficiencies in the sensitivity of the
GAD antibody or in the method of displaying it? Similar results
were obtained with three different samples of GAD antibodies.
b. Does the patchy labeling reflect the biology of the Purkinje
cells? Is it possible that not all Purkinje cells contain GABA
and GAD immunoreactivity? c. Does the GABA content of Purkinje
cells undergo cycles so that GAD and therefore GAD immunoreactivity is present in low and barely detectable levels at certain
phases in the cells' life? This question is made more pointed by
the fact that blockers of fast axonal transport effectively raised
levels of GAD immunoreactivity in materal obtained after in vivo
injections (Chan-Palay, unpublished data) as well as in material
prepared according to the more conventional postfixation immunocytochemical methods (Ribak et al, 1976).

        The other cerebellar cortical elements labeled by GAD anti-
body at the injection site included many stellate and basket cells
of the molecular layer, Golgi cells in the granular layer, and
the dendrites and axons belonging to these neurons throughout the
cortex. Golgi axons surrounding glomeruli were also labeled, but
not granule cells. A significant observation is that neuroglial
cells were not GAD immunoreactive (see Figs. 2a, c; compare with
Figs. 2b, d).

        Control injections with preimmune sera provided different
results (Figs. 2b, d). Within the injection sites no Purkinje
cells, stellate, basket, Golgi, or granule cells were immuno-
reative. Instead, intense nonspecific staining was found in neuroglial cells and their processes throughout the cortex (Figs. 2b,
d). The cell bodies of the Golgi epithelial neuroglial cells
(double arrows) between unstained Purkinje cell somata (arrows)
were intensely stained, as were their processes, the Bergmann fibers, in the molecular layer. Protoplasmic and velate astrocytes
and their processes were also well stained and their veil-like
sheets (Fig. 2b crossed arrows) defined the spaces occupied by
unreactive granule cells in the granule cell layer. Occasionally,
entire single neuroglial cells were delineated by the uptake of
injected preimmune sera (Fig. 2d crossed arrows). A comparison
of Figs. 2a, c with 2b, d shows the difference between GAD specific immunoreactivity and nonspecific staining at the injection
sites after in vivo injection of GAD antibody and preimmune sera
respectively.

        Injections of GAD antibody into the dentate nucleus resulted
in the labeling of approximately 5-10% of the neurons, mostly
multipolar or fusiform cell bodies ranging between 8 µm and 14 µm
in diameter. In the neuropil numerous boutons and fibers were
also GAD immunoreactive and these were probably the processes of
intrinsic dentate cells as well as terminals of Purkinje cell
axons from the cortex. Control injections with preimmune sera

into the dentate nucleus did not label neurons; only neuroglial elements were stained, providing data corresponding to that already presented above for the cortex.

Anterograde transport of GAD antigen-antibody complexes (Fig. 3a)
Injections of GAD antibody into the cerebellar cortex produced two distinct forms of specific labeling in the deep cerebellar and vestibular nuclei. There was an anterograde corticonuclear transport of label from GAD immunoreactive neurons. Since a vast literature shows that the major cortical projection GABA neuron is the Purkinje cell, the following description of the observations will presume that the GAD immunoreactive anterograde transport path is the Purkinje cell corticonuclear projection. A second, retrograde transport in the nucleocortical system also exists. Microinjections of GAD antibody unilaterally into the vermis on one side of the midline allowed anterograde transport into axons en route to the ipsilateral fastigial nucleus and consequent labeling of axons and terminal projectional fields of GAD immunoreactive Purkinje cells. Corresponding injections to the paravermal cortex and simple lobule allowed specific immunoreactive labeling of projection axons and terminal fields in the anterior and posterior interpositus complex and a small lateral portion of the fastigius nucleus. Injections into the folia of the lateral hemisphere (e.g., in Crus II) produced specific GAD immunoreactive labeling of axons en route to their terminal projections in the dentate nucleus and neighboring lateral portions of the interpositus nucleus. The GAD immunoreactive axons were individually and discretely labeled so that each could be followed separately, and in fascicles, on their corticonuclear trajectory among unlabeled axons in the white matter. The arrangement of the projections of GAD immunoreactive axons from Purkinje cells to deep cerebellar and vestibular nuclei conformed to the traditional topographic distribution patterns as described in detail for the cerebellum of many experimental species (Brodal, 1967; Voogd, 1954). These results are summarized schematically in Fig. 3a. An example of a GAD-labeled injection site in the cortex (lobulus simplex), the axonal trajectory, and the terminal projection fields in the fastigius and interpositus nucleus are illustrated in Fig. 3c.

The GAD immunoreactive terminals of Purkinje cells labeled by in vivo injections in the cortex were observed in the ipsilateral cerebellar and lateral vestibular nuclei. The GAD immunoreactive boutons and terminals, 1-4 μm in diameter, were found in the neuropil in large numbers directly applied to the somatic and dendritic surfaces (Fig. 3d, arrows) of large and medium-sized neurons. The boutons were intensely labeled with dense grains that could be resolved with the oil immersion lens in the light microscope. GAD immunoreactive boutons not directly applied against neuronal surfaces were found in groups (crossed

Figs. 2a and c, and Figs. 2b and D: Comparison of the injection
sites in cerebellar cortex 4 h after injections with 0.025 µl
undiluted GAD antibody (a,c) and preimmune control sera respectively (b,d). Immunofluorescence, 10 µm sections.

Fig. 2a: Photomicrograph of a section through the Purkinje cell
layer showing neuronal somata, excluding nuclei, intensely labeled
by GAD immunoreactivity (arrows), others lightly GAD labeled
(crossed arrows) and still others not reactive at all in between.
x 200.

Fig. 2c: Coronal section through the molecular (mol), Purkinje
cell (PC), and granule cell layers (gr l) of the cerebellar cortex showing intense GAD immunoreactivity in PC somata (arrows) and
Golgi cell somata, and light specific labeling in the neuropil
of the granular and molecular layers. x 100.

Fig. 2b:Photomicrograph through the Purkinje cell layer (PC) and
granular layers (gr l) of the cerebellar cortex showing unlabeled
Purkinje cell somata (arrows) surrounded by intense nonspecific
fluorescence with control preimmune sera in Golgi epithelial
neuroglial cells (double arrows). Nonspecifically labeled protoplasmic and velate astrocytes of the granular layer surround unlabeled granule cells (crossed arrows). x 200.

Fig. 2d: Coronal section through the molecular layer (mol),
Purkinje cell layer (PC), and granule cell layer (gr l) of the
cerebellar cortex showing no label within the cerebellar neurons
or Purkinje cells (arrow). Intense nonspecific staining is seen
in two Golgi epithelial neuroglial cells and their processes
(crossed arrows). x 100.

Fig. 2e: A group of GAD immunoreactive mossy fiber rosettes
(crossed arrows) and intervaricose segments (arrows) near the location of a GAD antibody injection into the cerebellar cortex.
Immunofluorescence with FITC, 4 h postinjection survival. x 150.

Fig. 2f: Cerebellar dentate neurons after retrograde labeling
by GAD immunoreactivity due to an injection of GAD antibody into
the cortical lateral hemisphere. Intensely labeled neurons
(crossed arrows) and moderately labeled neurons (arrow) intermingle with completely nonreactive ones. Vibratome section, 20 µm
thick, immuno-fluorescence method, 4 h post-injection survival.
x 60.

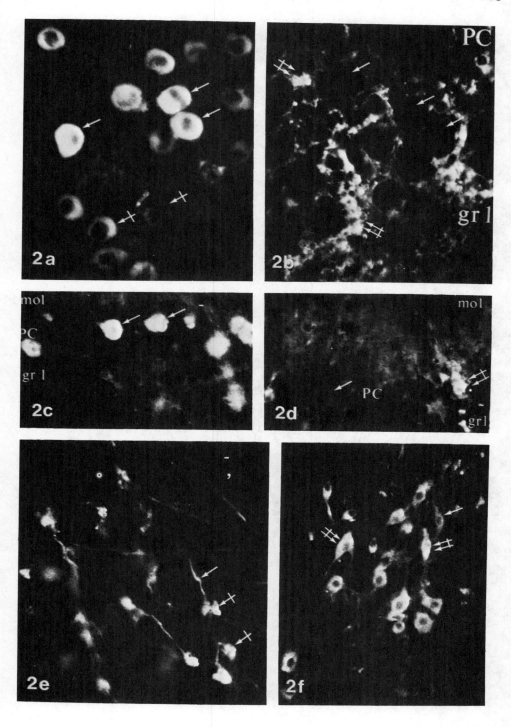

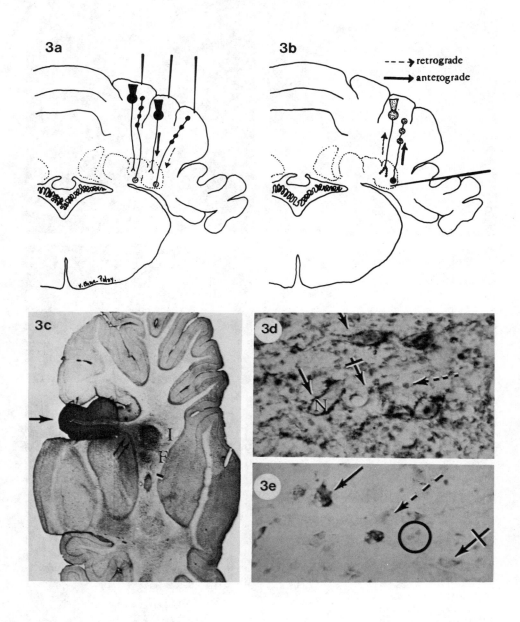

Figs. 3a and 3b: Schematic diagrams to summarize the results of anterograde and retrograde transport of GAD antigen-antibody complexes after in vivo injections of GAD antibody into the cerebellar cortex a and b. The concepts of reciprocity and topographic GABA projections are illustrated in these tracings of corticonuclear and nucleocortical projections. a Unilateral injections of GAD antibody into the cerebellar cortex produce GAD immunoreactive Purkinje cells (black), which project anterogradely and topographically to the ipsilateral dentate nucleus, indicated by numerous GAD immunoreactive boutons. GAD-immunoreactive mossy fiber rosettes cause a diffuse labeling in smaller cerebellar nuclear neurons (stipple circles) via retrograde transport. b Unilateral injections of GAD antibody into the dentate nucleus produces a number of diffusely labeled Purkinje cells ipsilaterally (stipple) by retrograde transport. GAD-immunoreactive neurons (black circles) in the dentate nucleus can effect labeling of small groups of mossy fibers in the overlying cerebellar cortex through anterograde axonal transport. Anterograde and retrograde transport in these systems does not appear to be inhibited by short term application of colchicine.

Fig. 3c: Low magnification photomicrograph to show injection sites of GAD antibody into the simple lobule on the right side (arrow) and the resulting labeled axonal tracts from cortex through the white matter (double arrows) to terminal projection fields in the ipsilateral fastigial nucleus (F) and interpositus nuclei (I) following a typical corticonuclear topographic distribution. 30 μm frozen section, treated with the PAP technique and counterstained with thionin. 4 h post-injection survival. Coronal section. Control injections with preimmune sera show injection sites (see Fig. 2a,c) without transport or terminal field labeling. x 80.

Fig. 3d: Anterograde transport of GAD antigen-antibody complexes after a GAD antibody cortical injection. Photomicrograph of unreactive neurons (N) in the cerebellar dentate nucleus showing numerous dark GAD-immunoreactive terminals and boutons upon the dendritic and somatic surfaces (arrows). Other GAD immunoreactive terminals are found in the neuropil (crossed arrows). Vibratome section, 20 μm thick, PAP technique, 4 h post-injection survival. The tissue has been lightly counterstained with creasyl violet to show non GAD-reactive neurons and neuroglial cells. x 120 (broken arrow).

Fig. 3e: Photomicrograph of neurons in the ventral posterior interpositus nucleus of the cerebellum labeled retrogradely after injection of GAD antibody into the cerebellar cortex. The labeled cells and dendrites (arrow) are usually smaller than the larger unlabeled ones (crossed arrow) and are readily differentiated from neuroglia (circle). Vibratome section 20 μm, 4 h post-injec-

arrow, Fig. 3d) in the neuropil participating in nucleocortical
connections. Conversely, injections of GAD antibody into the
dentate nucleus also resulted in anterograde labeling which was
detectable in approximately 25% of the cases studied. Small
groups of mossy fiber rosettes, intensely GAD immunoreactive, with
labeled intervaricose segments were seen in the cerebellar cortex
of the lateral hemispheres. These regions were not near or
within the track of the injecting micropipette and were not likely
artifacts of the injection itself. These GAD immunoreactive mossy
fiber rosettes may be part of the projections of the dentatocortical mossy fiber system (see Fig 2e). Nucleocortical axons that
terminate as mossy fibers in a topographic manner have been
described in a number of species (Chan-Palay, 1977; Tolbert et al,
1976). In addition, other investigators have contributed to
establishing the presence and organization of nucleocortical projections by means of HRP and amino acid autoradiography, without
specifically defining the terminal formations (Gould, 1977; Gould
and Graybiel, 1976). The present evidence suggests that some
dentatocortical mossy fibers are GAD-containing and GABA-synthesizing as well.

Retrograde Transport of GAD Antigen-Antibody Complexes (Fig. 3a)
Injections of GAD antibody into small, discrete zones of the
cerebellar cortex produced GAD immunoreactive labeling of
Purkinje cells, stellate, basket, and Golgi cells and their processes (see above), as well as intense GAD immunoreactivity in
small groups of mossy fiber rosettes and their intervaricose segments (Fig. 2e). GAD immunoreactive mossy fiber rosettes were
not found in control tissues from animals injected with preimmune
sera.

     In the cases in which injections into the vermis or paraver-
mal cortex resulted in GAD-immunoreactive mossy fibers, groups of
diffusely labeled GAD-immunoreactive cells were found in the fastigius and interpositus nuclei; most commonly in the ventral
posterior interpositus nucleus, in a thin band arranged above the
roof of the fourth ventricle. These cells (Fig. 3e, 2f, arrows)
were neuronal and not neuroglial. They measured 9-18 μm in
diameter and were either multipolar or fusiform with labeled perikarya and dendrites (arrow). Compared with the remaining unlabeled neurons (crossed arrow) these GAD laveled cells were small.

     Injections of GAD antibody into the lateral hemisphere
induced labeling in a small number of mossy fibers which transport
GAD immunoreactive material to cells in the dentate nucleus in
accordance with its expected topography (Chan-Palay, 1977; Tolbert
et al, 1976). These neurons were found in groups of 2 or 3 to 18.
They were usually diffusely labeled in their perikaryal cytoplasm
and dendrites. The intensity of GAD immunoreactivity ranged from
great (Fig. 2f, crossed arrows) to moderate (arrow) and they were

surrounded by numerous unlabeled cells. These GAD-immunoreactive nucleocortical neurons ranged from 8μm to 16 μm in diameter and were multipolar or fusiform. In some cases, these neurons occurred at the boundaries of the dentate nucleus, particularly within the rostral trabeculae (Chan-Palay, 1973a).

Thus GAD immunoreactive mossy fiber rosettes and preterminal segments apparently transport the GAD antigen-antibody complexes retrogradely and in an ipsilateral and topographic order to their neurons of origin in the deep cerebellar nuclei.

Corticonuclear Projections (Fig. 3b) Injections of GAD antibody into the dentate nucleus retrogradely labeled a small number of Purkinje cells in the overlying cerebellar cortex. The cells were identifiable as Purkinje cells because of their location in the cortex and the size of their somata. The GAD immunoreactivity was generally of low intensity and the cells were widely dispersed over the folium. This disposition may be due to a. the small amounts of GAD antigen-antibody complexes accumulated in the Purkinje cell body, b. the fact that not all neighboring Purkinje cells project to the same cerebellar nuclear area (Chan-Palay, 1973b), c. the fact that the Purkinje cells in general are difficult to domenstrate reliably by morphological techniques for the localization of GABA mechanisms. ^{3}H-GABA uptake studies do not consistently label Purkinje cells in adult animals (Ljungdahl et al, 1973; Sotelo et al, 1972). GAD immunocytochemistry reveals Purkinje cell somata irregularly (Barber and Saito, 1976) and more consistently if colchicine is applied. Similar observations have been made with studies using antibodies with GABA-transaminase (Chan-Palay et al, 1979).

Colchicine. In experiments in which GAD antibody was injected into animals pre-treated with colchicine, there was an apparent increase in the detectability of GAD immunoreactivity at injection sites and in terminal projection areas after retrograde and anterograde transport, with both immunofluorescence and the PAP method. Except for the enhanced levels of immunoreactivity, there was no difference in the localization or distribution of labeled cells and fibers. The increased intensity of immunoreactivity obtained indicates that colchicine treatment increased the accumulation GAD antigen-antibody complexes in neurons and their processes, but it did not block fast axonal transport to the point of preventing the phenomenon of retrograde and anterograde labeling. In general we suggest that experiments with antibody injections for afferent and efferent pathway tracing are best done without colchicine pretreatment. However, colchicine pretreated controls, as used here, are necessary in order to determine whether any negative results obtained are due a. to low sensitivity of the immunocytochemical detection method used and therefore reflect a technical inadequacy, or b. to a genuine

absence of afferent or efferent projections in the chemically
specific system studied.

Specificity. Throughout these studies it has been accepted that
detectable staining in neural structures by the purified, characterized GAD antibody indicates the presence of specific GAD
immunoreactive sites. Control studies with preimmune sera substantiate this by indicating no staining in the same neural structures in the absence of GAD specific antibodies.

The control studies with preimmune sera injections into the
cerebellum compared with injections of GAD antisera indicate that
whereas anti-GAD sera bind specifically to neurons with previously
demonstrated GAD and GABA-Tase immunoreactivity, ^{3}H-GABA uptake,
and ^{3}H-muscimol-GABA receptor binding properties, preimmune sera
bind nonspecifically to non-neuronal sites. Small localized
injections with the GAD antisera showed that immunoreactive neurons can bind and transport the antigen-antibody complex from
cortex to nuclei or vice versa, but injections with preimmune
control sera showed no comparable results. The present experiments indicate that when neurons in a specified location in the
cerebellum are injected with GAD antiserum, the antigen-antibody
complex can be detected in their projection targets or in cell
bodies at more distant sites away from the injection points. It
is presumed that these complexes are transported to these sites
in anterograde or retrograde fashion. No indication can be gained
from these studies as to whether this process is one of active
transport or of passive diffusion.

In conclusion, the present investigations utilized in vivo
injections of antibody against GAD to demonstrate reciprocal projections within the cerebellum between cortex and nuclei. Based
upon the retrograde and anterograde transport of GAD antigen-
antibody complexes taken up from the injection site, these
studies indicate that known corticonuclear and nucleocortical
projections within the cerebellum can be confirmed. In addition,
this technique imparts important information on the chemical
specificity of these pathways and suggests that some of the
nucleocortical projections are GABA-containing. The method
promises to be a significant means for investigation of chemically
specific connections in the central and peripheral nervous
systems.

Immunocytochemical localization of gamma-aminobutyric acid transaminase at cellular and ultrastructural levels. There is considerable interest in the identification of cellular sites of the
biosynthesis (McLaughlin et al, 1974, 1975) and metabolism of
GABA. Localization of GABA transaminase (GABA-Tase; 4-aminobu-
tyrate: 2-oxoglutarate aminotransferase), an enzyme involved in
GABA degradation, has been attempted by histochemical stains

(Hyde, 1978; Van Gelder, 1965), by light microscope, and by electron microscope immunocytochemistry (Barber and Saito, 1976;
Chan-Palay, 1979b). In our experiments we employed the indirect
immunofluorescence method (Coons, 1958), and the peroxidase-
antiperoxidase (PAP) method (Sternberger, 1979) for light and
electron microscopy. GABA-Tase was purified from mouse brain and
its purity was established by gel electrophoresis, high-speed
sedimentation equilibrium in dilute buffer, deuterium oxide, and
guanidine hydrochloride solution, and polyacrylamide gel electrophoresis as described by others (Schousboe et al, 1973, 1974;
Wu, ·1976). Antisera to GABA-Tase were produced in rabbits by
weekly infrascapular injections of 30 µg of enzyme in complete
Freund's adjuvant; serum was collected after the fourth injection.
GABA-Tase antisera were characterized by immunodiffusion micro-
complement fixation and immunoelectrophoresis as described
(Saito, 1976; Schousboe et al, 1974; Wong et al, 1974; Wu, 1976).
GABA-Tase antisera were used at dilutions of 1:100 or 1:200, and
normal rabbit preimmune sera served as the controls for cytochemical specificity in light and electron microscope studies.

     In the molecular layer, numerous stellate and basket cell
somata (greater than 80%) were immunoreactive. The neuroglial
somata surrounding Purkinje cells and their radial fibers (Palay
and Chan-Palay, 1974) displayed the most intense reaction. Purkinje cell somata were unreactive when glutaraldehyde was present
in the fixative but appeared as single immunoreactive cells or as
groups of up to 10 or 12 immunoreactive cells when formaldehyde
was used alone or after colchicine treatment, respectively
(Fig. 4a, b). These results indicate that the content of GABA-
Tase may differ from one Purkinje cell to another. In the granular layer, Golgi neurons were always intensely reactive, as were
neuroglial cells, but granule cells and axons were not. In the
deep nuclei, some large neurons and neuroglial cells were reactive
and this reactivity was most intense in large and small neurons
after harmaline treatment. The total amount of immunoreactivity
was considerably lower in the deep nuclei than in the cortex.
Labeled structures were randomly scattered in the cerebellum, and
no sagittal microzonation (Chan-Palay et al, 1979) in GABA-Tase
distribution was seen. Changes in the intensity of GABA-Tase
immunoreactivity were detectable on administration of various
drugs. Increased reactivity was obtained by treatment with
colchicine, GABA and oxamic acid, GABA, harmaline, norepinephrine
and glutamate, or diazepam in order of decreasing effectiveness.
Serotonin produced no detectable increase in GABA-Tase reactivity
above normal, and apomorphine and muscimol decreased it. No
specific staining was obtained in control tissues treated with
preimmune rabbit serum.

     Electron microscopy confirmed the light microscope results.
Labeled neurons included Golgi cells, basket and stellate cells,

and Purkinje cell somata and their dendrites. Neuroglial cells
between Purkinje cells were also labeled, as were their processes
surrounding neural elements in the molecular layer, other cells
in the granular layer, and blood vessels. In the labeled neuron
or neuroglial cell, two components were recognized--membranous
and cytoplasmic. The reactive material was detectable on the
plasma membranes, on outer nuclear membranes, on outer mitochondrial membranes, on membranes of the granular and smooth endoplasmic reticulu, and on microtubules and neurofilaments. The cytoplasmic matrix appeared as a dark reactive flocculent material
between the cellular organelles. Where the label occurred only
in neuroglial cells, the unlabeled neuronal elements were encir-
cled by reactive glial processes around Purkinje cells (Fig. 4d),
stellate cells, Purkinje cell dendrites, and mossy fibers. At
the synaptic interface, the presynaptic and postsynaptic membranes
alone could be specifically labeled (Fig. 4e).

    Evidence is provided for the presence of GABA-Tase in the
neuronal and neuroglial compartments of the cerebellum. In the
neuronal pool, cells that have been observed with GABA-Tase
immunoreactivity in their cytoplasm and membranes are cerebellar
GABA neurons previously shown to have glutamic acid decarboxylase
immunoreactivity (Barber and Saito, 1976), and ^{3}H-GABA uptake
(Chan-Palay, 1977; Ljungdahl et al, 1973). GABA-Tase immunoreactivity was also observed on postsynaptic membranes alone opposite
terminals of axons belonging to non-GABA-containing neurons
such as granule cells. This indicates that GABA-Tase is a major
cytoplasmic and membrane-related degradative enzyme in GABA-synthesizing neurons but is, in addition, selectively bound to the
postsynaptic membrane at synapses formed by non-GABA-containing
axons on GABA-containing neurons. Neuroglial cells, particularly
those enveloping GABA-containing neurons, have significant amounts
of cytoplasmic and membrane-bound GABA-Tase. Although many
Purkinje cells have GABA-Tase immunoreactivity, some have none.
All Purkinje cells and their dendrites, however, are ensheathed
by GABA-Tase immunoreactive neuroglial processes. The presence
of GABA-Tase in GABA neurons, neuroglia and non-GABA neurons
associated with GABA synapses indicates the participation of these
cells in important mechanisms for terminating transmitter action
--the uptake and degradation of GABA.

    GABA-Tase immunoreactivity was greater: a. in cerebella from
animals anesthetized with ether than with barbiturates; b. in
tissues treated by the PAP method than by the immunofluorescence
method; c. in tissues fixed in formaldehyde without glutaraldehyde than in unfixed frozen material (the presence of glutaraldehyde in the primary fixative enhanced morphological preservation
for electron microscopy but decreased immunoreactivity); and d.
in tissues obtained after colchicine administration. An increase
in GAGA-Tase immunoreactivity can be induced by application of

GABA and intensified with the use of oxamic acid and of glutamate.
These effects may be explained by increases in enzyme substrate
(GABA), in coenzyme-ligand interactions (oxamic acid) and in
enzyme product interactions (glutamate). Colchicine, a drug that
blocks axoplasmic transport of proteins, also increases demonstrable GABA-Tase. The finding that muscimol, a potent GABA
agonist, does not increase GABA-Tase levels suggests that binding
sites for GABA-Tase and transmitter receptor sites are separate.
With the exception of muscimol and apomorphine, the selective
changes elicited in levels of GABA-Tase reactivity by pharmacological treatments indicate that drugs and neurotransmitter substances that increase the activity of cerebellar GABA neurons directly
(GABA, norepinephrine, glutamate), or indirectly (diazepam, harmaline) increase immunologically detectable levels of the enzyme.
These studies indicate that the ability to localize the precise
sites of a degradative enzyme such as GABA-Tase provides a powerful means for investigation of neurotransmitter mechanisms at
cellular and subcellular levels.

In vivo injections of characterized antibody against glutamic acid decarboxylase (GAD), the enzyme responsible for the synthesis of γ-aminobutryric acid (GABA), into cerebellar cortex
produced labeled stellate, basket, Purkinje, and Golgi cells and
their processes at the injection site. Anterograde transport of
GAD antigen-antibody complexes in Purkinje cell axons caused
intense labeling of terminals in deep cerebellar and several vestibular nuclei. Small groups of mossy fiber rosettes labeled and
produced retrograde labeling and GAD immunoreactivity in a small
number of pleomorphic neurons in the deep cerebellar nuclei.
Injections into the dentate nucleus produced retrograde labeling
in Purkinje cell bodies and anterograde labeling in a small number
of mossy fiber rosettes. All projections conformed to previously
reported topographic distributions of corticonuclear and nucleocortical cerebellar pathways. These findings confirm the GABA
content of most Purkinje cell-deep nuclei connections and provide
new evidence for a GABA component in part of the nucleocortical
pathway in the cerebellum. Immunocytochemical controls for
specificity were conducted by injections of preimmune rabbit
serum as a substitute for GAD antibody which produced only nonspecific labeling. Colchicine caused a cumulative enhancement
of GAD immunoreactivity in all cases.

GABA-Tase immunoreactivity in the rat's cerebellum was studied by light and electron microscopy wit indirect immunofluorescence and peroxidase-antiperoxidase methods. Evidence is
presented for neuronal and neuroglial compartments of GABA-Tase.
Labeled neurons included stellate, basket, Purkinje, and Golgi
cells of the cortex and a few large neurons in the deep nuclei.
Labeled neuroglia included those surrounding Purkinje cells, their
radial fibers in the molecular layer, and astrocytes in the gran-

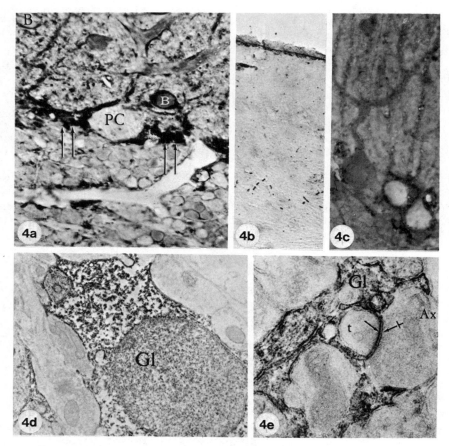

Figs. 4a, 4b, 4c: Light micrographs (a-b) of cerebellar cortex
       with immunoreactive neuronal and neuroglial elements
       visualized by GABA-Tase antisera using the PAP method.
       (a) Unlabeled Purkinje cell (PC) and primary dendrites
       surrounded by intensely immunoreactive neuroglial cells
       (arrows) and their processes. Labeled basket cells (B)
       are also present. x 480. (b) Control tissue treated
       with normal rabbit preimmune sera. x 120. (c) Normal,
       untreated, ether-anesthetized animal treated with cAMP
       antisera. x 100.

Figs. 4d, 4e: Electron micrographs of GABA-Tase immunoreactive
       cells in the cerebellar cortex from normal untreated
       animals anesthetized with ether and visualized by the
       PAP method without counterstains. (d) A neuroglial cell
       (GL) with immunoreactive surface membranes, organelles
       and cytoplasmic matrix and other unlabeled neuronal
       elements. x 6000. (e) GABA-Tase labeled glial (GL)
       process. x 25,000.

ular layer and deep nuclei. No evidence for sagittal microzonation was found. At the ultrastructural level, GABA-Tase immunoreactive sites were localized to cell surface membranes, intracellular organelles, and the cytoplasmic matrix. GABA-Tase
immunoreactivity at synapses could be localized precisely to pre-
and postsynaptic membranes in GABA-containing as well as non-GABA-
containing neurons. Specific label was absent from tissues
treated with normal rabbit preimmune sera.

ACKNOWLEDGEMENTS

     This work was supported in part by U.S. Public Health
Service Grants NS14740 and NS03659; Louise Harkness Ingalls
Fellowship on Parkinson's Disease from the Massachusetts General
Hospital; an Alfred P. Sloan Fellowship in Neuroscience. The
author thanks Mr. Howard Cook and Ms. Joyce Barton for photogra-
phic and technical assistance.

REFERENCES

Barber, R. & Saito, K., 1976. Light microscopic visualization of
GAD and GABA-T in immunocytochemical preparations of rodent CNS,
in 'GABA in Nervous System Function' (E. Roberts, T.N. Chase and
D.B. Tower eds.) p. 113, Raven Press, New York.

Chan-Palay, V., 1973a. Cytology and organization in the nucleus
lateralis of the cerebellum: the projections of neurons and their
porcesses into afferent axon bundles. A. Anat. Entwickl-Gesch.
141: 151-159.

Chan-Palay, V., 1973b. Afferent axons and their relations with
neurons in the nucleus lateralis of the cerebellum: a light
microscope study. A. Anat. Entwickl-Gesch. 142: 1-21.

Chan-Palay, V., 1977 in 'Cerebellar Dentate Nucleus, Organization,
Cytology, and Transmitters', Springer-Verlag, Berlin, Heidelberg,
New York.

Chan-Palay, V., 1978a. Autoradiographic localization of γ-aminobutyric acid receptors in the rat central nervous system using
^{3}H-muscimol. Proc. Natl. Acad. Sci. USA. 75: 1024-1028.

Chan-Palay, V., 1978b. Quantitative visualization of γ-aminobutyric acid receptors in the hippocampus and area dentata demonstrated by ^{3}H-muscimol autoradiography. Proc. Nat. Acad. Sci.
(Wash). 75: 6281-6284.

Chan-Palay, V., 1979a. Immunocytochemical detection of substance
P neurons, their processes and connections by in vivo microinjec-
tions of monoclonal antibodies: light and electron microscopy.
Anat. Embryol. (Berl). 156: 225-240.

Chan-Palay, V., 1979b. Combined immunocytochemistry and autoradiography after in vivo injections of monoclonal antibody to
Substance P and ^{3}H-serotonin: coexistence of two putative transmitters in single raphe cells and fiber plexuses. Anat. Embryol.
(Berl). 156: 241-254.

Chan-Palay, V. & Palay, S.L., 1978. Ultrastructural localization
of γ-aminobutyric acid receptors in the mammalian central nervous
system by means of ^{3}H-muscimol binding. Proc. Natl. Acad. Sci.
USA. 75: 2977-2980.

Chan-Palay, V., Wu, J-Y. and Palay, S.L., 1979. Immunocytochemical localization of GABA-transaminase at cellular and ultrastructural levels. Proc. Natl. Acad. Sci. USA. 76: 2067-2071.

Coons, A.G., 1958 in 'General Cytochemical Methods' (J.F. Danielli
ed.), pp. 399-422, Academic Press, New York.

Dahlstrom, A., 1968. Effect of colchicine on transport of amine
storage granules in sympathetic nerves of rat. J. Pharmacol.
5: 111-112.

Gould, B.B., 1977. Topographic organization of the cerevellar
nucleocortical projection in the cat. Anat. Rec. 187: 592.

Hokfelt, T. & Ljungdahl, A., 1970. Cellular localization of
labeled gamma-aminobutyric acid (^{3}H-GABA) in rat cerevellar cortex: an autoradiographic study. Brain Res. 22:391-396.

Hyde, J.C., 1978, Electron cytochemistry of GABA-transaminase in
rat cerebellar cortex, and evidence for multimolecular forms of
the enzyme, in 'Amino Acids as Chemical Transmitters' (F. Fonnum
ed.), p. 49, Plenum Press, New York.

Ljungdahl, A., Seiger, A., Hokfelt, T. and Olson, L., 1973.
(^{3}H)GABA uptake in growing cerebellar tissue: Autoradiography of
intraocular transplants. Brain Res. 61:379-384.

Matsuda, T., Wu, J-Y. and Roberts, E., 1973. Sodium dodecyl sulfate acrylamide gel electrophoresis of glutamic acid decarboxylase
from mouse brain. J. Neurochem. 21: 167-172.

McLaughlin, B., Wood, J.G., Saito, K., Barber, R., Vaughn, J.E.,
Roberts, E. and Wu, J-Y., 1974. The fine structural localization
of glutamate decarboxylase in synaptic terminals of rodent
cerebellum. Brain Res. 76: 377-391.

McLaughlin, B.J., Wood, J.G., Saito, K., Roberts, E. and Wu, J-Y., 1975. The fine structural localization of glutamate decarboxylase in developing axonal processes and presynaptic terminals of rodent cerebellum. Brain Res. 85: 355-371.

Palay, S.L. & Chan-Palay, V., 1974 in 'Cerebellar Cortex, Cytology and Organization', Springer-Verlag, Berlin, Heidelberg, New York.

Ribak, C.E., Vaughn, J.E. and Saito, K., 1976. Immunocytochemical localization of glutamic acid decarboxylase in neuronal somata following colchicine inhibition of axonal transport. Neurosci. Abstr. 11: 796.

Saito, K., 1976, Immunocytochemical studies of GAD and GABA-T, in 'GABA in Nervous System Function' (E. Roberts, T.N. Chase and D.B. Tower eds.), p. 103, Raven Press, New York.

Schousboe, A., Wu, J-Y. and Roberts, E., 1973. Purification and characterization of the 4-aminobutyrate-2-ketoglutarate transaminase from mouse brain. Biochem. 12: 2868-2873.

Schousboe, A., Wu, J-Y. and Roberts, E., 1974. Subunit structure and kinetic properties of 4-aminobutyrate-2-ketoglutarate transaminase purified from mouse brain. J. Neurochem. 23: 1189-1195.

Sotelo, C., Privat, A. and Drian, M.J., 1972. Localization of (^{3}H)GABA in tissue culture of rat cerebellum using electron microscopy radioautography. Brain Res. 45: 302-308.

Sternberger, L.A., 1979 in 'Immunocytochemistry. Basic and Clinical Immunology' (S. Cohen & R.T. McCluskey eds.), 2nd edition, John Wiley, New York.

Tolbert, D.L., Bantli, H. and Bloedel, J.R., 1976. Anatomical and physiological evidence for a cerebellar nucleocortical projection in the cat. Neuroscience 1: 205-218.

Van Gelder, N.M., 1965. The histochemical demonstration of γ-aminobutyric acid metabolism by reduction of a tetrazolium salt. J. Neurochem. 12: 231-237.

Voogd, J., 1964 in 'The Cerebellum of the Cat. Structure and Fibre Connexions', Van Gorcum & Co., Netherlands.

Wong, F., Schousboe, A., Saito, K., Wu, J-Y. and Roberts, F., 1974. Glutamate decarboxylase and GABA-transaminase from six mouse strains. Brain Res. 68: 133-139.

Wood, J.G., McLaughlin, B.J. and Vaughn, J.E., 1976, Immunocytochemical localization of GAD in electron microscopic preparations
of rodent CNS, in 'GABA in Nervous System Function' (E. Roberts,
N. Chase and D.B. Towers eds.), pp. 133-148, Raven Press,
New York.

Wu, J-Y., 1976, Purification, characterization, and kinetic
studies of GAD and GABA-T from mouse brain, in 'GABA in Nervous
System Function' (E. Roberts, T.N. Chase and D.B. Towers eds.),
p. 7, Raven Press, New York.

Wu, J-Y. & Roberts, E., 1974. Properties of brain L-glutamate
decarboxylase:Inhibition studies. J. Neurochem. 23: 759-767.

Wu, J-Y., Matsuda, T. and Roberts, E., 1973. Purification and
characterization of glutamate decarbosylase from mouse brain.
J. Biol. Chem. 248: 3029-3034.

THE ULTRASTRUCTURAL LOCALIZATION OF 5'-NUCLEOTIDASE

IN THE MOLECULAR LAYER OF THE MOUSE CEREBELLUM

E. Marani

Department of Anatomy and Embryology
University of Leiden, The Netherlands

INTRODUCTION

This paper describes the ultrastructural localization of the 5'-nucleotidase reaction product in the cerebellar molecular layer of mice, using a lead-salt enzymatic histochemical method (Scott, 1965, 1967). Light microscopically the localization of 5'-nucleotidase in longitudinal bands in the molecular layer, which alternate with negative regions is very characteristic (Marani, 1977, 1981; Marani and Boekee, 1975; Marani and Voogd, 1973; Scott, 1965, 1967). However, light microscopy alone cannot resolve the cellular localization of this enzyme. Light microscopy of the longitudinal band pattern was used to more specifically assess the influence of the fixatives used in our ultrastructural studies on 5'-nucleotidase. Histological criteria were also used to distinguish between 5'-nucleotidase and nonspecific phosphatases, since nonspecific phosphatases lack a band-like distribution. The ultrastructural determination of 5'-nucleotidase occurs at the narrow interval between optimal tissue fixation and maximal preservation of the enzyme. Much care, therefore, has been taken to identify and avoid adverse actions of fixatives, nonspecific phosphatase activity and artifacts due to lead precipitates and prolonged incubation. The numerous problems in establishing the procedure for demonstrating 5'-nucleotidase by electron microscopy with the lead-salt technique has been reviewed separately (Marani, 1981).

EXPERIMENTAL PROCEDURES

Mature female and male mice were anesthetized with chloroform or ether. Experiments were initiated late in the morning, thereby taking into account the circadian rhythms of nonspecific activity

reported for rats (Marani, 1980). The thorax was opened via the abdominal cavity and an intracardial injection (0,1 ml) of heparin (R)
5000 UI/ml: 1% and NaNO$_2$ (1:1) was given. The left ventricle was
opened, the perfusion needle inserted and clamped with a forceps.
After opening the right atrium, aortic perfusion was performed at
10-15 ml/min. Perfusion fixation was preceded by saline perfusion.
The perfusate contained 0.9% NaCl, 0.01% CaCl$_2$, 0.016 M cacodylate
buffer pH 7.4,300 m Osm and was injected at room temperature for
2-2.5 minutes. The first fixative (4% paraformaldehyde, freshly prepared in 0.16 M cacodylate buffer, with 0.01% CaCl$_2$, pH 7.4,1850 m
Osm, 0-4°C) was allowed to flow for 2-3 minutes. This first fixation
fluid was immediately followed by a 2 min (method A) or 5 min (method
B) perfusion fixation at room temperature with a 2.5% glutaraldehyde
solution (in 0.16 M cacodylate buffer with 0.01% CaCl$_2$, pH 7.4 containing 5.4 g/1 sucrose, 600 m Osm). Note that phosphate buffers are
omitted as in the solutions utilized by Rinvik and Grofova (1970).
Enzyme studies were carried out in two ways. Perfusion fixation
(method B) was followed by a 5 minute perfusion with the incubation
medium. The brain was then removed from the skull, vibratome chopped
(200 µm), and incubated. Alternatively, after perfusion fixation
(method A) the cerebellum may be quickly removed from the skull,
sectioned on the vibratome in 200 µm sections, and then incubated.
With the latter method the first sections for incubations were obtained within 10 minutes after the start of the perfusion fixation.
Sections obtained about 45 minutes after perfusion fixation no longer
revealed a band pattern of enzyme activity and were subsequently discarded.

The incubation media used are (1) Scott's (1967) medium for
5'-nucleotidase to which was sometimes added freshly prepared 1,3.c-
glyceromonophosphate (+ 10 mM) (Marani, in press), (2) Lake's medium
(Marani, 1977) for the determination of acid phosphatase. Nonspecific
phosphatase was determined by changing the pH of the buffer solution
of the Lake method (Marani, 1977) to pH 7.2. For light microscopic
purposes acid phosphatase was also determined by the method of Barka
and Anderson (1962). After incubation for 1-1.5 hours, the sections
were washed for 15 minutes in a cacodylate buffer of the same composition as the fixatives and postfixed in the 2.5% glutaraldehyde fixative for 30 minutes. Osmification was performed at room temperature
with OsO$_4$ (1%) in 0.16 M cacodylate buffer pH 7.4.

Dehydration was followed by 20 min in propyleneoxide and by one
hour in Epon-propylaneoxide (1:1). Sections were embedded in freshly
prepared Epon held at 60°C. Ultrathin sections were made and were contrasted and stained with lead hydroxyde and/or uranyl acetate. Adjacent uncontrasted sections were always examined.

RESULTS

Incubations omitting the capture agent Pb^{2+} in the Scott incubation medium (1965) did not produce localized reaction products. Perfusion fixation with the Scott medium, omitting the substrate AMP, showed non-specific lead-ion deposits at the surface membranes of endothelial cells. Acid phosphatase studies with the lead-β-glycerophosphate technique at pH 5.0 showed imperfect reaction product formation, even in lysosomal structures (Brederoo et al., 1968). This also was the case for nonspecific phosphatase activity (Figs. 1A, B and C). These lead-ion responses were rejected as being indicative of 5'-nucleotidase activity.

5'-Nucleotidase localization in the cerebellar molecular layer

A characteristic feature of 5'-nucleotidase is its arrangement in longitudinal zones of alternating positive bands (Figs 1E and 2A, C). The lateral borders of positive bands are sharply delineated from negative areas, while their medial borders sometimes show a gradual transition into the negative area bordering it (Fig. 2). The identification of these sharp lateral borders in ultrathin sections proves that the lead precipitates in these areas represent 5'-nucleotidase reaction products. Figure 3 shows one such border in the vermal part of lobule IV-V in the mouse cerebellar molecular layer. 5'-Nucleotidase reaction products are found within the dendritic tree of Purkinje cells in sections treated with and without a nonspecific phosphatase inhibitor. Reaction products for 5'-nucleotidase could not be demonstrated in the cell somata of Purkinje cells. They were absent from the rough endoplasmatic reticulum with all types of incubations used for 5'-nucleotidase demonstration. In the primary dendrites, 5'-nucleotidase reaction products are situated in structures comparable to the smooth endoplasmatic reticulum (Fig. 4), while just beneath the cell membrane they are found within the subsurface cisternae (Fig. 5). Reaction products were always within the lumen of the cisternae (Fig. 5). No connections of the 5'-nucleotidase-positive subsurface cisternae with the intra-dendritic smooth endoplasmic reticulum have been found, while our studies do not provide any findings suggestive of the origin of the 5'-nucleotidase producing system within Purkinje cell dendrites, it must be pointed out, however, that ribosome-like structures occur between the packed cisternae. The fine branches of the Purkinje cell dendritic tree are replete with spines. Dendritic spines are small protrusions onto which the axon of the granule cell (parallel fiber) synapses with the Purkinje cell. These spines contain a spine apparatus which is 5'-nucleotidase-positive (Marani, 1977, Fig. 6). The spine apparatus has the same ultrastructural appearance as the subsurface cisternae. The 5'-nucleotidase reaction product position appears to be identical in the subsurface cisternae and spine apparatus (compare Figs. 5 and 6). Parallel fibers are small caliber unmyelinated axons, which make synaptic contact with spines, stellate cells, basket cells and Golgi cells, by producing boutons en passage on these structures. The parallel fiber contains reaction products, which accumulate in tubular structures (i.e. microtubules). This electron density is absent from control incubations.

5'-Nucleotidase reaction products are not only found in the axon, but also in the parallel fiber boutons en passage (Figs. 6 and 7). In these boutons 5'-nucleotidase reaction products are localized in membrane bound spaces (cisternae?) always closely adjacent to a mitochondrion. Sometimes the mitochondrion is engulfed by cisternae containing the reaction product (Fig. 6). Cisternae containing reaction product have irregular contours that resemble buds (Fig. 8). As measured by the criteria developed in the introduction, stellate cells cannot be regarded as containing 5'-nucleotidase activity. In sections treated with 1,3.c-glyceromonophosphate, a specific inhibitor for inspecific phosphatase, these cells are negative for 5'-nucleotidase (Fig. 1D and E). However, some structures synapsing on stellate cells, or on stellate protrusions do show such a reaction. These structures have the characteristics of parallel fiber boutons, and contain 5'-nucleotidase reaction products in their mitochondria engulfing cisternae (Fig. 9).

The baskets around Purkinje cell somas were never found to be positive for 5'-nucleotidase reaction products. Basket cells themselves never contained 5'-nucleotidase activity in our experiments. In contrast, in sections treated for light microscopic purposes with chloroform: ether = 1:1, the baskets around Purkinje cells definitely became positive for localized reaction products. Profiles of Bergmann glia within the molecular layer were not found to be positive for 5'-nucleotidase activity. On one occasion, in a section not treated with an unspecific phosphatase inhibitor, these glial structures did contain some reaction product. In our material, the climbing fiber axon and the climbing fiber boutons were negative.

DISCUSSION

It should be clear from the introductory remarks that the lead products identified with our electron microscopic cytochemical method can only represent a small fraction of the activity of the enzyme 5'-nucleotidase, present in vivo. Inhibition by glutaraldehyde and Pb-ions further diminish 5'-nucleotidase activity, and the resolution of the method is diminished by its solubility. Nevertheless, since only one isoenzyme is present in the cerebellum of the mouse (Marani, 1981) all remaining activity must belong to the same type of 5'-nucleotidase. Still the question remains whether these results are representative of the overall 5'-nucleotidase localisation. It is obvious that negative results do not exclude the presence of 5'-nucleotidase. The positive results, however, consistently show localization in Purkinje cell dendrites and parallel fibers. The results of our study demonstrate an intracellular localization of 5'-nucleotidase in cisternae of both the pre- and post synaptic element of the parallel fiber (granular cell) - Purkinje cell synapse. Localizations for 5'-nucleotidase were deemed unacceptable when these coincided with nonspecific phosphatase activity. Arguments supporting the 5'-nucleotidase localizations are:

a) results from differential centrifugation studies show that 5'-nucleotidase activity is present in the synaptosomal fractions under biochemical optimal conditions (Marani, 1977).
b) destruction of climbing fibers with 3-acetylpyridine leaves the homologous 5'-nucleotidase pattern in rats unaltered, thereby excluding a primary localization of 5'-nucleotidase in climbing fibers (Marani, unpublished results).
c) light microscopic results are consistent with distribution in Purkinje cell dendrites (Scott, 1965, 1967, Fig. 2).
d) transection of the parallel fibers in the molecular layer of mice does not result in disappearance of the banding pattern (Marani, unpublished results). This indicates that other structures (i.e. Purkinje cells) must be involved in its generation.

One of the main results obtained from this study is evidence for the existence of two biochemically distinct populations of Purkinje cells in the cerebellum of the mouse, which differ with respect to the presence of 5'-nucleotidase in their dendrites. This difference may be related to the presence in the rat of two classes of Purkinje cells, those which react to the administration of various adenine derivatives with an increase in firing rate and those which do not respond to these agents (Kostopoulos, Limacher and Phillis, 1975). In mice the 5'-nucleotidase in positive Purkinje cells is contained in the dendrites. The somata of these cells are negative for 5'-nucleotidase, but possess nonspecific phosphatase activity at pH 7.2. The presence of 5'-nucleotidase both in the subsurface cisternae and in the spine apparatus of dendritic thorns, supports the notion of the continuity of these parts of the endoplasmatic reticulum (Palay and Chan-Palay, 1974). Because 5'-nucleotidase is thought to be a glycoprotein, the specific binding of concavelin A in subsurface cisternae of rat Purkinje cell dendrites (Wood, McLaughlin and Barber, 1974) closely agrees with our results.

It must be concluded from our observations that parallel fibers are 5'-nucleotidase positive only over part of their length. Although nothing definite is known about the length of parallel fibers in mice, it certainly exceeds the width of the 5'-nucleotidase positive bands, which varies between 0.1 and 0.4 mm. 5'-Nucleotidase reaction products appear to be present in the parallel fiber boutons in structures which look like synaptic vesicles. This would give the transmitter-modulator adenosine direct access to neurotransmitter at the parallel fiber - Purkinje cell synapse. We cannot conceive of a morphological experiment which could test this hypothesis.

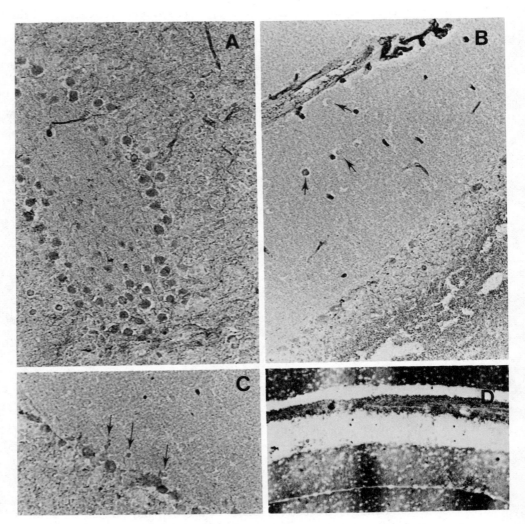

Fig.1 This figure demonstrates nonspecific phosphatase localization using beta-glycerophosphate activity in Purkinje cells and
basket cell axons.B demonstrates enzymatic activity in blood
vessels and in some stellate cells(arrows).In C nonspecific
phosphatase activity is present in basket cell somata.Arrows indicate nonspecific phosphatase activity in basket cell somata.
D shows an overall view of the experiment (H 8553) incubated for
2 hours in the Scott incubation medium with 1,3.c-glyceromono-
phosphate,demonstrating lack of 5'-nucleotidase in most cell
bodies present in the cerebellar molecular and granular layers.

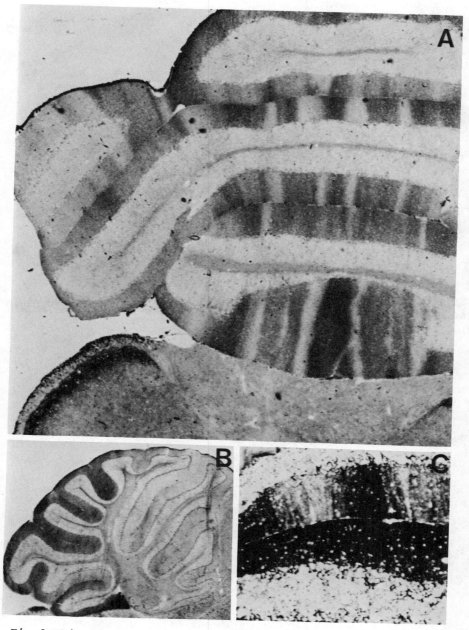

Fig.2 This figure demonstrates 5'-nucleotidase localization in
the mouse cerebellum(Scott 1965).A illustrates the longitudinal
pattern of 5'-nucleotidase in the posterior lobe.B reveals the
5'-nucleotidase location in a sagittal section.C shows the
striped appearance of the bands in a transverse section.

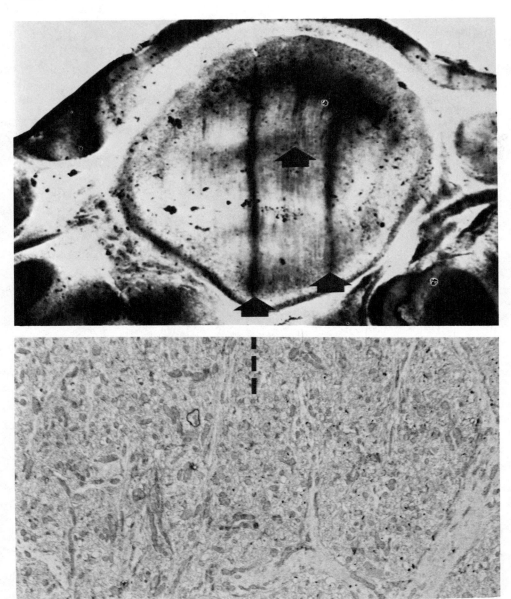

Fig.3 The top figure shows a vibratome section (200 mu) treated with sulfide after incubation in 5'-nucleotidase medium.Three parallel positive bands in the anterior lobe of the mouse cerebellum are seen(arrows).The bottom figure shows the sharp contrast even in E.M. photographs of the transition of 5'-nucleotidase positive to negative areas in an oblique section .The interrupted vertical line indicate the border.

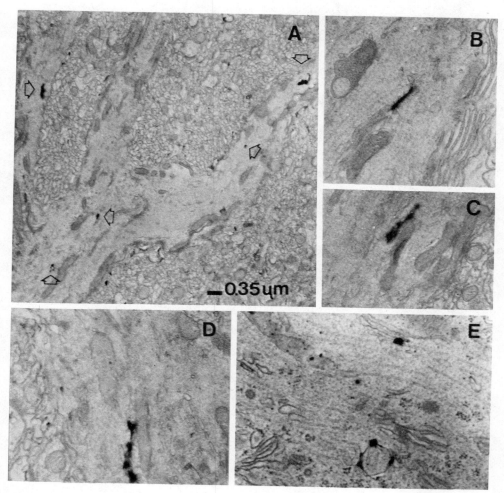

Fig.4 Localization of 5'-nucleotidase reaction products in the
smooth endoplasmic reticulum (SER) of Purkinje cell dendritic
trees are demonstrated in A to E.A shows a Purkinje cell dendrite
with 5'-nucleotidase reaction product located exclusively in the
SER,indicated by arrows.B and C show two cisternae of the SER that
are positive for 5'-nucleotidase.D is taken at the base of the
main Purkinje cell dendritic tree.E reveals a circular cisterna
of the SER filled with 5'-nucleotidase reaction product.Note that
in E ribosomes are present near this circular cisterna(method B,
see Experimental Procedures).

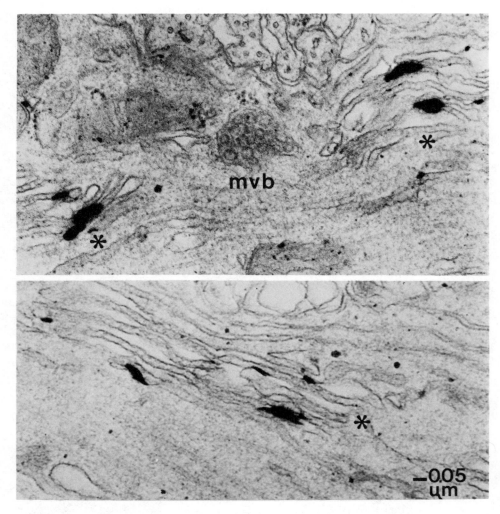

Fig.5 This figure shows two E.M.photographs of Purkinje cell dendritic subsurface cisternae(asterisks),in which 5'-nucleotidase
reaction products are localized.MVB:multi-vesicular body.

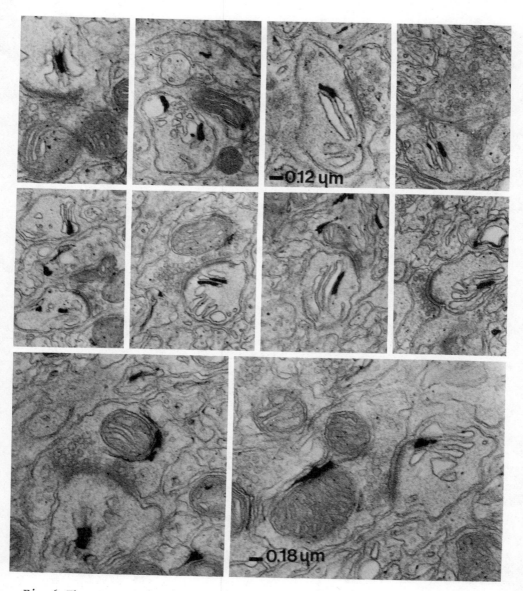

Fig.6 The upper eight electron micrographs demonstrate Purkinje cell dendritic spines,with or without synapting parallel fibers. 5'-Nucleotidase reaction products are confined to the cisternal spaces of the spine apparatus.The two micrographs at the bottom of the page reveal Purkinje cell dendritic spines positive for 5'-nucleotidase ,synapting on 5'-nucleotidase positive parallel fiber boutons(examples taken from method A and B).

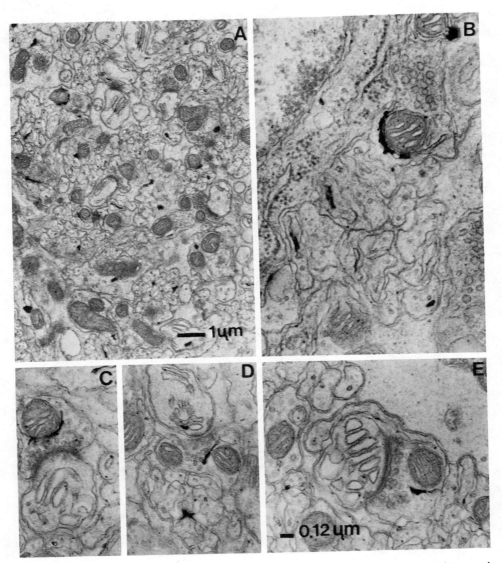

Fig.7 A demonstrates the overall localization of 5'-nucleotidase in
the molecular layer neuropil.B,C,D,E show parallel fiber boutons
synapting on Purkinje cell dendritic spines.These boutons are
5'-nucleotidase positive within the cisternal space surrounding
mitochondria.B also reveals that parallel fibers contain 5'-nucleo-
tidase activity(examples from method A and B),while the bouton is
localized near a stellate perikaryon.

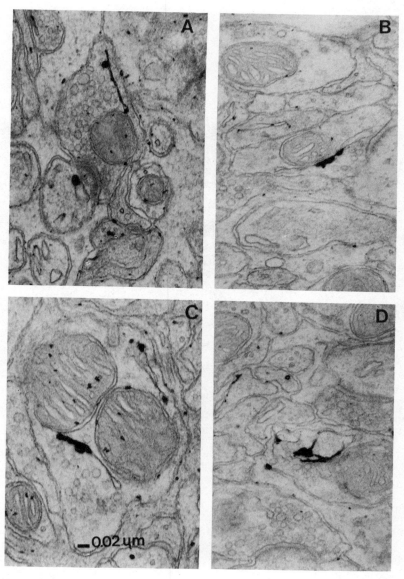

Fig.8 These four electron micrographs show 5'-nucleotidase reaction products within parallel fiber boutons.The fine cisternae,
located near mitochondria ,seem to be undergoing exocytosis.
A,B,and C demonstrates bulges that contain reaction products,
while D demonstrates that these cisternae are more complex than
would be expected from A,B,and C.Examples taken from methods A
and B

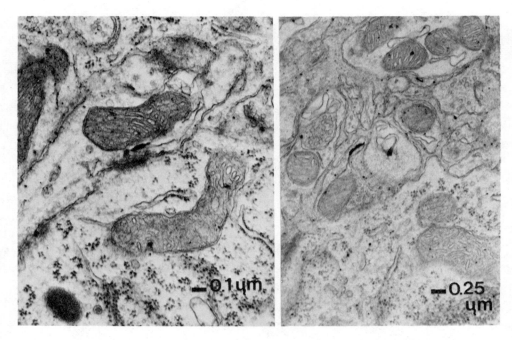

Fig.9 Two positive parallel fiber boutons are shown, synapting on
stellate cell soma. Examples taken from methods A and B.

Barka T., and Anderson, P.J., 1962, Histochemical methods for acid phosphatase using hexazonium pararosanilin as coupler. J. Histochem. Cytochem., 10: 741.

Brederoo, P., Daems, W. Th., Van Duyn, P., and Van der Ploeg, M., 1968, Quantitative investigations on the effect of aldehyde fixation on acid phosphatase activity, in: "Electron Microscopy", vol. 2, D.S. Bocciarelli, ed., Tipografia Poliglotta Vaticana, Roma.

Kostopoulos, G.K., Limacher, J.J., and Phillis, J.W., 1975, Action of various adenine derivatives on cerebellar Purkinje cells. Brain Res., 88: 162.

Marani, E., 1977, The subcellular distribution of 5'-nucleotidase activity in mouse cerebellum. Exp. Neurol., 57: 1042.

Marani, E., 1981, Enzymehistochemistry, in: "Methods in Neurobiology", vol. I, R. Lahue, ed., Plenum, New York.

Marani, E., 1980, 5'-Nucleotidase in der Molekularschicht des Rattenkleinhirns. Nur rhythmische Veränderungen der unspezifischen Phosphatasen, Acta Histochemica, Suppl. Band XXI, S. 237.

Marani, E., and Boekee, A., 1975, Aspects histoenzymologiques de la localisation de l'adenylcyclase, de la c.3',5'-nucléotide phosphodiestérase, de la 5'-nucléotidase et de l'alpha-glucanphosphorylase dans le cervelet de la souris, Bull. de l'Assoc. Anat. (Nancy), 57: 555.

Marani, E., and Voogd, J., 1973, Some aspects of the localization of the enzyme 5'-nucleotidase in the molecular layer of the cerebellum of the mouse, Acta Morphol. Neerl.-Scand., 11: 353.

Palay, S.L., and Chan-Palay, V., 1974, Cerebellar cortex. Cytology and Organization, Springer Verlag, Berlin, Heidelberg, New York.

Rinvik, E., and Grofová, J., 1970, Observations on the fine structure of the substantia nigra in the cat. Exp. Brain Res., 11: 229.

Scott, T.G., 1965, The specificity of 5'-nucleotidase in the brain of the mouse. J. Histochem. Cytochem., 13: 657.

Scott, T.G., 1967, The distribution of 5'-nucleotidase in the brain of the mouse, J. Comp. Neurol., 129: 97.

Wood, J.G., McLaughlin, B.J., and Barber, R.P., 1974, The visualization of concanavalin A binding sites in Purkinje cell somata and dendrites of rat cerebellum, J. Cell Biol., 63: 541.

MONOSODIUM GLUTAMATE (M.S.G.) EFFECTS ON ARCUATE CELLS AT PUBERTY

E. Marani[1], W.J. Rietveld[2] and M.E. Boon[3]

Laboratory of Anatomy[1] and Department of Physiology[2]
Leiden University, S.S.D.Z.[3] Delft, The Netherlands

The administration of M.S.G. results in the destruction of the arcuate dopaminergic cells in the hypothalamic area A_{12}. The M.S.G. effect on these cells was studied after the discovery that dopaminergic perikarya underwent a displacement from the median eminence (M.E.) towards the arcuate nucleus (ARC) similar to that, which has also been described for catalase positive cells in these areas (Marani et al. in press).

M.S.G. was administered intraperitoneally to female rats as described in a previous paper (Rietveld et al., 1979), and the brains studied at various survival times using a fluorescence technique (de la Torre et al., 1975). A new phenomenon was established, the migration of fluorescent perikarya from the ME towards the ARC. The fluorescence of dopaminergic and noradrenergic structures in normal rats starts in the E.M. at day 12 to 15 after birth. The fluorescent area is then displaced towards the lateral edge of the M.E. with an extension directed away from the pial surface into the hypothalamic area. This position is just beneath the ARC. At day 35 after birth the first cell bodies leave this area and are found just beneath the ARC. Between days 45 and 55 the perikarya are found within the arcuate nucleus, at 100 days and later a distinct subdivision can be noticed in the ARC. The fluorescence than exist in the dorsolateral part of this nucleus (A12).

In M.S.G. treated animals a brilliant fluorescence is already present at day 6 after birth. The described lateral shift takes place earlier in M.S.G. animals, around days 12 to 15 after birth. Between day 18 and 22 after birth the first somata are already leaving the lateral mitre shaped fluorescent area, at its extension towards

573

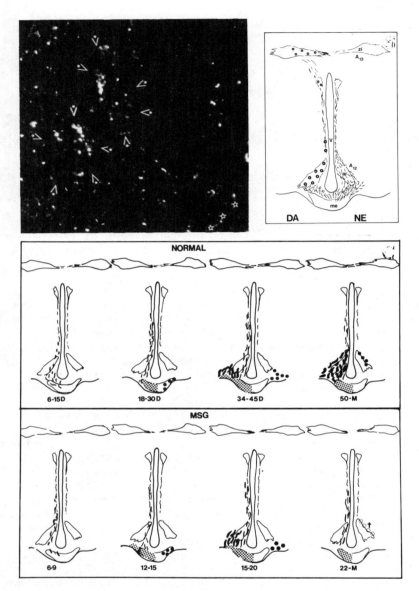

Figure 1.
This figure demonstrates in A. fluorescent cells just above the
mitre-like area, B. shows the topography of the involved dopaminergic (right side) and noradrenergic (left side) structures, C. gives
the time-comparison between normal and M.S.G. treated animals. The
final diagram shows at the left side the distribution of noradrenergic (fine lines) and dopaminergic (thick lines) varicosities.
The overall fluorescence is stippled. At the right side the displacement of cells (filled circles) is demonstrated.

the ARC. These fluorescent cells are never found in the ARC, presumably due to subsequent cell death as is also suggested by Nissl preparations.

These results indicate that the causation of death of fluorescent cells in the ARC has to be considered as a secondary effect. The primary effect of M.S.G. administered postnatally is the acceleration of the perikaryal migration due to the stimulation or de-inhibition of the normal processes before puberty. It can be argued that the neonatal M.S.G. administration effects the trigger mechanism of perikaryal migration in hypothalamic areas.

Marani, E., W.J. Rietveld, M.E. Boon and N.M. Gerrits. Fluores-
      displacement from the median eminence towards the arcuate
      nucleus at puberty.
      Accepted Histochemistry.
Rietveld, W.J., J.C. Osselton, N. Verwoerd and E.M. van Ingen,
      1979. The effect of monosodium glutamate on the endogenous
      peroxidase activity in the hypothalamic arcuate nucleus in
      rat. I.R.C.S. Medical Science 7, 573-574.
Torre, J.C. de la, and J.W. Surgeon, 1976. A methodological approach
      to rapid and sensitive M.A. histofluorescence using a modi-
      fied G.A. technique: The S.P.G. method.
      Histochemistry 49, 81-93.

THE AUTORADIOGRAPHIC LOCALIZATION OF BACLOFEN-SENSITIVE GABA$_B$

SITES IN RAT CEREBELLUM

G.P. Wilkin*, N.G. Bowery, D.R. Hill and A.L. Hudson

*Department of Biochemistry, Imperial College of
Science & Technology, London, SW7, England and
Department of Pharmacology, St. Thomas' Hospital
Medical School, London, SE1 7EH, London

The existence of a receptor for GABA on neurons of the mammalian peripheral and central nervous systems is now firmly established
and radiolabelled ligand binding studies have supported the view
that bicuculline prevents GABA from interacting with membrane
recognition sites (Zukin et al. 1974, Enna et al. 1978).   Such
studies have usually been performed using non-physiological media
and in the absence of divalent cations.   Recently, however, it has
been shown in one of our laboratories that the presence of either
Ca^{++} or Mg^{++} ions in the incubation media at an optimal concentration of 2.5mM reveals a second population of GABA binding sites
(Hill and Bowery, 1981).   These sites are insensitive to bicuculline and to the majority of accepted GABA-mimetics such as
3-aminopropanesulphonic acid (3-APS) or isoguvacine but sensitive
to the β-ρ-chlorophenyl derivative of GABA, baclofen.   The bicuculline-sensitive site has been designated as the GABA$_A$ receptor and
the baclofen sensitive site as the GABA$_B$ receptor (Hill and Bowery,
1981).   In vitro experiments have demonstrated that the interaction
of GABA with the B sites reduces the evoked release of certain
neurotransmitters in preparations of both peripheral and central
nervous tissue (Bowery et al. 1980 and Bowery et al. 1981) and these
data are compatible with a presynaptic location for GABA$_B$ receptors.
It was obviously of great interest to us to determine the morphological distribution of these receptor sites in the mammalian nervous
system and this report summarizes some of our preliminary findings.

A regional study of GABA binding to membrane preparations from
the rat CNS revealed that GABA$_A$ sites were present in greater
amounts than GABA$_B$ sites and interestingly that a relatively constant
ratio of GABA$_A$:GABA$_B$ sites of 3 or 4:1 were present in all regions
studied (Fig.1).   The highest concentration of GABA$_B$ sites was

577

found in the cerebellum and hence this region was chosen for our
initial morphological studies.

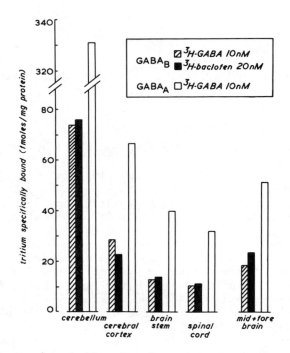

Fig.1.   The regional distribution of GABA binding sites in
rat brain preparations.   6% homogenates of separated brain
regions were made in 0.32M sucrose and centrifuged at 1000g
for 10min, and the supernatants recentrifuged at 2000g for
20min.   Pellets were then resuspended in the original volume
of distilled water and centrifuged at 4800g for 20min.   They
were then frozen at -15°C.   Prior to assay each pellet was
thawed at room temperature for about 30min before four washes
in 6ml tris-HCl buffer (pH 7.4, 50mM) containing $CaCl_2$ and
40μM isoguvacine (to prevent binding to the A site) for $GABA_B$
site, or tris-citrate buffer (pH 7.4, 50mM) for $GABA_A$ site
binding.   Pellets derived from the various regions were
suspended in the media (1-1.5mg protein per 0.8ml solution
determined by the method of Lowry et al) for the assay.   To
each 0.8ml aliquot 0.1ml of incubation medium with or without
1mM (±) baclofen ($GABA_B$ site) or 1mM isoguvacine ($GABA_A$ site)
was added.   A further 0.1ml containing [^{3}H]baclofen or [^{3}H]
GABA was added to provide final concentrations of 20nM or
10nM respectively.   Each tube was incubated for 10min at 20°C
and then centrifuged at 7000g for 10min.   The supernatant was
aspirated off and the pellet blotted dry before addition of
100μl of Soluene and then scintillation fluid.

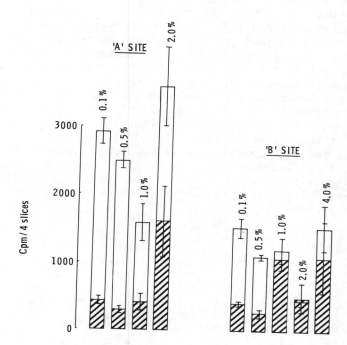

Fig.2. Binding of [³H]GABA to A and B sites in cryostat sections of cerebellum following perfusion fixation of rat brain with various concentrations of formaldehyde fixative. Rats were anaesthetised with pentobarbitone sodium (60mg/Kg ip) and the brains fixed by intracardiac perfusion with a number of concentrations of formaldehyde (shown over the histograms) in phosphate buffered saline (0.01M phosphate pH 7.4, 10min perfusion with 200ml). Saggital slices (10μm thick) of cerebellum were obtained by cryostat section and four slices placed on a single glass slide. The slices were dried at ambient temperature for 1h before freezing at -20°C. Prior to use slices were allowed to thaw and dry for approximately 45min and then washed for 50min by immersion in 250ml tris-HCl (50mM pH 7.4 containing 2.5mM CaCl₂, B sites) or tris-citrate (50mM pH 7.4, A sites) containing 190mM sucrose. Each slide was then air dried for 10-15min after removal of excess fluid. They were then incubated for 15min with 100μl (±) baclofen (B sites). Isoguvacine 40nM was added to those samples used for B site binding to suppress binding to A sites. The slides were then shaken separately to remove excess incubation solution and the bound radioactivity determined using liquid scintillation counting. Means and standard errors for 3 slices in each case are shown.
    Shaded areas = non-specific binding.

The method chosen for the localization of GABA binding sites was a modification of that described by Young and Kuhar (1979). This procedure utilizes lightly-fixed cryostat sections to which the radiolabelled ligand is bound and the disintegrations are detected through the application of an emulsion coated coverslip. This method allows measurement of the characteristics of ligand binding as well as autoradiography of adjacent cryostat sections. Preliminary experiments were performed to determine the effect of various concentrations of formaldehyde fixation (prepared from paraformaldehyde) on the binding of [^{3}H]GABA to A and B sites (Fig.2). At the concentrations below 0.5% formaldehyde saturable binding was readily detected and seemed to be independent of the fixative concentration, whereas above this concentration (up to 4%) it was markedly reduced and extremely variable. For all the further experiments described here perfusion was carried out using 0.1% formaldehyde.

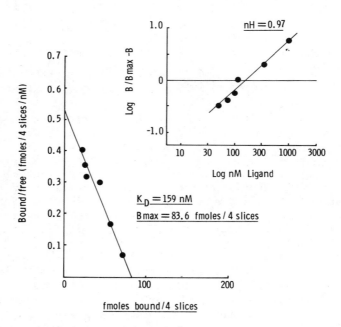

Fig.3. Scatchard analysis of [^{3}H]GABA binding to B sites in cerebellar slices. The binding experiments were performed as described in the legend to Fig.2. The Hill plot shown in the upper right hand of the figure indicates the non-cooperative nature of the binding.

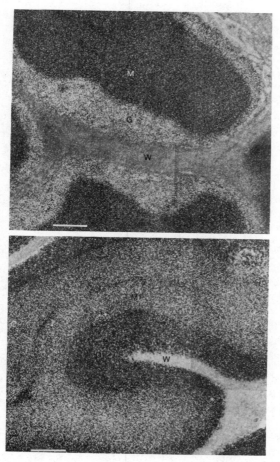

Fig. 4. Light microscopic darkfield autoradiograms of [^{3}H]
GABA binding to GABA$_A$ sites (above) and GABA$_B$ sites (below).
Binding was carried out as described in the legend to Fig.2.
The autoradiographic procedure was carried out by modification
of the method as described by Young and Kuhar (1979) using
Ilford K$_5$ emulsion.   The greatest concentration of GABA$_A$ binding sides can be seen over the granule cell layer whereas the
greatest concentration of GABA$_B$ sites is over the molecular
layer.   The greyish cast over the white matter in the upper
photograph and the stronger white colour over the white matter
in the lower photograph are due to a light scattering effect.
Grain counts over the white matter in these slides were found
to be very close to those obtained in control slides.
M = molecular layer, G = granule cell layer, W = White matter.
Autoradiographic exposure = 12 days.   Scale bar = 300µm.

A time course of [³H]GABA binding to B sites using a fixed (50nM) concentration of the ligand revealed that in excess of 85% of the specific binding had occurred by 15 min and this time was used in all subsequent experiments.

Scatchard analysis of specific [³H]GABA binding to GABA$_B$ sites in cerebellar slices showed a single saturable binding component Kd=159nM, B max 83.6 fmoles/4 slices (Hill coefficient = 0.97,Fig.3). The apparent affinity of this component was therefore a little lower in slices than previously found in homogenates (Kd=77nM, Hill and Bowery 1981).

[³H]GABA bound to GABA$_B$ sites in cryostat sections was displaceable by analogues shown previously to be active at GABA$_B$ sites in homogenates as well as whole tissue assays.   GABA and (-) baclofen displaced [³H]GABA with IC$_{50}$ values of 120nM.   The IC$_{50}$ values for other analogues were (±) baclofen 400nM, muscimol 2μM, 3APS 12.6μM and (+) baclofen 15.8μM.   The order of potency is in agreement with the analogue specificity observed previously in homogenates (Hill and Bowery 1981).   Bicuculline methobromide (100μM) was inactive as was the GABA transaminase inhibitor AOAA (100μM).   Three compounds which compete for the GABA uptake site DABA, nipecotic acid and cis-3-aminocyclohexane carboxylic acid (ACHC) had no effect on binding at a concentration of 10μM and reduced it by less than 20% at 100μM.   The IC$_{50}$ values were ≫1mM.

The good agreement between the pharmacological specificity found in slices and homogenates indicated that we could proceed with the autoradiography in slices.   The distribution of GABA$_A$ and GABA$_B$ sites was quite different (Fig.4).   The concentration of GABA$_A$ sites was highest in the granule cell layer and much less in the molecular layer whereas GABA$_B$ sites occurred mainly in the molecular layer.   The A site distribution was similar to that described by Palacios et al. (1980) who used [³H]muscimol as a ligand.   Grain counts revealed that there were equal numbers of A and B sites in the molecular layer 2.75 and 2.73 grains/100 sq.μm respectively, whereas there were more than three times this number of grains over the granule cell layer following GABA$_A$ binding (8.94 grains/100 sq. μm).

Concomitant experiments using slices from the same animal which were analyzed using scintillation spectrometry showed that when slices were incubated with [³H]GABA in the presence of Ca^{++} alone to obtain total GABA$_A$ and GABA$_B$ sites, the amount bound was the sum of the two figures obtained when the sites were analysed separately.

In summary this study has shown that Ca^{++} dependent GABA binding sites (GABA$_B$ sites) are found almost entirely within the molecular layer of rat cerebellum.   At the level of resolution obtained in the light autoradiographic technique used here, however, we are unable to determine the cellular location of these sites.   Further experimental approaches to determine their location are at present under way.

REFERENCES

Bowery, N.G., Doble, A., Hill, D.R., Hudson, A.L., Shaw, J.S., Turnbull, M.J., and Warrington, R. 1981. Bicuculline-insensitive GABA receptors on peripheral autonomic nerve terminals. Eur. J. Pharmac. 71, 53-70.

Bowery, N.G., Hill, D.R., Hudson, A.L., Doble, A., Middlemiss,D.N., Shaw, J. and Turnbull, M.J. 1980 (-) Baclofen decreases neurotransmitter release in the mammalian CNS by an action at a novel GABA receptor. Nature 283, 92-94.

Enna, S.J., Beaumont, K. and Yamamura, H.I. 1978 in Amino Acids as Neurotransmitters. (Ed. F. Fonnum). 487-492 Plenum New York

Hill, D.R. and Bowery, N.G. 1981 ^{3}H-baclofen and ^{3}H-GABA bind to bicuculline-insensitive GABA$_B$ sites in rat brain. Nature 290 149-152.

Palacios J.M., Young, W.S. and Kuhar, M.J. 1980 Autoradiographic localization of γ-aminobutyric acid (GABA) receptors in the rat cerebellum. Proc. Natn. Acad. Sci. U.S.A. 77 670-674.

Young, W.S. and Kuhar, M.J. 1979 A new method for receptor autoradiography : [^{3}H]opioid receptors in rat brain. Brain Research 179, 255-270.

Zukin, S.R., Young, A.B., Snyder, S.H. 1974. Gamma-aminobutyric acid binding to receptor sites in the rat central nervous system. Proc. Natn. Acad. Sci. U.S.A. 71 4802-4807.

EXCITATORY AMINO ACIDS IN THE CEREBELLUM:

RECEPTOR TYPES AND RECEPTIVE CELLS

John Garthwaite

Department of Veterinary Physiology and Pharmacology
University of Liverpool
Brownlow Hill, P.O. Box 147
Liverpool L69 3BX

INTRODUCTION

It now seems very likely that acidic amino acids (glutamate, aspartate and/or closely related compounds) are widely used as excitatory transmitters in the central nervous system (see Watkins & Evans, 1981). In the cerebellum, the evidence currently favours a role for glutamate as the transmitter of the granule cell parallel fibres while aspartate may operate as the climbing fibre transmitter (Young et al., 1974; Hudson et al., 1976; Sandoval & Cotman, 1978; Rea et al., 1980).

This article reviews results of some recent experiments aimed at further understanding certain aspects of excitatory amino acid action in the cerebellum, namely the association between activation of amino acid receptors and changes in the levels of cyclic GMP (cGMP) and the identification of the cell types on which the receptors are located.

EXCITATORY AMINO ACID RECEPTORS AND CYCLIC GMP

Of the different areas of the brain, the cerebellum is unusually enriched in cGMP and its associated enzymes (Steiner et al., 1972; Greengard, 1979). Previous evidence suggested that the levels of cerebellar cGMP could be markedly enhanced by activation of the parallel and climbing fibre pathways (Biggio & Guidotti, 1976; Rubin & Ferrendelli, 1977; Lundberg et al., 1979). Furthermore, glutamate injected intraventricularly (Mao et al., 1974; Briley et al., 1979) or added to slices in vitro (Ferrendelli et al., 1974; Garthwaite & Balazs, 1978) also induce an accumulation of cGMP. In

585

view of recent advances in the pharmacology of amino acid-mediated
excitation (Watkins & Evans, 1981), it seemed appropriate to examine
in more detail relationships between the activation of excitatory
amino acid receptors and changes in cGMP and to gain information on
the receptor types operating in the cerebellum.

Current evidence indicates that there may be at least three
pharmacologically distinct classes of excitant amino acid receptor
(Watkins & Evans, 1981; McLennan, 1981): receptors activated by
N-methyl-D-aspartate (NMDA) and, in some areas, by L-aspartate, and
blocked by the D-aminoadipate (DαAA) group of antagonists ("NMDA-
receptors"); receptors activated by quisqualate and L-glutamate and
antagonised by glutamate diethyl ester (GDEE) ("quisqualate-
receptors") and receptors activated by kainate, a structural analogue
of glutamate, but relatively resistant to the antagonists ("kainate-
receptors"). The excitants studied most thoroughly for their ability
to elevate cGMP levels were kainate, NMDA, L-glutamate and
L-aspartate (Garthwaite, 1982).

Adult Cerebellum

Application of the excitants to incubated slices of adult rat
cerebellum led to substantial increases in cGMP levels (Fig. 1a).
The dose-cGMP response curve to kainate, the most potent compound,
was biphasic, suggesting that two components (ED_{50} = 6 μM and 30 μM)
might be present. The next most effective agent was NMDA followed
by glutamate and aspartate. This order of potency conforms with the
relative excitatory potencies of these compounds in the central
nervous system (Watkins, 1978). Although the millimolar concentrations of glutamate and aspartate required to elevate cGMP may
seem rather high, they are similar to those required to elicit
excitation in cerebellar slices (Okamoto & Quastel, 1973). The concentrations in the vicinity of the receptors are likely to be much
less (Garthwaite & Balazs, 1981). Antagonist studies (Table 1a)
showed that responses to NMDA but not those to kainate, glutamate
and aspartate were inhibited significantly by DαAA. GDEE, on the
other hand, was most effective against glutamate with a lesser action
on responses to aspartate, NMDA and kainate.

These results indicate that the cGMP responses to the excitants
are receptor-mediated and that the receptor types operating in the
adult cerebellum fall into the same experimental categories as those
mediating central excitation as outlined above. The receptor type
activated predominantly by L-aspartate under these conditions appears
more GDEE-sensitive than DαAA-sensitive as found elsewhere in the
brain (McLennan, 1981) and conforming with its mode of excitation
of Purkinje cells (Crepel & Dhanjal, 1981).

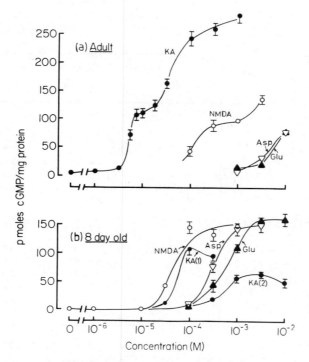

Fig. 1. Dose-response curves for cGMP accumulation in (a) adult and (b) immature (8 day old) cerebellar slices exposed to kainate(KA,●), NMDA (O), L-aspartate (Asp,▽) and L-glutamate (Glu, ▲). The slices were inactivated at the peaks of the responses (times given in Table 1); cGMP and protein were measured as described previously (Garthwaite & Balazs, 1978).

Immature Cerebellum

Responses were also examined in slices of the immature cerebellum in view of findings that glutamate could elicit surprisingly large increases in cGMP at an age (8 days) when the parallel fibres have largely to be developed and when the basal levels of cGMP are only about one tenth of their adult values (Garthwaite & Balazs, 1978).

Such large responses were not peculiar to glutamate (Fig. 1b). However, several differences in comparison with the adult cerebellum were apparent. Two components to kainate's action could be detected

TABLE 1.   EFFECTS OF ANTAGONISTS ON cGMP RESPONSES TO AMINO ACID
EXCITANTS IN ADULT AND IMMATURE RAT CEREBELLAR SLICES

Agonist	Exposure time[a] (min)	% Control cGMP levels	
		+DαAA (250 µM)	+GDEE (2.5mM)
(a) Adult cerebellum			
Kainate (30µM)	10	102	77*
NMDA (300µM)	5	45**	73
L-glutamate (10mM)	5	84	37****
L-aspartate (10mM)	5	88	60*
(b) Immature cerebellum			
Kainate (100µM)	1	99	41****
Kainate (1mM)	5	36****	57*
NMDA (100µM)	2	22****	66**
L-glutamate (1mM)	5	118	69*
L-aspartate (1mM)	2	96	50***

Asterisks indicate significant differences from control responses:
*$P<0.05$, **$P<0.02$, ***$P<0.002$, ****$P< 0.001$. N = 4 - 6.
[a] Exposure times correspond to the times giving peak cGMP responses
(Garthwaite 1982). Antagonists were added 5 min before the agonists.

kinetically: one was rapid (1 min to peak) and one slower (5 min)
and of lower amplitude (not shown). These two responses could be
further distinguished from each other by their different ED_{50} values
(60 µM and 400 µM; Fig. 1b) and by their differential antagonism:
the rapid response was inhibited strongly by GDEE but not by DαAA
whereas the slower component was most sensitive to DαAA (Table 1b).

Thus, in the immature cerebellum, kainate exhibited an overall
potency lower than in the adult and seemed to be exerting its effect,
directly or indirectly, via receptors other than the more conventional kainate receptors on which it acts primarily in the adult.

In contrast to kainate, the other excitants (glutamate, aspartate and NMDA) were all 5 to 10-fold more potent in the immature
tissue. This may relate to the larger extracellular spaces allowing
freer access to the receptors compared with the adult (Garthwaite et
al., 1980; Garthwaite & Balazs, 1981) although differences in the
numbers, distribution or kinetic properties of the receptors may
also be involved. DαAA retained its selectivity for NMDA responses

over those to glutamate and aspartate whereas GDEE produced a rather indiscriminate pattern of antagonism, with glutamate being the least affected (Table 1b) indicating that, despite its higher apparent potency, glutamate is not acting primarily by way of the GDEE-sensitive receptors instrumental in the adult. Aspartate responses were inhibited more by GDEE than DαAA, as in the adult, however.

IDENTIFICATION OF RECEPTIVE CELLS: NEUROTOXICITY

While the results discussed above allowed some understanding of the receptor types associated with increases in cGMP in the cerebellum, they provided little information on the identity of the cell types responding in this way. This was one of the chief reasons for examining the neurotoxic actions of the excitants.

The neurotoxicity of excitatory amino acids has received considerable interest both for producing selective neuronal lesions and for providing experimental models for various neurodegenerative disorders (see McGeer et al., 1978b). The precise mechanism of neurotoxic damage is presently uncertain but, like the cGMP responses, it does seem to be mediated through the activation of amino acid receptors (see McGeer et al., 1978b; Nadler, 1979; DiChiara & Gessa, 1981). Thus, identification of the cell types necrosed by the excitants combined with knowledge of the pharmacological properties of the receptors should yield information regarding the cellular distribution of the receptor types.

To examine the neurotoxicity of the excitants, cerebellar slices were employed. Compared with in vivo studies, slices offer many advantages. Notably, compounds can be applied in the absence of anaesthetic for known periods of time and in known concentrations which presumably bathe the cells uniformly. This approach should thus dispose of the many uncertainties associated with the application of kainate by micro-injection in vivo (McGeer & McGeer, 1978) and, furthermore, allow direct comparison with the cGMP data. Hitherto, the neurotoxic actions of kainate have been studied the most thoroughly.

Adult Cerebellum

In these experiments, a 30 min - 2 h exposure of the slices to kainate was found to be sufficient for the morphological changes to be monitored reliably. The patterns of necrosis at the different concentrations tested were unchanged if the exposure time was extended to 24 h.

At concentrations up to 3 μM, kainate produced no detectable cellular damage. At 5 μM (Fig. 2b) and more obviously at 10 μM (Fig. 2c), numerous swollen structures in the molecular layer could be seen and inhibitory interneurones were pyknotic with, frequently,

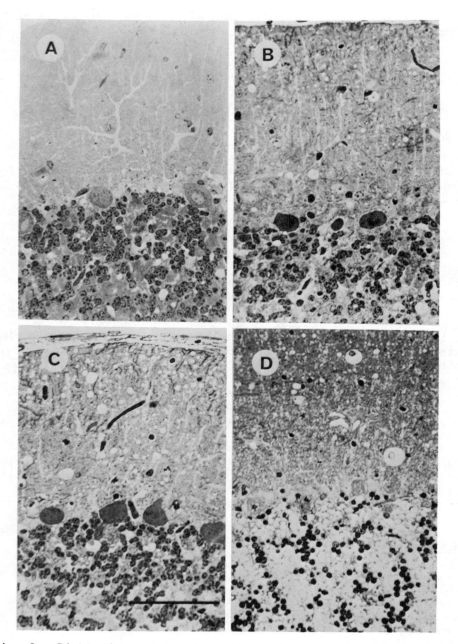

Fig. 2. Light micrographs of adult cerebellar slices incubated for
2 h. in the absence (a) or presence of 5 μM (b), 10 μM (c) or 30 μM
(d) kainate. Electron microscopy (Garthwaite & Wilkin, 1982) showed
the swelling in the granular layer in (d) to reside in the granule
cell dendritic digits.

highly expanded cytoplasms. Purkinje cell bodies and their dendrites
were darkly-staining. Under the electron microscope (not shown),
these cells were electron-dense, their endoplasmic reticulum and
Golgi apparatus expanded and nuclear chromatin clumped. Golgi cells
in the granule cell layer were similarly affected. Glial cells were
intact but their processes in the molecular layer were somewhat
swollen. In contrast to the other neurones, granule cell somata,
their axons (parallel fibres) and nerve terminals were normal in
appearance.

These morphological changes were reproduced if the concentration
of kainate was raised to 15 or 20 μM but at 30 μM additional effects
were evident (Fig. 2d). These consisted of a shrinkage of granule
cell bodies coupled with a massive dilatation of their dendrites
although the excitatory mossy fibre nerve endings in synaptic contact
with them appeared unaffected. Many of the Purkinje cells exposed to
this concentration had become extensively vacuolated.

Thus, over the concentration range 5 to 20 μM, kainate exerted
a selective toxic action on Purkinje cells and inhibitory interneurones in the slices while higher concentrations also affected the
granule cells. This pattern of vulnerability resembles closely that
found after microinjection of kainate in vivo (Herndon & Coyle,
1977). It should be stressed that the differences in concentration
producing no effect and selective damage (3 and 5 μM) and producing
selective damage and non-selective damage (20 and 30 μM) are rather
slight, which may help explain conflicting results obtained by
others in vivo (Lovell & Jones, 1980;   Foster & Roberts, 1980).

The concentration ranges inducing selective necrosis of Purkinje
cells and inhibitory interneurones on one hand and those affecting
granule cells on the other correlate remarkably well with the concentration ranges eliciting the two components to the dose-cGMP
response curve to kainate (Fig. 3a). This suggests that receptor
sites, differing in apparent affinity for kainate yet associated both
with cGMP increases and with neurotoxicity, are differentially located among the neuronal cell types in the cerebellum. This was
tested further by taking advantage of the fact that well-preserved
cells are required for the cGMP responses to the excitants to be
elicited (Garthwaite et al., 1979). If slices are exposed to 10 μM
kainate to induce selective necrosis of Purkinje cells and inhibitory
interneurones and are then allowed to 'rest' in kainate-free medium
for a further 2 h (no morphological recovery takes place), the higher
affinity component of the cGMP response is absent on subsequent exposure whereas the lower affinity response can still be elicited
(Table 2), supporting the postulate that this component is associated
with the granule cells.

The location of the most sensitive sites on Purkinje cells and
inhibitory interneurones would accord with the association of such

TABLE 2. KAINATE – INDUCED cGMP RESPONSES IN PRELESIONED
CEREBELLAR SLICES

| Kainate conc. | pmoles cGMP/mg protein | |
	Control	Prelesioned[a]
10 μM	104 ± 9	11 ± 5
100 μM	242 ± 30	106 ± 10

[a]Slices were exposed to 10μM kainate for 2 h in order to irreversibly
necrose Purkinje cells and inhibitory interneurones. After a 2 h
wash in kainate-free medium, the slices were further challenged for
10 min with kainate at the indicated concentrations. Results are
mean cGMP levels ± SEM.

receptors with cells receiving an excitatory amino acid-mediated
input, in this case the parallel fibres (cf. Biziere & Coyle, 1978;
Kohler et al., 1978; McGeer et al., 1978a; Malthe-Sorensen et al.,
1980; Streit et al., 1980). The transmitters for most of the mossy
fibres which excite granule cells, however, are presently unknown
and, given their diverse origins, different transmitters may well
operate in different fibres. Possibly, the receptors with a lower
affinity for kainate have a distribution which is less specific in
terms of the transmitter operating (Krammer et al., 1980) but which
may, nevertheless, be synaptically located (Foster et al., 1981) as
indicated by the most dramatic morphological changes being displayed
by the granule cell dendritic digits (c.f. Olney, 1981).

Immature Cerebellum

     The hypothesis that high vulnerability of specific cell types
to the neurotoxicity of kainate is dependent on the presence of
glutamate-containing nerve endings and that kainate and nerve ter-
minal-derived glutamate interact in some way to produce cellular
necrosis has received experimental support (Biziere & Coyle, 1978;
Kohler et al., 1978; McGeer et al., 1978a; Malthe-Sorensen et al.,
1980; Streit et al., 1980). It was of interest, therefore, to
examine the neurotoxicity of kainate in the immature cerebellum which
lacks a developed parallel fibre system (Altman, 1972) and, to judge
from the cGMP data, also lacks "true" kainate receptors (see above).

     Kainate neurotoxicity could still be demonstrated in the
immature tissue but higher concentrations were necessary: selective
damage to the Purkinje cells and inhibitory interneurones occurred
over the concentration range 30 to 300 μM and concentrations of 1mM

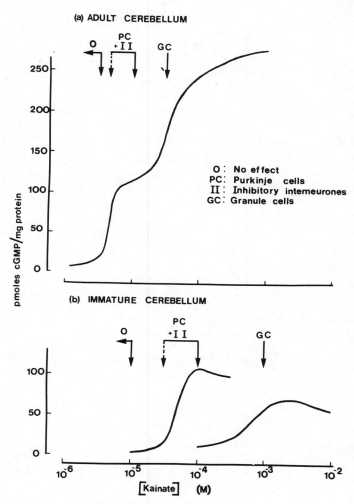

Fig. 3. Comparison between dose-cGMP response curves for kainate with concentrations exerting toxic effects on identified neuronal cell types in (a) adult and (b) immature cerebellar slices. Downward-pointing arrows show lowest concentrations at which necrosis was observed; broken arrows indicate partial effects.

or more were required to necrose granule cells in the internal layer (Fig. 4). The external (germinal) granule cell layer remained unaffected throughout except for some cells at its base which when exposed to 1 mM kainate exhibited a pattern of necrosis (pale nuclei and peripheral clumping of chromatin) similar to that seen in cells in the upper region of the internal granule cell layer.

Purkinje cells and inhibitory interneurones in the immature cerebellum were thus about 10-fold less sensitive to kainate neurotoxicity than in the adult while the reduction in vulnerability of the granule cells was even greater, about 30-fold. The cerebellum therefore appears similar to the striatum where high affinity kainate binding and neurotoxicity in the immature tissue is considerably less than in the adult and the development of these parameters correlates with the development of glutamatergic innervation in this region (Campochiaro & Coyle, 1978).

The concentration ranges exerting differential toxicity on the two groups of cells were again those eliciting two different components to the concentration-cGMP response curve (Fig. 3b). It seems likely, therefore, that in the immature cerebellum, the GDEE-sensitive receptors on which kainate acts are associated with Purkinje cells and inhibitory interneurones while the lower-affinity and more DαAA-sensitive sites are associated with the granule cells. The apparent relationship between excitatory amino acid receptors, cGMP responses and neurotoxicity was further strengthened by the observation that the replicating granule cells do not respond to kainate or other excitants with an increase in cGMP (Garthwaite & Balazs, 1978 and unpublished observations) and are highly resistant to kainate toxicity (Fig. 4). The susceptibility of the cells occupying the premigratory position in the external granule cell layer may then reflect the developmental timing of aquisition of receptors by these cells.

CONCLUSIONS

It seems clear that cGMP elevations occurring in the cerebellum on exposure to excitatory amino acids are mediated via the activation of receptor types showing properties expected of receptors eliciting excitation (Watkins & Evans, 1981). Recent pharmacological studies of the excitation of Purkinje cells in cerebellar slices by amino acid excitants (Crepel & Dhanjal, 1981) support this view. Thus, although cGMP responses might be remote from the primary event, their magnitude, the simplicity with which they can be measured and the faithfulness with which they reproduce electrophysiological data, make them a clear alternative to binding studies as a biochemical method for monitoring aspects of receptor activation.

The precise mechanism by which cGMP is elevated is, as yet, unclear but given the effectiveness of other agents such as K^+ and

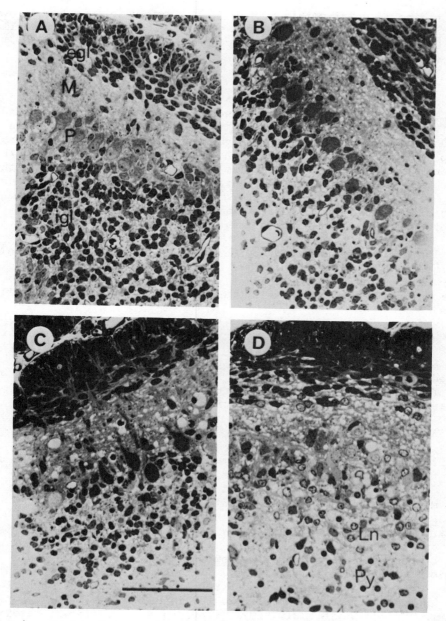

Fig. 4. Light micrographs of immature rat cerebellar slices incubated for 2 h. in the absence (a) or presence of 30 μM (b), 100 μM (c) or 1 mM (d) kainate. M: molecular layer; P: Purkinje cell layer; egl: external granule cell layer; igl: internal granule cell layer; Py: pyknotic cells; Ln: cells showing pale nuclei with peripheral clumping of chromatin.

veratridine in sharing this property, it is plausible that some event associated with neuronal depolarization (e.g. changes in intracellular Ca^{2+} concentrations) is involved (Ferrendelli et al., 1976; Ahnert et al., 1979).

By taking advantage of the neurotoxic properties of kainate, it proved possible to gain information regarding the cellular location of its sites of action. Thus, it seems likely that receptors sensitive to kainate are present on all the neuronal cell types in the cerebellum with those showing a higher apparent affinity for kainate being confined to Purkinje cells and inhibitory interneurones. While conventional kainate receptors seem to be little represented in the immature cerebellum, kainate appeared to be able to activate other receptor types, either directly or indirectly. The associated neurotoxic damage was consistent with these receptors also being differentially located amongst the different neuronal cell types.

The use of this approach can clearly be extended and is likely to prove valuable in examining the distribution of receptors for other related excitants as well as for probing the mechanism and possible prevention of excitatory amino acid-induced neuronal cell death.

ACKNOWLEDGMENTS

Most of the experiments described in this article were conducted at the M.R.C. Developmental Neurobiology Unit, London; I am grateful to Dr. R. Balazs for helpful discussions. The morphological studies were carried out in collaboration with Dr. G. P. Wilkin.

REFERENCES

Ahnert, G., Glossman, H. and Haberman, E., 1979. Investigations on the mechanism of cyclic guanosine monophosphate increase due to depolarizing agents as studied with sea anemone toxin II in mouse cerebellar slices. Naunyn-Schmiederberg's Arch. Pharmacol. 307: 159-166.

Altman, J.A., 1972. Postnatal development of the cerebellar cortex in the rat II. Phases in the maturation of Purkinje cells and of the molecular layer. J. Comp. Neurol., 145: 399-464.

Biggio, G. and Guidotti, A., 1976. Climbing fiber activation and 3', 5'-cyclic guanosine monophosphate (cGMP) content in cortex and deep nuclei of cerebellum. Brain Research 107: 365-373.

Biziere, K. and Coyle, J.T., 1978. Influence of cortico-striatal afferents on striatal kainic acid neurotoxicity. Neuroscience Lett. 8: 303-310.

Briley, P.A., Kouyoumdjian, J.C., Haidamous, M. and Gonnard, P., 1979. Effect of L-glutamate and kainate on rat cerebellar cGMP levels in vivo. Eur. J. Pharmacol. 54: 181-184.

Campochiaro, P. and Coyle, J.T., 1978. Ontogenetic development of kainate neurotoxicity: correlates with glutamatergic innervation. Proc. Nat. Acad. Sci. Wash. 75: 2025-2029.

Crepel, F. and Dhanjal, S.S., 1981. Sensitivity of Purkinje cell dendrites to glutamate and aspartate in cerebellar slices maintained in vitro. J. Physiol. in press.

DiChiara, G. and Gessa, G.L., 1981. "Glutamate as a Neurotransmitter", Raven Press, New York.

Ferrendelli, J.A., Chang, M.M. and Kinscherf, D.A., 1974. Elevation of cyclic GMP levels in central nervous system by excitatory and inhibitory amino acids. J. Neurochem. 22: 535-540.

Ferrendelli, J.A., Rubin, E.H. and Kinscherf, D.A., 1976. Influence of divalent cations on regulation of cyclic GMP and cyclic AMP levels in brain tissue. J. Neurochem. 26: 741-748.

Foster, A.C., Mena, E.E., Monaghan, D.T. and Cotman, C.W., 1981. Synaptic localization of kainic acid binding sites. Nature, Lond. 289: 73-75.

Foster, A.C. and Roberts, P.J., 1980. Morphological and biochemical changes in the cerebellum induced by kainic acid in vivo. J. Neurochem. 34: 1191-1200.

Garthwaite, J., 1982. Excitatory amino acid receptors and cyclic GMP in incubated slices of immature and adult rat cerebellum. Submitted for publication.

Garthwaite, J. and Balazs, R., 1978. Supersensitivity to the cyclic GMP response to glutamate during cerebellar maturation. Nature Lond. 275: 328-329.

Garthwaite, J. and Balazs, R., 1981. Excitatory amino acid-induced changes in cyclic GMP levels in slices and cell suspensions from the cerebellum, in: "Glutamate as a Neurotransmitter", G. DiChiara and G.L. Gessa, eds., pp. 317-326, Raven Press, New York.

Garthwaite, J. and Wilkin, G.P., 1982. Kainic acid-induced neurotoxicity in adult and immature rat cerebellar slices: correlation with cyclic GMP stimulation. Submitted for publication.

Garthwaite, J., Woodhams, P.L., Collins, M.J. and Balazs, R., 1979. On the preparation of brain slices: morphology and cyclic nucleotides. Brain Research 173: 373-377.

Garthwaite, J., Woodhams, P.L., Collins, M.J. and Balazs, R., 1980. A morphological study of incubated slices of rat cerebellum in relation to postnatal age. Devel. Neurosci. 3: 90-99.

Greengard, P., 1979. Cyclic nucleotides, phosphorylated proteins, and the nervous system. Federation Proc. 38: 2208-2219.

Herndon, R.M. and Coyle, J.T., 1977. Selective destruction of neurons by a transmitter agonist. Science 198: 71-72.

Hudson, D.B., Valcana, T., Bean, G. and Timiras, P.S., 1976. Glutamic acid, a strong candidate as the neurotransmitter of the cerebellar granule cell. Neurochem. Res. 1: 73-81.

Kohler, C., Schwarcz, R. and Fuxe, K., 1978. Perforant path transections protect hippocampal granule cells from kainate lesion. Neuroscience Lett. 10: 241-246.

Krammer,E.B., Lischka, M.F. and Sigmund, R., 1980. Neurotoxicity of kainic acid: evidence against an interaction with excitatory glutamate receptors in rat olfactory bulbs. Neuroscience Lett. 16: 329-334.

Lovell, K.L. and Jones, M.Z., 1980. Kainic acid neurotoxicity in the mouse cerebellum. Brain Research 186: 245-249.

Lundberg, D.B.A., Breese, G.R., Mailman, R.B., Frye, G.D. and Mueller, R.A., 1979. Depression of some drug-induced in vivo changes of cerebellar guanosine 3', 5'-monophosphate by control of motor and respiratory responses. Molec. Pharmacol. 15: 246-256.

Malthe-Sorensen, D., Odden, E. and Walaas, I., 1980. Selective destruction of neurons innervated by putative glutamatergic afferents in the septum and nucleus of the diagonal band. Brain Research 182: 461-466.

Mao, C.C., Guidotti, A. and Costa, E., 1974. The regulation of cyclic guanosine monophosphate in rat cerebellum: possible involvement of putative amino acid neurotransmitters. Brain Research 79: 510-514.

McGeer, E.G. and McGeer, P.L., 1978. Some factors influencing the neurotoxicity of intrastriatal injections of kainic acid. Neurochem Res. 3: 501-517.

McGeer, E.G., McGeer, P.L. and Singh, K., 1978a. Kainate-induced degeneration of neostriatal neurons: dependency upon cortico-striatal tract. Brain Research 139: 381-383.

McGeer, E.G., Olney, J.W. and McGeer, P.L., 1978b. "Kainic Acid as a Tool in Neurobiology", Raven Press, New York.

McLennan, H., 1981. On the nature of the receptors for various excitatory amino acids in the mammalian central nervous system, in: "Glutamate as a Neurotransmitter", G. DiChiara and G.L. Gessa, eds., pp. 253-262, Raven Press, New York.

Nadler, J.V., 1979. Kainic acid: neurophysiologic and neurotoxic actions. Life Sci. 24: 289-300.

Okamoto, K. and Quastel, J.H., 1973. Spontaneous action potentials in isolated guinea-pig cerebellar slices: effects of amino acids and conditions affecting sodium and water uptake. Proc. R. Soc. Lond. B. 184: 83-90.

Olney, J.W., 1981. Kainic acid and other neurotoxins, in: "Glutamate as a Neurotransmitter", G. DiChiara and G.L. Gessa, eds. pp. 375-384, Raven Press, New York.

Rea, M.A., McBride, W.J. and Rohde, B.M., 1980. Regional and synaptosomal levels of amino acid neurotransmitters in the 3-acetylpyridine deafferentated rat cerebellum. J. Neurochem. 34: 1106-1108.

Rubin, E.H. and Ferrendelli, J.A., 1977. Distribution and regulation of cyclic nucleotide levels in cerebellum, in vivo. J. Neurochem. 29: 43-51.

Sandoval, M.E. and Cotman, C.W., 1978. Evaluation of glutamate as a neurotransmitter of cereballar parallel fibres. Neuroscience 3: 199-206.

Steiner, A.L., Ferrendelli, J.A. and Kipnis, D.M., 1972. Radio-
    immunoassay for cyclic nucleotides. III Effect of ischaemia
    changes during development and regional distribution of adeno-
    sine 3', 5'-monophosphate and guanosine 3', 5'-monophosphate in
    mouse brain. J. Biol. Chem. 247: 1121-1124.
Streit, P., Stella, M. and Cuenod, M., 1980. Kainate-induced lesion
    in the optic tectum: dependency upon optic nerve efferents or
    glutamate. Brain Research 187: 47-57.
Watkins, J.C. and Evans, R.H., 1981. Excitatory amino acid trans-
    mitters. Ann. Rev. Pharmacol. Toxicol. 21: 165-204.
Young, A., Oster-Granite, M., Herndon, R. and Snyder, S.H., 1974.
    Glutamic acid: selective depletion by viral-induced granule
    cell loss in hamster cerebellum. Brain Research 37: 1-13.

PHYSIOLOGICAL AND CHEMICAL CONTROL OF HIPPOCAMPAL NEURONES

Per Andersen

Institute of Neurophysiology, U. of Oslo
Karl Johansgt. 47, Oslo 1, Norway

INTRODUCTION

The hippocampus is part of the limbic system.   It
represents the most simple of the cortical regions and
is comprised of several, strip-like cortical elements,
adjoining each other.   The overall position of the hippocampus in the rodent brain is indicated in Fig. 1A.   Here,
the outline of the hippocampus is drawn superimposed on
the lateral aspect of the brain.   In rodents, it has a
relatively large volume.   On ascending the phylogenetic
scale its relative size decreases.   The absolute volume
increases, however, and is highest in man and whales.
Dorsally and anteriorally it borders the septal region
whereas the amygdala nuclear complex is found anterior
and medial to its temporal pole.   Along its caudal border
lies the entorhinal area which is part of the hippocampal
gyrus.

In recent years, great interest has focused upon
the hippocampus for several reasons.   First, interference
with hippocampus or hippocampus-near structures have
given rise to memory deficits in man (Scoville and
Milner, 1957).   Second, animal experiments have indicated
that the hippocampus may be important for spatial memory
or tasks associated with handling of spatial coordinates
(O'Keefe and Nadel, 1978;   Olton and Feustle, 1981).
Thirdly, the hippocampus has been proposed to be involved
in certain mental disorders, notably those associated

601

with depression (MacLean, 1955). The basis for this has
been its connection with the amygdala and certain regions
and its contents of neuromodulators (Hökfelt et al., 1974).
Finally, a major reason for many researchers has been its
great degree of order which invites many experiments to
be done.

Overall Organization of the Hippocampal Formation

     Fig. 1B shows the temporal half of the hippocampal
cortex and how it is curved both around a longitudinal
and a transverse axis. The different cortical elements
which are bordering each other to compose the hippocampal
formation are indicated with different symbols. Comparing
these symbols with the unfolded cortical structure in Fig.
1C, one gets an idea how the cortex is composed of at
least five parallel and neighbouring strips. These strips
are further folded around a longitudinal axis (Fig. 1B,D).

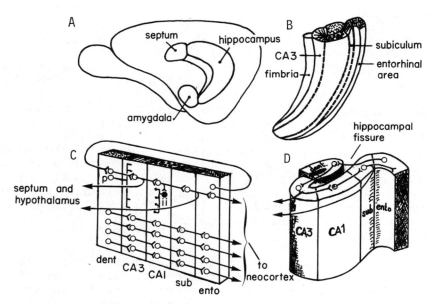

Fig. 1. Diagram of hippocampal position and connections.
A. Outline of hippocampus drawn on the contour of the
brain of a rodent, seen from the left side. B. Temporal
half of the left hippocampus to demonstrate its subdivisions. C. Diagram of the major cortical areas forming
the hippocampal formation. Symbols in Band C correspond.
D. As C, but now folded as in the animal. dent-dentate
area, ento-entorhinal area, sub-subiculum.

In Fig. 1D, I have tried to indicate how the input fibres
from the entorhinal area pass across the hippocampal
fissure which in the real brain is obliterated. The main
pathway for impulses in the hippocampal formation forms
a relay of four or five different elements as indicated
in Fig. 1D. These elements are in sequence: perforant
path fibres, mossy fibres, CA3 Schaffer collaterals, CA1
axons, and subicular axons. The outputs are collateral
branches from the CA3 cells which course to the fimbria
and fibres from the subiculum which run in the dorsal
fornix (Fig. 1C,D). These fibres reach the septal region
and various basal forebrain areas, notably different part
of the hypothalamus. Near the temporal end, certain output fibres also reach the amygdaloid nuclear complex. In
all parts of the hippocampal formation, the fibres comprising the main impulse system remain parallel to each
other, and transverse to the longitudinal axis to give
the system an orderly appearance (Fig. 1C,D). The axons
have, however, many collaterals which may excite other
neurones. One neurone is the polymorphic neurone (p)
which sends one axonal branch across the midline (Finch
and Babb, 1981). Another example is interneurones, one
which is drawn in Fig. 1C as a black structure (ii).
Because of this arrangement, a thin slice taken at right
angles to the septo-temporal axis, will contain all major
elements and thus comprise a micro-hippocampus or a
lamella (Blackstad et al, 1970; Andersen et al., 1971).

Principles of Organization

The hippocampus is a monolayered cortex with the dendrites normal to the cell layer and parallel to each other.

Major organizational principles in the hippocampus
are lamellation and stratification. The afferent fibres
do not only run parallel to each other across the structure, but also parallel to the main cellular layer. This
means that afferent fibres from a given source end on a
specific part of the dendritic tree with fibres crossing
it orthogonally. Excitatory fibres have en passage
boutons for every 3-5 μm, making synaptic contacts nearly
exclusively with spines (Andersen et al., 1966). Contacts
with interneurones are made directly upon their dendrites
which often have a beaded appearance. In contrast, interneurones, of which there are several in the hippocampal
cortex, tend to make synapses on the soma and shafts of
the primary and some of the secondary dendrites. The
excitatory synapses are of the asymmetric type, whereas
the interneurones seem to terminate with symmetrical

synapses. A particularly interesting synapse is the
coupling between the dentate granule cells and the CA3
pyramids. Here, the thin mossy fibres enlarge to large
globules into which finger-like spines burrow themselves.
These processes sit on the initial part of the apical dendrites. The synapse thus has multiple active sites inside one giant bouton (Hamlyn, 1963). Usually, excitatory synapses have round vesicles, whereas inhibitory
boutons often have pleomorphic vesicles, although there
are certain variations in the pattern.

Synaptic Effect

The arrival of the isolated hippocampal slice
(Yamamoto and McIlwain, 1966; Skrede and Westgaard, 1971),
meant a great advantage because many questions can now be
answered by a direct experimental test. Thus, we now
know that hippocampal synapses, both excitatory and inhibitory, mediate their effect chemically. Excitatory synapses
release transmitter(s), the identity of which is unknown as
yet. However, a good candidate for an excitatory transmitter in nearly all portions of the hippocampal cortex
is glutamate (Herz and Nacimiento, 1965; Biscoe and
Straughan, 1965; Storm-Mathisen, 1979; Storm-Mathisen
and Iversen, 1979; Schwartzkroin and Andersen, 1975).
In certain systems, aspartate may be the transmitter
(Nadler et al, 1976). Judged from the effect of iontophoretically applied glutamate (Dudar, 1974; Schwartzkroin
and Andersen, 1975) glutamate sensitive areas are found
in nearly all portions of the dendritic tree with the
possible exception of the very tips. Areas with equal
glutamate sensitivity are widespread even at considerable
distances from the soma.

Synaptic Efficiency

Because of the wide distribution of excitatory synapses, one would expect the most distal synapses to have
considerably less effect on the discharge probability
than more proximal synapses (Rall, 1962; 1967). However,
when afferent fibres located at various distances from
the soma were excited, the EPSPs produced were remarkably
similar in their time course. Furthermore, when experiments were made to ensure that a proximal and a distal
synaptic input had synaptic currents of equal magnitude,
the probability of discharge produced by these inputs
was very similar (Andersen et al., 1980b). Furthermore,
when lesions were made to abolish all synaptic inputs
except a small bundle of fibres crossing a tissue bridge

of known size and location, a small portion of activated fibres was sufficient to drive the cell, provided they were engaged synchronously. By comparing the size of the remaining tissue bridge with the total amount of afferent fibres, an estimate of 3 per cent of afferent fibres seemed necessary to drive the cell with a probability of 1.0. Furthermore, when such lesions were made at different levels relative to the soma, all bundles of fibres of the same magnitude were equally efficient (Andersen et al., 1980b). Such an estimation has only been made for the CA1 hippocampal pyramidal cells.

Such a remarkable synaptic efficiency could be explained if a large amount of transmitter was released at each bouton or by an effective summation of neighbouring activated synapses, or by a mixture of the two. Single fibre EPSPs have only been measured in the perforant path/granule cell synapses. Here, three different methods gave values around 0.1 mV (McNaughton et al., 1981). Because the summation of subsequent EPSPs is normally near in this system, the degree of non-linearity of EPSP summation was estimated from the relation between the size of extracellular EPSP and the input strength. With this correction, only about 400 synapses - of a total of 50-100 000 - needed to be activated simultaneously in order to discharge a granule cell which has a threshold of about 24 mV. If a similar figure applies for CA1 pyramidal cells, an even smaller number of synapses should be necessary since the voltage threshold for discharge is only about 6 mV from the resting potential. In addition, since EPSPs in CA1 pyramids add linearly, the remarkably small figure of 60 synapses seems necessary to drive the cell. Preliminary investigations have shown that a single fibre EPSP of about 0.1 mV also seems reasonable for CA1 pyramids.

Synaptic Summation

The cells of the hippocampal formation receive large numbers of synapses. They could conceivably summate non-linearly by reducing the driving potential for the synaptic current at subsequently activated synapses. However, direct observation of summation of EPSPs from two inputs on CA1 pyramidal cells showed that they summated linearly (Fig. 2) (Langmoen and Andersen, 1981). The averaged EPSPs of 15 trials to each of two inputs are seen in A and B. C shows the superimposed response when both inputs are activated simultaneously (observed sum) and D gives the algebraic summation of the individual EPSPs in A and B (algebraic sum). In 9 of 47 cells, these sums were per-

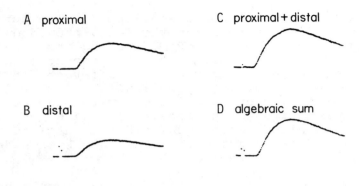

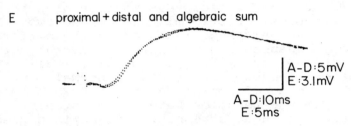

A-D:5mV
E:3.1mV

A-D:IOms
E:5ms

Fig. 2.   Linear summation of EPSPs in CAl pyramid.   A.
Average EPSPs (n=15) to a proximal input.   B.
As A, but from a distal input, same cell.   C.
Averaged EPSP to simultaneous activation of the
two inputs.   D. Algebraic summation of responses
seen in A and B.   E. Expanded versions of C and
D, superimposed.   From Langmoen and Andersen,
1981.

fectly similar. In the remaining 38 cells there was a
difference: the observed sum was less than the algebraic
sum. However, it turned out to be the addition of an
IPSP, probably of the recurrent variety. Thus, when the
experiment was repeated close to the equilibrium potential
for the IPSP, the observed sum was similar to the algebraic sum. In fact, the observed sum could be made larger
if the membrane potential was more negative than the equilibrium potential for the IPSP. The conclusion is that
synaptic potentials on CAl pyramids are summated linearly
whether they are of an excitatory or inhibitory nature.
Coupled with the observation that remarkably few afferent
fibres are necessary to drive a hippocampal pyramidal cell,
a new view of the synaptic control emerges. It does not

seem necessary to engage a large number of afferent fibres synchronously in order to drive the cell. Rather, because a small portion of simultaneously activated fibres can discharge the cell, the pyramidal cells may act as an output device for several sources, provided these sources activate their synapses synchronously.

Modification through Interneurones

There are many short axons or inter-neurones in the hippocampal formation (Ramon y Cajal, 1893; Lorente de Nó, 1934). Although only inhibitory inter-neurones have been found with certainty, the proposed excitatory variety remains a plausible arrangement (Dichter and Spencer, 1969). One type of the inhibitory inter-neurone, the basket cells, usually operates in a recurrent loop (Andersen et al., 1964). However, evidence for direct activation of these cells and, therefore, forward inhibition also exist. Judging from field potential distribution, the basket cell inhibition was located to the soma of the pyramidal cells. Later, Curtis et al. (1970) proposed that GABA is the inhibitory transmitter for the recurrent inhibition. Recently, we have recorded intracellularly while GABA has been applied near the soma of hippocampal pyramids and observed a hyperpolarization due to a conductance increase (Andersen et al., 1980a) (Fig.3). The inhibition is mediated by chloride ions (Allen et al., 1974). The equilibrium potential for this IPSP is 9-12 mV negative to the resting potential (Dingledine and Langmoen, 1980). Using immunofluorescence, Ribak et al. (1978) have shown that GAD (glutamate decarboxylase), the enzyme which produces GABA, is found in cells which are situated and terminate exactly like the basket cells.

In addition to the basket cell inhibition, there is evidence for another inhibitory mechanism on hippocampal pyramids. This is also mediated by GABA through a conductance mechanism. In this case, GABA has to be applied to the dendritic region at given specific places. GAD was found in large concentrations in dendritic areas (Storm-Mathisen and Fonnum, 1971). In accordance, GABA delivered at dendritic sites produced a conductance increase which gave rise to a depolarization. The depolarization may, in fact, be so large that it leads to cellular discharge (Andersen et al., 1980a). This effect is also sensitive to chloride concentration (Alger and Nicoll, 1979) but the equilibrium potential is not measured exactly. However, by extrapolation it looks to lie around -40 mV (Andersen et al., 1980a), making it unlikely that chloride is the

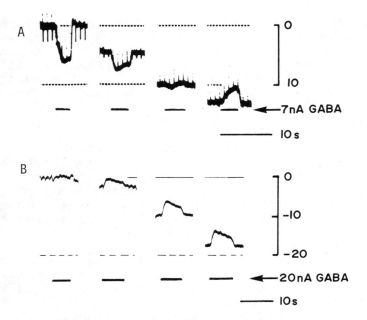

Fig. 3. A. Effect of membrane potential on responses of
         CAl pyramid to GABA applied near the soma. The
         response reverses about 10 mV negative to the
         resting level. Vertical lines are resistance
         pulses. The membrane potential was changed by
         passing current across the membrane. B. As A,
         but GABA applied in the dendritic area. Response
         now depolarizing, and increasing with more nega-
         tive membrane potential.

only ion involved. The major effect of this type of inhibition is probably to produce a localized and intense conductance increase in the dendritic tree. This leads to an
effective shunting of excitatory synaptic currents in the
vicinity. Remotely placed synapses, however, do not feel
this shunt and are indeed facilitated by the depolarization produced. The mechanism of inhibiting local excitatory synapses and facilitating the more remote has been
called discriminative inhibition and is proposed a new
mechanism for neuronal control. It remains to be seen
whether it operates under physiological circumstances.
In barbiturate—treated slices, Alger and Nicoll (1979)
have observed a long-lasting depolarizing potential to
afferent stimulation which has many characteristics similar
to that produced by GABA itself. The idea is that the

afferent impulse has excited GABA-containing inter-neurones, which can mediate an effect like the one produced by
iontophoretic application. Candidates for such interneurones   terminating on dendrites excist (Ramon y Cajal,
1893; Lorente de Nő, 1934; Ribak et al., 1978).

Other Modulatory Influences

From the nucleus of the diagonal band and the medial
septal nucleus, an important connection is distributed
to large portions of the dentate and the hippocampal
cortex. The fibres contain acetylcholinesterase and
probably release acetylcholine at their terminals. Stimulation of the system produces an increase in the amplitude
and frequency of the theta activity. In silent hippocampal cortex, it can induce the theta activity de novo.
Similarly, eserine will activate this activity, whereas
atropine may block at least one variety of this electro-
cortical graphic rhythm (Vanderwolf, 1975). In many
respects, the cholinergic theta activity is seen simultaneously with neocortical desynchronization. Iontophoretic application of acetylcholine to CAl pyramidal cells
gives a resistance increase and a slow depolarization
(Dodd et al., 1981). The most likely explanation is a
reduction of the resting potassium conductance produced
by acetylcholine, very similar to that proposed for the
neocortical synchronizing effect of acetylcholine
(Krnjević et al., 1971).

Modulation by Noradrenaline

The hippocampal cortex receives an important noradrenergic input (Blackstad et al., 1967; Storm-Mathisen and
Guldberg, 1974). Both locus coeruleus stimulation and
application of noradrenaline produce cessation of spontaneous and glutamate-driven discharges (Segal and Bloom,
1974a,b). By applying noradrenaline iontophoretically
to hippocampal pyramidal cells, two mechanisms were seen
which explain the inhibitory effect (Langmoen et al.,
1981). There was a moderate hyperpolarization (2.7 ± 1.7
mV) associated with a conductance increase (Fig. 4A). It
is likely that this is mediated by a chloride conductance
increase. In addition, there is another mechanism operating, which consists of reduction of the inward rectification seen in these cells. With depolarization close to the
threshold for the discharge, many CAl pyramidal cells show
a larger depolarization than expected. This so-called
inward anomalous rectification is most likely due to an
addition of an inward directed current, probably mediated

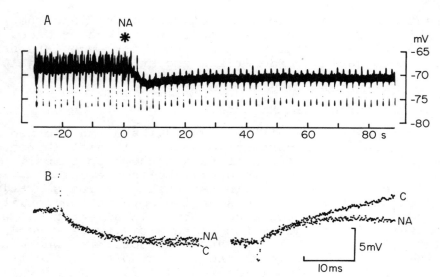

Fig. 4.   A. Effect on CA1 pyramid of a microdrop 1 nl
           10^{-3}M) noradrenaline (NA) applied on top of the
           slice (star).   Vertical lines are resistance
           pulses.   B. Responses to hyperpolarizing (left)
           and depolarizing (right) pulses before and after
           NA application.   From Langmoen et al., 1981.

by calcium ions (Hotson et al., 1979).   The reduction by
noradrenaline of this inward rectification has relatively
slow kinetics in that a noradrenaline only reduces the
plateau of the depolarizing potential, not the initial
portion (Fig. 4B, NA).   Thus, noradrenaline would be able
to block slowly occurring events, while fast events are
allowed.   Experiments with calcium blockers indicate that
noradrenaline has its main effect by blocking calcium
channels which probably are activated during the inward
rectification (Segal, 1981).

    A similar effect, although less dramatic, is seen by
the addition of ₅hydroxytryptamine.   Here, there is also
a hyperpolarization with a moderate conductance increase
(Segal, 1980).   Experiments with 4 AP and potassium superfusion indicate that potassium currents are activated
(Segal, 1980).

    No proper study of dopamine effects has been made on
hippocampal cells.   The few iontophoretic application

trials that have been made, have had a relatively meagre result.

Plasticity

Because of its possible relation to memory functions, the observation that hippocampal synapses change their efficiency over time with different training regimes is interesting. First, dentate granule cells may change their firing frequency in a conditioning paradigm. In behaving rats, Deadwyler et al. (1979) found dentate granule cells which increased their discharge rate when conditioned by an auditory signal. Following pairing of the auditory signal with a reward, the latency of the discharge decreased and the discharge duration increased. The response switched to an inhibitory one by starting to reward a tone of a different frequency. After a delay, the animal rearranged its reaction so that the dentate granule cells now responded again, but this time to the new tone being rewarded. Although the mechanism underlying this phenomenon is not clear, it shows that considerable plasticity is possible for the synapses involved.

More commonly observed is the phenomenon of habituation. In CA3 and CA1, the response to a novel stimulus is followed by an increased discharge (Vinogradova and Brazhnik, 1978). Following continued representations of a sensory stimulus with no consequence to the animal, there was a slow decline of the pyramidal cell response until no response was detectable. The cell could be dishabituated by a strong shock to the paw or by a loud noise.

A most interesting model for plastic changes in the nervous system is the long term potentiation described by Bliss and Lømo (1973). A relatively short tetanus within the physiological range (usually 10-20 Hz for 10-20 seconds creates a long-lasting (hours, even days) potentiation of synaptic transmission in the perforant path/granule cell synapse. Later, similar phenomena have been found for all synapses in the hippocampal formation where a proper search has been made. So far, only excitatory connections have been studied. The phenomenon appears to be homosynaptic in that the majority of investigators agree that only the tetanized pathways show the subsequent increased synaptic efficiency (Lynch et al., 1977; Andersen et al., 1977; 1980c; Wigström et al., 1979). There are, however, reports to the opposite effect (Misgeld et al., 1979). Trying to find out the mechanisms underlying the effect, studies have been made with intracellular recording from CA1 pyramids (Yamamoto, 1978;

Andersen et al., 1980c). The passive membrane properties
of the cells were not changed at all. Furthermore, the
input volley was not changed. However, there was a moderate, but clear increase of the EPSP amplitude, probably
indicating an increased amount of released transmitter.
There was also a clear reduction in the latency of discharge and a greatly increased probability of discharge.
These two parameters changed more than could be explained
by the moderate increase in the EPSP size. For this
reason it is possible that there are local postsynaptic
changes in addition to the presynaptic change of this
transmitter release. This possibility matches the
increased phosphorylation of proteins and the occurrence
of a specific protein following similar tetanization
(Brown et al., 1978; Duffy et al., 1981). Although the
changes at a given synapse may be moderate, the effect
along a series of synapses may be considerable. Whether
or not the long term potentiation is an essential element
or only an accompanying phenomenon to the major processes
underlying learning and memory, remains to be seen.

REFERENCES

Alger, B.E. and Nicoll, R.A., 1979, GABA-mediated biphasic
    inhibitory response in hippocampus. Nature, 281:
    315-317.
Allen, G.I., Eccles, J., Nicoll, R.A., Oshima, T. and
    Rubia, F.J., 1977, The ionic mechanisms concerned
    in generating the i.p.s.ps of hippocampal pyramidal
    cells. Proc. R. Soc. Lond. B., 198: 363-384.
Andersen, P., Blackstad, T.W. and Lømo, T., 1966, Location
    and identification of excitatory synapses on hippo-
    campal pyramidal cells. Exp. Brain Res.,1: 236-248.
Andersen, P., Bliss, T.V.P. and Skrede, K.K., 1971,
    Lamellar organization of hippocampal excitatory
    pathways. Exp. Brain Res., 13: 222-238.
Andersen, P., Dingledine, R., Gjerstad, L., Langmoen, I.A.
    and Mosfeldt Laursen, A., 1980a, Two different
    responses of hippocampal pyramidal cells to appli-
    cation of gamma-amino butyric acid. J. Physiol.,
    305: 279-296.
Andersen, P., Eccles, J.C. and Løyning, Y., 1964, Pathway
    of postsynaptic inhibition in the hippocampus.
    J. Neurophysiol., 27: 608-619.
Andersen, P., Silfvenius, H., Sundberg, S.H. and Sveen, O.,
    1980b, A comparison of distal and proximal dendritic
    synapses on CAl pyramids in hippocampal slices in
    vitro. J. Physiol., 307: 273-299.

Andersen, P., Sundberg, S.H., Sveen, O. and Wigström, H., 1977, Specific long-lasting potentiation of synaptic transmission in hippocampal slices. Nature, 266: 736-737.

Andersen, P., Sundberg, S.H., Swann, J.N. and Wigström,H., 1980c, Possible mechanisms for long-lasting potentiation of synaptic transmission in hippocampal slices from guinea pigs. J. Physiol., 302: 463-482.

Biscoe, T.J. and Straughan, D.W., 1966, Micro-electrophoretic studies of neurones in the cat hippocampus. J. Physiol., 183: 341-359.

Blackstad, T.W., Brink, K., Hem, J. and Jeune, B., 1970, Distribution of hippocampal mossy fibers in the rat. An experimental study with silver impregnation methods. J. comp. Neurol., 138: 433-450.

Blackstad, T.W., Fuxe, K. and Hökfelt, T., 1967, Noradrenaline nerve terminals in the hippocampal region of the rat and the guinea pig. Zellforsch., 78: 463-473.

Bliss, T.V.P. and Lømo, T., 1973, Long-lasting potentiation of synaptic transmission in the dentate area of the anaesthetized rabbit following stimulation of the perforant path. J. Physiol., 232: 331-356.

Browning, M., Dunwiddie, T., Bennett, W., Gispen, W. and Lynch, G., 1979, Synaptic phosphoproteins: specific changes after repetitive stimulation of the hippocampal slice. Science, 203: 60-62.

Curtis, D.R., Felix, D. and McLennan, H., 1970, GABA and hippocampal inhibition. Brit. J. Pharmacol., 40: 881-883.

Deadwyler, S.A., West, M. and Lynch, G., 1979, Activity of dentate granule cells during learning: differentiation of perforant path input. Brain Res., 169: 29-43.

Dichter, M. and Spencer, W.A., 1969, Penicillin-induced interictal discharges from the cat hippocampus. I. Characteristics and topographical features. J. Neurophysiol., 32: 649-662.

Dingledine, R. and Langmoen, I.A., 1980, Conductance changes and inhibitory actions of hippocampal recurrent IPSPs. Brain Res., 185: 277-287.

Dodd, J., Dingledine, R. and Kelly, J.S., 1981, The excitatory action of acetylcholine on hippocampal neurones of the guinea pig and rat maintained in vitro. Brain Res., 207: 109-127.

Dudar, J.D., 1974, In vitro excitation of hippocampal pyramidal cell dendrites by glutamic acid. Neuropharmacol., 13: 1083-1089.

Duffy, C, Teyler, T.J. and Shashoua, V.E., 1981, Long-
    term potentiation in the hippocampal slice:
    evidence for stimulated secretion of newly synthe-
    sized proteins. Science, 212: 1148-1151.
Finch, D.M. and Babb, T.L., 1981, Demonstration of
    caudally directed hippocampal efferents in the rat
    by intracellular injection of horseradish peroxi-
    dase. Brain Res.,214: 405-410.
Hamlyn, L.H., 1963, An electron microscope study of
    pyramidal neurones in the Ammon's Horn of the
    rabbit. J. Anat. (Lond.), 97: 189-201.
Herz, A. and Nacimiento, A., 1965, Über die Wirkung von
    Pharmaka auf Neurone des Hippocampus nach mikro-
    elektrophoretischer Verabfolgung. Naunyn-
    Schmiedebergs Arch. Exp. Pat. u. Pharmak.,251:
    295-314.
Hökfelt, T., Ljungdahl, Å., Fuxe, K. and Johansson, O.,
    1974, Dopamine nerve terminals in the rat limbic
    cortex: Aspects of the dopamine hypothesis of
    schizophrenia. Science, 184: 177-179.
Hotson, J.R., Prince, D.A. and Schwartzkroin, P.A.,
    1979, Anomalous inward rectification in hippocampal
    neurons. J. Neurophysiol., 42: 889-895.
Krnjević, K., Pumain, R. and Renaud, L., 1971, The
    mechanism of excitation by acetylcholine in the
    cerebral cortex. J. Physiol., 215: 247-268.
Langmoen, I.A. and Andersen, P., 1981, Summation of
    excitatory presynaptic potentials in hippocampal
    pyramidal cells. Submitted to J. Neurophysiol.
Langmoen, I.A., Segal, M. and Andersen, P., 1981, The
    mechanism of action of norepinephrine on hippocampal
    pyramidal cells in vitro. Brain Res.,208: 349-362.
Lorente de Nó, R., 1934, Studies on the structure of the
    cerebral cortex. II. Continuation of the study of
    the Ammonic system. J. Psychol. Neurol, (Lpz),46:
    113-177.
Lynch, G.S., Dunwiddie, T. and Gribkoff, V., 1977,
    Heterosynaptic depression: a postsynaptic corre-
    late of long-term potentiation. Nature,266: 737-739.
McLean, P.D., 1955, The limbic system "visceral brain"
    and emotional behaviour. Arch. Neurol. Psychiat.
    (Chicago), 73: 130-134.
McNaughton, B.L., Barnes, C.A. and Andersen, P., 1981,
    Synaptic efficacy and EPSP summation in granule
    cell of rat fascia dentata studied in vitro.
    J. Neurophysiol. , Submitted.
Misgeld, U., Sarvey, J.M. and Klee, M.R., 1979, Hetero-
    synaptic postactivation potentiation in hippocampal
    CA3 neurons: Long-term changes of the postsynaptic
    potentials. Exp. Brain Res.,37: 217-229.

Nadler, J.V., Vaca, K.W., White, W.F., Lynch, G.S. and Cotman, C.W., 1976, Aspartate and glutamate as possible transmitters of excitatory hippocampal afferents. Nature (Lond.), 260: 538-540.

O'Keefe, J. and Nadel, L., 1978, The hippocampus as a cognitive map. Clarendon Press, Oxford University Press, 570p.

Olton, D.S. and Feustle, W.A., 1981, Hippocampal function required for nonspatial working memory. Exp. Brain Res., 41: 380-389.

Rall, W., 1962, Electrophysiology of a dendritic neuron model. Biophys. J., 2: 145-167.

Rall, W., 1967, Distinguishing theoretical synaptic potentials computed for different somadendritic distributions of synaptic input. J. Neurophysiol., 30: 1138-1168.

Ramon y Cajal, S., 1893, Beiträge zur feineren Anatomie des grossen Hirns. I. Über die feinere Struktur des Ammonshornes. Z. wiss. Zool., 56: 615-663.

Ribak, C.E., Vaughn, J.E. and Saito, K., 1978, Immunocytochemical localization of glutamic acid decarboxylase in neuronal somata following colchicine inhibition of axonal transport. Brain Res., 140: 315-332.

Schwartzkroin, P.A. and Andersen, P., 1975, Glutamic acid sensitivity of dendrites in hippocampal slices in vitro, in:"Advances in Neurology", G.W. Kreutzberg Raven Press, New York, 12: 45-51.

Scoville, W.B. and Milner, B., 1957, Loss of recent memory after bilateral hippocampal lesions. J. Neurol. Neurosurg. Psychiat., 20: 11-21.

Segal, M., 1980, The action of serotonin in the rat hippocampal slice preparation. J. Physiol., 303: 423-439.

Segal, M., 1981, The action of norepinephrine in the rat hippocampus: intracellular studies in the slice preparation. Brain Res., 206: 107-128.

Segal, M. and Bloom, F.E., 1974, The action of norepinephrine in the rat hippocampus. I. Iontophoretic studies. Brain Res., 72: 79-97.

Segal, M. and Bloom, F.E., 1974, The action of norepinephrine in the rat hippocampus. II. Activation of the input pathway. Brain Res., 72: 99-114.

Skrede, K.K. and Westgaard, R.H., 1971, The transverse hippocampal slice: a well-defined cortical structure maintained in vitro. Brain Res., 35: 589-593.

Storm-Mathisen, J., 1979, Tentative localization of glutamergic and aspartergic nerve endings in brain. J. Physiol., Paris, 75: 677-684.

Storm-Mathisen, J. and Fonnum, F., 1971, Quantitative
     histochemistry of glutamate decarboxylase in the
     rat hippocampal region. J. Neurochem., 18: 1105-
     1111.
Storm-Mathisen, J. and Guldberg, H.C., 1974, 5-Hydroxy-
     tryptamine and noradrenaline in the hippocampal
     region: Effect of transection of afferent pathways
     on endogenous levels, high affinity uptake and some
     transmitter-related enzymes. J. Neurochem., 22:
     793-803.
Storm-Mathisen, J. and Iversen, L.L., 1979, Uptake of
     [^{3}H] Glutamic acid in excitatory nerve endings:
     Light and electronmicroscopic observations in the
     hippocampal formation of the rat. Neurosci., 4:
     1237-1253.
Vanderwolf, C.H., 1975, Neocortical and hippocampal
     activation in relation to behavior: effect of
     atropine, eserine, phenothiazines and amphetamine.
     J. comp. physiol. Psychol., 88: 300-323.
Vinogradova, O.S. and Brazhnik, E.S., 1978, Neuronal
     aspects of the septo-hippocampal relations, in:
     "Functions of the septo-hippocampal system",
     J. Gray, ed., Pp. 145-171, Ciba Found. Symp. 58,
     Elsevier, Amsterdam.
Wigström, H., Swann, J.W. and Andersen, P., 1979,
     Calcium dependency of synaptic long-lasting
     potentiation in the hippocampal slice. Acta physiol.
     scand., 105: 126-128.
Yamamoto, C., 1978, Long-term potentiation in thin
     hippocampal sections studied by intracellular
     recordings. Exp. Neurol., 58: 242-250.
Yamamoto, C. and McIlwain, H., 1966, Electrical activities
     in thin sections from the mammalian brain maintained
     in chemically-defined media in vitro. J. Neurochem.,
     13: 1333-1343.

THE POSTSYNAPTIC ACTION OF A VARIETY OF CONVENTIONAL AND

NON-CONVENTIONAL PUTATIVE NEUROTRANSMITTERS ON HIPPOCAMPAL NEURONES

J.S. Kelly, V. Crunelli & S.Y. Assaf

Department of Pharmacology
St. George's Hospital Medical School, London S.W.17.

INTRODUCTION

In the central nervous system, the analysis of the postsynaptic action of putative neurotransmitter substances on single neurones is based on the assumption that the action of many excitatory and inhibitory substances may be explained by supposing that they open channels or pathways through the membrane for one or more ions (see review by Ginsborg, 1967). For excitatory substances, the channels would be selective for Na^+ and perhaps one other ion species and for inhibitory substances K^+ or Cl^-. For the most part, the evidence comes from intracellular studies in which orthodromic stimulation of a particular pathway, or the extracellular iontophoresis of a particular substance is shown to alter both the excitability and electrical properties of the cell under study. It is convenient to describe the actions of putative transmitters in electrical terms.

The most widely used method is that first described by Fatt & Katz, (1951) and ideally consists of using one intracellular electrode to record the membrane potential and another to pass intracellular currents of varying magnitude and different polarities across the cell membrane. Using this method, at the neuromuscular junction, Fatt & Katz (1951) showed the amplitude of the endplate potential evoked by stimulation of the presynaptic nerve, to increase during the passage of hyperpolarizing current and to decrease during the passage of current of opposite polarity. The relationship between the amplitude of the endplate potential, e and the membrane potential, Vm, was a straight line, which could be extrapolated to a point, E, where the amplitude of the endplate was zero and the resting potential had a value of between zero and

617

-14mV. This straight line relationship can be explained on the
basis of the simple electrical model in which the resting membrane
is assumed to have a resistance, Rm and the opening of the ion
channels during the action of the transmitter to change this
resistance to a value Rm* so that:

$$e = (E - Vm) (1 - Rm^*/Rm)$$

Much in the same way, the depolarization evoked by the extracellular
application of acetylcholine (ACh) by iontophoresis (del Castillo &
Katz, 1954; Takeuchi, 1963) was shown to be linearly related to the
displacement of the membrane potential and to be zero at the transmitter equilibrium potential (E_{ACh}) for acetylcholine. This potential is also known as the reversal potential since the model predicts
that further depolarization will cause the transmitter-evoked
potential to change in sign and thereafter to increase linearly in
amplitude.

        This chapter described in some detail how we have used a
single intracellular electrode to examine the action of a variety
of putative neurotransmitters on hippocampal neurones, in order to
explore the underlying electrical events.

MATERIALS AND METHODS

Preparation of materials

        Hippocampal slices were prepared and maintained in vitro as
described previously (Dingledine et al, 1980; Dodd et al, 1981;
Assaf et al, 1981). Transverse slices were taken from
rats, 100-200 g in weight, and maintained in vitro in a superfusion
chamber at $37^{\circ}C$. The slices were perfused with a saline solution
comprising NaC1, 134 mM; KC1, 5 mM; KH_2PO_4, 1.24 mM; $MgSO_47H_2O$,
2 mM; $CaC1_2$, $2H_2O$ 2 mM; $NaHCO_3$, 16 mM; glucose, 10 mM (pH 7.2) and
oxygenated with a warmed, moistened O_2/CO_2 mixture (95 : 5).

Intracellular Recording

        Intracellular records from CA1 pyramidal and granule cells
were made using conventional techniques. Omega glass microelectrodes ('Kwik-fil'; Clark Electromedical Instruments) were
back-filled with 1 M potassium acetate, and had tip resistances of
80-120 MΩ. Under visual control the microelectrode was positioned
on the surface of the slice and driven slowly into the cell body
layer using a stepping microdrive unit.

        Potentials from the electrode were recorded with respect to a
silver/silver chloride pellet, embedded in the base of the superfusion chamber, through a precision electrometer (WP Instruments,
M-707). The electrometer was also used to inject current through
the recording microelectrode.

In each experiment the tip of the multibarrelled microiontophoretic pipette, containing glutamate and other putative
transmitters, was placed just below the surface of the hippocampal
slice in the region of the pyramidal cell body layer or the granule
cell body layer of the dentate gyrus, and a second, intracellular
micropipette was used to penetrate the soma of a nearby neurone.
Excitability was tested by passing depolarizing ramps of current
through the electrode of magnitude just sufficient to evoke one or
two action potentials during the control period. Membrane
resistance was monitored, using rectangular and ramp-shaped hyperpolarizing current pulses of similar amplitude and duration.

Subsequently, the data were analyzed on a computer and the
peak responses to each of the putative transmitters determined by
plotting against time the membrane potential, membrane resistance,
the number of spikes evoked by the depolarizing ramp, and the
latency and threshold of the first spike evoked by the ramp.

Individual barrels of microiontophoretic pipettes contained
acetylcholine chloride (ACh), 0.5 M, pH 4.5; sodium chloride (NaC1)
1 M; monosodium-L-glutamate (Glut), 1 M, pH 6.7; GABA 0.2 M, pH 4.5;
5 hydroxytryptamine 0.5 M, pH 4.0. Drugs were ejected by the
passage of current through the individual solution-filled barrels
using a circuit described previously by Kelly et al, (1975) and
at all other times a backing current of 25 nA and of appropriate
polarity was applied to each barrel. Although it was hoped that
the separation of the recording and microiontophoretic electrodes
would lead to the abolition of artifacts due to current coupling,
the appropriate controls were always carried out. On several
occasions, the current used to eject either ACh or glutamate was
counterbalanced automatically by the passage of a current of equal
amplitude and opposite polarity through a barrel containing 1 M
NaC1. At the end of each experiment, the intracellular electrode
was withdrawn and the effect of the iontophoretic application of
the drugs and control solutions was retested. On the few occasions
when the magnitude of the coupling response appeared to be
significant the data were discarded.

Peptides were dissolved in perfusion medium from which calcium
and glucose were omitted. Peptide solutions were ejected from the
tip of the pipette by the application of pressure (100-2000 kPa)
to individual barrels using a system described by Dingledine et al,
(1980).

Experiments were performed only on CA1 pyramidal cells and
granule cells with resting membrane potentials between 50-70mV.
Only cells able to fire a spike of short duration and of sufficient
magnitude to overshoot the resting potential of the cell in response
to direct stimulation through the electrode were selected for study.
The input resistance measured by injecting a hyperpolarizing

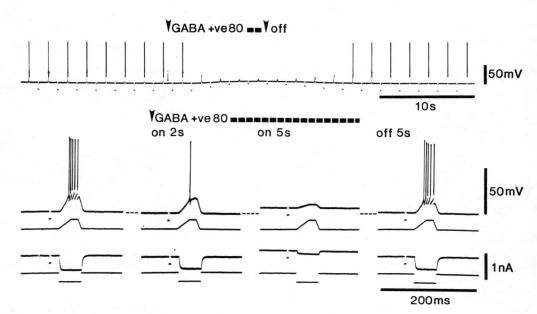

Fig. 1.   Intracellular recordings from a granule cell in the
hippocampal slice to show the response to the iontophoretic application of GABA. (A) Voltage record made on moving film to show
the way in which an intracellular injection of a depolarizing ramp
of current is used to test the cell's excitability. Each alternate
second a hyperpolarizing current pulse is used to measure the input
resistance. In B and C single shots show the application of GABA to
inhibit the spike discharge evoked by the ramp, to cause a substantial decrease in the input resistance to produce a small
depolarization with respect to resting membrane potential (dotted
line in B). From Assaf et al (1981).

current pulse (0.1-0.5nA) through the recording electrode had a
value between 50-100 MΩ.

RESULTS AND DISCUSSION

Actions of GABA on granule cells

When GABA was applied by iontophoresis using positive ejecting
currents between 4 and 160nA from an independently mounted electrode
positioned less than 100μm from the impaled cell body it produced
a marked depolarization accompanied by a substantial decrease in
input resistance (Fig. 1). At the peak of the response the ability
of the impaled cell to fire action potentials was completely
abolished even though the depolarization evoked by GABA occasionally
exceeded the threshold for spike initiation in the control
situation.

The latency to the onset of the response was extremely variable
and ranged between 250msec and 2 seconds after the onset of the
GABA application. However in every cell the magnitude of depolarization and concomitant increase in conductance was related to the
magnitude of the ejecting current (Fig. 1B) and the distance of the
independently mounted iontophoretic electrode from the impaled soma
(not shown). Bath application of GABA (1.0×10^{-6}M) at neutral pH
produced similar responses.

As predicted, on single cells ΔV was linearly related to
Rm*/Rm throughout the entire GABA application and from application
to application (Fig. 2). However, between cells E_{GABA} ranged
between -39 and -58mV and had a mean value of 17.5 ± 9mV depolarizing with respect to the resting membrane potential (Vm).
Presumably the difference between cells reflects either differences
in their internal ionic environment, differences in the distribution
of GABA receptors with respect to the position of the recording
electrode in the soma or the integrity of the electrode
impalement.

Postsynaptic Nature of the GABA Response

The responses described above occurred in the presence of a
low CA^{++} (0.25mM) and high Mg^{++} (16mM) media. Moreover an increase
in intracellular chloride caused by the leakage of anions from a
3M KCl filled recording pipette enhanced the GABA evoked depolarization and shifted E_{GABA} to a more positive value.

Thus the iontophoretic application of GABA in vitro appears in
some cells to be accompanied by a substantial depolarization and it
is the decrease in membrane resistance, which invariably leads to
a decrease in excitability (Scholfield, 1978a, b; Brown &
Scholfield, 1979). On the other hand on CA1 pyramidal cells GABA

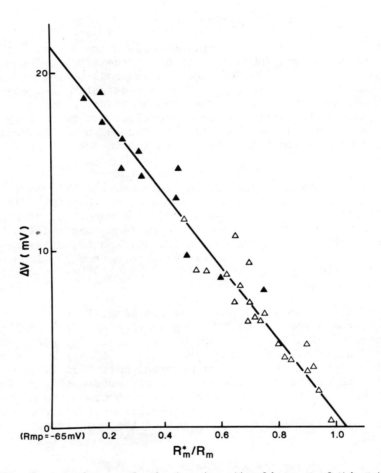

Fig. 2.   Regression analysis to show the linear relationship
between the depolarization (ΔV) evoked by two doses of GABA and
the associated decrease in resistance.   GABA was ejected with
currents of 160(▲) and 40(Δ) nA and the linear regression intersects
the voltage axis at -44mV and this was taken to be the reversal
potential for GABA.   From Assaf et al (1981).

has been shown to have both hyperpolarizing and depolarizing actions.
(Langmoen et al, 1978; Andersen et al, 1980; Thalman et al, 1979;
Jahnsen & Laursen, 1981).   Indeed, it appears that the two effects
are spatially separate, GABA depolarizing the dendritic membrane
while hyperpolarizing the soma.   Although both actions could result
in functional inhibition of orthodromically induced firing, the
depolarization evoked by GABA may facilitate excitation at distant
synapses (Andersen et al, 1980) and may occur solely at extra -
junctional sites (B.E. Alger & R.A. Nicoll - personal communication).

       Recently, Jahnsen & Laursson, (1981) have shown that both the
hyperpolarizing and depolarizing action of GABA on the CA1 pyramidal
cells of the hippocampal slice to be enhanced by the addition of
the water-soluble benzodiazepine, midazolam (10^{-7}M) to the
perfusion fluid.

Action of 5-hydroxytryptamine on granule cells.

       On many cells, iontophoretic 5HT caused a similar depolar-
ization, decrease in excitability and input resistance.   Indeed on
a number of occasions, as illustrated in Fig. 3 the reversal
potentials for the GABA and 5HT evoked inhibitions on the same cell
were virtually identical.   The onset of the inhibition, however,
was usually 2-3 times slower than that evoked by GABA on the same
cell.   In addition, GABA was always more potent than 5HT.   Although
these differences may be related to the ease with which GABA leaves
the pipette during iontophoresis, similar differences were observed
when GABA and 5HT were bath applied to the same cell (unpublished
observations of S.Y. Assaf and J.-M. Godfraind).

       In contrast, in the CA1 region of guinea-pig hippocampal
slices, 5HT have been shown to evoke a hyperpolarization accompanied
by a decrease in membrane resistance greatest when 5HT is applied
to the cell soma (Janssen, 1980).   Again the onset of the inhibition
was slower than that evoked by GABA.   The reversal potential was
13mV hyperpolarizing with respect to a resting potential of 60mV
and therefore the response could be mediated by either Cl^- or K^+
ions.   The response was unaltered by raising the concentration of
Mg^+ in the medium or the presence of Co^{++} or Mn^{++}.   In a few cells,
however, 5HT was excitatory and the depolarization accompanied by
an increase in membrane resistance.

       Segal (1980) has also shown the action of 5HT on CA1 neurones
to be hyperpolarizing.   Again the effect was rather slow in onset
and was maximal when a droplet containing a concentration of 100μm
was applied to the cell body layer or striatum pyramidalis, rather
than the dendrites of the striatum radiatum.   The effect was
blocked by the presence of the serotonin antagonist, methysergide
0.1mM.   However in this instance the hyperpolarization was
associated with an increase in resistance and Segal's attempts to

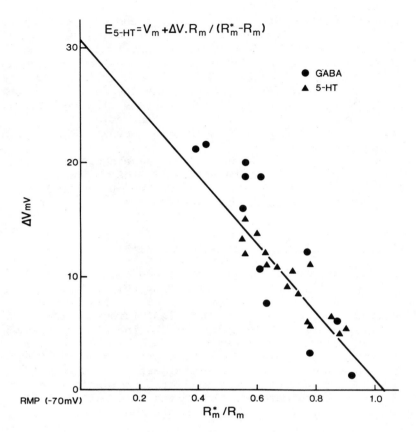

$$E_{5\text{-HT}} = V_m + \Delta V \cdot R_m / (R_m^* - R_m)$$

Fig. 3.   Regression analysis to show the linear way in which the depolarizations (ΔV) evoked by both GABA and 5-HT are correlated with an associated decrease in membrane resistance (Rm*/Rm).   The slope of the line is a measure of the difference between equilibrium potential of the putative neurotransmitter (E_{PNt}) and membrane potential (V_m).   In this instance, the difference is greater than 30mV in a depolarizing direction.

The similarity of the results obtained during iontophoretic applications of GABA and 5-HT raises at least two, equally, likely, possibilities.   Either the action of 5-HT is mediated by the opening of ionic channels similar to those activated by GABA, or a presynaptic action of 5-HT which causes GABA release.   From the work of Assaf et al, (1981).

prove the involvement of K^+ ions were only partially successful, since only partial reversal of the response was achieved by passing hyperpolarizing current through the electrode. However, on 2 cells, only a minimal hyperpolarization was evoked by 5HT when the cells was partially depolarized by raising the external K^+ concentration in the external media to 10mM. However the addition of 10mM TEA to the medium failed to block the hyperpolarization evoked by 5HT, even though the concentration was sufficient to increase the membrane resistance and cause substantial spike widening.

Thus we are left with the rather unsatisfactory situation in that 5HT is most effective in both the CA1 and dentate region when applied to the cell body layer, even though the dendrites seem to be a more likely target of the 5HT innervation (Azmita & Segal, 1978; Moore & Halaris, 1975; Conrad et al, 1974).   Rather surprisingly, the substantial decrease in the resistance caused by 5HT in the dentate is accompanied by a depolarization which is almost certainly mediated by the same ions as those responsible for the depolarization evoked by GABA, whereas in the CA1 region of the hippocampus, the responses are of strikingly different polarities and therefore unlikely to be mediated by the same ions. On the other hand as mentioned earlier, other workers have suggested that GABA does, in fact, evoke a hyperpolarization in the CA1 region when applied strictly to the cell body layer (Langmoen et al, Andersen et al, 1980; Thalman et al, 1979; Jahnsen & Laursen, 1981) and thus it is possible that GABA and 5HT also evoke potentials of the same polarity in the cell body of CA1 cells.

Action of Noradrenaline on CA1 Pyramidal Cells

The topical application of 0.1mM noradrenaline has been shown by Segal (1981) to cause a 3-4mV hyperpolarization associated with a 10-20% decrease in input resistance. The time-course of the potential and resistance changes however were substantially slower than those evoked by GABA and 5HT on other cells in the same slice preparation. The most pronounced effect of noradrenaline occurred when it was applied directly to the pyramidal layer close to the electrode in the soma. Although the hyperpolarization may in part be mediated by an increase in chloride permeability, the remainder of the effect was abolished by low temperature and by ouabain (50 μM). The hyperpolarization evoked by noradrenaline was mimicked by isoprotenal and blocked by the β-adrenergic blocker, sotalol. Cyclic AMP also produced a 3-4mV hyperpolarization associated with minimal changes in input resistance which could also be blocked by ouabain. The phospho-diesterase inhibitor, IBMX, potentiated the hyperpolarization evoked by small doses of noradrenaline.

In another study, however Langmoen et al (1981) have shown noradrenaline to cause a greater attenuation of the depolarizing,

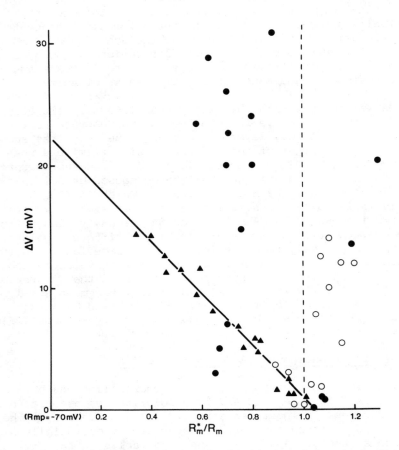

Fig. 4. Relationship between depolarization and input resistance
evoked by iontophoretic applications of glutamate. The depolarizations and changes in resistance evoked by iontophoretic
application of GABA (▲) and glutamate with 40 (●) or 160nA (○) near
the soma are compared. As is the case of most cells examined, a
linear regression can be drawn through the changes evoked by GABA.
However, the points for glutamate are widely dispersed and could be
on the left or right of the dotted line dividing decreases from
increases in input resistance. Note that the lower dose of
glutamate in the main evokes an increase in input resistance. From
Assaf et al (1981).

as opposed to hyperpolarizing pulses used to test the membrane resistance. Presumably this result could arise from a reduction in the Ca^{2+} and/or Na^+ current thought to be responsible for anomalous rectification (Hotson et al, 1979). However, the authors could not exclude an increase in Cl^- or K^+ conductance. In this particular study however the hyperpolarizing action of NE could not be completely blocked with the β-receptor antagonist, sotalol and thus the receptor involved may be different from that studied by Segal (1981).

Actions of Glutamate

On nearly every CA1 pyramidal neurone examined, a significant degree of excitation and depolarization could be evoked with glutamate-injecting currents in the region of 50nA applied for approximately 20s. The recovery from glutamate-evoked depolarizations and excitations was usually abrupt and often accentuated by a short period of reduced excitability. Occasionally, after particularly intense excitations evoked by small doses of glutamate, or after the use of larger doses of glutamate, this interval of decreased excitability was prolonged and clearly accompanied by a hyperpolarization and a reduction in membrane resistance.

In both CA1 pyramidal cells (Dodd et al, 1981) and the dentate, (Assaf et al, 1981) both large and small iontophoretic applications of glutamate produced dose-dependent depolarizations and increases in excitability and both increases and decreases in resistance were commonplace. However, in some cells, the excitation evoked by low-current was clearly associated with an increase in resistance, where as that evoked with high currents resulted in a decrease in input resistance. However in contrast to the depolarization evoked by GABA illustrated under the amplitudes of the depolarizations (ΔV) evoked by two different doses of glutamate were not related to the change in membrane resistance even though similar measurements made during the application of GABA to the same cell produced a typical linear relationship (Fig. 4).

During bath application, Constanti et al (1980) rather surprisingly found a 2-4 minute exposure of 1-3mM glutamate or aspartate was required to produce a relatively slowly developing depolarization of olfactory cortical neurones. Invariably the depolarization and increase in the number of spikes evoked by a depolarizing current pulse were accompanied by a marked decrease in membrane input resistance. During the washout, the depolarization was often followed by a pronounced hyperpolarization. Thus the response to bath applied glutamate in the olfactory cortex appears to be similar to our results obtained with "large," as opposed to "small" iontophoretic applications of glutamate.

In vivo Bernardi et al, (1972), Curtis et al, (1972) and

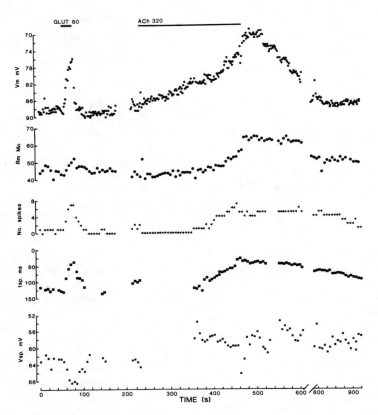

Fig. 5.   The time course of the responses evoked by glutamate and
acetylcholine.   Although the depolarization evoked by acetylcholine
is one of the fastest seen, the response to glutamate is very much
faster.   The acetylcholine-evoked depolarization is associated
with a slowly developing increase in membrane resistance and
excitability.   The threshold voltage (Vsp) at which the first
spike was evoked by the ramp was also determined and near the
peak of the ACh-evoked depolarization the excitability of the cell
suddenly declined, presumably due to an increase in sodium
inactivation.

Zieglgänsberger & Puil (1973) showed the depolarizations evoked by glutamate on cat motoneurones to be accompanied by a decrease in membrane resistance and Zieglgänsberger & Champagnat (1979) have suggested that the presence or absence of such a decrease in membrane resistance depends solely on whether the application site is somatic or dendritic. However, Engberg et al, (1975, 1979) and Sonnhof et al, (1975) have shown large and consistent decreases in membrane resistance only to occur when the application of glutamate is "large". Modest applications of glutamate resulted in small decreases, no change or small increases in membrane resistance. Similar increases and decreases in membrane resistance evoked by iontophoretic glutamate in isolated frog spinal cord has been attributed, by Shapovalov et al (1978) to the opening and closing of postsynaptic channels for Na^+ and K^+ respectively.

Although Dudar (1972) and Schwartzkroin and Andersen (1975) reported that the glutamate sensitivity of hippocampal neurones was preferentially located on proximal dendrites about 200μm from the soma, Spencer et al (1978) have suggested that the entire surface of the pyramidal cells is readily excited by small doses of glutamate.

The extremely rapid and abrupt recovery which followed the depolarization evoked by glutamate was often associated with a hyperpolarization of the membrane and could, therefore, be due to the spread of glutamate to nearby inhibitory interneurones. Recently however we have shown the decrease in resistance evoked by larger doses of glutamate to occur in the presence of either low Ca^{2+} and high Mg^{2+} or TTX. Thus the hyperpolarization could also be due to the activation of the sodium pump by the entry of sodium ions (Koike et al, 1972) during increased levels of firing.

Actions of Acetylcholine on CA1 pyramidal neurones

On CA1 neurones we (Dodd et al, 1981) have shown the depolarization of cortical neurones by ACh to be accompanied by an increase in membrane resistance and thus confirmed the original observations of Krnjević et al (1971) (Figs. 5 & 6). Furthermore, the value of -105mV, obtained for the reversal level of the ionic species involved is not significantly different from those obtained by these authors. The ACh evoked excitation, therefore, may be mediated by the closure of ionic channels normally open in the absence of ACh (Ginsborg, 1967; 1973; Krnjević et al, 1971; Ginsborg et al, 1974; Adams & Brown, 1975; Brown & Scholfield, 1979). Thus the action of ACh does not comply with the model we proposed in the introduction in that the closure as opposed to the opening of ion channels is involved.

Although the idea that the depolarizing action of ACh is primarily due to a closure of potassium channels, and there is a

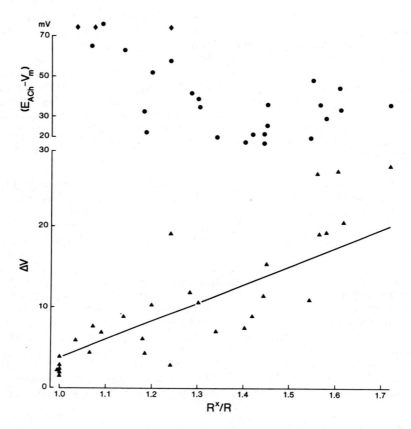

Fig. 6.   Regression analysis of the results from the cell in
Fig. 5 to show the linearity of the relationship of the depolarization evoked by ACh (ΔV), measured at 2 sec intervals throughout
the ACh application, to the corresponding increase in membrane
resistance (R^X) expressed as a function of the membrane resistance
measured before and after the response to ACh (R^X).   The linearity
of the line suggests that the reversal for ACh remained constant
throughout the entire application of ACh.   The correlation coefficient was 0.75 and the difference between the reversal
potential and the membrane potential was 38.1 mV. The upper graph
shows the individual values of the difference between the reversal
level and the membrane potential ($E_{ACh} - V_m$), ◆ signifies that the
value was greater than 70 mV.

substantial amount of evidence from sympathetic neurones to support this idea (see Brown & Constanti, 1980) there has always been others who believed that muscarinic agents promote anomalous rectification and that this may involve inward Na^+ and/or Ca^{2+} currents (Weight & Votava, 1970; Kuba & Kuketsu, 1976).   However, in a recent series of papers, Constanti & Brown (1980) argue against this possibility and suggest that the action of muscarinic agonists on rat sympathetic ganglia is due solely to an alteration in the rectifying properties in the cell, and not to the action of additional currents.   This view is strengthened by voltage-clamp studies (Brown & Adams, 1980) which show the depolarizing action of muscarine to be mediated by the specific depression of a time- and voltage-dependent outward potassium current.

        The depolarization evoked by acetylcholine is also unusual in that the onset and offset are very much slower than that evoked by glutamate, and are very much greater than would be explained by the diffusion of substance from the tips of the multibarrelled micro-pipette to different sites on the same neurone.   Presumably the slowness of the ACh response must therefore be explained by some intrinsic property of the ACh receptor, which involves a delay between the arrival of the ligand and closure of the K^+ channel. Indeed, the slowness is best explained by postulating sequential chemical reactions to follow the formation of the neurotransmitter receptor complex.   Thus the rate of depolarization evoked by ACh might be limited by the rate of formation of some intracellular product, and the long duration of the response by the time that would be required for its inactivation.   Indeed, a number of authors have investigated the possibility that the ACh-evoked depolarization involved the generation of an intracellular messenger, such as cyclic guanosine 3', 5'-monophosphate (cGMP) (Lee et al, 1972).

Action of peptides on CA1 pyramidal neurones

        Using pressure ejection we have shown gastrin 13 and 14 chole-cystokinin 4 and 8, caerulein, VIP and bombesin all to be rapid and potent excitants of pyramidal neurones in the CA1 region of the rat hippocampal slice.   In our most detailed study (Dodd & Kelly, 1981) depolarizations evoked by CCK-4 and CCK-8 were care-fully compared with that evoked by glutamate, released by micro-iontophoresis from an adjacent barrel of the same multibarrelled pipette.   On 15 cells both the latency of the onset (5.5 ± 0.9sec) and the rate at which the CCK-8 evoked depolarization developed (0.9 ± 0.2mV/sec) were as fast as that evoked by glutamate (6.6 ± 1.6sec and 0.7 ± 0.2mV/sec).   Indeed, on 8 cells, the depolarization evoked by CCK-4 appeared to develop more rapidly (3.0 ± 0.9s and 1.2mV/sec).   On a few occasions the onset of the depolarization evoked by gastrin was almost instantaneous, and much more rapid than the response of the same cell to glutamate (Fig. 7).

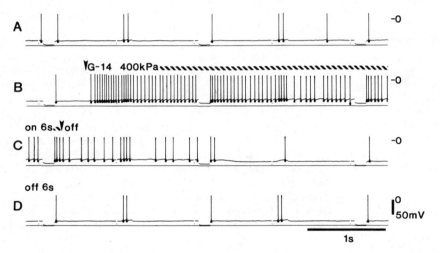

Fig. 7.   The excitation of a CA1 cell by the application of G-14
with a pressure of 400 kPa.   From Dodd & Kelly, 1981.

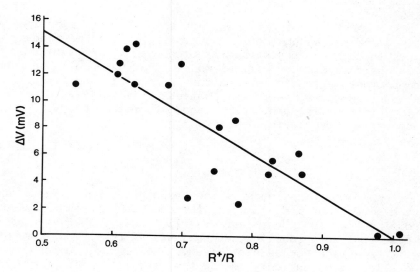

Fig. 8.   Graph to show the linear relationship between the
depolarization evoked by CCK-8 and the associated changes in
membrane resistance.   The correlation coefficient of the line
was 0.84 and the reversal potential was estimated to be -44.8mV
by extrapolation of the line to $R^+/R = 0$.   From Dodd & Kelly 1981.

As with a number of putative transmitters, on a number of occasions the excitation and depolarization evoked by CCK-8 was clearly accompanied by a decrease in membrane resistance and the amplitudes of the depolarization evoked by CCK-8 and CCK-4 through-out a single dose, or multiple doses, was linearly related to the change in membrane resistance (Fig. 8). Reversal potentials for CCK on 13 neurones thus suggests that the application of CCK results in a change in membrane permeability to one or more ionic species which have a net equilibrium potential closer to zero than resting membrane potential. Peterson and Philpott (1979) report a reversal potential of between -10 and -15mV for the action of a CCK-like peptide, caerulein, on pancreatic acinar cells.

CCK-8 and CCK-4 appear therefore to excite CA1 pyramidal neurones, and evoke substantial depolarization accompanied by a decrease in membrane resistance as predicted for conventional neurotransmitter by our original model. Furthermore these results are complementary to the observations of Phillis and Kirkpatrick (1979) on frog spinal neurones; Iwatsuki et al, (1977) on pan-creatic acinar cells, and Dockray and Hutchinson (1980), on neurones of the myenteric plexus.

CONCLUSIONS

Although the hippocampal slice preparation was introduced almost a quarter of a century ago (Li and McIlwain, 1957) it is only during the last three years (Ryall & Kelly, 1978) that its full potential as a tool for the analysis of postsynaptic neuro-transmitter action has been realised. This increased popularity of the slice is undoubtedly due to the ease with which high-quality, long-lasting intracellular recordings, can be made from the larger neurones of the slice. Only by recording intracellularly can the nature of the ionic events which underly the changes in excit-ability evoked by putative transmitters, be investigated in a meaningful way.

REFERENCES

Adams, P.R. and Brown, D.A. 1975. Actions of γ-aminobutyric acid on sympathetic ganglion cells. J. Physiol. 250: 85-120.

Andersen, P., Dingledine, R., Gjerstad, L., Langmoen, I.A. and Mosfeldt-Laursen, A. 1980. Two different responses of hippocampal pyramidal cells to application of gamma-aminol-butyric acid (GABA). J. Physiol. 305: 279-296.

Assaf, S., Crunelli, V, and Kelly, J.S. 1981. Electrophysiology of the rat dentate gyrus in vitro. in: Electrophysiology of isolated mammalian CNS preparations. Eds. G.A. Kerkut & H. Wheal. Academic Press. p 153-187.

Azmitia, E. and Segal, M. 1978. The efferent connections of the dorsal and median raphe nuclei in the rat brain. J. Comp. Neurol. 179: 641-668.

Bernardi, G., Zieglgänsberger, W., Herz, A. and Puil, E.A. 1972. Intracellular studies on the action of L-glutamic acid on spinal neurones of the cat. Brain Res. 39: 523-525.

Brown, D.A. and Adams, P.R. 1980. Muscarinic suppression of a novel voltage-sensitive K^+ -current in a vertebrate neurone. Nature 283: 673-676.

Brown, D.A. and Constanti, A 1980. Intracellular observations on the effects of muscarinic agonists on rat sympathetic neurones. Br. J. Pharmac. 70: 593-608.

Brown, D.A. and Scholfield, C.N. 1979. Depolarization of neurones in the isolated olfactory cortex of the guinea-pig by γ-amino-butyric acid. Br. J. Pharmacol. 65: 339-345

Conrad, L.C.A., Leonard, C.M. and Pfaff, D.W. 1974. Connections of the median and dorsal raphe nuclei in the rat: an autoradio-graphic and degeneration study. J. Comp. Neurol. 156: 179-206.

Constanti, A., Connor, J.D., Galvan, M. and Nistri. A. 1980. Intracellularly-recorded effects of glutamate and aspartate on neurones in the guinea-pig olfactory cortex slice. Brain Res. 195: 403-420.

Curtis, D.R., Duggan, A.W., Felix, D., Johnston, G.A.R., Tebécis, A.K. and Watkins, J.C. 1972. Excitation of mammalian central neurones by acidic amino acids. Brain Res. 41: 283-301.

Del Castillo, J. & Katz, B. 1954. The membrane change produced by the neuromuscular transmitter. J. Physiol. 125: 546-565.

Dingledine, R., Dodd, J. and Kelly, J.S. 1980. The in vitro brain slice as a useful neurophysiological preparation. J. Neurosci. Meth. 2: 323-362.

Dockray, G.J. and Hutchinson, J.B. 1980. Cholecystokinin octa-peptide in guinea-pig ileum myenteric plexus: localization and biological action. J. Physiol. (Lond.) 300: 28P.

Dodd, J., Dingledine, R. and Kelly, J.S. 1981. The excitatory
    action of acetylcholine on hippocampal neurones of the guinea-
    pig and rat maintained in vitro. Brain Res. 207: 109-127.

Dodd, J. and Kelly, J.S. (1981). The actions of cholecystokinin
    and related peptides on pyramidal neurones of the mammalian
    hippocampus. Brain Res. 205: 337-350.

Dudar, J.D. 1972. Glutamic acid sensitivity of hippocampal
    pyramidal cell dendrites. Act. Physiol. Scand. 84: 28A C6.

Engberg, I., Flatman, J.A. and Lambert, J.D.C. 1975. DL-Homo-
    cysteate-induced motoneurone depolarization with membrane
    conductance decrease. Br. J. Pharmacol. 55: 250-251P.

Engberg, I., Flatman, J.A. and Lambert J.D.C. 1979. The actions
    of excitatory amino acids on motoneurones in the feline spinal
    cord. J. Physiol. 288: 227-261.

Fatt, P. and Katz, B. 1951. An analysis of the end-plate potential
    recorded with an intracellular electrode. J. Physiol. 115:
    320-369.

Ginsborg, B.L. 1967. Ion movements in junctional transmission.
    Pharmac. Rev. 19: 289-316.

Ginsborg, B.L. 1973. Electrical changes in the membrane in
    junctional transmission. Biochim. Biophys. Acta. 300: 289-317.

Ginsborg, B.L., House, C.R. and Silinsky, E.M. 1974. Conductance
    changes associated with the secretory potential in the cockroach
    salivary gland. J. Physiol. 326: 723-731.

Hotson, J.R., Prince, D.A. and Schwartzkroin, P.A. 1979. Anomalous
    inward rectification in hippocampal neurones. J. Neurophysiol.
    42: 889-895.

Iwatsuki, N., Kato, N. and Nishiyama, A. 1977. The effects of
    gastrin and gastrin analogues on pancreatic acinar cell membrane
    potential and resistance. Brit. J. Pharmacol. 60: 147-154.

Jahnsen, H. and Laursen, A.M. 1981. The effects of a benzodiaz-
    epine on the hyperpolarizing and the depolarizing responses of
    hippocampal cells to GABA. Brain Res. 207: 214-217.

Janssen, H. 1980. The action of 5-hydroxytryptamine on neuronal
    membranes and synaptic transmission in area CA1 of the hippo-
    campus in vitro. Brain Res. 197: 83-94.

Kelly, J.S., Simmonds, M.A. and Straughan, D.W. 1975. Micro-electrode techniques. in: Methods in Brain Research, P.B. Bradley. Wiley, London. 333-377.

Koike, J., Mano, N., Okada, Y. and Oshima, T. 1972. Activities of the sodium pump in cat pyramidal tract cells investigated with intracellular injection of sodium ions. Expl. Brain Res. 14: 449-462.

Krnjević, K., Pumain, R. and Renaud, 1971. The mechanism of excitation by acetylcholine in the cerebral cortex. J. Physiol. 215: 247-268.

Kuba, K. and Koketsu, K. 1976. Analysis of the slow excitatory postsynaptic potential in bullfrog sympathetic ganglion cells. JAP. J. Physiol. 26: 647-664.

Langmoen, I.A., Andersen, P., Gjerstad, L., Mosfeldt-Laursen, A. and Ganes, T. 1978. Two separate effects of GABA on hippocampal pyramidal cells in vitro. Acta. Physiol. Scand. 102: 28-29A.

Langmoen, I.A., Segal, M. and Andersen, P. 1981. Mechanisms of norepinephrine actions on hippocampal pyramidal cells in vitro. Brain Res. 208: 349-362.

Lee, T.-P., Kuo, J.F. and Greengard, P. 1972. Role of muscarinic cholinergic receptors in regulation of guanosine 3', 5'-cyclic monophosphate content in mammalian brain, heart muscle, and intestinal smooth muscle. Proc. Natn. Acad. Sci. USA 69: 3287-3291.

Li. C.IL. and McIlwain, H. 1957. Maintenance of resting membrane potentials in slices of mammalian cerebral cortex and other tissues in vitro. J. Physiol. 139: 178-190.

Moore, R.Y. & Halaris, A.E. 1975. Hippocampal innervation by serotonin neurones of the mid brain raphe in the rat. J. Comp. Neurol. 164: 171-184.

Peterson, O.H. and Philpott, H.G. 1979. Pancreatic acinar cells: effects of microiontophoretic polypeptide application on membrane potential and resistance. J. Physiol. (Lond.) 290: 305-315.

Phillis, J.W. and Kirkpatrick, J.R. 1979. Actions of various gastrointestinal peptides on the isolated amphibian spinal cord. Canad. J. Physiol. Pharmacol. 57: 887-899.

Ryall, R.W. and Kelly, J.S. 1978.   Iontophoresis and Transmitter
    Mechanisms in the Mammalian Central Nervous System.   Elsevier/
    N. Holland, Amsterdam.

Scholfield, C.N. 1978a.   Electrical properties of neurones in the
    olfactory cortex slice in vitro.   J. Physiol. 275: 535-546.

Scholfield, C.N.   1978b.   Characteristics of CA1 neurones recorded
    intracellularly in the hippocampal in vitro slice preparation.
    Brain Res. 85: 423-436.

Schwartzkroin, P.A. and Andersen, P. 1975.   Glutamic acid sen-
    sitivity of dendrites in hippocampal slices in vitro.   Adv. In
    Neurology.12:   45-51.

Segal, M. 1980.   The action of serotonin in the rat hippocampal
    slice preparation.   J. Physiol. 303: 423-439.

Segal, M. 1981.   The action of norepinephrine in the rat hippocampus:
    Intracellular studies in the slice preparation.   Brain Res. 206:
    107-128.

Shapovalov, A.I., Shiriaev, B.I. and Velumian, A.A. 1978. Mechanisms
    of post-synaptic excitation in amphibian motoneurones.   J.
    Physiol. 279: 437-455.

Sonnhof, U., Linder, M., Grafe, F. and Krumnikl, G. 1975.   Post-
    synaptic actions of glutamate on somatic and dendritic membrane
    areas of the lumbar motoneurones of the frog.   Pflügers Arch.
    ges Physiol. 355: 171.

Spencer, H.J., Gribkoff, V.K., Cotman, C.W. and Lynch, G.S. 1976.
    GDEE antagonism of iontophoretic amino acid excitations in the
    intact hippocampus and in the hippocampal slice preparation.
    Brain Res. 105: 471-481.

Takeuchi, N. 1963.   Some properties of conductance changes at the
    end-plate membrane during the action of the transmitter.   J.
    Physiol. 167: 141-155.

Thalmann, R.H., Peck, E.J. and Ayala, G.F. 1979.   Biphasic response
    of pyramidal neurones to GABA iontophoresis in hippocampal
    slices.   Soc. Neurosci. Abst. 5: 74.

Weight, F.F. and Votava, J. 1970.   Slow synaptic excitation in
    sympathetic ganglion cells: Evidence for synaptic inactivation
    of potassium conductance.   Science. 170: 755-758.

Zieglgänsberger, W. and Champagnat, J. 1979. Cat spinal motoneurones exhibit topographic sensitivity to glutamate and
   glycine.   Brain Res. 160: 95-104.

Zieglgänsberger, W. and Puil, E.A. 1973. Action of glutamic acid
   on spinal neurones. Exp. Brain. Res. 17: 35-49.

SYNAPTIC EFFICACY AND RELIABILITY IN PERFORANT PATHWAY

B.L. McNaughton

Cerebral Functions Group, Department of Anatomy
University College London
London WC1E 6BT, England

This paper represents a summary of some experiments concerned with elucidating the factors contributing to the efficacy and reliability of synaptic transmission in the perforant path from the entorhinal cortex to the fascia dentata of the hippocampus. Not only is this system the major source of excitatory afferents to the fascia dentata, but it also appears to represent a large fraction of the total excitatory cortical input to the hippocampal system as a whole. A detailed understanding of the function of this major input stage is thus crucial for any overall model of hippocampal function.

The perforant pathway has been separated on anatomical and physiological grounds into two discrete components; the medial perforant pathway, arising in the medial entorhinal cortex and terminating in the middle one third of the molecular layer, and the lateral pathway which originates in lateral entorhinal cortex and terminates in the distal one third of the molecular layer (Hjorth-Simonsen, 1972; Steward, 1976). The two termination fields are biochemically distinct (Haug, 1973) and the synapses of the two zones exhibit markedly different responses to repetitive activation (McNaughton, 1980). For technical reasons, most of the work described here was carried out on the medial perforant pathway, although some information on the lateral input is provided for comparison.

Medial perforant path synapses have the classical morphological characteristics of chemically mediated synapses (Nafstad, 1967) and there is some evidence favouring glutamate as the transmitter (White, Nadler, Hamberger and Cotman, 1977). Since the overall granule cell electrotonic length is about .9 (Fricke, Prince and Brown, 1979), medial perforant path synapses are electrotonically rather close to the soma. This has permitted an estimate of the reversal potential

641

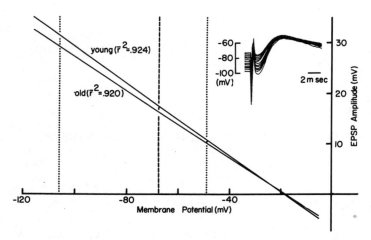

Fig. 1 Summary of an experiment carried out in collaboration with
C.A. Barnes in which the effect of experimentally altering granule
cell membrane potential in vitro on the amplitude of the intracellularly recorded medial perforant path e.p.s.p. in fascia dentata of
young and old rats. The old animals exhibited slightly smaller
e.p.s.p.s at a given stimulus level because of atrophy of afferent
fibres. Nevertheless, both groups showed the same apparent reversal
potential (-18 mV). The dashed line represents the mean resting
potential which was not different between groups whereas the dotted
lines represent the average levels within which the membrane potential
could be shifted with applied current. The solid lines represent the
mean regression lines for 62 old and 66 young granule cells.
Insert: example of the e.p.s.p. recorded at various membrane
potentials.

of the e.p.s.p. to be obtained by passing hyperpolarizing and
depolarizing current into the cell body (Fig. 1) via a balanced
bridge circuit. Since the granule cell membrane impedance falls
off with increasing current in both the hyperpolarizing and depolarizing direction (Barnes and McNaughton, 1980a) it has not been
possible to obtain complete reversal of the e.p.s.p. However, within
the range of -106 to -49 mV around resting potential, an almost
perfectly linear relationship between e.p.s.p. amplitude and resting
potential was obtained (average r^2 value .922 for 128 cells). The
extrapolation to 0 e.p.s.p. amplitude gave -18 mV as the reversal
potential. The actual reversal potential is probably somewhat more
negative than this because of the voltage attenuation between soma
and synapse.

The average size of the post-synaptic response to activation
of a single perforant path fibre is 0.1 mV ± .03 (S.D.). This has
been determined in vitro by carrying out a detailed study of the
threshold region of the e.p.s.p. vs. stimulus intensity curve.
A discrete transition occurs between the lowest response detectable,
and zero (Fig. 2).

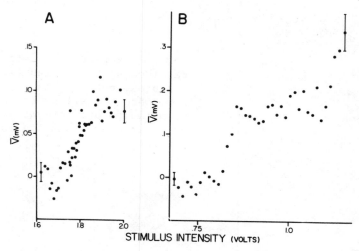

Fig. 2 Two examples of the relation between e.p.s.p. amplitude (V)
and stimulus intensity as the latter is varied in small steps in the
vicinity of threshold for a single afferent perforant path fibre.
Each data point represents the mean of 128 responses; error bars
represent one S.D. and, for clarity, are plotted only for the first
and last elements of each data set. An F test on the residuals
after removal of the linear component was used to test for a transition in the data set. Significant transitions, averaging 0.1 ±
.03 mV were found in 10 of 12 cells studied in this manner. These
data suggest that the average e.p.s.p. due to a single perforant
path fibre is 0.1 mV.

        The average height of the e.p.s.p. above resting potential
(-69 ± 8 mV) necessary to elicit granule cell discharge in vitro
is 24 ± 9 mV (McNaughton, Barnes, and Andersen, 1981). Thus, on
average, at least 240 perforant path fibres must co-operate to
discharge the granule cell. Using the assumption that the presynaptic
fibre potential is linearly related to the number of medial perforant
path fibres converging on a given cell, an approximate correction can
be made for the effects of non-linear summation of e.p.s.p.s. When
this correction is carried out one obtains a figure closer to 400
as the actual number of convergent perforant path fibres necessary
to discharge the granule cell in the absence of other influences.

        The amplitude of the intracellular e.p.s.p. exhibits consider-
able fluctuation. This fluctuation has been shown not to be due to
changes in the responses of individual afferent fibres, but to
fluctuation in the number of transmitter quanta released per impulse
per fibre. With low stimulus intensities which activate one or a
few fibres, response failures can be quite clearly observed (Fig. 3).

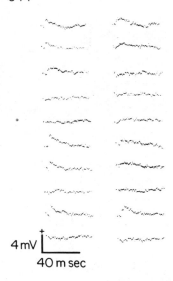

Fig. 3 Extract from a larger data
set showing the variability of the
perforant path - granule cell e.p.
s.p. when a small number of perforant
path fibres are activated. A number
of apparent response failures are
present.

4 mV

40 m sec

Using large data sets (of which Fig. 3 is an extract) which were
carefully selected for stationarity of response amplitude and resting
potential, 3 methods were applied to estimate the mean quantal content
(m) of the e.p.s.p. of a single fibre: the coefficient of variation
method, which assumes that m is equal to the ratio of the mean e.p.-
s.p. squared devided by the e.p.s.p. amplitude variance after the
subtraction of the variance due to thermal and membrane noise; the
method of failures, which assumes m to be equal to the natural
logarithm of the total number of trials divided by the number of
trials on which zero response occurs; and finally, a fourier
transform method which is independent of any assumptions about the
precise nature of the statistical process governing transmitter
release. The latter method essentially detected the most significant
periodicity component of the frequency histogram of e.p.s.p.
amplitudes. Again, an approximate correction, based on the assumption
of a linear relation between presynaptic fibre potential and number
of convergent active fibres was used to correct the values of m
determined by the coefficient of variation method for non-linear
summation. The three methods gave values of m of 0.9, 0.4, and 0.7
respectively. There is reason to believe that the failures method
is an underestimate because of the problem of erroneously counting
as failures a proportion of unusually small responses. Thus the
quantal content of the e.p.s.p. from a single fibre is likely to be
somewhere between 0.6 and 1. This has the interesting consequence
that, assuming Poisson statistics, a given perforant path synapse
is likely to fail to transmit approximately 50% of the time under
"normal" conditions. One is thus led to ask whether there might
not be conditions under which the probability of transmission can
be increased in perforant path synapses so as to make them more
reliable.

One method of determining the statistical probability of quantal release (p) is to deliver pairs of shocks over a range of intervals. In neuromuscular systems, the interpretation of such experiments has been that following a single shock the number of available quanta (n) is reduced because some are used up (Martin, 1966). Neglecting the early superimposed facilitation phase which decays rapidly, the depression curve relating e.p.s.p. magnitude on the second shock relative to the first can be extrapolated to zero interval to give a measure of p. In such an experiment the medial perforant pathway behaves both <u>in vivo</u> and <u>in vitro</u> much like a neuromuscular junction under normal release conditions with a value of p of about 0.3. The lateral perforant pathway, on the other hand, behaves like a neuromuscular junction bathed in low calcium medium with a p value of less than 0.1 (Fig. 4). In support of this interpretation, the depression seen on paired shocks to the medial perforant pathway is reduced in direct proportion to the magnitude of the initial response when the probability of transmitter release is reduced by lowering the Ca^{++} concentration in the bathing medium (Fig. 5).

Following relatively brief episodes of high-frequency stimulation, perforant path synapses can undergo rather pronounced increases in their efficacy. This has been of particular interest because of the possibility that such a change may be involved in various types of information storage in the brain. It has been

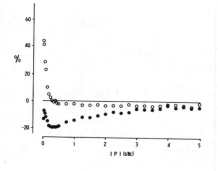

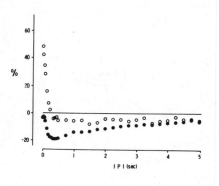

Fig. 4 Two examples of <u>in vivo</u> experiments in which the <u>lateral</u> (open circles) or medial (filled circles) were stimulated with pairs of shocks at various intervals. The medial pathway consistently showed considerably more paired shock depression than the lateral. Neglecting the early facilitation superimposed on the depression, extrapolation of the depression curve to zero interval gives 0.3 as an estimate of the release probability.

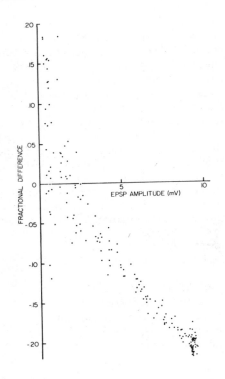

Fig. 5 In this in vitro experiment,
the normal bathing medium which
contained 2 mM Ca++ was exchanged
for a Ca++ free ringer over approximately 30 minutes. During this
time, paired shocks were delivered
to the medial perforant pathway.
The plot shows that paired pulse
depression was reduced in direct
proportion to the reduction in the
amplitude of the first e.p.s.p.
in each pair. Since Ca++ is known
to reduce transmitter release
probability this indicates that
the paired pulse depression method
gives a valid estimate of p in this
system. Restoration of Ca++ also
restored the control levels of
e.p.s.p. and paired pulse depression.

shown that following the high-frequency activation of relatively
few perforant path fibres, only short-term changes are involved.
The e.p.s.p. magnitude may be increased by as much as 3 fold but
invariably returns to baseline within several minutes (Fig. 6).
The decay function follows a double exponential time course with
parameters almost identical to the processes of augmentation and
potentiation at the neuromuscular junction as defined by Magleby
and Zengel (1976) who showed them to be due to an increase in the
number of quanta released per impulse. In the perforant pathway,
the depression seen on paired responses with short inter-stimulus-
intervals was increased in direct proportion to the combined
magnitudes of augmentation and potentiation. This leads to the
conclusion that short-term augmentation and potentiation are both
due to an increase in the probability of quantal release.

When increasing numbers of perforant path fibres are brought
into simultaneous high-frequency activity a different type of
synaptic change occurs with strikingly different properties. This
change was originally called long-lasting potentiation (Bliss and
Gardner-Medwin, 1973; Bliss and Lømo, 1973) but for reasons to be
described below, the term enhancement will be used here. Enhancement
can be elicited using the same stimulus train parameters as
augmentation and potentiation merely by increasing the stimulus

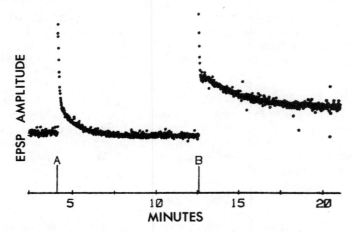

Fig. 6   Example of the effect of stimulating lateral perforant
pathway with low and high intensity.   The e.p.s.p. amplitude is
plotted against time, low intensity test shocks being delivered
once every three seconds.   Tetanization parameters were 100 pulses
at 250 Hz for both trains.   However, during the second train the
intensity was raised so as to activate more afferent fibres.
Following the train the stimulus intensity was returned to the
control level.   The first train elicited only short-term augmentation and potentiation.   During this period of raised e.p.s.p.
amplitude, paired shock depression is increased proportionally
and recovers the control level with the same time course.   This
indicates that short-term augmentation and potentiation involve an
increase in the probability of transmitter release.   Following the
high-intensity train, augmentation and potentiation were also
elicited.   However, a third process is also activated.   This
enhancement of synaptic efficacy is not a long-term form of
potentiation since it has no effect on paired shock depression,
and hence does not involve a change in transmitter release
probability.

intensity during the train (Fig. 6), or by activating two pathways
such as the medial and lateral perforant pathway simultaneously
rather than separately (McNaughton, Douglas and Goddard, 1978).
It is specific to those synapses on a given postsynaptic neuron
which were active together at high frequency (McNaughton and Barnes,
1977) and also to those synapses made by a given presynaptic fibre
which were in close proximity to other concurrently active presynaptic fibres (Levy and Steward, 1979).   It lasts, on the average,
about one week in chronically prepared rats following a single
stimulation session but can be considerably prolonged by several
repetitions at 24 hour intervals (Barnes, 1979; Barnes and
McNaughton, 1980b).   Unlike augmentation and potentiation it does

not involve an increase in p. Enhancement has no effect on the
relative depression seen on paired shocks, even though the absolute
magnitudes of the responses may be elevated by 30 to 50% (McNaughton,
1977, 1981). Enhancement is thus not a long-term form of potentiation.

In conclusion, a considerable body of information exists on the
factors governing synaptic efficacy and its modification in this
particular neural pathway. It will be of interest to see future
experiments designed to clarify the relation of these microphenomena
to actual information processing and storage in the fascia dentata
of intact, behaving animals.

REFERENCES

Barnes, C.A. 1979. Memory deficits associated with senescence:
A neurophysiological and behavioural study in the rat. J. Comp.
Physiol. Psychol., 93: 74-104.

Barnes, C.A. and McNaughton, B.L. 1980a. Spatial memory and
hippocampal synaptic plasticity in middle-aged and senescent rats.
in 'Psychobiology of aging: Problems and Perspectives' (D. Stein,
ed.) Elsevier, New York.

Barnes, C.A. and McNaughton, B.L., 1980b. Physiological compensa-
tion for loss of afferent synapses in rat hippocampal granule cells
during senescence. J. Physiol. (Lond.) 309: 473-485.

Bliss, T.V.P. and Gardner-Medwin, A.R., 1973. Long-lasting potentiation of synaptic transmission in the dentate area of unanaesthetized rabbit following stimulation of the perforant path.
J. Physiol. (Lond.) 232: 357-374.

Bliss, T.V.P. and Lømo, T. 1973 Long-lasting potentiation of synaptic
transmission on the dentate area of the anaesthetized rabbit
following stimulation of the perforant path. J. Physiol. (Lond.)
232: 334-356.

Fricke, R.A., Brown, R.H. and Prince, D.A., 1979. Electrotonic
structure of hippocampal neurons. Soc. Neurosci. Abst., 5: 502.

Haug, F.M.S., 1973. Heavy metals in the brain. Adv. Anat., Embryol.
and Cell Biol., 47:4.

Hjorth-Simonsen, A., 1972. Projection of the lateral part of the
entorhinal area to the hippocampus and fascia dentata. J. Comp.
Neurol., 147: 219-232.

Levy, W.B. and Steward, O., 1979. Synapses as associative memory
elements in the hippocampal formation. Brain Res., 175: 233-245.

Magleby, K.L. and Zengel, J.E.. 1976. Augmentation: a process that acts to increase transmitter release at the frog neuromuscular junction. J. Physiol. (Lond.) 257: 449-470.

Martin, A.R. 1966. Quantal nature of synaptic transmission. Physiol. Rev., 46: 51-66.

McNaughton, B.L., 1977. Dissociation of short- and long-lasting modification of synaptic efficacy at the terminals of the perforant path. Neurosci. Abst., 7.

McNaughton, B.L., 1980. Evidence for two physiologically distinct perforant pathways to the fascia dentata. Brain Res., 199: 1-19.

McNaughton, B.L., 1981. Long-term synaptic enhancement and short- term potentiation in rat fascia dentata act through different mechanisms. Under editorial review.

McNaughton, B.L., Barnes, C.A., and Andersen, P.,1980. Synaptic efficacy and EPSP summation in granule cells of rat fascia dentata studied in vitro. J. Neurophysiol., in press.

McNaughton, B.L., Douglas, R.M. and Goddard, G.V., 1978. Synaptic enhancement in fascia dentata: co-operativity among co-active afferents. Brain Res., 157: 277-293.

Nafstad, P.H.J., 1967. An electron microscope study on the termination of the perforant path fibers in the hippocampus and the fascia dentata. Zeit. für Zellforsch., 76: 532-542.

Steward, O.,   1976. Topographic organization of the projections from the entorhinal area to the hippocampal formation of the rat. J. Comp. Neurol., 167: 285-314.

White, W.F., Nadler, J.V., Hamberger, A. and Cotman, C.W., 1977. Glutamate as transmitter of hippocampal perforant path. Nature, 270: 356-357.

GONADAL STEROID ACTION ON

BRAIN SEXUAL DIFFERENTIATION AND SEXUAL BEHAVIOR

Bruce S. McEwen

The Rockefeller University
New York, NY 10021 USA

INTRODUCTION

One of the goals of research on the brain is to understand
how neurons are organized into systems which control behaviors
and how these systems are modified by factors in the external and
internal environment. Hormonal influences on the brain represent
one of the best paradigms for pursuing this goal. We have been
studying steroid hormone effects on the brain and have come to
recognize three unique opportunities offered by such studies.
First, by localizing putative receptors with radiolabeled hormones,
it is possible to localize potential sites of hormone action
within the brain. Second, by identifying putative receptors in
brain regions, one has access to a likely cellular mechanism by
which nerve cell function is modulated, namely, by a modification
of genomic activity. Third, steroids and particularly gonadal
steroids regulate both developing as well as adult neural targets
and thus provide access to two aspects of brain function:
"organizational", dealing with permanent establishment of neural
circuits and response capabilities, including sex differences;
and "activational", dealing with the reversible facilitation of
neural activity and neuronal properties which underlie reversible
changes of neuroendocrine status and behavior. One of the goals
of our research on this topic is to identify cellular events
triggered by hormones in neurons which are necessary and sufficient for "organizational" and "activational" effects. This
article is a progress report of efforts in this direction.

ORGANIZATIONAL EFFECTS

"Organizational effects" of hormones refer to actions during brain development which permanently alter neural circuitry or the response characteristics of neurons and lead, for example, to sex differences in brain function and behavior (cf. Goy and McEwen, 1980). Brain sex differences in mammals arise, like the morphological sex differences in the reproductive tract, through the developmental actions of testicular secretions. Male rats castrated at birth fail to develop a complete reproductive tract and also are deficient in masculine reproductive behavior, even after replacement with testosterone in adulthood (cf. Goy and McEwen, 1980).

Neonatally castrated male rats also display feminine sexual behavior and an LH "surge" after priming with estradiol plus progesterone in adulthood. Male rats castrated as adults and treated with estradiol plus progesterone rarely, if ever, show LH "surges" and display very little feminine sexual behavior. Female rats can be made to respond like adult castrated male rats if, as neonates, they are given a single testosterone injection. This suppression of feminine response characteristics is known as "defeminization", whereas the enhancement of masculine characteristics by testosterone is known as "masculinization" (Beach, 1975).

Defeminization in rats is also produced by estrogens given neonatally (cf. Plapinger and McEwen, 1978). This finding, together with the ineffectiveness of 5α reduced androgens, has led to the discovery that defeminization is mediated by estrogen receptors after the conversion of testosterone to estradiol within target cells of the brain (cf. Goy and McEwen, 1980). Pharmacological blockade of aromatization or of estrogen receptors antagonizes defeminization (Vreeburg et al., 1977; McEwen et al., 1977). Moreover, the androgen-receptor deficient Tfm mutant male rat shows signs of having undergone normal defeminization (Olsen, 1979a,b; Beach and Buehler, 1977); and it is known that Tfm males have normal testosterone secretion, as well as normal aromatase activity and neural estrogen receptor levels (Krey et al., 1981). In contrast to defeminization, masculinization in rats appears to occur through a combination of aromatization and estrogen receptors, on the one hand, and androgen receptor-mediated effects on the other (cf. McEwen, 1981).

Although for some years the brain and not the pituitary was presumed to be a primary site of testosterone action during development (Harris and Jacobsohn, 1952), it is only recently that there has been real progress in understanding what happens to the brain in the course of sexual differentiation. Neuroanatomical studies have led the way, beginning with the first observation of sex differences in nucleolar and cell nuclear size in brains of gonadally intact (Pfaff, 1966) and hormone-

treated adult rodents and primates (Bubenik and Brown, 1973).
The electron microscopic studies of Raisman and Field (1973),
showing a sex difference in adult rat preoptic area synaptic
patterns which is dependent on early testosterone exposure,
triggered a series of recent observations at the light and electron microscopic level revealing sex differences in central nervous system morphology in songbirds (Nottebohm and Arnold, 1976;
Gurney and Konishi, 1980) and rodents (Greenough et al., 1977;
Gorski et al., 1978; Rethelyi, 1979; Matsumoto and Arai, 1980;
Breedlove and Arnold, 1980; Loy and Milner, 1980; Arimatsu et al.,
1981; Nishizuka and Arai, 1981; Ross et al., 1981). Among the
more notable features of some of these sex differences are their
occurrence in neural pathways and brain regions related to
sexually-dimorphic and hormone-dependent neural events such as
song in birds (Nottebohm and Arnold, 1976; Gurney and Konishi,
1980), penis movement (Breedlove and Arnold, 1980), and gonadotropin secretion (Matsumoto and Arai, 1980) in rats. Differences
in cell number and cell size in addition to different patterns of
synapses are characteristic of these sex differences.

How do these sex differences arise during the critical
period of early perinatal neural development in mammals and birds?
One of the mechanisms currently under investigation is hormone-
stimulated neurite growth which has been demonstrated in organ
culture (Toran-Allerand, 1976) of mouse brain to be influenced by
testosterone or estradiol and which appears to emanate in those
cultures from developing neurons which contain estrogen receptors
(Toran-Allerand et al., 1980). From current information regarding the sequence of cellular events in neural development (Lund,
1978), neurite growth stimulated by gonadal hormones might be a
condition sufficient to produce differences in cell number and
cell size as well as patterns of synaptic connections which are
the major features of the sex differences already described in
the adult brain (see above). However, it would be premature to
overlook possible hormone effects on other aspects of neural
development, including the reinitiation of cell division or the
promotion of cell death, as well as the production of factors
which stabilize synaptic contacts. Furthermore, it is also
possible that testosterone may help to program the differentiation of groups of neurons with respect to neurotransmitter type
or other cellular characteristics. Glucocorticoids have been reported to have such effects on neurotransmitter expression in
developing neurons (McLennan et al., 1980; Fukada, 1980; Jonakait
et al., 1980).

Hormone stimulation of sexual differentiation occurs at a
stage of neuronal development when considerable cellular differentiation has already occurred, in that estrogen (MacLusky et al.,
1979; Vito and Fox, 1979) and androgen receptors (Vito et al.,
1979; Lieberburg et al., 1980) and enzymes involves in testoste-

rone metabolism to estradiol (Reddy et al., 1974) and 5α dihydrotestosterone (Denef et al., 1974) have already been laid down in
certain neural cells. These confer upon particular neurons the
ability to respond to the hormonal signal, and, as noted above, it
is now known that both androgens and oestrogens arising from testosterone participate in sexual differentiation (Goy and McEwen,
1980), albeit in differing degrees depending on the species (Baum,
1979). It is evident that some estrogen and androgen receptors are
already present in the fetal rodent hypothalamus in the last tri-
mester of gestation (Vito and Fox, 1979; Vito et al., 1979) from
around the time of final cell division (Ifft, 1972). However, estrogen receptor levels in the male and female rat brain increase
markedly beginning shortly before birth (MacLusky et al., 1979)
and androgen receptor levels increase markedly as of one week after birth (Lieberburg et al., 1980; Attardi and Ohno, 1976). A
major challenge for our further understanding of the origins of
brain sex differences will be to uncover the factors, hormonal or
otherwise, which govern the first appearance and subsequent perinatal increases of estrogen and androgen receptors and testosterone metabolizing enzymes in both male and female brains.

ACTIVATIONAL EFFECTS

"Activational effects" of hormones are reversible actions
which lead, for example, to ovulation and sexual behavior or ag-
gressive behavior and vocalization (e.g., song in birds). Such
effects operate on a neural substrate which may have been subject
to "organizing" actions of the same hormones. For example, testosterone acts in development to permanently organize the neural substrate for vocalization in songbirds (Nottebohm, 1980) and for masculine sexual behavior (e.g., in rats); and it also acts to activate these behaviors in the mature animal (cf. Goy and McEwen,
1980). And as noted above, testosterone, acting via estradiol, de-
feminizes the rat brain and suppresses its ability to respond to
estradiol and progesterone with respect to ovulation and feminine
sexual behavior. In this section, we shall examine some of the
characteristics of estradiol and progesterone action on the normal
female rat brain as an illustration of activational effects and
how they can be studied.

One of the major advantages of studying estradiol and progesterone action on feminine sexual behavior in rats is that both
hormones act within a few hours to activate behavior. The behavioral endpoint is highly reliable, clearcut, and quantitative. As
a result, there has been a great deal of recent progress in elucidating the mechanisms involved (Pfaff, 1980; McEwen, 1981).

Estradiol effects on feminine sexual behavior are manifested
after a lag period of 18h and become clearly evident by 24h

(Green et al., 1970; Parsons et al., 1980). Progesterone treatment is required, but it only is effective after estrogen priming.
Progesterone acts more rapidly than estradiol, with a latency of
only an hour (Meyerson, 1972; McGinnis et al., 1981). These
actions of exogenous estradiol and progesterone in ovariectomized
rats mimic the temporal pattern of hormone secretion in the estrus cycle of the rat: estradiol levels rise a day before the
onset of behavioral estrus, whereas a peak of progesterone secretion occurs at the time of the preovulatory LH surge which pre-
cedes behavioral estrus by only a few hours (Smith et al., 1975).

        Estradiol and progesterone action both appear to involve a
stimulation of protein synthesis. Estradiol action to facilitate
feminine sexual behavior is blocked by an RNA synthesis inhibitor,
actinomycin D (Quadagno et al., 1971) and by protein synthesis
inhibitors, cycloheximide (Quadagno and Ho, 1975) and anisomycin
(Rainbow et al., 1980a). When estradiol is applied continuously
via Silastic capsules, a 6h period of treatment is sufficient to
activate behavior (Rainbow et al., 1980a; Parsons et al., 1981).
Moreover, the critical protein synthesis appears to take place
within the 6h period (Rainbow et al., 1980a). If, however, the
estrogen stimulus is broken into two 1h segments, two such ex-
posures, which are not less than 4h or more than 14h apart, are
sufficient to activate sexual behavior measured at 24h (Parsons
et al., 1981). Under these conditions, the period of protein
synthesis, as defined by the susceptibility to protein synthesis
inhibitors, is prolonged after the first 1h exposure; however,
protein synthesis triggered by the second 1h estradiol stimulus
is completed within 2h of the second exposure (Parsons et al.,
1981). We interpret these findings to indicate that estradiol
triggers more than one phase of protein synthesis and that the
later phase may occur as little as 10h before behavior is manifested.

        Progesterone action to facilitate feminine sexual behavior
is also blocked by anisomycin (Rainbow et al., 1980). Besides
stimulating formation of protein involved in facilitating sexual
behavior, progesterone also appears to promote formation of proteins which have a delayed effect to inhibit sexual behavior.
This is revealed by experiments in which anisomycin treatment
3-10h after progesterone administration blocks the "sequential
inhibition" by progesterone of sexual behavior at 24h (Parsons
and McEwen, 1981).

        A crucial event linking estradiol and progesterone action
in the brain, pituitary and reproductive tract is the induction
of progestin receptors by estradiol (Parsons et al., 1980; McEwen
et al., 1982). In the rat brain this induction occurs in hypothalamus and preoptic area and is temporally correlated with the

activation of feminine sexual behavior. A "threshold" level of 30%
of maximal induction has been associated with the potential to display this behavior; below 30%, sexual behavior is not elicitable
by progesterone administration (Parsons et al., 1980). Progesterone receptor induction by estradiol is attenuated by treatment with
an anti-estrogen, CI628 (Roy et al., 1979), and a protein synthesis inhibitor, anisomycin (Rainbow et al., 1980a), under conditions
which also block activation of feminine sexual behavior.

      Estradiol and progesterone both produce their effects when in-
troduced locally into the ventromedial hypothalamus of ovariectomized rats. The ventromedial hypothalamic region is known to be
essential for lordosis: lesions abolish the behavior and electrical stimulation of this area facilitates lordosis responding
(Pfaff, 1980). Intrahypothalamic steroid administration has been
regined by diluting the hormone with cholesterol and by the use of
tritiated hormones, and a high degree of spatial localization has
been achieved (Davis et al., 1979). The ventrolateral portion of
the ventromedial nucleus of the hypothalamus appears to be the
most sensitive brain region, stimulation of which bilaterally by
estradiol (Davis et al., 1979) and by progesterone, after estrogen
priming (Rubin and Barfield, personal communication), leads to
activation of lordosis. Introduction of anisomycin into the ventromedial hypothalamus reversibly blocks the effects of systemically
administered estradiol and progesterone in activating feminine sexual behavior (Rainbow et al., 1980b).

                       CONCLUSIONS AND PROSPECTUS

      Beyond the temporal and spatial aspects of estradiol and pro-
gesterone action in brain lies the largely unexplored area of the
neurochemical aspects of hormone action: i.e., how hormone action
results in altered neural activity and what are the key events or
properties of neurons and synapses which are regulated by steroid
hormones. There are demonstrated steroid effects on neural electrical activity, monoamine turnover, release and reuptake of neurotransmitters, induction of neurotransmitter-related enzymes, and
regulation of neurotransmitter receptors (McEwen, 1981). Some of
these changes have been shown to occur in steroid-sensitive cell
groupings known to be involved in hormone-dependent behaviors. For
example, in the Zebra finch, testosterone induces cholinergic enzymes (choline acetyltransferase and acetylcholinesterase) in an-
drogen-sensitive motoneurons of the hypoglossal nucleus which innervate the syrinx, the song organ (Luine et al., 1980); song in
birds is influenced by androgens (Nottebohm, 1980). In the ventromedial nucleus of the female rat hypothalamus, an area which is

essential for estradiol and progesterone action on feminine sexual behavior, estradiol treatment increases progestin receptor levels (Rainbow and Parsons, unpublished) and muscarinic cholinergic receptors (Rainbow et al., 1980c) and decreases glutamic acid decarboxylase (GAD)(Wallis and Luttge, 1980) and monoamine oxidase (Luine, unpublished) activity. Progestin receptor induction is clearly relevant to the synergistic action of progesterone on feminine sexual behavior in this brain region (see above); and induction of muscarinic receptors may be related to the fact that muscarinic transmission in hypothalamus appears to be involved in facilitation of feminine sexual behavior (Clemens and Dohanich, 1980; Clemens et al., 1980). Decreased ventromedial hypothalamic activity of GAD resulting from estradiol exposure might result in lesser gabaminergic influence, presumably inhibitory (Al Satli et al., 1980), on feminine sexual behavior and thus contribute to behavioral facilitation. What emerges from this kind of analysis is that the behaviorally-relevant neurochemical changes evoked by estrogen treatment even in one brain region may be plural rather than singular, i.e., both potentiation of facilitatory pathways and suppression of inhibitory pathways may be involved in the activation of behavior.

As noted above, studies of feminine sexual behavior in rats are fruitful for the understanding of brain sexual differentiation. The "organizing" action of testosterone on the developing rat brain results in the suppression of the capacity to display lordosis behavior in normal males and neonatally testosterone-treated females. The consequences of these suppressive actions of testosterone might manifest themselves as a deficit in particular brain regions of males of particular cellular constituents (e.g., neurotransmitters; steroid receptors) or by a deficit in males of particular steroid-dependent events (e.g., choline acetyltransferase induction by estradiol, which occurs in female but not in male, rat preoptic area; Luine et al., 1975). Further information regarding the neurochemical aspects of brain sex differences will be extremely useful in the further understanding and analysis of the normal control of sexual behavior in females as well as the location and mechanism of brain sexual differentiation.

ACKNOWLEDGMENT

Research in the author's laboratory is supported by research grant NS07080 from the USPHS and by an Institutional grant RF 70095 from the Rockefeller Foundation for research in reproductive biology.

REFERENCES

Al Satli, M., Ciesielski, L., Kempf, D., Mack, G. and Aron, C. 1980. Involvement of serotonin and γ-aminobutyric acid in the timing of estrous receptivity in the cyclic female rat. Psychoneuroendocrinology 5:319-328.

Arimatsu, Y., Seto, A., and Amano, T., 1981. Sexual dimorphism in α-bungarotoxin binding capacity in the mouse amygdala. Brain Research 213:432-437.

Attardi, B. & Ohno, S., 1976. Androgen and estrogen receptors in the developing mouse brain. Endocrinology 99:1279-1290.

Baum, M.J., 1979. Differentiation of coital behavior in mammals: a comparative analysis. Neurosci. Biobehav. Rev. 3:265-284.

Beach, F.A., 1975. Hormonal modification of sexually dimorphic behavior. Psychoneuroendocrinology 1:3-23.

Beach, F.A. & Buehler, M.G., 1977. Male rats with inherited insensitivity to androgen show reduced sexual behavior. Endocrinology 100:197-200.

Breedlove, S.M. & Arnold, A.P., 1980. Hormone accumulation in a sexually dimorphic motor nucleus of the rat spinal cord. Science 210:564-566.

Bubenik, G.A. and Brown, G.M., 1973. Morphologic sex differences in primate brain areas involved in regulation of reproductive activity. Experientia 29:619-621.

Clemens, L.G. & Dohanich, G.P., 1980. Inhibition of lordotic behavior in female rats following intracerebral infusion of anticholinergic agents. Pharmac. Biochem. Behav. 13:89-95.

Clemens, L.G., Humphrys, R.R. and Dohanich, G.P., 1980. Cholinergic brain mechanisms and the hormonal regulation of female sexual behavior in the rat. Pharmac. Biochem. Behav. 13:81-88.

Davis, P.G., McEwen, B.S. & Pfaff, D.W., 1979. Localized behavioral effects of tritiated estradiol implants in the ventromedial hypothalamus of female rats. Endocrinology 104:898-903.

Denef, C., Magnus, C. & McEwen, B.S., 1974. Sex-dependent changes in pituitary 5α-dihydrotestosterone and 3α-androstanediol formation during postnatal development and puberty in the rat. Endocrinology 94:1265-1274.

Fukada, K., 1980. Hormonal control of neurotransmitter choice in sympathetic neuron cultures. Nature 287:553-555.

Gorski, R.A., Gordon, J.H., Shryne, J.E. & Southam, A.M., 1978. Evidence for a morphological sex difference within the medial preoptic area of the rat brain. Brain Research 148:333-346.

Goy, R.W. & McEwen, B.S. eds., 1980. 'Sexual Differentiation of the Brain'. Based on a Work Session of the Neurosciences Research Program, MIT Press, Cambridge, 211 pp.

Green, R., Luttge, W.G. & Whalen, R.E., 1970. Induction of receptivity in ovariectomized female rats by a single intravenous injection of estradiol-17 β. Physiol. Behav. 5:137-141.

Greenough, W.T., Carter, C.S., Steerman, C. & DeVoogd, T., 1977. Sex differences in dendritic patterns in hamster preoptic area. Brain Research 126:63-72.

Gurney, M.E. & Konishi, M., 1980. Hormone-induced sexual differentiation of brain and behavior in zebra finches. Science 208:1380-1382.

Harris, G.W. & Jacobsohn, D., 1952. Functional grafts of the anterior pituitary gland. Proc. Royal Soc. London B. 139: 263-276.

Ifft, J.D., 1972. An autoradiographic study of the time of final division of neurons in rat hypothalamic nuclei. J. Comp. Neurol. 144:193-204.

Jonakait, G.M., Bohn, M.C. & Black, I.B., 1980. Maternal gluco-corticoid hormones influence neurotransmitter phenotypic ex-pression in embryos. Science 210:551-553.

Krey, L.C., Lieberburg, I., MacLusky, N.J. & Davis, P.G., 1981. Aromatization in the brain of the Stanley-Gumbreck pseudoherma-phrodite male rat: implications for testosterone modulation of neuroendocrine activity. Endocrinology (submitted).

Lieberburg, I., MacLusky, N.J. & McEwen, B.S., 1980. Androgen receptors in the perinatal rat brain. Brain Research 196:125-138

Loy, R. & Milner, T.A., 1980. Sexual dimorphism in extent of axonal sprouting in rat hippocampus. Science 208:1282-1283.

Luine, V.N., Khylchevskaya, R.I. & McEwen, B.S., 1975. Effect of gonadal steroids on activities of monoamine oxidase and choline acetylase in rat brain. Brain Research 78:293-306.

Luine, V.N., Nottebohm, F., Harding, C. & McEwen, B.S., 1980. Androgen effects cholinergic enzymes in syringeal motor neurons and muscle. Brain Research 192:89-107.

Lund, R.D., 1978. 'Development and Plasticity of the Brain' pp. 370, Oxford University Press, New York.

MacLusky, N.J., Lieberburg, I. & McEwen, B.S., 1979. The development of estrogen receptor systems in the rat brain: perinatal development. Brain Research 178:129-142.

Matsumoto, A. & Arai, Y., 1980. Sexual dimorphism in 'wiring pattern' in the hypothalamic arcuate nucleus and its modification by neonatal hormonal environment. Brain Research 190: 238-242.

McEwen, B.S., 1981. Neural gonadal steroid actions. Science 211:1301-1311.

McEwen, B.S., 1981. Sexual differentiation of the brain: gonadal hormone action and current concepts of neuronal differentiation in 'Molecular Approaches to Neurobiology' (I. Brown ed.), Academic Press, New York.

McEwen, B.S., Davis, P.G., Gerlach, J.L., Krey, L.C., MacLusky, N.J., McGinnis, M.Y., Parsons, B. & Rainbow, T.C., 1982. Progestin receptors in the brain and pituitary gland in 'Progesterone and Progestins' (C.W. Bardin, P. Maivais-Jarvis and E. Milgrom eds.) Raven Press, New York, in press.

McEwen, B.S., Lieberburg, I., Chaptal, C. & Krey, L.C., 1977. Aromatization: important for sexual differentiation of the neonatal rat brain. Horm. Behav. 9:249-263.

McGinnis, M.Y., Parsons, B., Rainbow, T.C., Krey, L.C. & McEwen, B.S., 1981. Temporal relationship between cell nuclear progestin receptor levels and sexual receptivity following intravenous progestin administration. Brain Research.

McLennan, I.S., Hill, C.E. & Hendry, I.A., 1980. Glucocorticoids modulate transmitter choice in developing superior cervical ganglion. Nature 283:206-207.

Meyerson, B., 1972. Latency between intravenous injection of progestins and the appearance of estrous behavior in estrogen-treated ovariectomized rats. Horm. Behav. 3:1-10.

Nishizuka, M. & Arai, Y., 1981. Sexual dimorphism in synaptic organization in the amygdala and its dependence on neonatal hormone environment. Brain Research 212:31-38.

Nottebohm, F., 1980. Brain pathways for vocal learning in birds: a review of the first 10 years in 'Progress in Psychobiology and Physiological Psychology' (J.M. Sprague and A.N. Epstein eds.) pp. 85-124, Academic Press, New York.

Nottebohm, F. & Arnold, D.P., 1976. Sexual dimorphism in vocal control areas of the songbird brain. Science 194:211-212.

Olsen, K.L., 1979a. Androgen-insensitive rats are defeminized by their testes. Nature 279:238-239.

Olsen, K.L., 1979b. Induction of male mating behavior in androgen-insensitive (Tfm) and normal (King-Holtzman) male rats: effect of testosterone propionate, estradiol benzoate, and dihydrotestosterone. Horm. Behav. 13:66-84.

Parsons, B., MacLusky, N.J., Krey, L.C., Pfaff, D.W., and McEwen, B.S., 1980. The temporal relationship between estrogen-inducible progestin receptors in the female rat brain and the time course of estrogen activation of mating behavior. Endocrinology 107:774-779.

Parsons, B. & McEwen, B.S., 1981. Sequential inhibition of sexual receptivity by progesterone is not causally related to decreased hypothalamic progestin receptors in the female rat. J. Neurosci. 1:527-531.

Parsons, B., Rainbow, T.C., Pfaff, D.W. & McEwen, B.S., 1981. A discontinuous schedule of oestradiol binding in rat hypothalamus is sufficient to activate lordosis behaviour and to increase cytosol progestin receptors. Nature (in press).

Pfaff, D.W., 1966. Morphological changes in the brains of adult male rats after neonatal castration. J. Endocrinol. 36:415-416.

Pfaff, D.W., 1980. 'Estrogens and Brain Function' pp. 281, Springer-Verlag, New York.

Plapinger, L. & McEwen, B.S. 1978. Gonadal steroid-brain interactions in sexual differentiation in 'Biological Determinants of Sexual Behavior' (J. Hutchinson ed.), pp. 193-218, J. Wiley, New York and London.

Quadagno, D.M. & Ho, G.K.W., 1975. The reversible inhibition of steroid-induced sexual behavior by intracranial cycloheximide. Horm. Behav. 6:19-26.

Quadagno, D.M., Shryne, J. & Gorski, R.A., 1971. The inhibition of steroid-induced sexual behavior by intrahypothalamic actinomycin D. Horm. Behav. 2:1-10.

Rainbow, T.C., Davis, P.G. & McEwen, B.S., 1980a. Anisomycin inhibits the activation of sexual behavior by estradiol and progesterone. Brain Research 194:548-555.

Rainbow, T.C., Davis, P.G., McGinnis, M. & McEwen, B.S., 1980b. Application of anisomycin to the lateral ventromedial nucleus blocks the activation of sexual behavior by estradiol and progesterone. Soc. Neurosci. Abst. 293.4, p. 862.

Rainbow, T.C., DeGroff, V., Luine, V.N. & McEwen, B.S. 1980c. Estradiol 17β increases the number of muscarinic receptors in hypothalamic nuclei. Brain Research 198:239-243.

Reddy, V.V.R., Naftolin, F. & Ryan, K.J., 1974. Conversion of androstenedione to estrone by neural tissues from fetal and neonatal rats. Endocrinology 94:117-121.

Raisman, G. & Field, P.M., 1973. Sexual dimorphism in the neuropil of the preoptic area of the rat and its dependence on neonatal androgen. Brain Research 54:1-29.

Rethelyi, M., 1979. Regional and sexual differences in the size of the neuro-vascular contact surface of the rat median eminence and pituitary stalk. Neuroendocrinology 28:82-91.

Ross, D.A., Glick, S.D. & Meibach, R.C., 1981. Sexually dimorphic brain and behavioral asymmetries in the neonatal rat. Proc. Nat. Acad. Sci. USA 78:1958-1961.

Roy, E.J., MacLusky, N.J. & McEwen, B.S., 1979. Antiestrogen inhibits the induction of progestin receptors by estradiol in the hypothalamus-preoptic area and pituitary. Endocrinology 104:1333-1336.

Smith, M.S., Freeman, M.E. & Neill, J.D., 1975. The control of progesterone secretion during the estrous cycle and early pseudo-pregnancy in the rat: prolactin, gonadotropin and steroid levels associated with rescue of the corpus luteum of pseudopregnancy. Endocrinology 96:219-226.

Toran-Allerand, C.D., 1976. Sex steroids and the development of the newborn mouse hypothalamus and preoptic area in vitro: implications for sexual differentiation. Brain Research 106: 407-412.

Toran-Allerand, C.D., Gerlach, J.L. and McEwen, B.S., 1980. Autoradiographic localization of ^{3}H estradiol related to steroid responsiveness in cultures of the newborn mouse hypothalamus and preoptic area. Brain Research 184:517-522.

Vito, C.C. & Fox, T.O., 1979. Embryonic rodent brain contains estrogen receptors. Science 204:517-519.

Vito, C.C., Wieland, S.J. & Fox, T.O., 1979. Androgen receptors exist throughout the "critical period" of brain sexual differentiation. Nature 282:308-310.

Vreeburg, J.T.M., van der Vaart, P.D.M. & van der Schoot, P., 1977. Prevention of central defeminization but not masculinization in male rats by inhibition neonatally of oestrogen biosynthesis. J. Endocrinol. 74:375-382.

Wallis, C.J. & Luttge, W.G., 1980. Influence of estrogen and progesterone on glutamic acid decarboxylase activity in discrete regions of rat brain. J. Neurochem. 34:609-613.

INTRACELLULAR COMPARTMENTATION OF THE OESTROGEN RECEPTOR IN THE FEMALE RAT HYPOTHALAMUS

Louis Lim, John White, Sean Thrower,
Christine Hall and Stephen Whatley

Miriam Marks Department of Neurochemistry
Institute of Neurology, National Hospital
London University, Queen Square, WC1N 3BG

In recent years the role of intracellular receptors in mediating the action of sex steroids has been clarified as a result of experiments on the oviduct and uterus. Sex steroids complex with specific receptors which then bind to the chromatin in the nucleus and activate specific transcription, eventually resulting in the appearance of new proteins (O'Malley & Birnbaumer, 1977, 1978). Although direct interaction of the receptor with the chromatin has been demonstrated in these target tissues, there is increasing interest in the interaction of oestrogens with membranes, and in the brain there is electrophysiological data for this latter aspect of steroid action (Dufy & Vincent, 1980). Nevertheless, there is good circumstantial evidence that oestrogens also operate via intracellular receptors and that these receptors, present specifically in hypothalamic neurones, mediate genomic activity within the brain (McEwen, 1978). In this communication we discuss our own work on factors involved in the intracellular distribution of the oestrogen receptor in the female rat hypothalamus and also the interactions of the receptor complex in the nuclear compartment.

INTRACELLULAR DISTRIBUTION OF THE OESTROGEN RECEPTOR

All target tissues for oestrogens contain apparently similar specific receptors with high affinity for the hormone in cytosolic and nuclear compartments. We have shown that in the hypothalamus of female rats undergoing the oestrous cycle, cyclic changes in the content of nuclear receptors parallel those in the uterus, a classical target organ (White et al, 1978). These changes are the result of oestradiol-induced translocation of the cytosol receptors into the nucleus; accordingly, maximal concentrations of

665

these nuclear receptors occur at the appropriate phase when the
level of circulating oestradiol is highest i.e. at pro-oestrus.
The nuclear receptor increase in the hypothalamus is associated
with increased gonadotrophin secretion, ovulation and sexual receptivity, responses all probably resulting from enhanced hypothalamic production of LH-RH. There are differences in the behaviour
of the oestrogen receptors between the hypothalamus and the uterus.
Whether they are pertinent to differences in tissue responsivity
(the uterine response of proliferation never being expressed by
the hypothalamus) remains to be established. Some of these receptor differences relate to depletion of cytosol receptors and the
low extent of nuclear binding of receptor in the hypothalamus compared with the uterus.

     As far as we know, receptors in the cytosol do not appear to
have any other function apart from ligand (oestrogen) binding.
Once this is achieved translocation of the oestrogen-receptor complex into the nucleus occurs; co-incident with the translocation
the receptor is transformed from a 4S cytosol form to a 5S nuclear
form. The 4S and 5S designations refer to the apparent size of
the receptor and are based on sucrose density centrifugation measurements.

MEDIATORY ROLE OF A BINDING FACTOR

     Transformation in vitro of the cytosol receptor from a 4S to a
5S form can also occur on binding to DNA-cellulose or oligo(dT)-
cellulose, which serves as a binding matrix (Thrower et al, 1976).
Oligo-(dT) cellulose is used routinely instead of DNA-cellulose
since the latter is subject to nuclease activity and may also contain polysaccharides and other contaminants which interfere with
receptor binding to the polydeoxyribonucleotide matrix. This receptor binding to the matrix in vitro mimics its binding to the
nucleus in vivo (Yamamato & Alberts, 1976) where DNA has been
shown to be an obligatory element in the binding process. The 5S
receptor can be extracted from nuclei using 0.4 M KCl-buffer which
is also effective in eluting the 5S receptor from the DNA- or
oligo (dT)-cellulose matrix. In uterine and hypothalamic preparations a cytosol factor mediates the binding of the receptor to the
oligo-(dT)-cellulose and its transformation. Extensive experiments on uterine preparations have shown that the characteristics
of the binding factor are widely different from the receptor itself (Thrower et al, 1976; Myatt et al, 1981). In the transformation step it is possible that the two components combine with
one another irreversibly since we have difficulty separating the
components once the 5S form is established.

     In the uterus, the binding factor appears to be present in
sufficient quantities to support extensive nuclear binding of the
receptor which is 3 to 4 fold higher than in the brain, as estima-

ted from receptor concentrations in the cytosol and nuclear compartments at different phases (White et al, 1978; Lim et al, 1981).
The factor is also present as a constant proportion of the cytosol
receptor at all phases. This suggests that in the uterus the factor is replenished to the same extent as the cytosol receptor
throughout the cycle (White et al, 1978; Myatt et al, 1978). This
is not the case in the hypothalamus where the concentration of the
factor, relative to receptor, in the cytosol is not only lower but
is also depleted at pro-oestrus with the concomitant increase of
the nuclear content of receptor (White et al, 1978). It should be
noted that this nuclear binding of receptor in both tissues is dependent on initial translocation brought about by increases in the
circulating concentrations of oestradiol.

We have also obtained evidence for an inhibitor of the binding
factor in hypothalamic cytosol (Shen et al, 1979). This finding
emphasizes the complexity of receptor interactions and points out
that receptor-mediated events in the brain may be subject to regulation exerted at diverse levels.

SIGNIFICANCE OF RECEPTOR TRANSLOCATION INDUCED BY EXOGENOUS OESTRA-
DIOL

In intact adult females the content of nuclear receptors can be
increased in the hypothalamus upon injection of oestradiol (White
et al, 1977; White & Lim, 1980). The content was increased maximally within 1 hour and then fell so that the content after 6 hours
was only about 2-fold higher. Nevertheless, this represented a
significant increase and is in keeping with other studies on immature and ovariectomized animals. In these animals it has been
demonstrated that oestradiol administration leads to translocation
of cytosol receptors into the nucleus of uterine cells, the initial rapid nuclear increase being followed by a slow decrease but
with the content still elevated 6-9 hours later. The decrease represents the disappearance of receptor translocated in excess of
the long-term nuclear binding sites. The increase in nuclear receptor at the 6-9 hours period (i.e. long-term nuclear receptor)
could be correlated with increases in wet weight of tissue and
other true uterotrophic responses such as growth and differentiation (Clark et al, 1973). However our recent studies suggest that
oestradiol administration does not lead to increases in long-term
nuclear receptors in the uteri of adult, intact animals (Thrower
& Lim, 1981). At each phase of the cycle although oestradiol administration led to nuclear increases within 60-90 minutes the
subsequent decrease in nuclear receptors (fall-out) was such that
by 8 hours the content had returned to normal uninjected values.
It seems that in the uteri of intact adults nuclear binding of the
so-called 'long-term' or active receptors was already saturated
at each phase, the maximal values for this saturation being different for each individual phase. These experiments suggested

that factors other than oestradiol were responsible for determining the extent of nuclear binding of receptor. {This suggestion
finds support from our observations that despite exposure to the
same concentration of oestrogens, either in vivo or in vitro and
the presence of similar quantities of binding factor and cytosol
receptors, there was a much lower concentration of nuclear oestrogen receptors in the uterine horn bearing an intra-uterine device compared with the contralateral control horn in the same
uterus (Myatt et al, 1978; 1980)}. These experiments also indicate that different regulatory mechanisms exist for the hypothalamus since we were able to increase the hypothalamic content of
long-term nuclear receptors by administration of oestradiol (White
& Lim, 1980).

The regulatory mechanisms may include those that ensure an attenuated intracellular exposure of the brain to oestradiol throughout the cycle. Such an attenuation, involving metabolic conversion
of oestrogens, is seen in the liver. In this organ, which also
contains significant concentrations of cytosol oestrogen receptors,
the content of nuclear oestrogen receptors remains constant at all
phases of the oestrous cycle (Marr et al, 1980b), presumably to
prevent excessive phasic oestrogenic stimulation of the liver. The
content of long-term nuclear receptors can be increased upon administration of the synthetic oestrogen, ethynyl oestradiol, which by-
passes the normal metabolic pathways responsible for inactivating
oestradiol (Marr et al, 1980a). However because the hypothalamic
nuclear oestrogen receptor content does increase, albeit to a
slight extent, at pro-oestrus, it may be that if such regulatory
mechanisms exist, they are only partially effective and need to be
so in view of the phasic requirement for oestrogenic stimulation
of hypothalamic activity leading to ovulation and sexual activity.

REGULATION OF NUCLEAR COMPARTMENTATION OF RECEPTOR

There are therefore a variety of factors which act to limit the
concentration of presumptive physiologically active nuclear receptors within the hypothalamus. These include (a) the non-replenish-
ment of cytosol receptors,as opposed to the uterus (b) the presence only in low concentrations of a cytosol factor which may be
obligatory for long-term nuclear binding of receptor (and which
is also not replenished) and (c) the occurrence of inhibitors of
the factor. Another factor which also operates to limit nuclear
binding in the hypothalamus is progesterone. We have found that
an injection of progesterone 24 hours before peak concentrations
of oestradiol are achieved in the cyclic rat (i.e. injection at
late dioestrus and examining at pro-oestrus) prevented the normal
cyclic increase at pro-oestrus in nuclear oestrogen receptor content in the hypothalamus but not in the uterus (Thrower & Lim,

1981). This finding should be viewed in the context of a progesto-
genic inhibition of sexual activity (Feder & Marrone, 1977).
{Although, progesterone receptors are present in the hypothalamus
(Thrower & Lim, 1980a) it is still unclear whether they are involved in potentiating the action of this hormone}. Compartmentation of the oestrogen receptor thus appears to regulate its activity. There are constraints which prevent the nuclear compartment
from being increased, except at specific times and then only for
a limited period, with progesterone perhaps ensuring the nuclear
fall-out process. The increase which occurs at pro-oestrus sets
in motion other processes which lead to sexual activity and ovulation.

    An increase in the hypothalamic nuclear receptor compartment
is also seen in the postnatal developmental period (White et al,
1979; Lim & Davison, 1980), at a time when final hypothalamic
differentiation occurs. This increase, relative to the nuclear
content in the first 3 weeks, occurs concomitantly with changes
in hypothalamic RNA metabolism (Hall & Lim, 1978) which coincide
with pre-pubertal changes in gonadotrophin levels. However it
must be pointed out that the hypothalamic responses even during
this developmental period, which are presumably dependent on nuclear binding of receptors, are limited when compared with the re-
spones of other target tissues; for example, even in the mature
uterus oestradiol promotes cellular proliferation. In the hypothalamus, these oestrogen receptors have been demonstrated to be
localized in neurones (McEwen, 1978) which have lost the ability
to divide. There is evidence in other tissues that the major responses induced by the hormone are dependent on nuclear receptor
concentration (Buller & O'Malley, 1976). The restricted response
of neurones to the potentially proliferative effect of the hormone
may lie in carefully regulated mechanisms which ensure that only a
small proportion of the oestrogen receptors is bound to the chromatin. Another factor to be considered is the unique chromatin
organisation of forebrain neurones. The chromatin of these neurones in the adult differ from chromatin of other cells in that
the DNA repeat length of the nucleosomes (chromatin subunits) is
shorter (Thomas & Thompson, 1977). Hypothalamic neurones also
show this short DNA repeat length (Whatley et al, 1980a) and it is
conceivable that this unique nuclear organization is involved in
ensuring that receptor binding in the nucleus does not trigger off
the extensive cellular responses seen in other target tissues, such
as proliferation. Exposure of foetal hypothalamic neurones cultured in vitro (Whatley et al, 1981b) to oestradiol was also without detectable morphological effect although oestrogen receptors
are known to be present in foetal rodent hypothalamus (Vito & Fox,
1979). It is noteworthy that neurones from the foetal hypothalamus but not cerebrum, already display the short DNA repeat length
in chromatin (Whatley et al, 1981a).

OCCURRENCE OF UNOCCUPIED OESTROGEN RECEPTORS IN THE NUCLEUS

Although in the hypothalamus the presence of nuclear oestrogen receptors is necessary to initiate genomic events the continued presence of oestrogen itself is not essential once translocation has been achieved. Thus, sexual receptivity in ovariectomized rats can be elicited only some considerable period after administration of the oestradiol during which time (20-30 hours later) there is little trace of the steroid itself, based on experiments with radio-active oestradiol (McEwen, 1978). The requirement for genomic activity was shown by using specific inhibitors of transcription which were effective in blocking the sexual responses when administered a few hours before or after the initial injection of the sex steroid. We have found that the majority of hypothalamic nuclear receptors are unoccupied i.e. free of the ligand throughout the cycle (Thrower & Lim, 1980b). We performed extensive experiments to rule out the presence of contaminating cytosol receptors or artefactual dissociation (White & Lim, 1980; Thrower et al, 1981). Moreover, the content of long-term, presumably active nuclear receptors that was increased on oestradiol administration was also predominantly unoccupied (White & Lim, 1980). This increase in unoccupied receptors occurred linearly after steroid administration, although the content of occupied receptors was sequentially increased and decreased (the latter representing fall-out). This suggests a processing of a pool of nuclear oestrogen receptors to unoccupied receptors. Whether loss of ligand represents metabolic processing of the active nuclear receptors or whether unoccupied receptors themselves are active and ligand loss is obligatory for activation of this class of nuclear receptor is unresolved. Nevertheless, unoccupied receptors must have a physiological significance since in neonatally androgenised anovulatory rats not only are they present in lower proportions, their content is not markedly increased on oestradiol injection (White & Lim, 1980). These rats do not respond to oestradiol administration either by ovulation or by increased sexual activity. However they can become both sexually active and fertile when given regulated injections of LH-RH suggesting that there is defective hypothalamic LH-RH synthesis in the androgenised rats (Hahn & McGuire, 1978). It could well be that this defect is associated with defective processing of hypothalamic nuclear oestrogen receptors. These rats also have an abnormally low hypothalamic content of both binding factor and nuclear receptor (White, 1978).

The androgenised rats have also proved useful in investigations on uterine nuclear oestrogen receptors. The rats are deficient in progesterone and display uterine epithelial hyperplasia and metaplasia (White et al, 1981). The abnormal morphology is associated with an abnormally high content of nuclear oestrogen receptors; both features are restored to normalcy upon progesterone therapy (White et al, 1982). In androgenised rats, the proportion of unoccupied nuclear receptor in the uterus is lower than normal and is increased on progesterone therapy. Interestingly, in normal rats at all phases, unoccupied receptors constitute the majority of the oestrogen receptors, and also form a constant proportion of the nuclear receptors in most target tissues (Thrower & Lim, 1980b).

FINAL REMARKS

Our interest in hypothalamic oestrogen receptor mechanisms has been stimulated in part by the extensive and elegant work of Bruce McEwen and his associates on the relationship of the oestrogen receptors to hypothalamic functions and sexual receptivity, summarized by McEwen (1978). Our own work suggests that in the hypothalamus, nuclear compartmentation of oestrogen receptors is restricted, occuring to a more limited extent than in other target tissues where the nuclear receptors initiate vigorous cellular responses. Evidence for a possible mediatory role of a cytosol protein in the nuclear binding of the receptor has been presented as well as for the presence of unoccupied nuclear receptors with possible physiological functions. This binding protein could itself be involved in the formation of the unoccupied nuclear receptor component since in androgenised rats a lower content of binding protein is associated with a decreased ability to form unoccupied receptors. Has the protein any other role ?

We have previously commented (Lim et al, 1981) on the similarities between the operations of the oestrogen receptor system and of neurotransmitter receptor systems involving adenylate cyclase, as outlined in the model by Rodbell (1980). Features in common include (a) specific ligand binding (b) receptor translocation (in the case of the neurotransmitter receptor intramembrane translocation occurs) and (c) interaction of the receptor with a regulatory protein. The regulatory protein involved in the neurotransmitter response, rather than the receptors themselves, activates specific enzymes. Whether in the case of the hypothalamus it is the cytosol binding/regulatory protein(s) that ultimately specifies the appropriate hormonal response and the ligand-receptor interaction serves only to introduce this protein(s) into the nuclear compartment is an interesting question. The multitude of responses in a variety of target tissues evoked by oestradiol binding to an apparently uniform cytosol receptor (Greene et al, 1980) obviously must be regulated by different nuclear binding sites on the chromatin for the translocated receptor. It is an intriguing possibility that genomic activation at these sites may be specified by cytosol regulatory proteins selectively transported into the nucleus only after association with the hormone-receptor complex.

Louis Lim acknowledges the generous support of the Brain Research Trust and the Wellcome Trust.

REFERENCES

Buller, R.E. and O'Malley, B.W., 1976, The biology and mechanism of steroid hormone receptor interaction with the eukaryotic nucleus. Biochem.Pharmacol., 25:1.

Clark, J.H., Anderson, J.N. and Peck, E.J., 1973, Nuclear receptor oestrogen complexes of rat uteri, in:"Advances in Experimental Medicine and Biology," B.W.O'Malley, A.R.Means, eds., Plenum Press, New York. Vol.36, p.15.

Dufy, B. and Vincent, J.D., 1980, Effects of sex steroids on cell membrane excitability: a new concept for the action of steroids on the brain, in:"Hormones and the Brain," D.De Wied, P.A.van Keep, eds., MTP Press Ltd., England. p.29.

Feder, H.H. and Marrone, B.L., 1977, Progesterone: its role in the central nervous system as a facilitator and inhibitor of sexual behaviour and gonadotrophin release. Ann.NY.Acad.Sci., 286:331

Greene, G.L., Fitch, F.W. and Jensen, E.V., 1980, Monoclonal antibodies to estrophilin - probes for the study of estrogen receptors. Proc.Natl.Acad.Sci., 77:157.

Hahn, D.W. and McGuire, J.L., 1978, The androgen-sterilised rat: induction of ovulation and implantation by luteinising hormone-releasing hormone. Endocrinology, 102:1741.

Hall, C. and Lim, L., 1978, The metabolism of high-molecular-weight ribonucleic acid in hypothalamic and cortical regions of the developing female rat brain. Biochem.J., 176:511.

Lim, L. and Davison, A.N., 1980, Nutrition and amino acid imbalance as factors influencing brain development. in:"Biochemistry of Brain," S.Kumar, ed., Pergamon Press, Oxford.p.323.

Lim, L., White, J.O., Thrower, S. and Hall, C., 1981, Nucleocyto-solic relationships of the oestrogen receptor in brain function and differentiation, in: "Chemisms of the Brain," R.Rodnight, H.Bachelard, W.Stahl, eds., Churchill Livingstone, London.

McEwen, B.S., 1978, Gonadal steroid receptors in neuroendocrine tissues. in:"Receptors in Hormone Action II", B.W.O'Malley, L.Birnbaumer, eds., Academic Press, London.

Marr, W., Elder, M.G. and Lim, L., 1980a, The effects of oestrogens and progestogens on oestrogen receptors in female rat liver. Biochem.J., 190:563.

Marr, W., White, J.O., Elder, M.G. and Lim, L., 1980b, Nucleocyto-plasmic relationships of oestrogen receptors in rat liver during the oestrous cycle and in response to administered natural and synthetic oestrogen. Biochem.J., 190:17.

Myatt, L., Chaudhuri, G., Elder, M.G. and Lim, L., 1978, The oes-trogen receptor in the rat uterus in relation to intra-uterine devices and the oestrous cycle. Biochem.J., 176:523.

Myatt, L., Chandhuri, G., Elder, M.G. and Lim, L., 1980, Effect of an intra-uterine device on intracellular relationships of the uterine oestrogen receptor, particularly during pregnancy. J.Endocrinology, 87:357.

Myatt, L., Elder, M.G., Neethling, C. and Lim, L., 1981, The binding of rat uterine cytosol oestrogen receptors to oligo-deoxy-
thymidylate cellulose; its relationship to a stable form of receptor complex with separate ligand and oligo-nucleotide binding sites. Biochem.J., in press.
O'Malley, B.W. and Birnbaumer, L. (eds.), 1977, 1978, Receptors
in Hormone Action, Volumes 1 and 2, Academic Press, New York.
Rodbell, M., 1980, The role of hormone receptors and GTP-regulatory proteins in membrane transduction. Nature, 264:17
Shen, G., Thrower, S. and Lim, L., 1979, Uterine oestrogen-receptor binding to oligo(dT)-cellulose: an inhibitor from hypothalamic cytosol. Biochem.J., 182:241.
Thomas, J.O. and Thompson, R.J., 1977, Variation in chromatin
structure in two cell types from the same tissue: A short DNA
repeat length in cerebral cortex neurons. Cell, 10:633.
Thrower, S., Hall, C., Lim, L. and Davison, A.N., 1976, The selective isolation of the uterine oestradiol receptor complex
by binding to oligo(dT)-cellulose. The mediation of an essential activator in the transformation of cytosol receptor. Bio-
chem.J., 160:271.
Thrower, S. and Lim, L., 1980a, Characterisation of rat hypothalamic progestin binding by spherodial hydroxylapatite chromatography. Biochem.J., 186:295.
Thrower, S. and Lim, L., 1980b, A comparison of the relationships
between progestin receptors and oestrogen receptors in neural
and non-neural target tissues of the rat during the oestrous
cycle. Biochem.J., 190:691.
Thrower, S. and Lim, L., 1981, The nuclear oestrogen receptor in
the female rat. Effects of oestradiol administration during
the oestrous cycle on the uterus and contrasting effects of
progesterone on the uterus and hypothalamus. Biochem.J., 198:
385.
Thrower, S., Neethling, C., White, J.O. and Lim, L., 1980, The
unoccupied nuclear oestradiol receptor in the rat uterus and
hypothalamus during the oestrous cycle. Biochem.J., 194:667.
Vito, C.C. and Fox, T.O., 1979, Embryonic rodent brain contains
estrogen receptors. Science, 204:517.
Whatley, S.A., Hall, C. and Lim, L., 1981a, Chromatin organisation in the hypothalamus during early development. Biochem.
J., 196:115.
Whatley, S.A., Hall, C. and Lim, L., 1981b, Hypothalamic neurons
in dissociated cell culture: Mechanism of increased survival
times in the presence of non-neuronal cells. J.Neurochem.,
36:2052.
White, J.O., 1978, The oestrogen receptor of rat brain: Intracellular relationships in the developing and adult female.
Ph.D. Thesis, University of London.
White, J.O., Hall, C. and Lim, L., 1979, Developmental changes
in the content of oestrogen receptors in the hypothalamus of
the female rat. Biochem.J., 184:465.

White, J.O. and Lim, L., 1980, Unoccupied nuclear oestrogen recep-
    tors in the female rat hypothalamus: increases on oestrogen
    administration. Biochem.J., 190:833.
White, J.O., Moore, P.A., Elder, M.G. and Lim, L., 1981, The re-
    lationships of the oestrogen and progestin receptors in the
    abnormal uterus of the adult anovulatory rat. Biochem.J.,
    196:557.
White, J.O., Moore, P.A., Elder, M.G. and Lim, L., 1982, Proge-
    sterone therapy results in partial reversibility of uterine
    abnormalities of the adult anovulatory rat. Biochem.J.,
    submitted.
White, J.O., Thrower, S. and Lim, L., 1977, The oestrogen recep-
    tor of the female rat hypothalamus: Relationship between nu-
    clear content and oligothymidylate-cellulose binding to cytosol
    receptor. Biochem.Soc.Trans., 5: 1558.
White, J.O., Thrower, S. and Lim, L., 1978, Intracellular rela-
    tionships of the oestrogen receptor in the rat uterus and hypo-
    thalamus during the oestrous cycle. Biochem.J., 172:37.
Yamamoto, K.R. and Alberts, R.A., 1976, Steroid receptors: ele-
    ments for modulation of eukaryotic transcription. Ann.Rev.
    Biochem., 45:721.

VASOPRESSIN AND OXYTOCIN, CHEMICAL MESSENGERS IN THE BRAIN

R.M. Buijs

Netherlands Institute for Brain Research
Ijdijk 28, 1095 KJ Amsterdam, the Netherlands

The neurohypophyseal hormones vasopressin and oxytocin are synthesized in the supraoptic (SON) and paraventricular nuclei (PVN),
while the suprachiasmatic nucleus (SCN) contains vasopressin only
(Swaab and Pool, 1975; Vandesande et al., 1975). These peptides are
transported to the median eminence and the neurohypophysis where
release into the blood occurs, where vasopressin acts primarily as
an antidiuretic hormone on the kidney, while only in high doses it
is effective on blood pressure. Oxytocin acts in the female on the
mammary gland for the milk ejection and on the uterus especially
during labor. In the male no clearcut peripheral function for oxytocin
has been established up till now. Already in the thirties central
effects for these hormones were suggested by Cushing (1932), in
addition to the peripheral endocrine actions of vasopressin and
oxytocin. He demonstrated pronounced central effects of an extract
of the neurohypophysis following an injection into the cerebral
ventricles of hypophysectomized patients. It was de Wied, however,
who opened up the experimental field on the effects of pituitary
hormones on the brain. It was demonstrated, e.g., that injection
of vasopressin, either peripherally (de Wied, 1971) or centrally
(Kovacs et al., 1979) resulted in the consolidation of acquired

675

behavior. In addition, vasopressin might be involved in the central
regulation of water balance (Raichle and Grub, 1978), temperature
(Cooper et al., 1979) or brain development (Boer et al., 1980).

   By means of specific and sensitive immunocytochemical methods,
a wide-spread vasopressin and oxytocin fiber system is demonstrated
arising from the above mentioned hypothalamic nuclei. These peptidergic fibers reach brain regions ranging from the olfactory bulb
to the spinal cord. In addition, from immunoelectronmicroscopical
observations it appeared that these peptidergic fibers terminate
on neurons and dendrites in the limbic system by means of synapses
indistinguishable from the classical aminergic ones. These and
other recent observations led to the conclusion that vasopressin
and oxytocin most probably execute their central action via exohypothalamic fibers and might be regarded as peptidergic neurotransmitters.

Localization of vasopressin and oxytocin

Antisera against these peptides were raised and purified using
agarose beads coupled with the heterologous peptide (Swaab and
Pool, 1975). Rat brains were fixed by perfusion with 2.5% glutaraldehyde, 1% paraformaldehyde in 0.1 M cacodylate buffer pH 7.2
and sectioned on a vibratome for immunolight- or immunoelectronmicroscopy, using the unlabeled antibody enzyme method (Sternberger,
1974). For further details of fixation, staining and specificity
controls see Buijs et al. (1978); Buijs and Swaab (1979).

   In the adult rat, vasopressin or oxytocin was demonstrated in
cell bodies of the PVN and SON and in fibers running towards the
neurohypophysis, as well as in cell bodies scattered throughout
the hypothalamus. From the PVN or SON a great number of vasopressin
or oxytocin fibers were found to run into many regions in the
brain. It appeared that oxytocin fibers dominated in the caudal
brain regions as the brain stem and spinal cord while mostly vasopressin fibers were demonstrated in the more rostral brain regions

of which especially the limbic system is densely innervated. In
addition, also from the SCN a large number of only vasopressin
containing fibers fan out into various directions (fig. 1).

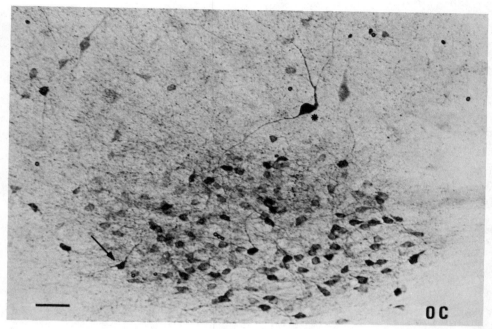

Fig. 1 - Sagittal 100 µm thick vibratome section of the vasopressin
containing parvocellular suprachiasmatic nucleus with fibers
fanning out, (OC)= rostral part of the optic chiasm. Note the bipolar parvocellular neuron (arrow) and the magnocellular one (*)
(Bar=25µm).

However, as it appeared from lesion studies of the SCN (Hoorneman
and Buijs, 1982) it is extremely difficult by immunocytochemical
techniques alone to establish the source of the exohypothalamic
fibers to a certain hypothalamic nucleus. From this lesion experiment followed by the immunocytochemical localization of vasopressin,
it appeared that the SCN projects only to the organum vasculosum
lamina terminalis, dorsomedial nucleus of the hypothalamus and
periventricular nucleus (Hoorneman and Buijs, 1982). Consequently,

projections formerly ascribed to the SCN as the lateral septum,
lateral habenular nucleus, diagonal band of Broca (Buijs et al.,
1978; Buijs, 1978; Buijs, 1980; Sofroniew and Weindl, 1978a,b),
amygdala, dorsal raphe nucleus and nucleus tractus solitarius

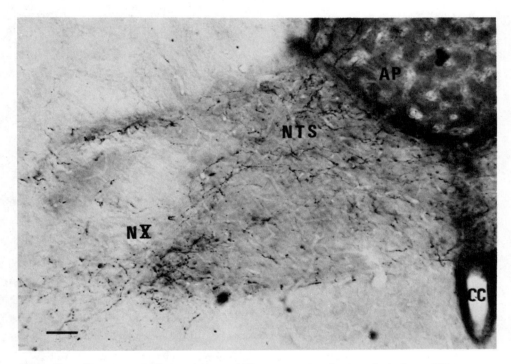

Fig. 2 - Transversal section with vasopressin containing fibers
terminating in the region of the nucleus of the solitary tract
(NTS)(AP=area postrema; NX=dorsal motor nucleus of the vagus; cc=
central canal)

(Sofroniew and Weindl, 1978b) will be derived from the PVN or SON.
Fig. 3 summarizes the main vasopressin pathways derived from the
PVN or SON. In addition, it appeared that vasopressin fibers in
the lateral septum terminate in a sex-dependent way, resulting in
a much less innervation of this area in the female rat (de Vries
et al., 1981).

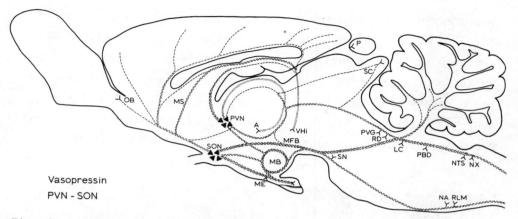

Vasopressin
PVN - SON

<u>Fig. 3</u> - illustrates pathways and possible sites of termination of
vasopressin containing fibers in the rat brain projected in the
sagittal plane. Paraventricular (PVN) and supraoptic nucleus (SON)
are indicated by large triangles. 1, 2 or 3 interrupted lines are
an indication for an increasing number of fibers in the pathway,
while a λ indicates a possible site of termination.
A=amygdala; DBB=diagonal band of Broca; LC=locus coeruleus; LH=
lateral habenular nucleus; MB=mammillary body; ME=median eminence;
MFB=medial forebrain bundle; MS=medial septal nucleus; NA=nucleus
ambiguus; NTS=nucleus of the solitary tract; NX=dorsal motor nucleus
of the vagus; OB=olfactory bulb; P=pineal; PBD= dorsal parabrachial
nucleus; PVG=periventricular grey; RD=dorsal raphe nucleus; RLM=
lateral magnocellular reticular nucleus; SC=superior colliculus;
SN=substantia nigra; VHi=ventral hippocampus

The synaptic localization of vasopressin and oxytocin

In order to verify whether vasopressin and oxytocin fibers really
terminate in these brain regions, immunoelectronmicroscopy was
performed on the most densely innervated structures, i.e. the
lateral septum, lateral habenular nucleus and amygdala (Buijs and
Swaab, 1979). In all three regions synaptic structures containing

vasopressin were found to terminate mostly on dendrites (fig. 4) but also on cell bodies. These synapses contained largely clear vesicles and infrequently dense core vesicles, the latter with a diameter of approximately 100 nm. These structures containing neurohypophyseal "hormones" were indistinguishable from classical neurotransmitter containing synapses, as visualized with a similar pre-embedding staining technique (e.g. Pickel et al., 1979).

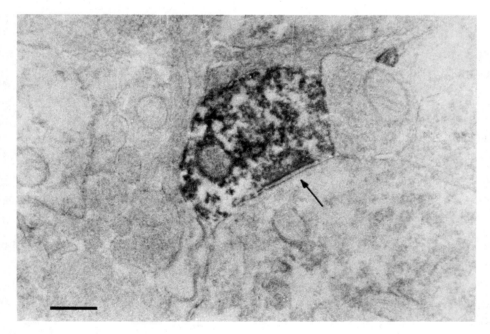

Fig. 4 - Vasopressin containing terminal forming a synapse (arrow) with an unlabelled dendrite in the lateral septum. Note the DAB deposit around the clear vesicle-like structures. (Bar=0.25 μm)

The observation that vasopressin and oxytocin are present in granules of 100 nm, does not fit in with the observation that the PVN and SON (where these fibers originate) contain granules of a larger size (140 nm)(van Leeuwen et al., 1978). Since in the neuro-hypophysis using this technique a granular size was found of 150 nm, it seems obvious that different cells project towards the neuro-

hypophysis and the brain or that a different release mechanism exists
in central brain regions and neurohypophysis. Vasopressin immunoreactivity was frequently found at the surface of clear vesicle-
like structures (fig. 4). This might fit in with the idea that the
smooth endoplasmatic reticulum serves as an alternative vehicle for
intra-axonal transport of non-granular neurosecretory material
(Droz et al., 1973) that gives rise to clear vesicles in the axonal
terminal (Alonso and Assenmacher, 1978).

Vasopressin and oxytocin; two peptide neurotransmitters?

The criteria for identification of a substance as a transmitter
in the central nervous system as formulated by Werman (1966), were
recently extended with criteria for neuromodulators, neuromediators,
neurohumours etc. (Barchas et al., 1978; Bloom, 1979; Dismukes,
1979; Siggins, 1979). Arguments will be given for which points
these two neuropeptides fulfil the criteria for being a neurotransmitter.

The wide-spread distribution of these two peptides throughout
the central nervous system and their presence in synaptic structures is the fulfilment of a major criterium to establish a substance as a neurotransmitter. Equally important is the ability of
these synapses to release their transmitter upon a depolarizing
stimulus. Recent in vitro experiments (R.M. Buijs, unpubl. obs.)
demonstrated a Ca^{2+}-dependent K^+ stimulated release of vasopressin
from the lateral septum and oxytocin release in the nucleus of the
solitary tract. In addition, the central release of AVP upon a
physiological stimulus was demonstrated by Cooper et al. (1979),
who found that using a push-pull canule in the sheep septal region
vasopressin release was negatively correlated with induced changes
in body temperature. Receptor binding for vasopressin and oxytocin
is still undemonstrable. However, often a good correlation is
found between the central sites of action and the distribution of
the areas where these peptidergic fibers appear to terminate

(Kovacs et al., 1979; Cooper et al., 1979; Buijs, 1978; Buijs and Swaab, 1979).

Finally the ability of neurohypophyseal peptides to change membrane potentials was demonstrated by Morris et al. (1980), who found an inhibition of glutamate induced or spontaneous firing after iontophoretically applied oxytocin to brain stem neurons in a region that is densely innervated by oxytocin containing fibers, the nucleus of the solitary tract.

It will thus be clear that these two neuropeptides are very good candidates for a function in the central nervous system as neurotransmitters. Although not all criteria are fully met, the arguments for such a role for the much longer studied aminergic or aminoacid neurotransmitters are often not better.

The ubiquitous presence of these peptides throughout the animal kingdom, even in insects, molecules closely related to neurophysins have been demonstrated (Friedel et al., 1980), while the human brain is also densely innervated by these peptidergic fibers, suggests important central functions of vasopressin and oxytocin. However, at present the limited data available are mostly from studies in rats (de Wied and Bohus, 1979); it seems likely from the latter physiological or behavioral observations in combination with the anatomical data, that these peptides might be involved in the integration of (stressful) stimuli and influence important autonomic functions like the regulation of temperature (Cooper et al., 1979), bloodpressure (Bohus, 1980; le Moal et al., 1981) and water balance (Raichle and Grub, 1978). Dysfunctioning of these processes in older individuals seems to coincide with a change in the staining of the vasopressin cells in the aged human brain (E. Fliers, unpubl. obs.), suggesting that these peptides may be essential compounds for the functioning of the central nervous system in development, adulthood and aging.

REFERENCES

Alonso, G., Assenmacher, I., The smooth endoplasmic reticulum in
    neurosecretory axons of the rat neurohypophysis. Biol. Cell 32
    203-206 (1978)

Barchas, J.D., Akil, H., Elliott, G.R., Holman, R.B., Watson, S.J.:
    Behavioral neurochemistry: Neuroregulators and behavioral
    states. Science 200, 964-973 (1978)

Bloom, F.E., Contrasting principles of synaptic physiology:
    peptidergic and non-peptidergic neurons. In: K. Fuxe, T.
    Hökfelt, and R. Luft (eds.), Central Regulation of the Endocrine
    System, pp. 173-187, Plenum Press, New York (1979)

Boer, G.J., Swaab, D.F., Buijs, R.M., Uylings, H.B.M., Velis, D.N.,
    and Boer, K., Neuropeptides in rat brain development. In: P.S.
    McConnell, G.J. Boer, H.J. Romijn, N.E. van de Poll, and M.A.
    Corner (eds.), Adaptive Capabilities of the Nervous System,
    Progress In Brain Research, Vol. 53. Elsevier, Amsterdam (in
    press)(1980)

Bohus, B., Effects of neuropeptides on adaptive autonomic processes.
    In: D. de Wied and P.A. van Keep (eds.), Hormones and the Brain,
    pp. 129-139, MTP Press, Lancaster (1980)

Buijs, R.M., Intra- and extrahypothalamic vasopressin and oxytocin
    pathways in the rat. Pathways to the limbic system, medulla
    oblongata and spinal cord. Cell Tiss. Res. 192, 423-435 (1978)

Buijs, R.M., Vasopressin and oxytocin innervation of the rat brain.
    A light- and electronmicroscopical study. Ph.D. thesis,
    Amsterdam (1980)

Buijs, R.M., and Swaab, D.F., Immunoelectron microscopical demon-
    stration of vasopressin and oxytocin containing synapses in
    the limbic system of the rat. Cell Tiss. Res. 204, 355-365
    (1980)

Buijs, R.M., Swaab, D.F., Dogterom, J., and van Leeuwen, F.W.,
    Intra- and extrahypothalamic vasopressin and oxytocin pathways

in the rat. Cell Tiss. Res. 186, 423-433 (1978)

Cooper, K.E., Kasting, N.W., Lederis, K., and Veale, W.L., Evidence supporting a role for endogenous vasopressin in natural suppression of fever in sheep. J. Physiol. 295, 33-45 (1979)

Cushing, H., Paper relating to the pituitary body, hypothalamus and parasympathetic nervous system. C.C. Thomas (ed.), Springfield, Ill. U.S.A. (1932)

Dismukes, R.K., New concepts of molecular communication among neurons. Behav. Brain Sci. 2, 409-448 (1979)

Droz, B., Koenig, H.L., Giaumberardino, L.J., Axonal migration of protein and glycoprotein to nerve andings. I. Radioautographic analysis of the renewal of protein in nerve endings of chicken ciliary ganglions after intracerebral injection of ^{3}H-lysine. Brain Res. 60, 93-127 (1973)

Friedel, T., Laughton, B.G., Andrew, R.D., A neurosecretory protein from Locusta migratoria. Gen. Comp. Endocr. 41, 487-498 (1980)

Hoorneman, E.M.D., Buijs, R.M., Exohypothalamic vasopressinergic fibre pathways in the rat brain after lesioning of the suprachiasmatic nucleus (submitted)

Kovacs, G.L., Bohus, B., Versteeg, D.H.G., de Kloet, E.R., and de Wied, D., Effect of oxytocin and vasopressin on memory consolidation: sites of action and catecholaminergic correlates after local microinjection into limbic midbrain structures. Brain Res. 175, 303-314 (1979)

Leeuwen, F.W. van, Swaab, D.F., and de Raay, C., Immunoelectronmicroscopic localization of vasopressin in the rat suprachiasmatic nucleus. Cell Tiss. Res. 193, 1-10 (1978)

Le Moal, M., Koob, G.F., Koda, L.Y., Bloom, F.E., Manning, M., Sawyer, W.H., and Rivier, J., Vasopressor receptor antagonist prevents behavioural effects of vasopressin. Nature 291, 491-493 (1981)

Morris, R., Salt, T.E., Sofroniew, M.V., and Hill, R.G., Actions of microiontophoretically applied oxytocin, and immunohistochemical localization of oxytocin, vasopressin and neurophysin in the rat caudal medulla. Neurosci. Lett. 18, 163-168 (1980)

Pickel, V.M., Joh, T.H., Reis, D.J., Leeman, S.E., and Miller, R.J., Electron microscopic localization of substance P and enkephalin in axon terminals related to dendrites of catecholaminergic neurons. Brain Res. 160, 387-400 (1979)

Raichle, M.E., Grubb, R.L., Regulation of brain water permeability by centrally released vasopressin. Brain Res. 143, 191-194 (1978)

Siggins, G.R., Neurotransmitters and neuromodulators and their mediation by cyclic nucleotides. In: Y.H. Ehrlich, J. Volavka, L.G. Davis and E.G. Brungraber (eds.), Modulators, Mediators and Specifiers in Brain Function, pp. 41-64, Plenum Press, New York (1979)

Sofroniew, M.V., and Weindl, A., Extrahypothalamic neurophysin containing perikarya, fiber pathways and fiber clusters in the rat brain. Endocrinology 102, 234-237 (1978a)

Sofroniew, M.V., and Weindl, A., Projections from the parvocellular vasopressin and neurophysin containing neurons of the suprachiasmatic nucleus. Amer. J. Anat. 153, 391-430 (1978b)

Sternberger, L.A., Immunocytochemistry, New York: Prentice Hall, Englewood Cliffs (1974)

Swaab, D.F., Pool, C.W., Specificity of oxytocin and vasopressin immunofluorescence. J. Endocrinol. 66, 263-272 (1975)

Vandesande, F., Dierickx, K., and de Mey, J., Identification of the vasopressin neurophysin producing neurons of the rat suprachiasmatic nuclei. Cell Tiss. Res. 156, 377-380 (1975)

Wied, D. de, Long-term effect of vasopressin on the maintenance of a conditioned avoidance response in rats. Nature 232, 58-60 (1971)

Wied, D. de, Bohus, B., Modulation of memory processes by neuropeptides of hypothalamic neurohypophyseal origin. In: M.A.B. Brazier (ed.), Brain mechanisms in memory and learning: from the single neuron to man, pp. 139-149, New York, Raven Press (1979)

A PROCEDURE FOR THE CHARACTERISATION OF IDENTIFIED NEURONAL PATHWAYS

J.V.Priestley, P.Somogyi, A.Consolazione and
A.C.Cuello

University Departments of Pharmacology and Human
Anatomy, South Parks Road, Oxford;
1st Department of Anatomy, Semmelweis University
Medical School, Budapest (PS).

Recently several groups have published procedures which combine the retrograde transport of horseradish peroxidase (HRP) with peroxidase-antiperoxidase (PAP) immunohistochemistry (Bowker et al.,1981; Sofroniew and Schrell,1981; Priestley et al.,1981). This allows a projection neuron identified on the basis of HRP retrograde labelling to be also stained immunohistochemically for a particular transmitter marker. We describe here one such procedure and illustrate its application for the exploration of rostral serotonin (5-HT) projections from the dorsal raphe nuclei.

Unilateral injections of 0.1μl 20% HRP were made into the striatum of rats and after 24 hours the animals were perfused through the abdominal aorta with 4% paraformaldehyde 0.1% glutaraldehyde. The brains were removed, kept in fixative for a further 4 hours and then transferred to 0.1M phosphate buffer containing 5% sucrose. Subsequently 20μ cryostat sections were cut at various levels of the dorsal raphe. Sections were first stained to localise HRP (LaVail,1978), then washed thoroughly and stained by PAP immunohistochemistry using a monoclonal antibody raised against a serotonin bovine serum albumin conjugate (Consolazione et al.,1981). DAB and hydrogen peroxide were used as substrates for the peroxidase reaction in both cases. Full details of various controls and of the distribution of stained cells have been reported previously (Priestley et al.,1981). More recently we have also examined the pattern of staining obtained following the injection of HRP into various areas of the thalamus. The retrogradely HRP labelled cells in the dorsl raphe show a distinct punctate pattern of staining when examined in the light microscope, probabley because the HRP is concentrated in multivesicular and dense bodies (LaVail,1978).

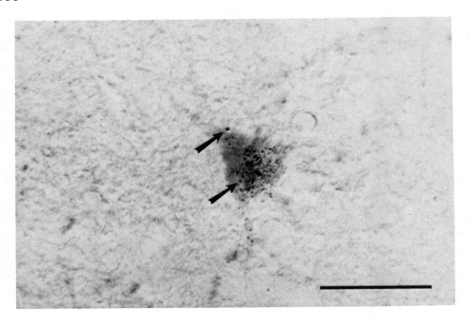

Fig.1. A cell in dorsal raphe retrogradely labelled from the
        thalamus with HRP and immunostained for 5-HT. Staining for
        HRP appears as distinct granules (arrows) which are super-
        imposed on the diffuse immunostaining. Interference contrast
        illumination.   Scale bar = 20μ

In contrast the 5-HT PAP immunostained cells in the same area have
diffuse homogeneous staining, probabley due to diffusion of the 5-HT
prior to fixation (Priestley and Cuello,1981). Thus it is possible
to distinguish the retrogradely transported peroxidase and the
immuno-localised peroxidase (PAP) simply on the basis of their
appearance in the light microscope. A number of dually stained cells
were observed in which punctate retrogradely transported HRP staining was superimposed on diffuse PAP staining (Fig.1) and such cells
represent 5-HT containing cells which project to the site of HRP
injection. Following injection of HRP into the striatum it was
possible to identify retrogradely labelled cells in the dorsal raphe
which showed no immunostaining as well as the dually labelled cells,
indicating the presence of both non-serotonergic and serotonergic
components in this pathway.

    The procedure described here has so far only been used to
identify serotonin pathways but it should be applicable to any
system in which a transmitter, neuropeptide or transmitter marker

can be localised immunohistochemically in cell bodies. In addition, since the DAB reaction product is an osmiophilic insoluble polymer it should be possible to extend these studies to the electron microscopic level and such work is now in progress.

Acknowledgements

J.V.P. is an M.R.C. Scholar. P.S. was supported by the Wellcome Trust and A.C. by the Italian Labour Department and the E.E.C. Support to A.C.C. from the Royal Society, the Medical Research Council (UK) and the Wellcome Trust is gratefully acknowledged.

REFERENCES

Bowker, R.M., Steinbusch, H.W.M., and Coulter, J.D., 1981, Serotonergic and peptidergic projections to the spinal cord demonstrated by a combined retrograde HRP histochemical and immunocytochemical staining method, Brain Research, 211:412-417

Consolazione, A., Milstein, C., Wright, B., and Cuello, A.C., 1981, The immunohistochemical detection of serotonin with monoclonal antibodies, J.Histochem.Cytochem., In press

LaVail, J.H., 1978, A review of the retrograde transport technique, in: "Neuroanatomical Research Techniques," R.T.Robertson, ed., Academic Press, New York.

Priestley, J.V., Somogyi, P., and Cuello, A.C., 1981, Neurotransmitter specific projection neurons revealed by combining PAP immunohistochemistry with retrograde transport of HRP, Brain Research, 220:231-240

Priestley, J.V., and Cuello, A.C., 1981, Electron microscopic immunocytochemistry: CNS transmitters and transmitter markers, in: "IBRO Handbook-Immunohistochemistry", A.C.Cuello, ed., John Wiley, London. In press

Sofroniew, M.V., and Schrell, U., 1981, Evedence for a direct projection from oxytocin and vasopressin neurons in the hypothalamic paraventricular nucleus to the medulla oblongata: immunohistochemical visualization of both the horseradish peroxidase transported and the peptide produced by the same neurons, Neuroscience Letters, 22:211-217

FUNCTIONAL MORPHOLOGY OF RETINAL NEURONS WITH MONOAMINE OR AMINO ACID NEUROTRANSMITTERS

B. Ehinger

Department of Ophthalmology
University of Lund, Lund, Sweden

INTRODUCTION

In the analysis of how the central nervous system works it is desirable to link morphology with function, also for a comparatively simply built part like the retina. We have therefore chosen to try to identify the neurotransmitters of the retina, to establish which neurons they are used in and to find out how these neurons are connected to each other. About a dozen proven or presumed neurotransmitters have so far been identified (including certain peptides) but it is at the same time clear that there are many more to be discovered. Most of the so far discovered neurotransmitters are in amacrine cells which must be presumed to have various control functions in the retina but only little is yet known about the transmitters in the synapses directly engaged in the transmission of information from the photoreceptors to the brain. It has further been shown that cells which morphologically seem to belong to the same type may have different neurotransmitters and that not only are the non-mammalian retinas more complex than the mammalian ones, but there are also variations between species as close as different primates. This review will deal with the most recent developments in identification, localization and possible function of amino acid and primary monoamine neurotransmitters in the retina. Graham (1974) has given an excellent review of the older literature. Other reviews on various aspects of the topic have been presented by Neal (1976), Ehinger (1978), Voaden, Morjaria and Oraedu (1980), Lam, Marc, Sarthy, Chin, Su, Brandon and Wu (1980) and Osborne (1981).

PHOTORECEPTORS

The photoreceptor synapses are characterized by an accumulation

691

of small synaptic vesicles in the presynaptic part and a synaptic
ribbon which makes it very likely that they operate with chemical
neurotransmission. Horizontal cells and bipolar cells are very sensitive to aspartate or glutamate (Dowling and Ripps 1972, Murakami,
Ohtsu and Ohtsuka 1972, Cervetto and McNichol 1972, Murakai, Ohtsuka
and Shimazaki 1975). More recently it was found that cone horizontal
cells are in the carp retina more sensitive to aspartate than glutamate; that the effects of both the natural photoreceptor transmitter
and exogenously applied aspartate are blocked by an aspartate antagonist, alpha-aminoadipic acid, and that exogenously applied aspartate has much greater effects on horizontal cells when the retina
is treated with Co^{2+}, an agent which depresses the spontaneous dark
release of transmitter from the photoreceptors (Wu and Dowling 1978,
Negishi and Drujan 1979c). Moreover, aspartate and glutamate are
present in significant concentrations (about 20-80 nmoles/mg
protein) in the photoreceptors in a number of species (Berger,
McDaniel, Carter and Lowry 1977, Voaden 1978), as required of a
photoreceptor neurotransmitter. Further, Thomas and Redburn (1978)
reported high affinity uptake of glutamate and aspartate in a photoreceptor cell preparation, and such high affinity uptakes are often
seen where these substances are transmitters. These observations
suggest that either glutamate or, particularly, aspartate could be
the transmitter of photoreceptors.

(^{3}H)-aspartate or (^{3}H)-glutamate are not very useful for labelling glutamate or aspartate neurons because both substances or their
metabolites are taken up by all nerve cells and by glia to such an
extent that specific uptake is disguised. However, the isomer,
(^{3}H)-D-aspartate, has been shown to be accumulated by brain neurons
likely to use glutamic acid as their neurotransmitter (Balcar and
Johnston 1972, see Ehinger 1981a for further references). D-aspartate is not significantly metabolized by brain tissue (Davies and
Johnston 1976, Takagaki 1978) and metabolites are therefore not
likely to influence the results. Intraocular injections of (^{3}H)-D-
aspartate were not very effective in labelling the photoreceptors
(Ehinger 1981a). Incubating retinas attached to the pigment epithe-
lium and choroid also resulted in rather poor labelling, but incubating detached retinas gave strong labelling of about 10 per cent
of the photoreceptors in rabbits and guinea-pigs (Fig. 1). The
perikarya of these cells were situated in the outermost part of the
outer nuclear layer, and the terminals in the outer plexiform layer
were seen to be large. The labelled cells thus have the characteristics ascribed to cones in these animals. The results are compatible with aspartate or glutamate being the transmitter of these
cells. Neal, Collins and Massey (1979) and Neal and Massey (1980)
reported a fall in the endogenous aspartate release upon light
stimulation, precisely the expected effect if aspartate is transmitter in photoreceptors. Glutamate showed no such decrease. Since
aspartate thus seems to be present presynaptically, to be released
by the appropriate stimulus (darkness) and since it has striking

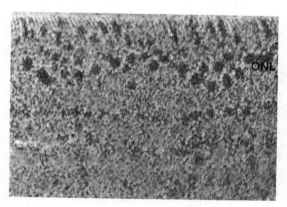

Fig. 1.　Guinea-pig retina incubated in (^{3}H)-D-aspartate. Heavily labelled cones can be seen at the top of the picture. They are about 10 per cent of the photoreceptors. ONL, outer nuclear layer. Phase contrast micrograph, X 180.

postsynaptic effects, indistinguishable for the effect of the physiological stimulation, it is a strong candidate as a photo-receptor neurotransmitter, presumably in cones in rabbit and guinea-pig.

Species variations in the types of neurotransmitters used by what appears to be morphologically identical classes of neurons are now well known in the retina, with perhaps the interplexiform cell as the most notable example. (^{3}H)-D-aspartate labelling shows similar variability. In humans it labels rods but not cones very much (Fig. 2). A similar labelling of rods but not cones was noted

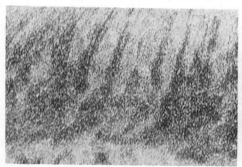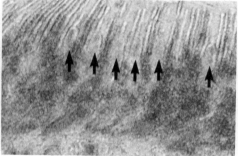

Fig. 2.　Photoreceptor layer from a human retina incubated in (^{3}H)-D-aspartate. Rods are heavily labelled and cones (arrows) only little. Left, focus on the grains; right, focus on the section. Phase contrast micrograph, X 830.

also with (^{3}H)- L-glutamate (Bruun and Ehinger 1974, Lam and Hollyfield 1980) but in this case it was not known to what extent it
could have been the result of metabolism of the (^{3}H)- L-glutamate.
(^{3}H)-D-aspartate does not label the photoreceptors in goldfish
retina very well after either intraocular injections or in incubations (Ehinger, unpublished). However, kainic acid strongly affects
cone bipolar cells and rod and cone horizontal cells in goldfish
(Yazulla and Kleinschmidt 1980) and since this acid is supposed to
act by overstimulating receptors on the cells (Olney 1978) it seems
that aspartic or glutamic acid may nevertheless be photoreceptor
transmitters also in this species. This is also suggested by the
responses in cone horizontal cells discussed above (Wu and Dowling
1978). Kainic acid was in rabbit seen to destroy cone horizontal
cells (Hampton, Garcia and Redburn 1981) which agrees with a role
for aspartic acid or glutamic acid as a cone neurotransmitter in
this species.

HORIZONTAL CELLS

      Horizontal cells have a very special type of synaptic contact
with the photoreceptors in the triads and it is not known how this
synapse works. However, they also make contacts with other cell
processes with synapses of conventional appearance with small synaptic vesicles and membrane specializations, and it is therefore
reasonable to assume that they may to some extent operate with conventional chemical neurotransmission. In most species, the transmitters of horizontal cells are unknown, but in goldfish, pigeons,
chicken, and frogs horizontal cells accumulate (^{3}H)-GABA (Lam,
Marc, Sarthy, Chin, Su, Brandon and Wu 1980, Marshall and Voaden
1974a, Voaden, Marshall and Murani 1974, Hollyfield, Rayborn,
Sarthy and Lam 1979), (^{3}H)-muscimol (Yazulla and Brecha 1981) and
(^{3}H)-isoguvacine (Agardh and Ehinger, unpublished, see further
below) which suggests they may use GABA as their transmitter. They
have in goldfish also been shown to contain the GABA synthesizing
enzyme, GAD, both by biochemical assay of isolated cells (Lam 1975)
and immunohistochemistry (Lam, Su, Swain, Marc, Brandon and Wu
1979). The GABA accumulating cells have been identified as H1 cells
(Marc, Stell, Bok and Lam 1978) connected to red-sensitive cones
(Stell, Ishida and Lightfoot 1975). It was also reported (Lam and
Steinman 1971, Marc, Stell, Bok and Lam 1978, Lam, Marc, Sarthy,
Chin, Su, Brandon and Wu 1980) that the (^{3}H)-GABA uptake into goldfish horizontal cells was stimulated by light, but this has proven
difficult to verify (Agardh and Ehinger 1981). Electrophysiologically, Wu and Dowling (1980) have demonstrated a direct hyperpolarizing effect by GABA on cones, suggesting direct feedback in the
synapses between cone horizontal cells and cones. Similarly,
Murakami, Shimoda and Nakatani (1979) found evidence for a GABA-
mediated feedback from horizontal cells to cones in the dark. In
another teleost, the channel catfish, the cones are all of the red-
sensitive type and it has correspondingly been found that all cone

horizontal cells accumulate (^{3}H)-GABA (Lam, Lasater and Naka 1978). Electrophysiological analysis of the effect of bicuculline suggested that in the catfish, GABAergic horizontal cell feedback to the cones serves to improve the frequency response of the system. However, other functions have not been excluded.

INTERPLEXIFORM CELLS

Dopaminergic terminals were first observed around horizontal cells with the formaldehyde fluorescence histochemical method of Falck and Hillarp (Ehinger, Falck and Laties 1969) and have subsequently been studied in several laboratories both by fluorescence microscopy and autoradiography (Dowling and Ehinger 1975, 1978a, Negishi, Hayashi, Nakamura and Drujan 1979, Sarthy and Lam 1979b, Dowling, Ehinger and Florén 1980, Hayashi 1980, Negishi, Nakamura and Hayashi 1980). When it was noted that labelling them with 5,6-DHT makes them identifyable in the electron microscope, it was soon discovered that they make conventional synapses on both horizontal cells (mainly the GABAergic type H1) and bipolar cells in the outer plexiform layer. However, they receive no observable input in that layer, only in the inner plexiform layer from where they originate. Hence it is assumed that they send information centrifugally in a feedback loop from the inner to the outer plexiform layer, and this formed the basis for identifying them as a special class of cells (Dowling and Ehinger 1975, 1978a, Dowling, Ehinger and Florén 1980). Both horizontal and bipolar cells are sensitive to dopamine (Hedden and Dowling 1978, Negishi and Drujan 1979 a and b) and the evidence suggests that the dopaminergic neurons diminish the inhibitory effect of the surround on the center response of both bipolar and horizontal cells, a kind of contrast enhancing mechanism. Dopamine affected the non-color coded L-type cone horizontal cells (which correspond to the morphologically defined H1 cells discussed above), but had variable effects on the color coded C-type horizontal cells.

Interplexiform cells have dopamine as their transmitter only in teleost fish and certain New World monkey retinas (Dowling and Ehinger, 1975, 1978a, Dowling, Ehinger and Florén 1980), but exist also in a number of other species (Gallego 1971, Dawson and Perez 1973, Boycott, Dowling, Fisher, Kolb and Laties 1975, Oyster and Takahashi 1977, Kolb 1977, Kolb and West 1977, Fisher 1979) and both GABA and glycine have been proposed as possible neurotransmitters. In cats, (^{3}H)-GABA was reported to be accumulated in cells with processes extending into both plexiform layers (Nakamura, McGuire and Sterling 1980). A few of the cells were reconstructed in electron microscopical autoradiographs of serial sections. Input to them was found only in the inner plexiform layer. They correspond to the interplexiform cells previously described by Kolb and West (1977) in cats. In the outer plexiform layer they were found to be presynaptic to rod bipolar cells and, less frequently, to cone bipolar cells. They did not contact horizontal cells. In the inner plexiform layer they were presynaptic to amacrine cells and to rod and cone bipolar cells. Three input synapses from presumed amacrine cell processes were seen in the inner plexiform layer. Pourcho (1980) did not see these cells, but this could be because she used lower concentrations of (^{3}H)-GABA.

Marshall and Voaden (1976) noted that (^{3}H)-glycine labelled processes in the outermost part of the outer plexiform layer in frog retinas. With sufficiently high concentrations of (^{3}H)-glycine, this can be seen also in goldfish and rabbit retinas (Ehinger 1981b, Marc and Lam 1981, Dowling, Ehinger and Mossinger, unpublished), together with some cell bodies among the horizontal cells. At times such cell bodies were also found displaced to the innermost part of the outer nuclear layer. Marc and Lam (1981), using very high (^{3}H)-glycine concentrations found labelled processes traversing the inner nuclear layer and therefore regarded these cells as a glycinergic variety of interplexiform cells, labelled "I2 cells". However, they receive input from H1 horizontal cells, and therefore do not fit with the original identification of interplexiform cells as neurons that have input only in the inner plexiform layer and output in the outer plexiform layer (Ehinger and Dowling 1975). The number of the glycine accumulating cells in and at the outer plexiform layer is comparatively small, and does not compare with the number of dopaminergic interplexiform cells in the cyprine retina.

Previously, Murakami, Ohtsu and Ohtsuka (1972) noted that both L- and C-type horizontal cells hyperpolarize in response to glycine and, similarly, Wu and Dowling (1980) found that glycine hyperpolarized L-type horizontal cells and about 20% of the H2 (or C-type) horizontal cells and selectively abolished their depolarizing responses to red light. Negishi and Drujan (1979c) noted a similar variability in the response of C-type horizontal cells. There is, however, no more detailed evidence available on the function of the very recently detected glycine accumulating cells in the outer plexiform layer.

BIPOLAR CELLS

Bipolar cells have a special arrangement of their synapses, the dyads. There is a presynaptic ribbon with numerous synaptic vesicles associated with it and also some membrane specializations both on the pre- and postsynaptic side. The postsynaptic processes can be either two amacrine cells or one amacrine and one ganglion cell. This type of synapse is likely to be chemical. However, there are hardly any indications as to what their transmitters are. In chicken, Baughman and Bader (1977) found that certain cells which they tentatively identified as bipolar cells accumulated (^{3}H)-choline with a high-affinity mechanism. However, there was only very little (^{3}H)-choline uptake in the outer plexiform layer where the bipolar cells have their dendrites and acetylcholine esterase

was not found in pigeon bipolar cells (Nichols and Koelle 1968).
Pourcho (1980) found that in cats, certain cell bodies identified
as cone bipolar cells accumulated glycine. This is somewhat unexpected because glycine is usually thought to be an inhibitory neurotransmitter, and the bipolar cells are usually assumed to be excitatory (sign-conserving) neurons (Naka 1977, Frumkes and Miller 1979).
However, there is no proof that either of these two assumptions
must be universally valid and the possibility remains that glycine
is the transmitter of some bipolar cells in the cat.

AMACRINE CELLS

   Dopamine. Dopamine was the first neurotransmitter to be firmly
established in the retina. It was originally demonstrated in the
amacrine cells with the formaldehyde histofluorescence method of
Falck and Hillarp (Malmfors 1963) and the procedure has subsequently
been used to demonstrate them in many different laboratories, most
recently by Törk and Stone (1979), Kato, Nakamura and Negishi
(1980), Adolph, Dowling and Ehinger (1980) and Wyse and Lorscheider
(1981). They have also been shown by autoradiography in a number of
species (Ehinger and Falck 1971, Kramer, Potts and Mangnall 1971,
Sarthy and Lam 1979b, Sarthy, Rayborn, Hollyfield and Lam 1981,
Pourcho 1981). The results with the two techniques agree. Dopamine
fulfills most of the criteria of a retinal neurotransmitter, including release by light stimulation or depolarization with potassium
(Kramer 1971, Sarthy and Lam 1979b, Bauer, Ehinger and Åberg 1980,
Dowling and Watling 1981) and ranks as one of the best proven
neurotransmitters in the retina.

   Dopaminergic neurons can be seen in the electron microscope
after labelling with either 5,6-dihydroxytryptamine or (^{3}H)-
dopamine, and their synaptic contacts have been analysed in a
number of species. In rabbits (Dowling and Ehinger 1978b), cats
(Pourcho 1981), and cynomolgus monkeys (Holmgren 1981) they exclusively contact other amacrine cells, forming a set of interamacrine
neurons (Fig. 3). In cats (Pourcho 1981), the postsynaptic amacrine
cell is the bistratified AII type which links rod bipolar cells to
ganglion cells (Famiglietti and Kolb 1975, Kolb 1979). At least
some of the AII cells are likely to use glycine as neurotransmitter
(Pourcho 1980). Dopamine release could thus be expected to inhibit
the presumed inhibitory effects of the glycinergic AII neurons on
some ganglion cells (Fig. 4). However, such disinhibition remains
to be demonstrated.

   Dopamine is also the likely transmitter of the interplexiform
cells seen in the goldfish and Cebus monkey retina, forming feedback loops from the inner plexiform to the outer plexiform layers
(Fig. 5). They receive input mainly from other amacrine cells in
the inner plexiform layer, and in carp Hayashi (1980) found ace-
tylcholesterase containing fibres in close apposition to the dopa-

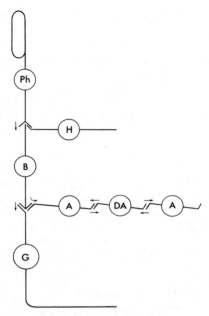

Fig. 3.   Simplified scheme of the contacts made by dopaminergic
           cells (DA) in rabbit, cat and cynomolgus monkey retina.

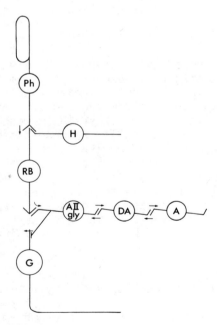

Fig. 4.   Simplified scheme of the contacts made by dopaminergic
           and glycinergic neurons in the cat.

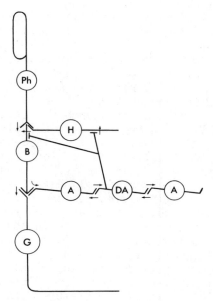

Fig. 5.   Scheme of the contacts made by the dopaminergic interplexiform cells in goldfish and Cebus monkey retina.

minergic neurons, suggesting a cholinergic input into them. There
are also electrophysiological results suggesting that acetylcholine
may activate the interplexiform cells (Negishi and Drujan 1979b).
However, a cholinergic agonist was with an indirect technique not
found to release endogenous dopamine (Dowling and Watling 1981) so
that the cholinergic input remains speculative.

Since the dopaminergic cells receive information from other
amacrine cells, it seems likely that they should display receptors
for transmitters found in amacrine cells. Depolarizing the neurons
with 40 mM potassium will release substantial amounts of (^3H)-dopa-
mine, but a number of known and putative neurotransmitters (GABA,
muscimol, glutamic acid, kainic acid, glycine, and carbachol, all
$10^{-4}M$) were found to be without effect in rabbits (Bauer, Ehinger
and Åberg 1980). Similarly, serotonin, aspartate, glutamate,
carbachol, substance P, 2-D-ala, 5-D-leu-enkephalin, GABA and
glycine failed to induce any endogenous dopamine release from the
carp retina, measured as failure to increase the dopamine sensitive
adenylate cyclase (Dowling and Watling 1981). It therefore seems
unlikely that any of these substances could have any direct excitatory influence on the dopaminergic neurons.

GABA. (^3H)-GABA was first shown to be accumulated by certain
amacrine cells in the rabbit retina (Ehinger 1970, Ehinger and

Falck 1971). It is also to a considerable extent taken up by glial cells which in many mammalian species disguise the neuronal uptake (Ehinger 1977). Attempts have therefore been made to analyze the uptake of other possible GABA neuron markers. (^{3}H)-ACHC was found to label neurons in the frog retina (Neal, Cunningham and Marshall 1979) but not in the rabbit, rat or guinea-pig retina (Cunningham, Marshall and Neal 1981, Agardh and Ehinger 1981). (^{3}H)-muscimol has been found to be accumulated and stored by retinal neurons which are likely to use GABA as neurotransmitter (goldfish and chicken: Yazulla and Brecha 1980, 1981, rabbit, guinea-pig and goldfish: Agardh and Ehinger 1981) but again, the localization is in the mammals not as clear as is desirable. (^{3}H)-isoguvacine has recently been found to give much better labelling (Agardh and Ehinger 1981). It is in the retina of all species tested so far (goldfish, frogs, chicken, rats, guinea-pigs, rabbits and humans) accumulated in cells with the position of amacrines and in the inner plexiform layer. In the submammalian species it is also accumulated in horizontal cells. Glial labelling is negligible. The uptake is not very striking in terms of tissue to medium ratio (about 2.5 with 60 min incubations) but is nevertheless a high-affinity system with Km at about 1.2×10^{-7}M. It is temperature dependent and inhibitable with ouabain. The binding of isoguvacine to the cellular storage sites seems strong because the labelling remains for more than 24 hours and it is not readily released with for instance light flashes or depolarization with potassium.

There is only little glial labelling by (^{3}H)-GABA in birds, amphibians and fish (Marshall and Voaden 1974a, Voaden, Marshall and Murani 1974, Marc, Stell, Bok and Lam 1978, Hollyfield, Rayborn, Sarthy and Lam 1979, Bonaventure, Wioland and Roussel 1980) so that in these species it can be used for labelling neurons. As noted above, horizontal cells become labelled in birds, amphibians and goldfish (H1 cells in goldfish). In the inner plexiform layer, (^{3}H)-GABA labels several types of amacrines. One of them is in goldfish a large pyriform type (called Ab) which sends its process to sublamina b of the inner plexiform layer where it is both pre- and postsynaptic to red-sensitive center-depolarizing (ON-type) bipolar cells (Marc, Stell, Bok and Lam 1978). The Ab cells are morphologically similar to the red-depolarizing sustained amacrine cells (Famiglietti, Kaneko and Tachibana 1977). In cats, four types of amacrine cells were consistently labelled with (^{3}H)-GABA (Pourcho 1980), two of which were more heavily labelled than the others. A total of 38% of the amacrine cells were labelled. This a high proportion, and it should be remembered that uptake of a substance into a cell does not necessarily always mean that the substance is the transmitter of the cell. This is particularly dangerous when high concentrations of the label are used.

GABA neurons can be observed by demonstrating immunohistochemically the enzyme synthesizing GABA, GAD, and this has been done in rat, rabbit, frog and goldfish (Vaughn, Barber, Saito, Roberts and Famiglietti 1978, Brandon, Lam and Wu 1979, Brandon, Lam, Su and Wu, 1980. In rabbit, five strata of GAD positive processes were found in the inner plexiform layer, together with amacrine cell bodies in the innermost cell row of the inner nuclear layer. In the electron microscope, GAD positive processes were most often found to be presynaptic to amacrine and bipolar cells, and synapses to ganglion cells were seen far less often. The input into the GAD positive processes was not found. In the rat retina, the output synapses were similar and GAD positive processes were also found to be postsynaptic to both bipolar and amacrine cell processes (Vaughn, Barber, Saito, Roberts and Famiglietti 1978). Light-induced acetylcholine release was in rats found to be inhibited by GABA (Massey and Neal 1978) and some of the amacrine cells which are postsynaptic to GABA neurons may therefore be cholinergic.

GABA receptors have been shown in the retina with biochemical methods (Redburn, Kyles and Ferkany 1979, Redburn and Mitchell 1980, Redburn, Clement-Cormier and Lam 1980), as well as autoradiographically with (^{3}H)-muscimol labelling (Yazulla and Brecha 1981). Benzodiazepine receptors, presumed to be related to the GABA receptors, have also been demonstrated in the retina (Howells, Hiller and Simon 1979, Borbe, Müller and Wollert 1980, Osborne 1980b, Howells and Simon 1980, Regan, Roeske and Yamamura 1980). A benzodiazepine, oxazepam, was in humans found to prolong the ocular readaptation time, which was tested as the time it took for the eye to regain its ability to detect moving stripes (Bergman, Borg, Högman, Larsson, Linde and Tengroth 1979). Since the GABA blocker, picrotoxin, inhibits the directional sensitivity of rabbit ganglion cells (Wyatt and Daw 1976) it is possible that movement detection is mediated by GABA neurons sensitive to benzodiazepines.

Light flashes can release (^{3}H)-GABA from rabbit retina (Bauer 1978) as can depolarization with potassium (Redburn 1977, Lopez-Colomé, Salceda and Pasantes-Morales 1978, Hollyfield, Rayborn, Sarthy and Lam 1979). However, it is remarkably difficult to elicit any release with aspartic or glutamic acid or acetylcholine (Bauer, unpublished), suggesting that GABA neurons either lack excitatory receptors to these substances or that stimulation with them activates excitatory and inhibitory processes that precisely inhibit each other at the level of the amacrine cells. Since the latter alternative is somewhat unlikely, it seems reasonable to assume that rabbit GABA neurons lack excitatory input from neurons releasing aspartate, glutamate or acetylcholine. It is perhaps significant that it was difficult to find input synapses on rabbit GABA neurons (Brandon, Lam, Su and Wu 1980).

Glycine. Glycine is present in the retina in significant amounts (see tables in Voaden 1976 or Ehinger 1978) and there is a very active uptake system that can be used for labelling neurons

in all species investigated (goldfish: Marc and Lam 1981, Ehinger
1981b, frog: Voaden, Marshall and Murani 1974, Marshall and Voaden
1975, 1976, Bonaventure, Wioland and Roussel 1980, chicken and
pigeon: Marshall and Voaden 1974a, rat: Marshall and Voaden 1974b,
Bruun and Ehinger 1974, guinea-pig: Bruun and Ehinger 1974, rabbit:
Ehinger and Falck 1971, Ehinger 1972a, Bruun and Ehinger 1972, 1974,
cat: Bruun and Ehinger 1974, Pourcho 1980, man: Ehinger 1972b, Lam
and Hollyfield 1980). The cell bodies are usually located in the
innermost cell rows of the inner nuclear layer and the processes
extend into the inner plexiform layer. With fluid fixation sublamina
a of the inner plexiform layer becomes somewhat more labelled than
sublamina b (Pourcho 1980, Chin and Lam 1980, Marc and Lam 1981)
but with freeze-drying and formaldehyde gas fixation this is less
evident (Ehinger 1981b). As noted above, some glycine accumulating
cells can also be seen at the outer plexiform layer and, perhaps,
among the bipolar cells. In cats, some of the (^3H)-glycine accumulating cells have been identified as AII amacrine cells (Pourcho
1980), which receive input from, among others, the dopaminergic
neurons (Fig. 4), and which link bipolar cells to ganglion cells
(Famiglietti and Kolb 1975, Kolb 1979). In goldfish (Marc and Lam
1981), glycinergic amacrine cells (called Aa cells) receive input
from other amacrine cells and send output to other such cells, at
times in reciprocal synapses. Synapses were also seen on some bipolar cells. Red light was found to decrease the uptake of (^3H)-
glycine and the (^3H)-glycine accumulating cells were therefore
suggested to be identical with the red-hyperpolarizing, sustained
amacrine cells in cyprine retinas (Marc and Lam 1981).

Kainic acid and glutamic acid have both been shown to release
(^3H)-glycine from rabbit retinas, and the glutamic acid receptor
blocker, nuciferine, is able to block the effect of glutamic acid.
The release is Ca^{2+}-dependent (Bauer 1981). Aspartic acid and
cysteic acid were without effect as were the GABA agonists muscimol
and THIP. The results suggest presence of glutamic acid receptors
in the pathways to glycinergic neurons in the rabbit but absence of
aspartic acid receptors on them and a difference between the receptors for kainic acid and glutamic acid.

(^3H)-glycine has been shown to be released by light stimulation in cats, rabbits, and rats (Ehinger and Lindberg 1974, Ehinger
and Lindberg-Bauer 1976, Coull and Cutler 1978) and by depolarizing
with potassium in rabbit, chicken, frog and goldfish (Kong, Fung and
Lam 1980, López-Colomé, Salceda and Pasantes-Morales 1978, Rayborn,
Sarthy, Lam and Hollyfield 1981, Chin and Lam 1980). Since it is
present in significant amounts in the retina (see, e.g., Voaden
1976 or Ehinger 1978), which also has glycine receptors (Borbe,
Müller and Wollert 1981) it is a likely retinal neurotransmitter.

Indoleamines. Indoleamine accumulating amacrine neurons occur
in the retina of a number of species (Ehinger and Florén 1976, 1980,

Florén 1979a and b, Ehinger and Holmgren 1979, Osborne 1980a, 1981, Dowling, Ehinger and Florén 1980). In contrast to the 5-hydroxytryptamine containing neurons in the brain, they are not demonstrable with formaldehyde fluorescence histochemistry in normal animals but only after the injection of an indoleamine into the eye or incubating the retina in the indoleamine. This procedure will show the indoleamine accumulating neurons in lamprey, mudpuppy, goldfish, pigeon, chicken, rabbit, cat and Cebus monkeys but does not show any such neurons in rat, pig, cow, baboons, cynomolgus monkey or humans. In guinea-pig the fluorescence histochemistry is ambiguous (Ehinger and Florén 1980). However, in cow and pig autoradiography demonstrated uptake of (^{3}H)-5-hydroxytryptamine into neurons not observable with formaldehyde histochemistry (Osborne 1980a, Ehinger, Florén and Tornqvist 1981). Dopaminergic neurons have some ability to accumulate 5-hydroxytryptamine and might be a source of error, but it was shown that the radioactivity was not to any significant extent found in these cells. Autoradiography fails to demonstrate any indoleamine-accumulating neurons in cynomolgus monkeys, baboons, rats, and humans. Very recently, a set of indoleamine-accumulating neurons has been discovered among the horizontal cells of squirrel monkeys (Florén and Hendrickson 1981).

When demonstrable, the indoleamine-accumulating neurons have their cell bodies in the inner half of the inner nuclear layer and their terminals in the inner plexiform layer, at times in definite sublayers.(Fig. 6). No branches have been seen to reach out to the outer plexiform layer.

It is currently debated what the actual neurotransmitter of the indoleamine-accumulating neurons is. Obviously, 5-hydroxytryptamine has been suspected, and there are several studies showing uptake and storage of exogenously applied 5-hydroxytryptamine as well as 5-hydroxytryptamine receptors in the retina (Ehinger and Florén 1978, Florén 1979a, Thomas and Redburn 1979, 1980, Thomas, Buckholtz and Zemp 1979, Osborne 1980a and b, Osborne and Richardson 1980). Potassium induced release of (^{3}H)-5-hydroxytryptamine from the retina has also been demonstrated (Thomas and Redburn 1979, 1980, Osborne 1980a, 1981) as well as a slight light-induced release (Fig. 7). However, the indoleamine-accumulating uptake system is in rabbits not identical with the 5-hydroxytryptamine uptake system in the brain (Florén 1979a) and the 5-hydroxytryptamine concentration is very low in mammals. It is higher in some non-mammalian species (Table 1). Fluorimetric methods have often given higher values than the more recent techniques. Given that indoleamine accumulating neurons are much more numerous than the dopaminergic ones (about fifteen to twenty times more in rabbits and mudpuppies, Ehinger and Åberg 1981, Adolph, Dowling and Ehinger 1980) it seems that on a molecular basis, the concentration of 5-hydroxytryptamine in the indoleamine accumulating neurons in rabbits is in the order of 50 to 200 times less than the dopamine

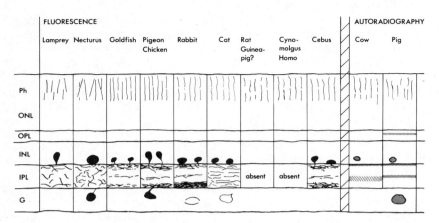

Fig. 6.   Indoleamine accumulating neurons in different species.
Note that in some species (cow, pig) they are demonstrable
with autoradiography only and in others (rat, primates)
they are not demonstrable at all.

concentration in the dopaminergic neurons (Ehinger and Åberg 1981).
This readily explains why the indoleamine-accumulating neurons are
not demonstrable by formaldehyde fluorescence histochemistry.
Osborne (1981) has suggested that perhaps the 5-hydroxytryptamine
neurons in the retina can work with very low transmitter concentrations. There is no previous evidence for the existence of such
neurons anywhere and it is not apparent why then some neurons in
the brain should have higher concentrations in order to function.
The possibility that the 5-hydroxytryptamine concentration is low
because there is a high turnover does not exist, because even
though there is some capacity of the retina to form 5-hydroxytryp-
tamine from 5-hydroxytryptophan (Osborne 1980a), the rate is at
least twenty times less than in the brain (Florén and Hansson
1979). Therefore, at present the weight of evidence seems to favour
some other indoleamine than 5-hydroxytryptamine as the transmitter
of most indoleamine-accumulating neurons in mammals. However,
attempts to isolate this presumed indoleamine have so far not been
successful (Osborne 1981). This raises the question whether the
transmitter is not an indoleamine but perhaps one of the peptides
now known to exist in neurons with indoleamine uptake and storage
systems (Hökfelt, Johansson, Ljungdahl, Lundberg and Schultzberg
1980).

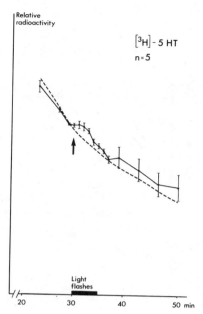

Fig. 7.   Release of (^{3}H)-5-hydroxytryptamine from rabbit retina.
Light flashes (2 Hz) induce a slight but probably significant ($p<0.05$) increase in the release of radioactive
5-hydroxytryptamine (Bauer, Ehinger and Tornqvist, unpublished).

Antibodies directed against 5-hydroxytryptamine have recently
become available and have shown immunofluorescence in chicken,
goldfish and frog retinas (Osborne 1981, Ehinger and Tornqvist unpublished). The morphology of the 5-HT immunoreactive neurons is
identical with that seen with formaldehyde histofluorescence after
injections of indoleamines. It has not been possible to see any
such immunofluorescence in the retina of pig, cow, rabbit, rat,
guinea-pig and humans. This agrees with the observation that the
5-hydroxytryptamine concentration of chicken retina is higher than
in other species (Table 1) and it is possible that 5-hydroxytrypta-
mine is the transmitter of the indoleamine-accumulating neurons in
chicken, goldfish and frog.

The indoleamine-accumulating neurons are readily demonstrable
not only in the fluorescence microscope but also in the electron
microscope because of the characteristic changes induced by 5,6-DHT
when accumulated by the neurons. The synaptic connections have been
analysed in goldfish (Dowling and Holmgren-Taylor 1981a), rabbit
(Ehinger and Holmgren 1979), Cebus monkey (Dowling, Ehinger and

Table 1.   5-Hydroxytryptamine in the retina (ng/g wet weight)

	Häggendal and Malmfors 1965 (Fluorimetry)	Suzuki and co-workers 1977 (Fluorimetry)	Thomas and Redburn 1979 (Fluorimetry)	Florén and Hansson 1979 (HPLC) (Radioenzym. method)		Ehinger, Hansson and Tornqvist (HPLC)	Osborne 1980,1981 (DANSYL) (HPLC)	
Normal rabbits	not detectable (< ~50 ng/g)			24 ± 5	36 ± 6		30 ± 6	
Perfused rabbits						3.8 ± 0.9	20 ± 6	
Cow			100.3 ± 10.1			26.2 ± 7.2	31 ± 7	39 ± 4
Pig						5.9 ± 0.8		
Guinea-pig						6.0 ± 2.6		
Chicken		176 ± 12		34 ± 4	67 ± 17			
Chicken (newborn)				71 ± 5	90 ± 8			80 ± 8
Frog							290 ± 18	500 ± 80
Lizard							96 ± 8	

Florén 1980) and cat (Dowling and Holmgren-Taylor 1981b). Common to all the mammalian species investigated is that the input comes from bipolar cells, in the cat mainly rod bipolar cells in sublamina b. There is in cats also in sublamina a an exchange of information with flat cone bipolar cells and amacrine cells throughout the inner plexiform layer. In all species, there are numerous short feedback loops in reciprocal synapses on the bipolar cells (Fig. 8). In goldfish and carp, however, the indoleamine-accumulating neurons mainly form interamacrine links, much like the dopaminergic neurons do in mammals. The indoleamine-accumulating cells do not have processes reaching out to the outer plexiform layer (Dowling and Holmgren-Taylor 1981b).

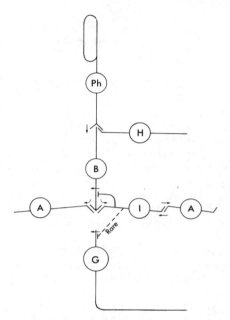

Fig. 8.   Simplified diagram of the synapses of indoleamine accumulating neurons in rabbit, cat, and Cebus monkey.

GANGLION CELLS

The transmitters of ganglion cells have largely remained elusive. A number of studies have shown that none of the transmitters known or presumed to operate in the brain are likely to be the transmitter of the majority of ganglion cells. However in the marine toad, Bufo marinus, there is some recently reviewed evidence (Oswald and Freeman 1980) that acetylcholine is the transmitter of some of the ganglion cells.

Glutamic acid has been proposed as a transmitter of ganglion cells because retinal ablation caused a decrease in glutamate and aspartate and in the high affinity uptake of glutamate in the optic tectum (Cuénod and Henke 1978, Fonnum and Henke 1979). In the monkey retina, the glutamate and aspartate concentrations show an increase in the innermost layer (Berger, McDaniel, Carter and Lowry 1977) and both substances are present in significant concentrations in the ganglion cell layer in rats and frogs (see Voaden 1978, Voaden, Morjaria and Oraedu 1980). Finally, (^{3}H)-D-aspartate, presumed to be a marker for glutamate and/or aspartate neurons, was found to be accumulated by about 5 to 10% of the ganglion cells of pigeon, guinea-pig and rabbit (Ehinger 1981a). Cuénod and collaborators have recently seen a similar labelling of pigeon ganglion cells, irregularly dispersed in the retina (Cuénod, Brandt, Canzek, Streit and Reubi 1981). It is thus possible that a fraction of the mammalian ganglion cells use glutamate or aspartate as their neurotransmitter. However, in the majority of cells, the transmitter remains unknown.

Ganglion cells show complex response patterns and can be classified in a multitude of types. Y cells integrate non-linearly within their receptive fields and GABA receptor blockers (picrotoxin and bicuculline) inhibit their surround response more than their centre in both cats and rabbits (Kirby and Enroth-Cugell 1976, Caldwell and Daw 1978). Similar results were seen in frogs (Bonaventure, Wioland and Roussell 1980). The glycine receptor blocker, strychnine, does not affect Y cells. X cells integrate linearly within their receptive fields and strychnine was in cats reported to affect their surround more than their centre (Kirby 1979). This was not seen in rabbits (Caldwell and Daw 1978).

Miller, Dacheux and Frumkes (1977) demonstrated that about one half of the ganglion cells in mudpuppy retina have inhibitory postsynaptic potentials which are blocked by strychnine while the remainder have such potentials which are blocked by picrotoxin or bicuculline. Glycine and GABA were both found to hyperpolarize ganglion cells in the presence of Co^{2+}, suggesting these cells have receptors for both substances.

The effect of picrotoxin and strychnine was in rabbits studied on five types of more complex cells (Caldwell, Daw and Wyatt 1978). Picrotoxin abolished the special properties of directionally sensitive cells, orientation specific cells, large field units and uniformity detectors. Strychnine abolished the size specificity of local edge detectors. These effects suggest that GABA and glycine neurons form parts of the circuits generating the characteristics of the cells, although it is not yet possible to specify the network in more detail. Nevertheless, it is clear that drugs interfering with, for instance, GABA neurotransmission may adversely affect important visual functions such as movement detection.

Precise knowledge of the synapse functions will enable us to tell which visual tasks different drugs are likely to interfere with and thus facilitate the design of adequate tests to assess how detrimental the drugs may be to demanding visual tasks.

ACKNOWLEDGEMENTS

Work reported in this paper was supported by the Swedish Medical Research Council (project 14X-2321), the Herman Järnhardts Stiftelse, by the Trygg-Hansa Foundation and by the Torsten och Elsa Segerfalks stiftelse.

REFERENCES

Adolph, A., and Dowling,.J. E., 1980, Monoaminergic neurons of the mudpuppy retina, Cell Tiss. Res., 210:269.

Agardh, E., and Ehinger, B., 1981, (^{3}H)-muscimol, (^{3}H)-nipecotic acid and (^{3}H)-isoguvacine as autoradiographic markers for GABA neurotransmission, In preparation.

Balcar, V. J., and Johnston, G. A. R., 1972, The structural specificity of the high affinity uptake of L-glutamate and L-aspartate by rat brain slices, J. Neurochem., 19:2657.

Bauer, B., 1978, Photic release of radioactivity from rabbit retina preloaded with (^{3}H)-GABA, Acta Ophthalmol. (Copenhagen), 56:270.

Bauer, B., 1981, Stimulated release of (^{3}H)-glycine from retina, Albr. v. Graefe's Arch. klin. exp. Ophthalmol., In press.

Bauer, B., Ehinger, B., and Åberg, L., 1980, (^{3}H)-dopamine release from the rabbit retina, Albr. v. Graefe's Arch. klin. exp. Ophthalmol., 215:71.

Baughman, R., and Bader, C., 1977, Biochemical characterization and cellular localization of the cholinergic system in the chicken retina, Brain Res., 138:469.

Berger, S. J., McDaniel, M. L., Carter, J. G., and Lowry, H., 1977, Distribution of four potential transmitter amino acids in monkey retina, J. Neurochem., 28:159.

Bergman, H., Borg, S., Högman, B., Larsson, H., Linde, C. J., and Tengroth, B., 1979, The effect of oxazepam on ocular readaptation time, Acta Ophthalmol. (Copenhagen)., 57:145.

Bonaventure, N., Wioland, N., and Roussel, G., 1980, Effects of some amino acids (GABA, glycine, taurine) and of their antagonists (picrotoxin, strychnine) on spatial and temporal features of frog retinal ganglion cell responses, Pflügers Arch., 385:51.

Borbe, H. O., Müller, W. E., and Wollert, U., 1980, The identification of benzodiazepine receptors with brain-like specificity in bovine retina, Brain Res., 182:466.

Boycott, B. B., Dowling, J. E., Fisher, S. K., Kolb, H., and Laties, A. M., 1975, Interplexiform cells of the mammalian retina and their comparison with catecholamine containing retinal cells,

      Proc. Roy. Soc. Lond. Series B, 191:353.

Brandon, Ch., Lam, D. M. K., and Wu, J-Y., 1979, The γ-aminobutyric
      acid system in rabbit retina: Localization by immunocyto-
      chemistry and autoradiography, Proc. Natl. Acad. Sci.,
      U.S.A., 76:3557.

Brandon, Ch., Lam, D. M. K., Su, Y. Y. T., and Wu, J-Y., 1980,
      Immunocytochemical localization of GABA neurons in the rabbit
      and frog retina, Brain Res. Bull., Suppl. 2: GABA neuro-
      transmission, 5:21.

Bruun, A., and Ehinger, B., 1972, Uptake of the putative neurotrans-
      mitter, glycine, into the rabbit retina, Invest. Ophthalmol.,
      11:191.

Bruun, A., and Ehinger, B., 1974, Uptake of certain putative neuro-
      transmitters into retinal neurons of some mammals, Exp. Eye
      Res., 19:435.

Caldwell, J. H., and Daw, N. W., 1978, Effects of picrotoxin and
      strychnine on rabbit retinal ganglion cells: changes in
      centre surround receptive fields, J. Physiol., 276:299.

Caldwell, J. H., Daw, N. W., and Wyatt, J. H., 1978, Effects of
      picrotoxin and strychnine on rabbit retinal ganglion cells:
      lateral interactions for cells with more complex receptive
      fields, J. Physiol., 276:277.

Cervetto, L., and MacNichol, E. F., 1972, Inactivation of horizon-
      tal cells in turtle retina by glutamate and aspartate,
      Science, 178:767.

Chin, C-A., and Lam, D. M. K., 1980, The uptake and release of (^{3}H)-
      glycine in the goldfish retina, J. Physiol., 308:185.

Coull, B. M., and Cutler, W. P., 1978, Light-evoked release of
      endogenous glycine into the perfused vitreous of the intact
      rat eye, Invest. Ophthalmol., 17:682.

Cuénod, M., Beaudet, A., Canzek, V., Streit, P., and Reubi, J. C.,
      1981, Glutamatergic pathways in the pigeon and the rat
      brain, in: "Glutamate as a Neurotransmitter," G. DiChiara
      and G. L. Gessa, eds., Raven Press, New York.

Cuénod, M., and Henke, H., 1978, Neurotransmitters in the avian
      visual system, in: "Amino Acids as Chemical Transmitters,"
      F. Fonnum, ed., Plenum Press, New York-London.

Cunningham, J., Marshall, J., and Neal, M. J., 1981, The radioauto-
      graphical localization in the vertebrate retina of (^{3}H)-(±)-
      Cis-aminocyclohexane carboxylic acid (ACHC); a selective
      inhibitor of neuronal GABA transport, Exp. Eye Res., 32:445.

Davies, L. P., and Johnston, G. A. R., 1976, Uptake and release of
      D- and L-aspartate by rat brain slices, J. Neurochem., 26:
      1007.

Dawson, W. W., and Perez, J. M., 1973, Unusual retinal cells in the
      dolphin, Science, 181:747.

Dowling, J. E., and Ehinger, B., 1975, Synaptic organization of the
      amine-containing interplexiform cells of the goldfish and
      Cebus monkey retinas, Science, 188:270.

Dowling, J. E., and Ehinger, B., 1978a, The interplexiform cell

    system. I. Synapses of the dopaminergic neurons of the gold-
    fish retina, Proc. Roy. Soc. Series B, 201:7.
Dowling, J. E., and Ehinger, B., 1978b, Synaptic contacts of dopa-
    minergic neurons in the rabbit retina, J. Comp. Neurol.,
    180:203.
Dowling, J. E., Ehinger, B., and Florén, I., 1980, Fluorescence and
    electron microscopical observations on the amine accumulating
    neurons of the Cebus monkey retina, J. Comp. Neurol., 192:665.
Dowling, J. E., and Holmgren-Taylor, I., 1981a, Synaptic organiza-
    tion of the indoleamine-accumulating neurons in the cyprine
    retina, In preparation.
Dowling, J. E., and Holmgren-Taylor, I., 1981b, Electron microsco-
    pical observations on the indoleamine-accumulating neurons
    and their synaptic connections in the retina of the cat,
    In preparation.
Dowling, J. E., and Ripps, H., 1972, Adaptation in skate photore-
    ceptors, J. Gen. Physiol., 60:698.
Dowling, J. E., and Watling, K. J., 1981, Dopaminergic mechanisms
    in the teleost retina. II. Factors affecting the accumula-
    tion of cyclic AMP in pieces of intact carp retina, J. Neuro-
    chem., 36:569.
Ehinger, B., 1970, Autoradiographic identification of rabbit retinal
    neurons that take up GABA, Experientia, 26:1063.
Ehinger, B., 1977, Glial and neuronal uptake of GABA, glutamic acid,
    glutamine and glutathione in the rabbit retina, Exp. Eye Res.,
    25:221.
Ehinger, B., 1978, Biogenic monoamines and amino acids as retinal
    neurotransmitters, in: "Frontiers in Visual Science," S. J.
    Cool and E. L. Smith III, eds., Springer Series in Optical
    Sciences, New York-Heidelberg-Berlin.
Ehinger, B., 1981a, (^{3}H)-D-aspartate accumulation in the retina of
    pigeon, guinea-pig and rabbit, Exp. Eye Res., In press.
Ehinger, B., 1981b, Cells accumulating (^{3}H)-glycine in the goldfish
    retina, Albr. v. Graefe's Arch. klin. exp. Ophthalmol., In
    press.
Ehinger, B., and Falck, B., 1971, Autoradiography of some suspected
    neurotransmitter substances: GABA, glycine, glutamic acid,
    histamine, dopamine, and L-dopa, Brain Res., 33:157.
Ehinger, B., Falck, B., and Laties, A. M., 1969, Adrenergic neurons
    in teleost retina, Z. Zellforsch., 97:285.
Ehinger, B., and Florén, I., 1976, Indoleamine-accumulating neurons
    in the retina of rabbit, cat and goldfish, Cell Tiss. Res.,
    175:37.
Ehinger, B., and Florén, I., 1978, Quantitation of the uptake of
    indoleamines and dopamine in the rabbit retina, Exp. Eye
    Res., 26:1.
Ehinger, B., and Florén, I., 1980, Retinal indoleamine accumulating
    neurons, in: "Neurochemistry of the Retina," N. Bazan, ed.,
    Neurochemistry International, In press.
Ehinger, B., Florén, I., and Tornqvist, K., 1981, Autoradiography

of (^{3}H)-5-hydroxytryptamine uptake in the retina of some mammals, In preparation.

Ehinger, B., and Holmgren, I., 1979, Electron microscopy of the indoleamine accumulating neurons in the rabbit retina, Cell Tiss. Res., 197:175.

Ehinger, B., and Lindberg, B., 1974, Light-evoked release of glycine from the retina, Nature, 251:727.

Ehinger, B., and Lindberg-Bauer, B., 1976, Light-evoked release of glycine from cat and rabbit retina, Brain Res., 113:535.

Ehinger, B., and Åberg, L., 1981, Density of amine accumulating neurons in rabbit and guinea-pig retina, Acta Physiol. Scand., 112:111.

Famiglietti, E. V., Kaneko, A., and Tachibana, M., 1977, Neuronal architechture of on and off pathways to ganglion cells in carp retina, Science, 198:1267.

Famiglietti, E. V., and Kolb, H. Jr., 1975, A bistratified amacrine cell and synaptic circuitry in the inner plexiform layer of the retina, Brain Res., 84:293.

Fisher, L. J., 1979, Interplexiform cell of the mouse retina - a Golgi demonstration, Invest. Ophthalmol., 18:521.

Florén, I., 1979a, Arguments against 5-hydroxytryptamine as neurotransmitter in the rabbit retina, J. Neural. Transm., 46:1.

Florén, I., 1979b, Indoleamine accumulating neurons in the retina of chicken and pigeon, Acta Ophthalmol. (Copenhagen), 57:198.

Florén, I., and Hansson, Ch., 1980, Aspects on 5-hydroxytryptamine as a neurotransmitter in the retina of rabbit and chicken, Invest. Ophthalmol., 19:117.

Florén, I., and Hendrickson, A., 1980, Indoleamine accumulating horizontal cells in the squirrel monkey retina, Invest. Ophthalmol., Suppl. April 1980:72.

Fonnum, F., and Henke, H., 1979, Effects of retinal ablation on the pool of some amino acids in different layers of pigeon tectum, Experientia, 35:919.

Frumkes, T. E., and Miller, R. F., 1979, Pathways and polarities of synaptic interaction in the inner retina of the mudpuppy. II. Insight revealed by an analysis of latency ant threshold, Brain Res., 161:13.

Gallego, A., 1971a, Horizontal and amacrine cells in the mammal's retina, Vision Res., Suppl. 3:33.

Graham, L. T. Jr., 1974, Comparative aspects of neurotransmitters in the retina, in: "The eye," H. Davson and L. T. Graham Jr., eds., Academic Press, New York-London.

Hampton, C. K., Garcia, C., and Redburn, D. A., 1981, Localization of kainic acid-sensitive cells in mammalian retina, J. Neurosci. Res., 6:99.

Hayashi, T., 1980, Histochemical localization of dopamine and acetylcholinesterase activity in the carp retina, Acta Histochem. Cytochem., 13:330.

Hedden, W. L., and Dowling, J. E., 1978, The interplexiform cell system. II. Effects of dopamine goldfish retinal neurons,

Proc. Roy. Soc. Series B, 201:27.

Hollyfield, J. G., Rayborn, M. E., Sarthy, P., and Lam, D. M. K.,
    1979, The emergency, localization and maturation of neuro-
    transmitter system during development of the retina in
    xenopus laevis, J. Comp. Neurol., 188:587.

Holmgren, I., 1981, Synaptic organization of the dopaminergic
    neurons in the retina of cynomolgus monkeys, Invest. Ophthal-
    mol., In press.

Howells, R. D., Hiller, J. M., and Simon, E. J., 1979, Benzodiaze-
    pine binding sites are present in retina, Life Sci., 25:2131.

Howells, R. D., and Simon, E. J., 1980, Benzodiazepine binding in
    chicken retina and its interaction with γ-aminobutyric acid,
    Eur. J. Pharmacol., 67:133.

Hökfelt, T., Johansson, O., Ljungdahl, A., Lundberg, J., and Schultz-
    berg, M., 1980, Peptidergic neurons, Nature, 284:515.

Ishida, A. T., Stell, W. K., and Lightfoot, D. O., 1980, Rod and
    cone inputs to bipolar cells in goldfish retina, J. Comp.
    Neurol., 191:315.

Kato, S., Nakamura, T., and Negishi, K., 1980, Postnatal develop-
    ment of dopaminergic cells in the rat retina, J. Comp. Neu-
    rol., 191:227.

Kirby, A. W., 1979, The effect of strychnine, bibuculline, and pic-
    rotoxin on X and Y cells in the cat retina, J. Gen. Physiol.,
    74:71.

Kirby, A. W., and Enroth-Cugell, C., 1976, The involvement of gamma-
    aminobutyric acid in the organization of cat retinal gang-
    lion cell receptive fields. A study with picrotoxin and bi-
    cuculline, J. Gen. Physiol., 68:465.

Kolb, H., 1977, The organization of the outer plexiform layer in the
    retina of the cat: electron microscopic observations, J. Neu-
    rocytol., 6:131.

Kolb, H., 1979, Inner plexiform layer in the retina of the cat -
    electron microscopic observations, J. Neurocytol., 8:295.

Kolb, H., and West, R. W., 1977, Synaptic connections of the inter-
    plexiform cell in the retina of the cat, J. Neurocytol.,
    6:155.

Kong, Y-C., Fung, S-C., and Lam, D. M. K., 1980, Postnatal develop-
    ment of glycinergic neurons in the rabbit retina, J. Comp.
    Neurol., 193:1127.

Kramer, S. G., 1971, Dopamine: A retinal neurotransmitter. I. Reti-
    nal uptake, storage, and light-stimulated release of H^3-
    dopamine in vivo, Invest. Ophthalmol., 10:438.

Kramer, S. G., Potts, M., and Mangnall, Y., 1971, Dopamine: A reti-
    nal neurotransmitter. II. Autoradiographic localization of
    H^3-dopamine in the retina, Invest. Ophthalmol., 10:617.

Lam, D. M. K., 1975, Biosynthesis of γ-aminobutyric acid by isolated
    axons of cone horizontal cells in the goldfish retina,
    Nature, 254:345.

Lam, D. M. K., and Hollyfield, J. G., 1980, Localization of putative
    amino acid neurotransmitters in the human retina, Exp. Eye

Res., 31:729.

Lam, D. M. K., Lasater, E. M., and Naka, K. I., 1978, Gamma-aminobutyric acid-neurotransmitter candidate for cone horizontal
cells of the catfish retina, Proc. Natl. Acad. Sci., U.S.A.,
75:6310.

Lam, D. M. K., Marc, R. E., Sarthy, D. V., Chin, C. A., Su, Y. Y. T.,
Brandon, C., and Wu, J-Y., 1980, Retinal organization: neurotransmitters as physiological probes, Neurochem. Internat.,
1:183.

Lam, D. M. K., and Steinman, L., 1971, The uptake of γ-^{3}H-amino-
butyric acid in the goldfish retina, Proc. Natl. Acad. Sci.,
U.S.A., 68:2777.

Lam, D. M. K., Su, Y. Y. T., Swain, L., Marc, R. E., Brandon, C.,
and Wu, J-Y., 1979, Immunocytochemical localization of L-
glutamic acid decarboxylase in the goldfish retina, Nature,
278:565.

López-Colomé, A. M., Salceda, R., and Pasantes-Morales, H., 1978,
Potassium-stimulated release of GABA, glycine and taurine
from the chick retina. I. γ-aminobutyric acid, J. Neurochem.,
3:431.

Malmfors, T., 1963, Evidence of adrenergic neurons with synaptic
terminals in the retina of rats demonstrated with fluorescence and electron microscopy, Acta Physiol. Scand., 58:99.

Marc, R. E., and Lam, D. M. K., 1981, Glycinergic pathways in the
goldfish retina, J. Neurosci., 1:152.

Marc, R. E., Stell, W. K., Bok, D., and Lam, D. M. K., 1978, GABA-
ergic pathways in the goldfish retina, J. Comp. Neurol.,
182:221.

Marshall, J., and Voaden, M., 1974a, An autoradiographic study of
the cells accumulating ^{3}H- γ-aminobutyric acid in the isolated retinas of pigeons and chickens, Invest. Ophthalmol.,
13:602.

Marshall, J., and Voaden, M., 1974b, An investigation of the cells
incorporating (^{3}H)-GABA and (^{3}H)-glycine in the isolated
retina of the rat, Exp. Eye Res., 18:367.

Marshall, J., and Voaden, M., 1975, Autoradiographic identification
of the cells accumulating ^{3}H-γ-aminobutyric acid in mammalian
retinae: a species comparison, Vision Res., 15:459.

Marshall, J., and Voaden, M. J., 1976, Further observations on the
uptake of (^{3}H)-glycine by the isolated retina of the frog,
Exp. Eye Res., 22:189.

Masland, R. H., and Mills, J. W., 1979, Autoradiographic identification of acetylcholine in the rabbit retina, J. Cell Biol.,
83:159.

Massey, S. C., and Neal, M. J., 1979, The light evoked release of
acetylcholine from the rabbit retina in vivo and its inhibition by γ-aminobutyric acid, J. Neurochem., 32:1327.

Miller, R. F., Dacheux, R. F., and Frumkes, T. E., 1977, Amacrine
cells in Necturus retina: Evidence for independent γ-amino-
butyric acid- and glycine-releasing neurons, Science, 198:748.

Murakami, M., Ohtsu, K., and Ohtsuka, T., 1972, Effects of chemicals on receptors and horizontal cells in the retina, J. Physiol., 227:899.

Murakami, M., Ohtsuka, T., and Shimazaki, H., 1975, Effects of aspartate and glutamate on the bipolar cells in the carp retina, Vision Res., 15:456.

Murakami, M., Shimoda, Y., and Nakatani, K., 1979, Effects of GABA on neuronal activities in the distal retina of the carp, Sensory Proc., 2:334.

Naka, K. I., 1977, Functional organization of catfish retina, J. Neurophysiol., 40:26.

Nakamura, Y., McGuire, B. A., and Sterling, P., 1980, Interplexiform cell in cat retina: Identification by uptake of γ-(^{3}H)-aminobutyric acid and serial reconstruction, Proc. Natl. Acad. Sci., U.S.A., 77:658.

Neal, M. J., 1976, Amino acid transmitter substances in the vertebrate retina, Gen. Pharmacol., 7:321.

Neal, M. J., Collins, G. G., and Massey, S. C., 1979, Inhibition of aspartate release from the retina of the anaesthetised rabbit by stimulation with light flashes, Neurosci. Lett., 14:241.

Neal, M. J., Cunningham, J. R., and Marshall, J., 1979, The uptake and radioautographical localization in the frog retina of (^{3}H)-($\pm$)-aminocyclohexane carboxylic acid, a selective inhibitor of neuronal GABA transport, Brain Res., 176:285.

Neal, M. J., and Massey, S. C., 1980, The release of acetylcholine and amino acids from the rabbit retina in vivo, Neurochem. Internat., 1:191.

Negishi, K., and Drujan, B.D.,1979a, Effects of catecholamines and related compounds on horizontal cells in the fish retina, J. Neurosci. Res., 4:311.

Negishi, K., and Drujan, B. D., 1979b, Similarities in effects of acetylcholine and dopamine on horizontal cells in the fish retina, J. Neurosci. Res., 4:335.

Negishi, K., and Drujan, B. D., 1979c, Effects of some amino acids on horizontal cells in the fish retina, J. Neurosci. Res., 4:351.

Negishi, K., Hayashi, T., Nakamura, T., and Drujan, B. D., 1979, Histochemical studies on catecholaminergic cells in the carp retina, Neurochem. Res., 4:473.

Negishi, K., Nakamura, T., and Hayashi, T., 1980, Spatial density of catecholaminergic cells in the carp retina, Exp. Eye Res., 31:711.

Nichols, C. W., and Koelle, G. B., 1968, Comparison of the localization of acetylcholinesterase and non-specific cholinesterase activities in mammalian and avian retinas, J. Comp. Neurol., 133:1.

Olney, J. W., 1978, Neurotoxicity of excitatory amino acids, in: "Kainic acid as a tool in neurobiology," E. G. McGeer, J. W. Olney and P. L. McGeer, eds., Raven Press, New York.

Osborne, N. N., 1980a, In vitro experiments on the metabolism, uptake and release of 5-hydroxytryptamine in bovine retina, Brain Res., 184:283.

Osborne, N. N., 1980b, Benzodiazepine binding to bovine retina, Neurosci. Lett., 16:167.

Osborne, N. N., 1981, Evidence for serotonin being a neurotransmitter in the retina, in: "Biology of Serotonergic Transmission," N. N. Osborne, ed., Wiley and Sons, London.

Osborne, N. N., and Richardson, G., 1980, Specificity of serotonin uptake by bovine retina: Comparison with tryptamine, Exp. Eye Res., 31:31.

Oswald, R. E., and Freeman, J. A., 1980, Minireview: Optic nerve transmitters in lower vertebrate species, Life Sci., 27:527.

Oyster, C. W., and Takahashi, E. S., 1977, Interplexiform cells in the rabbit retina, Proc. Roy. Soc. Lond. Series B, 197:477.

Parthe, V., 1972, Horizontal, bipolar and oligopolar cells in the teleost retina, Vision Res., 12:395.

Pourcho, R. G., 1980, Uptake of (^{3}H)-glycine and (^{3}H)-GABA by amacrine cells in the cat retina, Brain Res., 198:333.

Pourcho, R. G., 1981, Dopaminergic amacrine cells in the cat retina, In: ARVO abstracts, Invest. Ophthalmol., 20:203.

Rayborn, M. E., Sarthy, P. V., Lam, D. M. K., and Hollyfield, J. G., 1981, The emergence, localization and maturation of neurotransmitter systems during development of the retina in Xenopus laevis. II. Glycine., J. Comp. Neurol., 195:585.

Redburn, D. A., 1977, Uptake and release of (^{14}C)-GABA from rabbit retina synaptosomes, Exp. Eye Res., 25:265.

Redburn, D., Clement-Cormier, Y., and Lam, D. M. K., 1980, GABA and dopamine receptor binding in retinal synaptosomal fractions, Neurochem. Internat., 1:167.

Redburn, D. A., Kyles, C. B., and Ferkany, J., 1979, Subcellular distribution of GABA receptors in bovine retina, Exp. Eye Res., 28:525.

Redburn, D. A., and Mitchell, C. K., 1980, GABA receptor binding in bovine retina, Brain Res., 5:189.

Regan, J. W., Roeske, W. R., and Yamamura, H. I., 1980, ^{3}H-flunitrazepam binding to bovine retina and the effect of GABA thereon, Neuropharmacol., 19:413.

Ross, C. D., and McDougal Jr., D. B., 1976, The distribution of choline acetyltransferase activity in vertebrate retina, J. Neurochem., 26:521.

Sarthy, P. V., and Lam, D. M. K., 1979a, Endogenous levels of neurotransmitter candidates in photoreceptor cells of the turtle retina, J. Neurochem., 32:455.

Sarthy, P. V., and Lam, D. M. K., 1979b, The uptake and release of (^{3}H)-dopamine in the goldfish retina, J. Neurochem., 32:1269.

Sarthy, P. V., Rayborn, M. E., Hollyfield, J. G., and Lam, D. M. K., 1981, The emergence, localization and maturation of neurotransmitter systems during development of the retina in Xenopus laevis. III. Dopamine., J. Comp. Neurol., 195:595.

Scholes, J. H., 1975, Colour receptors and their synaptic connexions, in the retina of a cyprinid fish, Phil. Trans. Roy. Soc. London B, 270:61.

Stell, W.K., Ishida, A.T., and Lightfoot, D.O., 1977, Structural basis for on- and off-center responses in retinal bipolar cells, Science, 198:1269.

Thomas, T.N., Buckholtz, N.S., and Zemp, J.W., 1979, 6-methoxy-1, 2,3,4-tetra hydro-β-carboline effects on retinal serotonin, Life Sci., 25:1435.

Thomas, T.N., and Redburn, D.A., 1978, Uptake of (^{14}C)-aspartic acid and (^{14}C)-glutamic acid by retinal synaptosomal fractions, J. Neurochem., 31:63

Thomas, T.N., and Redburn, D.A., 1979, 5-hydroxytryptamine - a neurotransmitter of bovine retina, Exp. Eye Res., 28:55.

Thomas, T.N., and Redburn, D.A., 1980, Serotonin uptake and release by subcellar fractions of bovine retina, Vision Res., 20:1

Törk, T., and Stone, J., 1979, Morphology catecholamine-containing amacrine cells in the cat's retina, as seen in retinal whole mounts, Brain Res., 169:261.

Vaughan, J.E., Barber, R.P., Saito, K., Roberts, E., and Famiglietti Jr., E.V., 1978, Immunological identification of GABAergic neurons in rat retina, Anat. Rec., 190-571.

Voaden, M.J., 1976, Gamma aminobutyric acid and glycine as retinal neurotransmitters, in: "Transmitters in the Visual Process", S.L. Bonting, ed., Pergamon Press, Oxford-New York-Toronto-Sydney-Frankfurt.

Voaden, M.J., 1978, The localization and metabolism of neuroactive amino acids in the retina, in: "Amino acids as chemical neurotransmitters," F. Fonnum, ed., Plenum Press, New York.

Voaden, M. J., Marshall, J., and Murani, N., 1974, The uptake of (^{3}H)-γ-aminobutyric acid and (^{3}H)-glycine by the isolated retina of the frog, Brain Res., 67:115.

Voaden, M. J., Morjaria, B., and Oraedu, A. C. I., 1980, The localization and metabolism of glutamate, aspartate and GABA in the rat retina, Neurochem. Internat., 1:151.

Wu, S. M., and Dowling, J. E., 1980, Effects of GABA and glycine on the distal cells of the cyprinid retina, Brain Res., 199:401.

Wyatt, H. J., and Daw, N. W., 1976, Specific effects of neurotransmitters antagonists on ganglion cells in rabbit retina, Science, 191:204.

Wyse, J. P. H., and Lorscheider, F. L., 1981, Low retinal dopamine and serum prolactin levels indicate an inherited dopaminergic abnormality in B W rats, Exp. Eye Res., 32:541.

Yazulla, S., and Brecha, N., 1980, Binding and uptake of GABA analogue, ^{3}H-muscimol, in the retina of goldfish and chicken, Invest. Ophthalmol., 19:1415.

Yazulla, S., and Brecha, N., 1981, Localized binding of (H^3)-muscimol to synapses in chicken retina, Proc. Natl. Acad. Sci., U.S.A., 78:643.

Yazulla, S., and Kleinschmidt, J., 1980, The effects of intraocular
    injection of kainic acid on the synaptic organization of the
    goldfish retina, Brain Res., 182:287.

NEUROPEPTIDES IN THE VERTEBRATE RETINA

H.J. Karten and N. Brecha

Dept. of Psychiatry and Neurobiology
SUNY Stony Brook
Stony Brook, NY 11790
and
Center for Ulcer Research
UCLA
Los Angeles, California 90073

The vertebrate retina has been the object of extensive study both as a structure of considerable interest in its own right as well as a model for the study of a laminated neural system. Each band of the retina contains a specific population of cells of defined functional nature, and any given cell type may be found in only a restricted laminar zone of the retina, with only a few notable exceptions. The precisely organized and laminated cell populations, of defined functional nature, form an anatomical structure that lends itself to an analysis of the unique morphology and biochemistry of identified cell types.

All the photoreceptors occupy the outermost layer of the retina, their synaptic endings restricted to the outer (synaptic) plexiform layer. Horizontal cells lie more internally and are disposed in a single band of cells with the adjacent remaining portions of the inner nuclear layer occupied by bipolar and amacrine cells. The bipolar and amacrine cells extend their terminals into the complex and poorly understood inner plexiform layer (IPL) where they come into synaptic contact with the processes of the ganglion cells. The ganglion cells and their centrally directed axons lie most internally, facing the optic media of the eye.

The few notable exceptions in this orderly arrangement include occasional bipolar cells and displaced ganglion cells that may intermingle with the amacrine cells, as well as occasional displaced amacrine cells that may be found in the ganglion cell layer.

Any of the five major types of cells (photoreceptors, horizontal cells, bipolar cells, amacrine cells and ganglion cells) can therefore reliably be found to occupy a similar position in the retina of all vertebrates. Presumably each of these types of cells also perform similar general categories of operations in all vertebrate retinae. (See last chapter by Prof. B.Ehinger).

As outlined by Professor Ehinger, such a stable pattern of organization is particularly attractive as it may permit the identification of the transmitter(s) of each specific cell type. Initially students of the retina anticipated that each cell type might possess a distinctive transmitter unique to that general type of cell. Given the limited numbers of cell types, the task of identifying the transmitters of each cell type thus appeared to be reasonably simple and straightforward. Unfortunately the discovery of multiple putative transmitters, and the even larger number of nontraditional compounds involved in intercellular communication such as the neuropeptides, have greatly complicated the task of accomplishing the "simple" goal of assigning a particular transmitter to each particular cell type.

Dr. Ehinger has reviewed the considerable progress that has been accomplished in the analysis of retinal transmitters, and has demonstrated the value of the retina as a suitable model for attempting the ambitious goal of characterizing the transmitters of each major cell type. As he has pointed out, however, we are still far from a comprehensive picture of the pharmacological-biochemical nature of the retina to match the anatomical descriptions provided by contemporary anatomists employing various light and electron microscopic methods. His review has stressed the importance of acetylcholine, GABA, glycine, glutamate/aspartate, catecholamines and indoleamines in various discrete retinal cell populations.

As Dr. Ehinger has also pointed out, however, despite the efforts of many investigators, we are still bereft of likely transmitter candidates for many of the cells of the retina. We have putative transmitters for only a limited population of photoreceptors, horizontal cells, possibly for some of the bipolar cells, and only most recently, a likely candidate (Aspartate/Glutamate) for only 5-7% of the ganglion cells. Surprisingly, the cells for which the greatest number of putative transmitters have been identified are the amacrine cells— those cells whose functional contribution to the physiological operations of the retina are least well understood.

Amacrine cells have proven exceedingly heterogeneous not only in their size and dendritic morphology, but also in the diversity of their chemical contents. Amacrine cells have been shown to contain Acetylcholine (Baughmann and Bader 1977), GAD/GABA (Vaughn, et al, 1978, Brandon, et al, 1979), Dopamine (Ehinger 1967),Indolamines (Ehinger and Floren, 1976) as well as other amino acid transmitters. In addition to the variety of amino acid and aminergic transmitters, amacrine cells have also recently been found to contain a rich storehouse of a variety of recently identified transmitters/modulators, the neuropeptides.

The presence of neuropeptides within the vertebrate retina, including Substance P(Duner, et al, 1954), Somatostatin (Rorstad, et al, 1979)and TRF (Schaefer, et al, 1977), was first recognized biochemically using bioassay or radioimmunoassay. Their precise histochemical localization, however, has only been described more recently. Within only the past two years the presence of Enkephalin-like (ENK), Substance P-like (SP), Glucagon-like (GLU), Vasoactive Intestinal Polypeptide-like (VIP), Cholecystekinin-like (CCK), Neurotensin- like (NT), Beta-Endorphin-like (END), LHRH-like and Somatostatin-like (SS) immunoreactivity has been localized in the retina of various vertebrates. In all instances these peptides have been found either predominantly or exclusively in amacrine cells. However, not all of the above mentioned peptides have necessarily been found in the retina of any single species.

In our own studies (Brecha, Karten and Laverack 1979, Karten and Brecha 1980, Stell, et al, 1980, Brecha, Karten and Schenker 1980) in pigeons and chickens, six of these peptides (ENK, SP, NT, SS, VIP and GLU) were localized to morphologically distinctive types of amacrine cells and are distinguished by the unique arborization pattern of their processes within the inner plexiform layer (IPL). Within a selected single species such as the pigeon, the laminar arborization pattern was found to be distinct for each type of peptide. In several instances, the arborization pattern of the peptidergic amacrine cell was found to match specific cell types described by Cajal using the Golgi method. These observations lend further credence to Cajal's (1933) earlier classification of morphologically distinct amacrine cells on the basis of their unique arborization patterns within the IPL.

Figure 1 is a schematic summary showing the pattern of arborization of amacrine cells for each of several neuropeptides in the pigeon retina. There appears to be little overlap in the dendritic morphology and laminar distribution of each cell type.

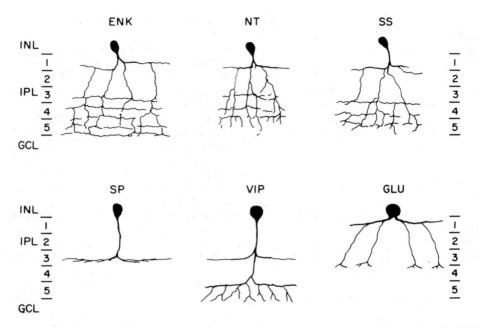

Figure 1. Schematic representation of peptidergic amacrine cells in
          the pigeon retina.

        The virtually exclusive distribution of neuropeptides within
amacrine cells of the pigeon retina raises several questions regarding the variety of different morphological and biochemical
types of amacrine cells that are found within this retina.

        1) Do any two or more peptides co-occur with each   other   in
the retina as they do in some other parts of the brain?

        2) How many amacrine cells of each type may be found in   the
retina and what is their regional density?

        3) Do peptides co-occur with any of the traditional putative
transmitters?

        4) Does the apparent morphology of any particular type of
peptidergic   amacrine   cell match the complex morphology as
demonstrated with the Golgi method?

        5) Are peptidergic amacrine cells, in any   particular
species, of constant morphology?

6) Is the pattern of arborization of peptidergic amacrine cells constant between species?

7) What is the functional significance of multiple peptides within amacrine cells as group?

8) What is the functional purpose of such diverse morphology and multiple chemical transmitters in amacrine cells?

Co-Occurrence of Peptides:

The multiplicity of peptides found within amacrine cells raises the question as to whether more than one peptide occurs in the same amacrine cell. We have been able to obtain some limited information on this issue on the basis of our concentration upon the retina of a single species, the pigeon (Columba livia). As shall be described in a subsequent section of this paper, cross-species comparisons pose special problems of interpretation and consequently an analysis of co-occurrence must be performed on only a single species at a time.

In the investigation of co-occurrence of peptidergic amacrine cells, as well as in the subsequent studies comparing peptidergic and nonpeptidergic cells, we employed three major criteria to examine retinae for the possible co-occurrence of substances within a single cell: a) The distinctive morphology of cell and its dendrites, b) Double labelling methods using different fluorophores such as FITC and Rhodamine and c) Quantitative measures of cell density.

On the basis of the cell size, relative location within the inner nuclear layer, and the laminar disposition of dendritic morphology of peptidergic amacrine cells, there does not appear to be any joint occurrence of ENK, SP, NT, SS, VIP or GLU (Fig 1). Despite the similarity of laminar disposition of dendrites of NT and SS cells within layers 1, 3 and 4, the specific pattern of arborization and relative density of dendrites within layer 3 provides clear morphological distinction between NT and SS containing amacrine cells. This was further confirmed in a series of quantitative and double label studies. The number of cells labeled for NT and for SS was counted in two adjacent sections stained for only NT or only for SS. A third section was simultaneously stained for both NT and SS. The total number of stained cell bodies was approximately equal to the cumulative total of cells stained for either NT or SS individually. The distinctiveness of these two separate populations was finally conclusively established by means of a double label method that distinguished NT from SS on the same section. There was some

slight resemblance between VIP and GLU containing amacrine cells
in that both of these types of peptidergic amacrine cells had
large cell bodies with come slight overlap in the pattern of
their dendrites.   VIP dendrites form a thin band between layers
2- 3 and another thin band between layers 4-5 with a rare process
in layer 1. GLU cells have a prominent plexus in layer 1, a thin
band between layers 2-3 and the isolated appearance of a thin
band between layers 4-5. The prominence of the layer 1 pattern
of GLU cells as well as a most unusual circumferential band of
GLU staining processes in the ora serrata assure little prospect
of co-occurrence of VIP and GLU in the same cell, though a proper
double label study would provide the definitive evidence of their
non-overlapping distribution.   Thus, we have found no clear
evidence of co-occurrence of any two peptides in a single retinal
amacrine cell, to date.

Co-Occurrence of Peptides with Nonpeptidergic Transmitters:

        Investigation of peptidergic mechanisms in the both the
central and peripheral nervous system has revealed that peptides
frequently co-occur with the more traditional substances that
mediate intercellular synaptic interactions. Amacrine cells of
the vertebrate retina have been reported to contain
Acetylcholine, GABA, Glycine, Dopamine and possibly Serotonin or
a related indoleamine. In light of the large numbers of amacrine
cells and their diverse morphology we may wonder as to 1) whether
any of the peptides co- occur in their distribution with these
more traditional transmitters, as they do in other neuronal
systems, 2) the total number of amacrine cells per square mm., 3)
what percentage of amacrine cells contain each of the peptides,
and 4) what percentage of amacrine cells contain ACh, GABA, Gly,
Dopamine or 5- HT.

        Within the last several years improvements in biochemical
methods and in immunology has permitted the development of
antibodies against either specific transmitters such as
Serotonin, or against the enzymes involved in their synthesis of
substances such as GABA (Glutamic Acid Decarboxylase-GAD),
Dopamine (Tyrosine Hydroxylase -TyOH) and Acetylcholine (Choline
Acetyl Transferase- CAT). Unfortunately we have not had occasion
to examine our preparation with CAT antibody, but comparison of
the peptidergic amacrines with those containing Serotonin, TyOH
and GAD has proven of value.

        Serotonin containing amacrine cells were localized
immunohistochemically with an antibody directed against a
Serotonin-BSA conjugate (Steinbusch, et al, 1978). Serotonergic

neurons were found to be small cells lying within the INL with prominent processes extending into the IPL. They could be readily distinguished from the much more faintly staining Serotonin positive bipolar cells both on the basis of their position within the INL, and the thin and faint staining internal and external processes of the bipolar cells. Unlike the peptidergic amacrine cells described above, the Serotonin amacrine cells showed an intensely staining plexus of dendrites in layers 1 and 5. Individual dendrites could regularly be followed in continuity from the cell body to their branches in both layers 1 and 5. On the basis of the unique dendritic morphology of the Serotonergic cell, we felt assured that it in no way corresponded to the morphology of any of the peptidergic cells thus far identified. These cells were identical in appearance to the indoleamine accumulating neurons of Floren (1979). Some portion of the plexus in layers 1 and/or 5 may also contain central processes of the bipolar cells.

Dopamine containing cells were identified by means of an antibody against Tyrosine Hydroxylase. TyOH is the first step rate limiting enzyme in the synthesis of Dopamine, Norepinephrine and Epinephrine. The presence of TyOH may therefore indicate the possible presence of either of these three amines. However, only Dopamine has been found in the retina of birds and most other vertebrates, hence TyOH may be used to directly determine the localization of presumptive Dopaminergic cells. These cells were found to be relatively large, with cell bodies generally lying at the margin of the INL and IPL. Following colchicine treatment, a limited number of additional positive cells were found in the ganglion cell layer. We presume this to be a small proportion of the displaced amacrine cell population. The pattern of dendritic arborization was as described by Professor Ehinger (1976), with prominent dendrites in layer 1, and with a thin band of dendrites at boundary between layers 2-3 and an occasional thin band at the boundary of layers 4-5. The size of the somata, and general morphology of dendrites was somewhat similar to that of the GLU cells. In contrast to GLU cells, however, there were no circumferential processes running in the ora serrata, and the number of such cells was significantly less than of the GLU cells(See section on Quantitative Studies). It is possible that the Dopamine amacrines in the INL proper are a subset of the GLU containing amacrine cells. No GLU staining displaced amacrine cells were found either with or without colchicine.

GABA and GAD: In a collaborative study with Dr. Wolfgang Oertel we have successfully obtained intense staining of GAD containing cell bodies and processes in the INL and IPL in the pigeon. No staining was found of somata in the ganglion cell layer(displaced amacrine cells) either with or without colchicine. As described below, the number of GAD positive cell bodies in the INL vastly exceeded that seen containing any of the other putative transmitters/modulators. Though the dendrites of many cells could be followed into the IPL, the density of staining of the IPL was so intense that individual dendritic profiles could not be readily discerned. Three broad prominent bands of GAD immunoreactivity was found. These bands occupied layers 1, 3, 5 and part of 4. Although occasional individual dendrites could be followed into the IPL, the overall density of dendrites in the IPL was so great that morphologic comparisons with the peptidergic cells could not be readily accomplished. Our current research is directed towards obtaining a more accurate assessment of the possible co- occurrence of GAD with either peptidergic or aminergic amacrine cells. Thus at the present time we are unable to confirm or deny the possible joint presence of GAD with any of these other substances.

        ACh and CAT: Baughmann and Bader (1977) and Masland and Mills(1979) localized ACh synthesizing cells in the chicken and rabbit retinae using an autoradiographic method. They observed moderate numbers of amacrine and displaced amacrine cells to be positive for ACh. We have not been able to combine the technology required in their procedures with immunohistochemistry. The lack of a readily available antibody against the enzyme CAT has limited our ability to directly examine the possible co-occurrence of ACh with either the peptides or amines. Hopefully the availability of antibodies against CAT (Kimura, et al, 1981, McGeer and McGeer, this volume) will soon permit us to accomplish this comparison.

Number and Density of Peptidergic and Other Amacrine Cells

        No adequate estimate has been suggested regarding the total number of amacrine cells in the pigeon or the retina of most other vertebrates. Bingelli and Paule (1969), and more recently Ehrlich (1981), have suggested that the displaced amacrine cells lying in the ganglion cell layer may occur in a density of approximately 10,000/sq.mm in the chick retina. Our very rough approximation in the pigeon retina suggest that the number of amacrine cells in the INL of the Red Field may be in the range of 40,000 cells/sq.mm. Thus the total number of amacrine cells/sq.mm. in the Red Field may be approximately 50,000 cells/sq.mm.(The measurement is expressed in sq.mm. in accord with the traditional means of describing cell density in the retina. The term refers to the number of cells of a particular type found underlying 1 sq.mm. of vitreal surface. Investigators using this concept are aware of the ambiguous use of the measure of area to indicate density of cells in three dimensional space.) The marked regional variation in thickness and differentiation of the retina results in substantial differences in the number of cells/sq.mm. in central versus more peripheral portions of the retina(Bingelli and Paule 1969). In order to minimize errors in measurement we confined our analysis to the Red Field of the pigeon retina, a zone of high density for all types of cells.

Table 1.   Estimated Numbers and Spacing of Various Types of Amacrine Cells (Pigeon — Red Field)

Content	Density	Spacing	% Identified Am Cells (9130)
ENK	2600/mm	20um	28%
SS	2500/mm	20um	27%
NT	1736/mm	24um	19%
5-HT	1600/mm	25um	17%
GLU	400/mm	55um	4%
VIP	244/mm	64um	3%
Ty-OH	50/mm	150um	0.5%

Table 1 is a summary of the estimated numbers of each of the cell types found in horizontal sections of the retina, including the Dopamine and Serotonin cells. The cells are listed in decreasing order of density. No estimate is given as to the number of SP containing cells as we were unable to obtain a reliable count of their density within the Red Field. The Table includes data on aminergic amacrines as well as peptidergic amacrine cells. Within this limited sampling of cells we estimate that we have accounted for no more than 20% of all the amacrine cell types in the Red Field. We were unable to obtain a reasonable estimate of the number of GAD positive cells for several reasons. The GAD positive cells in the amacrine cells layer were extremely numerous, and their density so great they presented many overlapping profiles rendering them difficult to count. In addition, the intensity of immunoreactive staining for GAD in any single cell body was much less than for the peptides or amines, often resulting in only light stippling within GAD positive cell bodies. We can only guess that the percentage of GAD positive cells may be three to four times as great as the number of peptidergic and aminergic cells combined, but no reasonable estimate can be made at this time. We have not been able to assess the density of ACh synthesizing cells.

On the basis of these measurements, however, several interesting points may be noted: The ENK and SS containing cells are amongst the most numerous. Despite some similarity in dendritic appearance of the GLU, VIP and Ty-OH (Dopamine) containing amacrine cells, the quantitative data indicates marked differences in density of each of three cell types. Perhaps the most notable consequence of these observations pertains to the Dopamine cells. Professor Ehinger's earlier studies with the Falck-Hillarp method did not readily lend themselves to quantitative measures of cell density. The uncertainties associated with the Falck-Hillarp methods inevitably led to an overestimate of the total number of Dopaminergic amacrine cells. The data also demonstrates that despite the widely ramifying dendrites of the Dopamine cells, they are only a very small proportion of the total number of amacrine cells (0.125-0.5%). They may yet prove to be a portion of a small subset of VIP and/or GLU cells, since all three substance show a prominent action on the synthesis of cyclic AMP in the avian retina. Clarification of their possible co- occurrence, however, must await further studies with double label methods.

Although the density of labelled amacrine cells was found to be fairly high, and the intercell spacing somewhat regular for several substances studied, no obvious mosaic pattern in their intercell spacing was found.

Regional Density of ENK Amacrine Cells Across the Retina:

The measurements shown in Table 1 were confined to the Red Field, a region of extremely high cell density of all major cell types. The density of all cell types, however, decreases within increasing distance from the central visual regions. We have measured the regional density of ENK containing amacrines as shown in Figure 2. ENK containing amacrines are found in highest density in the Red Field and with another zone reasonably high density in the region of the fovea. The density of cells diminishes markedly in more peripheral portions of the retina. The density of ENK amacrines approximately parallels the density of ganglion cells as described in Bingelli and Paule (1969). The measurement of the remaining populations of labelled cells is still in progress. The majority of cell types appear to follow

the general trend of density gradients of the ganglion cells and
of the ENK cells, but with the notable exception of the SP cells.
Though our measurements of the SP cells are still incomplete,
they appear to differ in their differential distribution from the
pattern found for ENK and others. SP containing amacrine cells
seem to occur in highest density in the more ventral portions of
the retina, and have a much lower density in the Red Field.

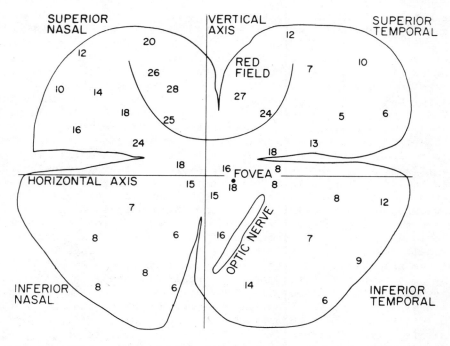

Figure 2. Regional variation in the density of Enkephalin-like
           immunoreactive amacrine cells in the pigeon retina.

        The specific relationship of different peptidergic cells to
each other requires further attention, particularly with the
electron microscope, in order to determine whether these cells
tend to form preferential amacrine-amacrine cell interactions.
The most difficult analysis, however, is likely to be that which
attempts to determine the particular types of ganglion cells
contacted by peptidergic amacrines, and if specific sets of
amacrines terminate as defined co-populations upon specific
ganglion cells.

Morphology of Peptidergic Amacrines- Comparison of Golgi Methods
and Immunohistochemistry:

      Cajal's analysis of the retina using Golgi methods provided
detailed illustrations of the dendritic arborizations of amacrine
cells within discrete laminae of the IPL. On the basis of his
studies with the Golgi method Cajal described many distinct types
of   amacrine   cells.   Direct   comparison   of   our   data using
immunohistochemistry also indicates the usefulness of this latter
method in the characterization of amacrine cell types.   However,
results   obtained   with   these   two   methods   are   not   readily
comparable. These difficulties are consequent to fundamental
differences in the nature of the data generated by each method.
The Golgi method stains only isolated cells but often provides an
image of the full extent of their dendritic arborizations. The
deficiency of the Golgi method is that it provides no indication
of the density or regional variation of   any particular cell
type. In contrast, the Immunohistochemical methods are more
reliable and consistent, and provide information on the density
and regional variations of any particular type of cell.   This is
particularly valuable in an analysis of variation in density of a
particular cell type as a function of eccentricity within the
retina.   The deficiency of the Immunohistochemical method,
however, is that it will often stain the dendrites of all members
of a set of any single type of cell with sufficient success that
the lateral extent of dendrites of any single cell cannot be
readily separated from those of adjacent cells. Thus the radius
of the effective dendritic arbors cannot be reliably established
and it is often difficult to ascertain the presence of multiple
morphologic cell types if they contain the same antigen.
Nontheless we have been able to match some of the peptidergic
cells with some of Cajal's Golgi impregnated cells.   As an
example, the Substance P containing amacrine cell of the pigeon
bears a marked resemblance to the Type J amacrine of Cajal.
Further comparison of the results of these two methods should
permit additional juxtaposition of cells types.

      Consequent to the some of the disadvantages of the
Immunohistochemical method stated above, there are inevitable
uncertainties in our attempts to establish the constancy of
morphology of peptidergic amacrine cells even within a single
retina. In the instance of a strictly monostratified cell, such
as the pigeon SP amacrine, this is obviously not a problem.
However, the occurrence of numerous multistratified cells may
obscure the presence of isolated cells of different types but
with partially overlapping dendritic morphologies. Thus in
strictest terms, we cannot be certain that e.g., all the ENK
cells of the pigeon retina are of a single type of dendritic
morphology.

In several other species, however, such as the toad (Bufo), the Macaque monkey and the rabbit, there are several different morphological types of SP containing cells in any single retina. Thus we must conclude that peptidergic amacrine cells of any particular species need not have a constant single morphology. Similarly, the presence of the same peptide in amacrine cells of two different species does not allow the proposition that such a peptidergic amacrine cell makes a similar contribuiton to overall retinal functions in both species, even though the peptide itself may be acting in the same manner at the level of the synapse.

Perhaps the most puzzling aspect of our findings is that so many different types of transmitters and modulators are found in amacrine cells. What is the functional significance of multiple peptides within amacrine cells as a group? Why are amacrine cells so diverse in morphology and chemical transmitters? Are these various peptides all necessarily involved in synaptic actions, or may they be playing some role in stabilizing the specific morphology of the cells, acting as second messengers or as one of the elusive trophic factors in growth and plasticity of the nervous system?

Acknowledgements: We wish to express our special thanks to our many colleagues who have so graciously provided us with the antibodies so vital to this effort. This research was made possible by support of the National Institutes of Health, Grant NEI 02146 and NS 12078.

REFERENCES

1. Binggeli, R.L. and W.J. Paule (1969)
The pigeon retina: Quantitative aspects of the optic nerve and ganglion cell layer.
J. Comp. Neurol., 137: 1-18.

2. Baughman, R.W. and C.R. Bader (1977)
Biochemical characterization and cellular localization of the cholinergic system in the chicken retina.
Brain Res., 138: 469-486.

3. Brandon, C., D.M.K. Lam and J. -Y. Wu (1979)
The gamma-aminobutyric acid system in rabbit retina - localization by immunocytochemistry and autoradiography.
Proc. Natl. Acad. Sci., U.S.A. 76: 3357-3361.

4. Brecha, N., H.J. Karten and C. Laverack (1979)
Enkephalin containing amacrine cells in the avian retina: immunohistochemical localization.
Proc. natn. Acad. Sci. U.S.A. 76: 3010-3014.

5. Brecha, N., H.J. Karten and C. Schenker (1981)
Neurotensin-like and somatostatin-like immunoreactivity within
amacrine cells of the retina.
Neurosci. 6: 1329-1340.

6. Cajal, S.R. (1933)
The Structure of the Retina
Translated from the original by S.A. Thorpe and M.Glickstein.
Publisher, Charles C. Thomas, Springfield, Illinois.(1972).
Originally published in Trav.Lab.Rech.Biol.Univ.Madrid, 28:
1-141 plus plates (1933).

7. Duner, H., U.S. von Euler and B. Pernow (1954)
Catecholamines and substance P in the mammalian eye.
Acta Physiol. Scand. 31: 113-118

8. Ehinger, B. (1967)
Adrenergic nerves in the avian eye and ciliary ganglion.
Z. Zellforsch. Mikrosk. Anat. 82: 577-588.

9. Ehinger, B. (1976)
Biogenic monoamines as transmitters in the retina.
In Transmitters in the Visual Process (ed. Bonting, S.L.)
pp. 145-163.

10. Ehinger, B. and I. Floren (1976)
Indoleamine-accumulating neurons in the retina of rabbit, cat
and goldfish.
Cell Tiss. Res. 175: 37-48.

11. Ehrlich, D. (1981)
Regional specialization of the chick retina as revealed by
the size and density of neurons in the ganglion cell layer.
J. Comp. Neurol., 195: 643-657.

12. Floren, I. (1979)
Indoleamine-accumulating neurons in the retina of chicken and pigeon.
Acta ophthalmol.(Kph.), 57: 198-210.

13. Karten, H.J. and N. Brecha (1980)
Localization of Substance P immunoreactivity in amacrine cells
of the retina.
Nature, Lond. 283: 87-88.

14. Kimura, H., P.L. McGeer, J.H. Peng and E.G. McGeer (1980)
The central cholinergic system studied by choline acetyltransferase
immunohistochemistry in the cat.
J. Comp. Nuerol. 200: 151-201.

15. Masland, R.H. and J.W. Mills (1979)
Autoradiographic identification of acetylcholine
in the rabbit retina.
J. Cell Biol. 83 159-178.

16. Rorstad, O.P., M. Brownstein and J.B. Martin (1979)
Immunoreactive and biologically active somatostatin-like
material in rat retina.
Proc. Natl. Acad. Sci. U.S.A. 76: 3019-3023.

17. Schaeffer, J. M., M. Brownstein and J. Axelrod (1977)
Thyrotropin-releasing hormone-like material in rat retina:
changes due to environmental lighting.
Proc. Natl. Acad. Sci. U.S.A. 74: 3579-3583

18. Steinbusch, H.W.M., A.A.J. Verhofstad and H.W.J. Joosten (1978)
Localization of serotonin iin the central nervous system by
immunohistochemistry: description of a specific and sensitive
technique and some applications.
Neuroscience, 3: 811-819.

19. Stell, W., D. Marshak, T. Yamada, N. Brecha and H.J. Karten (1980)
Peptides are in the eye of the beholder.
Trends in Neurosciences, 3: 292-295.

20. Vaughn, J.E., R.P. Barber, K. Saito, E. Roberts and
E.V. Famiglietti, Jr. (1978).
Immunocytochemical identification of GABAergic neurons in rat retina.
Anat. Rec. 190: 571-572.

EXCITATORY, INHIBITORY AND PEPTIDERGIC PATHWAYS IN THE MUDPUPPY RETINA

R.F. Miller, M.M. Slaughter and E. Dick

Departments of Ophthalmology, Physiology & Biophysics
Washington University School of Medicine, St. Louis
Mo., USA

The vertebrate retina contains a variety of neuronal connections which depend on chemical communication. Both excitatory
and inhibitory synapses are present: A substantial list of
putative transmitter agents has been expanded in recent years by
techniques which have localized several peptides to the retina
(Brecha and Karten, 1979; Stell et al., 1980). The physiologist
who attempts to define transmitter action in the retina does not
suffer from an abbreviated list of agents which may subserve
secretory transmission. We have studied the action of several
transmitter candidates and their antagonists using intracellular
recording techniques in the perfused retina-eyecup preparation
of the mudpuppy (Necturus maculosus). We have also studied the
effects of several peptides which have been localized to the
mudpuppy retina through immunohistochemical techniques of Brecha
and Karten. Our findings support the concept that excitatory
and inhibitory amino acids, as well as some peptides may be
involved in synaptic transmission.

PHOTORECEPTOR NEUROTRANSMISSION

In the outer retina, photoreceptors appear to communicate
with a dark released agent (Trifonov and Byzov, 1965; Dowling
and Ripps, 1973) which provides excitatory input at both the
onset and termination of a light stimulus (Kaneko and Shimazaki,
1975; Dacheux and Miller, 1976). Two post-synaptic elements
(horizontal cells (HCs) and OFF-bipolars) are depolarized in the
dark. A third cell type (ON-bipolar) is hyperpolarized in the
dark. A light stimulus which hyperpolarizes the photoreceptors
causes a reduction in the rate of transmitter release resulting
in a depolarization of ON-bipolars and a hyperpolarization of

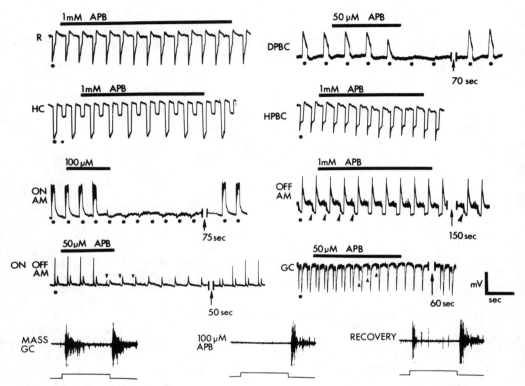

Fig. 1.   The effects of APB on intracellularly recorded responses
of a receptor (R), ON–bipolar (DPBC), horizontal cell (HC),
OFF–bipolar (HPBC), three types of amacrine cells (ON AM,
OFF AM, ON–OFF AM), a ganglion cell (GC) and extracellularly recorded mass ganglion cell discharge (MASS GC). In
the outer retina APB action blocks light modulation of the
ON–bipolar. In the inner retina ON responses and response
components are blocked (from Slaughter and Miller, 1981).

HCs and OFF-bipolars. Horizontal cells feedback onto cones
through a secretory pathway, and this feedback may account for
the center surround organization of bipolars (Werblin and Dowling,
1969; Kaneko, 1970).

Murakami et al. (1975) first described the effects of exogenously applied aspartate and glutamate on second order neurons.
These agents mimick the photoreceptor transmitter and since that
time these excitatory amino acids have been widely viewed as
likely photoreceptor transmitters. More recently, Wu and Dowling
(1979) have suggested that aspartate is a likely cone transmitter
in the carp retina. In the mudpuppy retina we have attempted to
characterize the synaptic receptors of second order neurons and
distinguish between direct and indirect actions of putative
transmitters and transmitter agonists. These studies have led to
an evaluation of a highly selective agonist (2-amino 4-phospho-
nobutyrate, APB) which appears to interact with the synaptic
receptors of ON-bipolars (Slaughter and Miller, 1980a, 1981a).
Figure 1 summarizes the effects of low levels of bath applied
APB on the different neuronal elements identified in the mudpuppy retina. In low concentrations APB action in the outer
retina is restricted to ON-bipolars. In the inner retina ON
responses or response components are eliminated but OFF responses
persist. Presumably the loss of ON activity in the inner retina
reflects the action of APB at the bipolar cell level. We have no
evidence to suggest that APB directly effects third order neurons.
It is interesting that in fairly high concentrations (10-20 mM)
APB (Slaughter and Miller, 1980b) acts as an antagonist to horizontal cells. The selective effect of APB on the ON-bipolar cell
is probably due to the L form; the D form is substantially less
active (we are indebted to J.C. Watkins for providing the D and L
forms of this compound).

One question raised by the observations in Fig. 1 is whether
APB acts on the synaptic receptors of the bipolar or whether it
depresses ON-bipolar cell activity by some other means. Since
HCs and OFF-bipolars are unaffected by low levels of APB it is
unlikely that this agent effects release of synaptic transmitter
from photoreceptors. One possibility is that APB may cause a
shunt at the bipolar cell level and thereby diminish the size of
light-evoked synaptic potentials. Figure 2 illustrates a test
of this possibility and an additional feature of APB action; the
upper trace shows a measurement of input resistance changes during the application of APB. A -0.1 nA current pulse balanced
through a bridge followed each light flash. As APB blocked the
light response the current pulse gave a more negative deflection
indicating that the input resistance had increased. The shunt
theory would require a decrease in input resistance. The lower
trace of Fig. 2 shows that APB caused a hyperpolarization of
the bipolar following a block of synaptic transmission with 3 mM

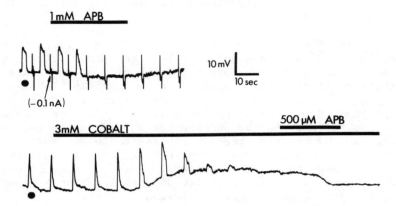

Fig. 2. Intracellular recordings from ON-bipolar cells exposed
to a 2-second, diffuse light stimulus once every 10 seconds
(irradiance = 3×10^{-8} watt/cm^2). In the top trace, a 0.1 nA
negative current pulse (arrow) was applied between light stimuli
to monitor relative changes in input resistance. With 1 mM APB
the light response was eliminated and the input resistance of the
cell was increased. In the bottom trace, a second ON-bipolar cell
was exposed to 3 mM cobalt which depolarized the cell and blocked
the light response. When 500 μM APB was superimposed on the
cobalt the cell hyperpolarized. These observations suggest that
APB is an agonist that mimics the action of the endogenous photoreceptor transmitter (from Slaughter and Miller, 1981a).

cobalt. This clearly shows that APB produces its effects by
activating the same conductance mechanism as that which underlies
the photoreceptor transmitter. Thus, APB is a highly selective
agonist. Presumably the synaptic receptors of ON-bipolars are
different than those of HCs or OFF-bipolars and APB readily distinguishes this difference. We have also tried 2-amino-3-
phosphonopropionic acid, an aspartate analog, and did not find
noticeable effects of this agent in concentrations up to 1 mM.
In fact, we have tried several amino acids and generally find
that "glutamate-like" agents are more effective than "aspartate-
like" analogs (Slaughter and Miller, 1981b). One exception is
that aspartate itself is usually more effective than glutamate,
although millimolar concentrations are needed to see these differences. The aspartate antagonist DL-α-aminoadipate does not
antagonize the exogenously applied apartate, and quite commonly
adipate synergizes externally applied aspartate (Slaughter and

Miller, 1980b). Thus, we have no evidence that the aspartate
action is mediated by an "aspartate receptor" as defined by the
use of aminoadipate.

Additional studies have attempted to characterize second
order neuronal activity by contrasting the effects of kainic
acid (KA) vs N-methyl-D-aspartate (NMDA) or N-methyl-DL-aspartate
(NMDLA). McCulloch et al. (1974) have suggested that these two
agents are more selective for the "glutamate" and "aspartate"
receptors, than either glutamate or aspartate per se.

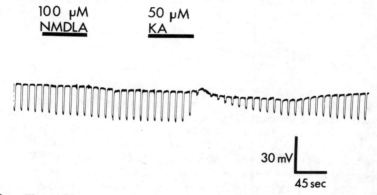

Fig. 3. The effects of bath applied NMDLA and KA on an intracellularly recorded horizontal cell in the mudpuppy retina.
Each downward deflection was evoked by a 2-second light stimulus.
KA resulted in a large decrease in the light response associated
with a small depolarization, whereas NMDLA at twice the KA dose
did not effect light activity.

Figures 3 and 4 show the effects of exogenously applied KA and
NMDLA on a HC recording before (Fig. 3) and after (Fig. 4) synaptic transmission is blocked by cobalt. It is clear that KA
is more effective and that this action persists in the presence
of cobalt suggesting that KA receptors are intrinsic to the

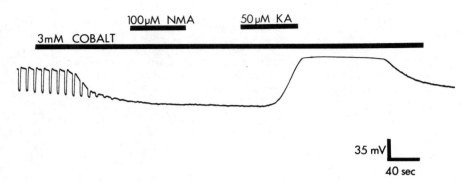

Fig. 4. Intracellular recording from a horizontal cell in the mudpuppy retina. Light responses (downward deflections) were blocked by 3 mM cobalt, as the cell hyperpolarized. In the presence of continuous cobalt, NMDLA was without effect, but KA resulted in a significant depolarization, followed by a prolonged recovery phase.

horizontal cell. The control experiments were done without Mg added to the Ringer solution in order to eliminate Mg suppression of the "aspartate" receptors (Watkins et al., 1980). We have found that KA is a much more effective agent than NMDA or NMDLA on all second order neurons. Recently, Ruck et al. (1981) have suggested that KA receptors and "folic acid" receptors are identical. We have tried folic acid and found it to be without effect at concentrations up to 1 mM. At the present time we do not know whether KA acts on synaptic or non-synaptic receptors. In summary, our findings are consistent with the idea that an amino acid or amino acid derivative may be the photoreceptor transmitter. Of the two popular candidates, glutamate vs aspartate, glutamate is favored by our experimental observations. One might reasonably ask whether glutamate itself is the transmitter. Application of fairly high levels of glutamate (1-10 mM) results in a transient loss of light responses of horizontal cells followed by a rapid desensitization and recovery of the light response, in the presence of continuous glutamate perfusion. Obviously, if continuous glutamate is present at the synaptic region, then light modulation of the synaptic receptor occurs in the face of fairly high glutamate levels, and this argues against glutamate as the transmitter. However, since we are applying glutamate at the vitreal surface glutamate could conceivably cause swelling of the inner retina, and reduce our ability to perfuse the distal retina. Further work is needed to clarify

the "desensitization" mechanism of glutamate application onto
second order neurons.

BIPOLAR NEUROTRANSMISSION

In the mudpuppy retina transmission from bipolar cells to
third order neurons is excitatory (Dacheux et al., 1979). At
light onset the ON-bipolars release an agent which depolarizes
ON and ON-OFF ganglion and amacrine cells, while at light off,
OFF-bipolars release an excitatory agent to OFF and ON-OFF
ganglion and amacrine cells. What transmitter candidates might
subserve bipolar transmission? We have recently explored this
problem using iontophoretic and bath applied agonists and antagonists. Acetylcholine does not appear to be a major transmitter
candidate in the mudpuppy retina. Iontophoretically applied
Ach has no effect on ganglion cell discharge and bath applied
Ach or carbachol does not influence bipolar, amacrine or ganglion
cells. Furthermore, muscarinic and nicotonic blocking agents do
not block excitatory light responses of the inner retina. One
finding, however, is that high doses of atropine block IPSPs at
the ganglion level, but these are much more effectively blocked
by GABA and glycine antagonists and we assume this high dose
atropine effect is a pharmacological action restricted to relatively high concentrations (mM range). Thus, while Ach is a
likely excitatory transmitter in some species, such as the rabbit
(Masland and Mills, 1979) it is probably not a transmitter of
either amacrine or bipolar cells in the mudpuppy.

Alternative candidate(s) for bipolar cell transmitters are
the excitatory amino acid agents glutamate and aspartate. Relatively small iontophoretically applied glut/asp evoke powerful
excitation to all ganglion cell types (Fig. 5). Intracellular
recordings from amacrine and ganglion cells (Slaughter et al.,
in prep.) show that these neurons are effectively excited by bath
applied excitatory amino acids and that the excitation persists
after transmission is blocked by cobalt. Thus, excitatory amino
acid receptors are intrinsic to amacrine and ganglion cells. It
is interesting to note that some ganglion cells are inhibited by
bath applied excitatory amino acids, but this effect is converted
to an excitatory action after synaptic transmission is blocked by
cobalt. It seems likely that the inhibitory effect results from
activation of an amacrine to ganglion cell inhibitory pathway
which is eliminated in cobalt, so that the intrinsic excitatory
effect is unmasked. We do not yet know whether the excitatory
receptors of third order neurons prefer KA or NMDA, but our
preliminary evidence suggests that NMDA is much more effective in
the inner retina than it is in the outer retina. In summary, our
studies of third order neurons are consistent with the idea that
an excitatory amino acid or amino acid derivative could be the
transmitter of ON and OFF bipolars.

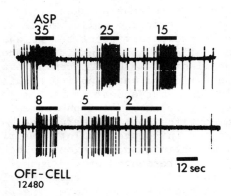

Fig. 5. Photographic reproduction of an oscilloscope record
from an off-ganglion cell in the absence of light stimuli.
Aspartate, ejected anionically (100 mM, pH 7.8) evokes spike
activity in a dose-dependent fashion. Iontophoretic currents
are indicated in nA. Note that the highest ejection level of
35 nA evoked high frequency positive-going spikes without the
negative spike component. This probably reflects an accommoda-
tion of the somatic spike component (from Slaughter et al., in
preparation).

INHIBITORY TRANSMISSION

The inhibitory agents gamma amino butyric acid (GABA) and
glycine have been implicated as possible transmitters in the
retina. We have extensively studied the effects of these two
agents (Miller et al., 1977, 1981a, 1981b; Frumkes et al., 1981).
Our evidence suggests that "GABAnergic" and "glycinergic" mechanisms play an important role in the inner retina, and more
specifically, that amacrine to ganglion cell inhibition plays
a dominant role in the determination of receptive field properties of some ganglion cell types. However, candidates other

than GABA or glycine have similar actions, including β-alanine, alanine, serine and taurine. More specifically, the actions of β-alanine and GABA are blocked by picrotoxin and bicuculline, whereas the actions of serine, taurine and glycine are blocked by strychnine (Slaughter and Miller, in preparation). Thus, on the basis of our experiments any or all of these agents could mediate inhibitory responses and for this reason we prefer the general terms GABA- and glycinergic to define a group of two distinct inhibitory inputs which can be distinguished on the basis of differential blocking effects of picrotoxin/bicuculline vs strychnine.

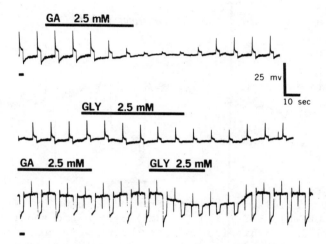

GA   2.5 mM

GLY   2.5 mM

25 mv

10 sec

GA   2.5 mM   GLY 2.5 mM

Fig. 6. Intracellular recordings from an ON-bipolar (two upper traces) and an OFF-bipolar (lowest trace). GABA application had a relatively greater effect than glycine (GLY) in suppressing the ON-bipolar whereas the opposite was observed for the relative GABA vs glycine sensitivity of the OFF-bipolar. Initial 2-second light flashes indicated by dark bar. Input resistance measurements were carried out with the OFF-bipolar; the glycine application was associated with a decreased input resistance (from Miller et al., 1981a).

One interesting observation related to GABA/glycine action is the fact that the ON and OFF channels show differential sensitivity to these two agents. Figure 6 shows the effects of GABA and glycine administered to an ON (upper two traces) and OFF

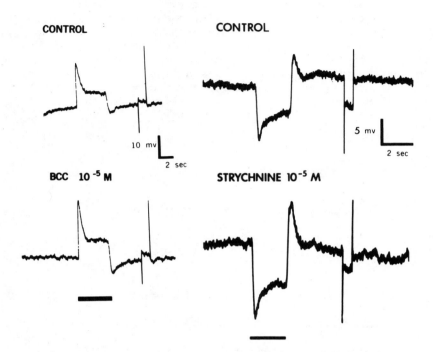

Fig. 7.   Intracellular recordings from an ON-bipolar (left column) and an OFF-bipolar (right column) before and about 1 minute
after bicuculline methiodide and strychnine were applied in the
indicated concentration. A positive (0.1 nA) current pulse was
applied to the electrode and a bridge to measure the relative
change in input resistance. The antagonists resulted in an
increase in the light response of each bipolar cell type, associated with an increased input resistance, as indicated by the
more positive going current pulse in the lower records. Bicuculline did not have an effect on OFF-bipolars, whereas strychnine either did not effect ON-bipolars or resulted in response
decline. Diffuse light stimulation (from Miller et al., 1981a).

(lowest trace) bipolar. The ON-bipolar shows a distinctly
greater sensitivity to GABA, while the OFF-bipolar is more glycine sensitive. GABA and glycine effects persist after synaptic
transmission is blocked so that these actions are largely direct
(Miller et al., 1981a). In addition, the GABA antagonists picrotoxin and bicuculline enhance depolarizing bipolars, but have
very little effect on hyperpolarizing bipolars, whereas strych-

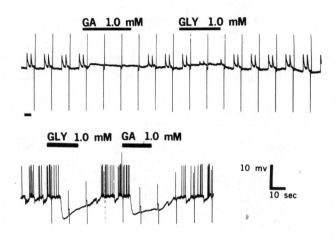

Fig. 8.   Intracellular recordings from an ON-OFF amacrine cell
(upper trace) and an OFF ganglion cell (lower trace) in response
to GABA and glycine application (1 mM levels).   In the amacrine
cell recordings both GABA and glycine caused a loss of the light
response associated with a decrease in input resistance (+0.1 nA
current pulse), but relatively small changes in membrane potential.   The ganglion cell showed a large decrease in input resistance (-0.1 nA current pulse), loss of spike activity and a
large hyperpolarization.   This was a major difference between
amacrine and ganglion cells.   Duration of diffuse light stimuli
indicated by initial bar under each trace.   Light stimulation
was maintained during GA/GLY application.   Modified from Miller
et al., 1981a.

nine enhances hyperpolarizing bipolars but either has no effect
or decreases response amplitude of ON-bipolars (Miller et al.,
1981a).   We have previously explained this phenomenon by suggesting that both GABA and glycine may be tonically released in
the dark, and cause a low level inhibition of the bipolars.   Consistent with this idea we find that the actions of agonist and
antagonist have opposite effects on the input resistance.
Figure 7 shows the increase in input resistance of an ON and OFF

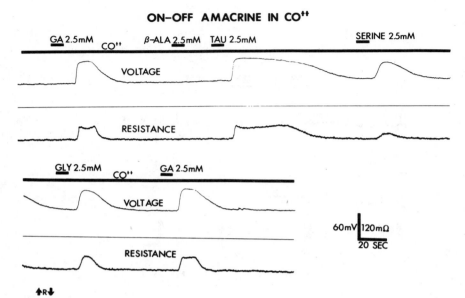

Fig. 9.   Intracellular recording from an ON–OFF amacrine using a
KCL-filled micropipette. The light response was previously
blocked with cobalt which continuously perfused the retina during
the course of this study.   Brief applications of GABA, β–
alanine, taurine (tau), serine, glycine (GLY) are indicated by
the dark bars above the traces.   The membrane potential was
recorded in the trace labelled voltage, and the input resistance
was monitored from the in–phase detector output of the lock–in
amplifier.   Note that with a KCL-filled pipette, inhibitory
amino acids depolarized the amacrine, in contrast to the normally
non-polarizing effects when K-acetate electrodes are used for
recording.   The depolarizing effects are associated with a
decrease in the input resistance of the cell.   The only amino
acid which did not have an effect was β–alanine, although this
agent proved effective in other cells (from Slaughter and
Miller, in preparation).

bipolar in response to bicuculline and strychnine application.
Response enhancement is associated with an increase in input
resistance, as indicated by the more positive going voltage
evoked by a +0.1 nA pulse through a bridge device.   The observation that GABA may be intimately associated with the ON pathway
and glycine with the OFF pathway may help to explain why both
mechanisms are operational at the same synaptic level.   We assume
that the GABA- and glycinergic pathways are from amacrines and
not from horizontal cells.   It is generally accepted that hori-

zontal cells underlie antagonistic- center-surround organization
(Werblin and Dowling, 1969; Kaneko, 1970). Although some horizontal cells in mudpuppy take up labelled GABA (D. Lam, personal
communication), we have been unable to show a loss of center-
surround organization of bipolars using GABA antagonists (Miller
et al., 1981a). Our evidence favors the idea that the major
GABA- and glycinergic neurons are subpopulations of amacrine
cells. Amacrine and ganglion cells are sensitive to both GABA
and glycine, although the ratio of sensitivities is highly variable. There appear to be a few ON ganglion cells which are
almost exclusively GABA sensitive, whereas a few OFF ganglion
cells show a much greater preference for gylcine (Miller et al.,
1981b). Most ganglion cells, however, were quite sensitive to
both agents. The action of GABA and glycine differed when
ganglion cells were compared to amacrines; amacrines experienced
a large conductance increase without an obvious change in membrane potential, whereas a large increase in conductance in
ganglion cells was associated with a substantial hyperpolarization (Fig. 8). Both mechanisms may depend on chloride.
Figure 9 illustrates a recording from an ON-OFF amacrine using a
KCL-filled electrode, after synaptic transmission had been
blocked with cobalt. Under these conditions inhibitory amino
acids cause a large depolarization, associated with a conductance
increase detected with a lock-in device (0.2 nA 50 ops current
injection). Filtering of the lock-in output slows the response
time of the conductance recording. Presumably the KCl electrode
resulted in an increase in intracellular chloride, so that
chloride dependent responses are now depolarizing. A similar
phenomenon has been observed in ganglion cell recordings when
IPSPs were converted to depolarizing responses by Cl^- injection.
There appears to be a major difference between amacrine and
ganglion cells with respect to chloride distribution: Chloride
is passively distributed in amacrines, but maintained at a
negative value in ganglion cells. This has been confirmed with
intracellular measurements of chloride, using chloride selective
microelectrodes (Miller and Dacheux, 1976).

IPSPS AT GANGLION CELL LEVEL INDICATE TYPES OF INHIBITORY AMACRINE CELL INPUT

A preliminary study of IPSPs at the ganglion cell level
suggested that two types of ON-OFF inhibition were present,
including both a GABA- and glycinergic pathway (Miller et al.,
1976). A more extensive analysis (Miller et al., 1981a,b;
Frumkes et al., 1981) has revealed two additional types of inhibitory phenomena. Figure 10 illustrates several types of
inhibitory responses. In addition to the two types of ON-OFF
inhibition we have found evidence for an ON inhibition which is
GABAnergic and an OFF inhibition which is glycinergic. To date,
however, we have not observed an OFF inhibition in the absence

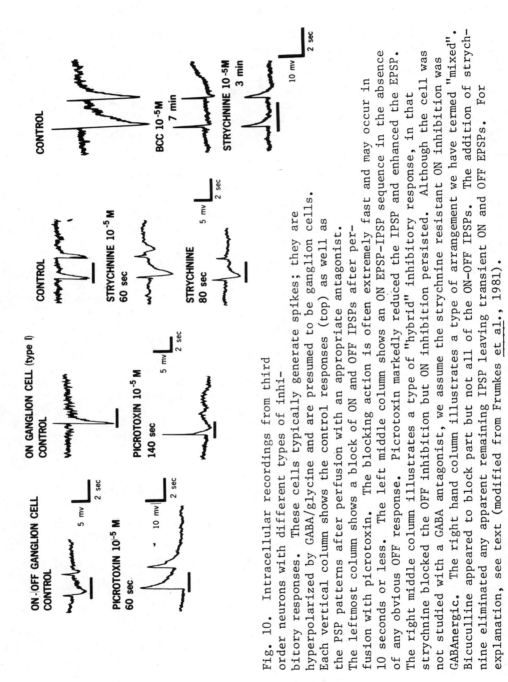

Fig. 10. Intracellular recordings from third
order neurons with different types of inhi-
bitory responses. These cells typically generate spikes; they are
hyperpolarized by GABA/glycine and are presumed to be ganglion cells.
Each vertical column shows the control responses (top) as well as
the PSP patterns after perfusion with an appropriate antagonist.
The leftmost column shows a block of ON and OFF IPSPs after perfusion with picrotoxin. The blocking action is often extremely fast and may occur in
10 seconds or less. The left middle column shows an ON EPSP-IPSP sequence in the absence
of any obvious OFF response. Picrotoxin markedly reduced the IPSP and enhanced the EPSP.
The right middle column illustrates a type of "hybrid" inhibitory response, in that
strychnine blocked the OFF inhibition but ON inhibition persisted. Although the cell was
not studied with a GABA antagonist, we assume the strychnine resistant ON inhibition was
GABAnergic. The right hand column illustrates a type of arrangement we have termed "mixed".
Bicuculline appeared to block part but not all of the ON-OFF IPSPs. The addition of strychnine eliminated any apparent remaining IPSP leaving transient ON and OFF EPSPs. For
explanation, see text (modified from Frumkes et al., 1981).

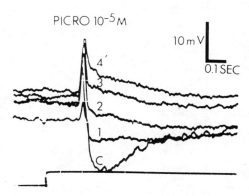

PICRO 10^{-5}M

10 mV

0.1 SEC

Fig. 11.   Intracellular recordings from an ON ganglion cell during the application of picrotoxin. The control record (C) showed
a small EPSP followed by a somewhat larger IPSP. The displaced
responses were recorded at 1,2,3 and 4 minutes after introducing
the picrotoxin. A progressive loss of the IPSP is associated
with progressive enhancement of the EPSP. The onset of the
diffuse light stimulus is indicated by the upward deflection of
the lowest trace (modified from Frumkes et al., 1981).

of any ON component. In some cases we see evidence of both
GABA- and glycinergic input to the same cell but in many instances one or the other predominates.

Conclusions about inhibitory input into ganglion cells are
based on the disappearance of hyperpolarizing response components (IPSPs) associated with the application of inhibitory amino
acid antagonists; often this results in the emergence of substantial depolarizing EPSPs. We originally interpreted this
sequence of events (illustrated in Fig. 11) as a progressive
loss of an inhibitory conductance change which normally masked
the excitatory drive. Since GABA and glycine antagonists did
not block light responses of amacrines (Miller et al., 1977) we

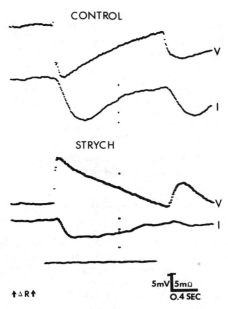

Fig. 12. Intracellular recording from a cell (presumed ganglion cell) showing prominent ON–OFF IPSPs. The upper trace in each pair of records is the signal averaged (n=4) voltage recording, while the lower record (I) is the in-phase detector output of a lock-in amplifier (PAR 5204) which provides an independent

continuous trace for monitoring changes in input resistance. For this measurement a 0.1 nA (P.P) 50 Hz current was applied to the electrode and balanced through a bridge. Filtering of the in-phase output slowed the conductance record in comparison to the voltage trace. In the control record, the IPSPs are associated with a decreased input resistance. The lower pair of records were signal averaged a few minutes after introducing strychnine 10^{-5} M into the bathing medium. Strychnine changed the voltage recording into ON and OFF EPSPs, but the conductance measurement showed that the EPSP was associated with a reduced conductance change compared to that observed in the control. This observation suggests that the EPSP did not block the IPSP by masking, but that strychnine caused a loss of an input conductance change at the ganglion cell level. Diffuse light stimulation.

assumed that the action of the antagonists was at the level of
the ganglion cell. We also demonstrated that the GABA and glycine antagonists were effective blocking agents of exogenously
applied GABA and glycine (Miller et al., 1981a). One additional
possibility however, is that the antagonists enhance the conductance changes of the excitatory pathways, and thereby mask
the still intact IPSPs at the ganglion cell level. Figure 12
illustrates a test of this possibility using the lock-in amplifier to provide a continuous measure of changes in input resistance (lower trace in each pair of records). These responses
were signal averaged (n=4) and photographed from an oscilloscope.
In the upper pair, the voltage recording is dominated by IPSPs
associated with a large conductance increase (lower trace indicated as I for in-phase detection). The lower pair of records
illustrates that after the IPSPs are blocked with strychnine,
EPSPs persist but the conductance changes are smaller than those
observed when IPSPs are present. These experiments argue against
the enhanced EPSP masking the IPSPs, and favor our previous
conclusions that IPSPs are in fact blocked by the antagonists.
With few exceptions, we find that the conductance changes associated with EPSPs are much smaller than those associated with
IPSPs. It appears that under the conditions of our experiments,
light stimuli activate more powerful inhibitory inputs compared
to excitatory drives. It is not difficult to see how some
ganglion cells can be inexcitable in response to diffuse light
stimulation (Lettvin et al., 1959).

In order to account for our observations on the selective
blocking action of GABA/glycine antagonists at the ganglion cell
level, we have proposed four different types of amacrine cells
(Frumkes et al., 1981). These include an ON type amacrine which
releases GABA (Fig. 10 left, middle column), an OFF type amacrine
which releases glycine (Fig. 10 right, middle column) and two
ON-OFF amacrines one of which releases glycine while the other
releases GABA (Fig. 10 left column, right column). In addition,
our findings suggest that both GABA and glycine are tonically
released in the dark and interact with bipolar, amacrine and
ganglion cells. With the exception of HCs our findings suggest
that all post-receptor neurons may be continuously influenced by
dark released inhibitory transmitters. In addition, the use of
the lock-in technique to provide continuous on-line measurement
of resistance, suggests that in many cells the application of
GABA antagonists enhances the conductance changes associated with
synaptic input. Thus far, this has been much more apparent with
GABA antagonists compared to strychnine. Whether this reflects
changes in the integrative properties of dendrites, or whether
this indicates a block of presynaptic inhibitory effects of GABA
is not presently clear, but it is possible that in addition to
segregation of GABA vs glycinergic mechanisms associated with ON
and OFF pathways, GABA may play an additional role controlling
presynaptic inputs not shared by the glycinergic system.

Do the results obtained in the mudpuppy retina relate to
those obtained in other species? With respect to the GABA/glycine
ON vs OFF association, two observations suggest that mudpuppy
results may be generally applicable to other species. Cunningham
and Miller (1976) showed that taurine application in the perfused
rabbit retina blocked OFF responses in the inner retina but not
ON responses. Since taurine acts like glycine (Cunningham and
Miller, 1980a,b), these observations support the idea that the
OFF pathway may be more glycine sensitive. In addition, Berger
et al. (1977) have done a chemical layer analysis of the monkey
retina and showed that glycine distribution was more distally
localized within the IPL when compared to GABA. If one accepts
the idea that ON and OFF inputs into the inner retina are
segregated respectively into proximal and distal IPL sublamina
(Famiglietti and Kolb, 1976; Famiglietti et al., 1977) then the
more distal glycine distribution is compatible with a preferential "glycine-OFF" association and the more proximal GABA distribution could reflect a preferential GABA-ON channel interaction. One of us (E.D.) has recently completed this type of
analysis in the rabbit retina working in Dr. O. Lowry's lab with
results similar to those reported in the monkey.

PEPTIDERGIC PATHWAYS IN THE MUDPUPPY RETINA:
IONTOPHORESIS AND INTRACELLULAR RECORDING

In recent years several peptides have been localized to the
retina by immunohistochemical and radioimmunoassay techniques.
In collaboration with N. Brecha and H. Karten, we have initiated
a study of possible peptidergic pathways in the mudpuppy retina.
Peptides which have localized to the mudpuppy include neurotensin,
substance P, enkephalin, vasoactive intestinal peptide, somatostatin, and cholecystokinin. The immunoreactive material shows
up in the inner retina, and cell body fluorescence has thus far
been confined to the amacrine cell layer. These agents therefore
should be considered as additional transmitter or "modulator"
candidates which mediate cell communication in the inner retina.
Our initial approach to the special problems associated with
peptides was to use iontophoretic techniques at the ganglion cell
level to determine whether well defined modulations of impulse
generating activity were associated with peptide application.
The initial experiments (Dick and Miller, 1980, 1981) have indicated that most ganglion cells in the mudpuppy retina are excited
by neurotensin and substance P (Figs. 13 and 14), while enkephalin (enkephalinamide) application (as well as morphine) depressed
ganglion cell firing (Fig. 15). The action of morphine, however,
was not blocked by iontophoretically applied naloxone. In fact,
naloxone itself tended to block ganglion cell firing. We do not
know whether the naloxone insensitivity of the morphine/enkepha-
lin action represents a local anesthetic action (in many instances the spike depression is associated with a diminished spike

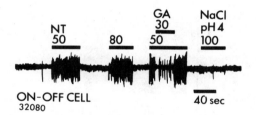

Fig. 13. Penwriter spike record from an OFF-center unit in the absence of light stimulation. Neurotensin (NT), ejected cationically (1.0 mM in 10 mM NaCl, pH 5) evokes spike activity in a dose-dependent fashion. Successively higher ejecting currents are associated with a reduction in the latency of the excitatory affects of the peptide and an increase in the frequency of the evoked spike activity. A 60 nA cationic current applied to a NaCl solution (10 mM, pH 4) had no effect (from Dick and Miller, in preparation).

amplitude) or whether a naloxone insensitive receptor could mediate this action. Intracellular recordings from ganglion cells in our laboratory (R. Zalutsky) show that morphine application is not associated with a large increase in membrane potential so that its effects are unlike those of the inhibitory amino acids. It is possible that the iontophoretic effect on spike generation is at the level of the spike generating mechanism itself.

We have initiated intracellular recording experiments to examine peptide actions on cells more distal than the ganglion cell level. Figure 16 illustrates an intracellular recording from a horizontal cell in the perfused axolotyl retina. Substance P 4-11 fragment was added to the bathing medium (10 μm): Note that the cell was depolarized, light responses were larger. The output from the lock-in (lower trace) indicates that the depolarization is associated with an increased input resistance. While our investigation into the problem of peptide usage as putative neurotransmitters is still preliminary, we find that most of these agents have transmitter-like effects and that their action is not confined to the ganglion cells. Preliminary observations in our laboratory (R. Zalutsky) also indicate that

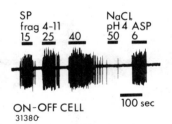

Fig. 14. A penwriter spike record from an ON-OFF ganglion cell
in the absence of light stimuli. The substance P 4-11 octapeptide fragment (SP 4-11), ejected cationically (2.5 mM, pH 5)
evokes spike activity in this unit. Larger ejecting currents
are associated with longer persistence of the excitatory actions.
A 50 nA cationic ejecting current applied to a NaCl solution
(10 mM, pH 4) had no effect while a 6 nA anionic ejecting current
applied to a solution of sodium aspartate (100 mM, pH 7.8) also
evoked spike activity (from Dick and Miller, in preparation).

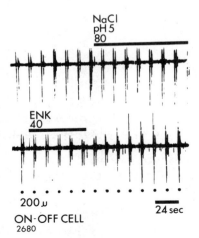

Fig. 15. Photographic reproduction of an oscilloscope record
from an ON-OFF cell during intermittent small spot illumination
(200 micron spot, 2 seconds on/10 seconds off) and during the
iontophoretic application of $(D-ala^2-met^5)$-enkephalinamide.
Met-enkephalinamide (ENK), ejected cationically (10 mM, pH 5)
caused a reduction in the amplitude of the extracellularly
recorded spikes. This effect was not due to current artifacts
as demonstrated by the lack of any effect of a 80 nA cationic
ejecting current applied to a NaCl solution (100 mM, pH 5) in an
adjacent barrel. Higher levels of met-enkephalinamide application are further associated with a loss of light-evoked spike
activity (from Dick and Miller, in preparation).

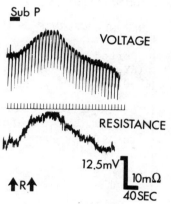

Fig. 16.   An intracellular recording from a horizontal cell in
the perfused axolotyl retina.   A brief application of Sub P
resulted in a depolarization and slight enhancement of the light
response.   The lower continuous monitor of input resistance used
the in-phase output of a lock-in amplifier with a 0.1 nA (P-P)
50 Hz current pulse applied to the electrode and subsequently
balanced out by a bridge and filtering.   The depolarizing effect
of Sub P was associated with an increased input resistance.

Substance P and neurotensin are excitatory agents at the amacrine and ganglion cell level. An essential step in our understanding of the role of peptides in neuronal communication will be to utilize effective blocking agents for the action of different peptides to determine whether physiologically evoked synaptic responses are modified by antagonists. Until experiments such as these can be directed at the single cell level we will be uncertain about the magnitude of peptide contribution to synaptic function. It is nevertheless clear that with the limited number of peptides we have studied so far, we have candidates for both excitatory (neurotensin and substance P) and inhibitory (enkephalin) mechanisms, and these agents should be included in the list of possible chemical agents subserving important roles in synaptic transmission and retinal homeostasis.

ACKNOWLEDGEMENTS

This research was supported by NIH grant EY-00844 to R.F.M., NIH Fellowship to M.M.S. (EY-05338), and E.D. received support from NIH Training Grant EY-07057.

We thank Judy Dodge for the figure illustrations and photographic work. We are especially grateful to Dr. J.C. Watkins for supplying us with N-methyl-D-aspartate and the D and L forms of 2-amino-4-phosphono butyric acid.

REFERENCES

Baylor, D.A., Fuortes, M.G.F. and O'Bryan, P., 1971. Receptive fields of cones in retina of the turtle. J. Physiol. (Lond.) 214: 265-294.

Berger, S.J., McDaniel, M.L., Carter, J.G. and Lowry, O., 1977. Distribution of four potential transmitter amino acids in monkey retina. J. Neurochem. 2: 159-164.

Brecha, N. and Karten, H.J., 1979. Enkephalin containing amacrine cells in the retina. Invest. Ophthal. Vis. Sci. Suppl. 19: 85.

Cunningham, R.A. and Miller, R.F., 1976. Taurine: Its selective action on the rabbit retina. Brain Research 117: 341-345.

Cunningham, R.A. and Miller, R.F., 1980a. Electrophysiological analysis of taurine and glycine action on neurons of the mudpuppy retina. I. Intracellular recording. Brain Research 197: 123-138.

Cunningham, R.A. and Miller, R.F., 1980b. Electrophysiological analysis of taurine and glycine action on neurons of the mudpuppy retina. II. ERG, PNR, and Müller cell recordings. Brain Research 197: 139-151.

Dacheux, R.F. and Miller, R.F., 1976. Photoreceptor bipolar cell transmission in the mudpuppy retina. Science 191: 963-964.

Dacheux, R.F., Frumkes, T.E. and Miller, R.F., 1979. Pathways and polarities of synaptic interactions in the inner retina of the mudpuppy. I. Synaptic blocking studies. Brain Research 161: 1-12.

Davies, J. and Watkins, J.C., 1981. Pharmacology of glutamate and aspartate antagonists on cat spinal neurones, in "Glutamate as a Neurotransmitter", Ed. by DiChiara and Gessa, pp. 275-284, Raven Press, New York.

Dick, E., Miller, R.F. and Behbehani, M., 1980. Opioids and substance P influence ganglion cells in amphibian retina. Invest. Ophthal. Vis. Sci. Suppl. 19: 132.

Dick, E. and Miller, R.F., 1981. Peptides influence retinal ganglion cells. Neurosci. Letters (in press).

Dowling, J.E. and Ripps, H., 1973. Effects of magnesium on horizontal cell activity in the skate retina. Nature 242: 963-964.

REFERENCES

Famiglietti, E.V. and Kolb, H., 1976. Structural basis for on and off-center responses in retinal ganglion cells. Science 194: 193-195.

Famiglietti, E.V., Kaneko, A. and Tachibana, M., 1979. Neuronal architecture of on and off pathways to ganglion cells in carp retina. Science 198: 1267-1269.

Frumkes, T.E., Miller, R.F., Slaughter, M.M. and Dacheux, R.F., 1981. Physiological and pharmacological basis of GABA and glycine action on neurons of mudpuppy retina. III. Amacrine-mediated inhibitory influences on ganglion cell receptive field organization: A model. J. Neurophysiol. 45: 783-804.

Kaneko, A., 1970. Physiological-morphological identification of horizontal, bipolar and amacrine cells in goldfish retina. J. Physiol. (Lond.) 207: 623-633.

Kaneko, A. and Shimazaki, H., 1975. Synaptic transmission from photoreceptors to bipolar and horizontal cells in the carp retina. Cold Spring Harb. Symp. Quant. Biol. 40: 537-546.

Lettvin, J.Y., Maturana, H.R., McCulloch, W.S. and Pitts, W.H., 1959. What the frog's eye tells the frog's brain. Proc. Inst. Radio Engrs. 47: 1940-1951.

Masland, R.H. and Mills, J.W., 1979. Autoradiographic identification of acetylcholine in the rabbit retina. J. Cell Biol. 83: 159-178.

McCulloch, R.M., Johnston, G.A.R., Game, C.J.A. and Curtis, D.R., 1974. The differential sensitivity of spinal interneurones and Renshaw cell to kainate and N-methyl-D-aspartate. Exp. Brain Res. 21: 515-518.

Miller, R.F. and Dacheux, R.F., 1976. Intracellular chloride activity in neurons of the mudpuppy retina. ARVO Meeting, Sarasota, Florida.

Miller, R.F., Dacheux, R.F. and Frumkes, T., 1977. Evidence for independent GABA- and glycine-releasing amacrine cells in mud-puppy retina. Science 198: 748-749.

Miller, R.F., Frumkes, T.E., Slaughter, M.M. and Dacheux, R.F., 1981a. Physiological and pharmacological basis of GABA- and glycine action on neurons of mudpuppy retina. I. Receptors, horizontal cells, bipolars and G-cells. J. Neurophysiol. 45: 743-763.

Miller, R.F., Frumkes, T.E., Slaughter, M.M. and Dacheux, R.F., 1981b. Physiological and pharmacological basis of GABA and gly- cine action on neurons of mudpuppy retina. II. Amacrine and gang- lion cells. J. Neurophysiol. 45: 764-782.

Murakami, M., Ohtsuka, T. and Shimazaki, H., 1975. Effects of aspartate and glutamate on the bipolar cell in the carp retina. Vision Res. 15: 456-458.

Ruck, A., Kramer, S., Metz, J. and Brennan, M.J.W., 1980. Methyltetrahydrofolate is a potent and selective agonist for kainic acid receptors. Nature 287: 852-853.

Slaughter, M.M. and Miller, R.F., 1980a. A unique action of 2- amino-4-phosphonobutyrate on the ON pathway in the mudpuppy retina. Soc. for Neurosci. 6: 7.

Slaughter, M.M. and Miller, R.F., 1980b. Is aspartate or gluta- mate a photoreceptor transmitter? Invest. Ophthal. Vis. Sci. Suppl. 19: 131.

Slaughter, M.M. and Miller, R.F., 1981a. 2-Amino-4-phosphono- butyric acid: A new pharmacological tool for retina research. Science 211: 182-185.

Slaughter, M.M. and Miller, R.F., 1981b. Pharmacological studies of the photoreceptor-on bipolar synapse in the mudpuppy retina. Invest. Ophthal. Vis. Sci. Suppl. 20: 44.

Stell, W., Marshak, D., Yamada, T., Brecha, N. and Karten, H., 1980. Peptides are in the eye of the beholder. TINS 3: 292-295.

Trifonov, J.A. and Byzov, A.L., 1965. The response of the cells generating S-potential on the current passed through the eyecup of the turtle. Biofizika 10: 673-680.

Watkins, J.C., Davies, J., Evans, R.H., Francis, A.A. and Jones, A.W., 1981. Pharmacology of receptors for exhibitory amino acids, in "Glutamate as a Neurotransmitter", Ed. by DiChiara and Gessa, pp. 263-284, Raven Press, New York.

Werblin, F.S. and Dowling, J.E., 1969. Organization of retina of the mudpuppy, Necturus maculosus. II. Intracellular recording. J. Neurophysiol. 32: 339-355.

Wu, S.M. and Dowling, J.E., 1978. L-aspartate: Evidence for a role in cone photoreceptor transmission in the carp retina. Proc. Natl. Acad. Sci. 75: 5205-5209.

TRANSMITTER RELEASE FROM THE RETINA

Michael J. Neal

Department of Pharmacology, The School of
Pharmacy, University of London, 29/39
Brunswick Square, London WC1N 1AX, UK.

INTRODUCTION

Studies on the release of transmitters from the
retina have involved many of the techniques used in
other areas of the CNS. For example, many studies have
used isolated superfused retinae in which the transmitter pool has been radiolabelled by previous incubation with precursors or the transmitter itself. In a
few cases, endogenous transmitter release has been
measured. A technique which is unique to the retina is
the eye-cup preparation, in which the entire retina is
exposed to superfusion with minimal disturbance.

In the retina, even greater care than usual must
be taken in using exogenously added transmitters,
because a given compound may be accumulated in different
types of cell in different species. For example, ^3H -
GABA is accumulated mainly by glia in the rat retina
(Neal and Iversen, 1972) but by horizontal cells in the
frog (Neal et al., 1979b). On the other hand, by
suitably varying the lighting conditions during the
incubation period with ^3H GABA in the goldfish retina,
either horizontal cells or amacrine cells can be
selectively labelled, enabling the release of ^3H GABA
to be studied from both these cell types (Marc et al.,
1978).

It must be admitted that release studies of transmitters in the retina have not kept pace with the ever
increasing number of retinal transmitter candidates, but

761

they are important because the release of a substance in
response to a physiological stimulus (light in the
present case) is a major criterion in establishing a
neurotransmitter role for a substance.

In this paper, the literature on transmitter
release from the retina will be reviewed, concentrating
on studies in which light rather than potassium
depolarization was used as the stimulus. (For
references on anatomical and electrophysiological
aspects of retinal transmitters, the reader should
consult the papers by Ehinger, Lam, Karten and Miller in
this volume). It will be apparent that only in the case
of ACh have release studies progressed much further than
a simple demonstration of light evoked release. The
remainder of the paper will describe some of our recent
experiments on the modulation of the light evoked
release of ACh from the rabbit retina by GABAergic and
glycinergic drugs and by ω-phosphonic derivatives of
α-amino acids. For convenience I have usually referred
throughout to "transmitters", rather than to "putative
transmitters", but for some substances the evidence for
their transmitter role is certainly not conclusive.

Only ten years ago, Kramer (1971) demonstrated the
first light evoked release of a transmitter (dopamine)
from the superfused retina of the anaesthetised cat.
His results and the results of subsequent studies on
the light release of transmitters from the retina are
summarised in Table 1. It is clear that far more is
known about factors affecting retinal ACh release than
any other transmitter, reflecting the relative ease in
obtaining reproducible light evoked releases of this
transmitter. Only two reports concern dopamine, and
although the results in cats seem quite convincing,
those from the rabbit are somewhat less so. In two
preliminary experiments using the rabbit eye-cup
preparation we failed to obtain a light-evoked release
of dopamine. We do not know whether this failure is
due to technical deficiences in our experiments or to a
genuine species difference between cats and rabbits.

Of the putative amino acid transmitters, the light
evoked release of taurine (radiolabelled and endogenous)
is the largest and most reproducible, but the cellular
origin of the released amino acid is not yet known. It
may be released from a sub-population of amacrine cells,
the photoreceptors, or both. A small but significant
release of ^{3}H glycine from amacrine cells of the

Table 1. Transmitter Release From The Retina.

"Transmitter"	Endogenous/ Labelled	Preparation	Photic Stimulation	K+ Stimulation	Notes and references
GABA	^{3}H	Isolated rabbit retina	↑		Ca-dependent. Blocked by AOAA and pentobarbitone. Bauer & Ehinger (1977); Bauer (1978).
GABA	^{3}H	Isolated rabbit retina in vivo			Release increased by α-M.S.H. Bauer & Ehinger (1980).
GABA	^{3}H	Goldfish retina in vitro		↑	Inhibited by enkephalin. Djamgoz et al (1981).
Glycine	^{3}H	Isolated rabbit retina, cat retina in vivo	↑ ↑		Cat results variable. Ehinger & Lindberg (1974); Ehinger & Lindberg-Bauer (1976).
Glycine	^{14}C	Chick in vitro & synaptosomes		↑ ↑	Ca-dependent. Lopez-Colome et al (1978).
Glycine	Endog.	Rat retina in vivo	↑		Pigmented rats only Coull & Cutler (1978).
Glycine	Endog.	Rat retina in vitro	0	↑	Kennedy & Neal (1978)
Glycine	Endog.	Rabbit eye-cup in vivo	0		Neal et al (1979)

(continued)

Table 1. (Continued).

"Trans-mitter"	Endogenous/ Labelled	Preparation	Photic Stimulation	K+ Stimulation	Notes and references
Aspartate	Endog.	Rabbit eye-cup in vivo	↓		Neal et al (1979a)
Glutamate	Endog.	Rabbit eye-cup in vivo	0		Neal et al (1979a)
Glutamate	Endog.	Isolated chick retina	0		Pasantes-Morales et al (1974)
Taurine	35S	Chick retina in vitro	↑		Pasantes-Morales et al (1973)
Taurine	Endog.	Chick retina in vitro	↑		Pasantes-Morales et al (1974)
Taurine	35S	Chick retina in vitro			Release coupled with Ca. Salceda & Pasantes-Morales (1975).
Taurine	35S	Chick retina & synaptosomes		↑	No release from synaptomes. Lopez-Colome et al (1978).
Taurine	Endog.	Rabbit eye-cup in vivo	↑		Neal et al (1979).
Taurine	35S	Rat & cat retina in vitro	↑		No release in retinal degeneration. Schmidt (1978).
T.R.H. Somato-statin Substance P	Endog.	Bullfrog retina in vitro		↑	Ca-dependent. Eskay et al (1980).

Transmitter	Label	Preparation		Notes / References
Dopamine	^3H	Cat eye-cup in vivo	↑	Max. release 3Hz. Continuous light ineffective. Kramer (1971)
Dopamine	^3H	Rabbit retina in vitro	↑	Release not affected by kainate, GABA, carbachol, glycine, muscimol, α-M.S.H. caused release. Bauer & Ehinger (1980). Bauer, Ehinger & Aberg (1980).
5-HT	^3H	Bovine retinal synaptosomes	↑	Thomas & Redburn (1980).
5-HT	^{14}C	Bovine retina in vitro	↑	Osborne (1980).
ACh	^3H	Rabbit retina in vitro	↑	Ca-dependent. Masland & Livingstone (1976).
ACh	^3H	Rabbit eye-cup in vivo	↑	Max. release 3Hz, Ca-dependent. Massey & Neal (1978; 1979). Inhibited by GABA, increased by bicuculline, Neal & Massey (1980).

(continued)

Table 1. (Continued).

"Trans-mitter	Endogenous/Labelled	Preparation	Photic Stimulation	K$^+$ Stimulation	Notes and references
ACh	^{3}H	Rabbit eye-cup in vivo	↑		Inhibited by GABA agonists, glycine and taurine. Not by peptides, 5-HT dopamine or morphine. Neal & Cunningham (1981).
					Abolished (90%) by 2-amino-4-phosphonobuty-rate (APB) and APV (+) LAPB more potent than (-) DAPB, Collins et al (1981).

isolated rabbit retina has been described by Ehinger &
Lindberg (1974), and in a proportion of their experiments, a light evoked release of ^{3}H glycine from cat
retina in vivo was demonstrated. In addition, Coull &
Cutler, found a light evoked release of endogenous
glycine using the rat retina in vivo. Thus, glycine
release has been demonstrated, although with some
difficulty, in three species.

The present situation for GABA is less satisfactory,
with only one demonstration of a light evoked release of
^{3}H GABA from the isolated rabbit retina (Bauer &
Ehinger, 1977). The use of labelled GABA is complicated
in these experiments by the fact that much of the amino
acid is accumulated by glial cells. Fortunately, 4 hr
following intravitreal injection, the ^{3}H GABA has been
largely metabolised in the glial cells, and the radioactivity after this time is found largely in a sub-
population of (GABAergic) amacrine cells. This explains
why the presence of AOAA, which blocks GABA metabolism,
abolishes the light evoked release of ^{3}H GABA (Bauer &
Ehinger, 1977). As far as I am aware, there has been no
report of a light evoked release (or decrease) of
endogenous GABA from the retina of any species.

Glutamate and aspartate may be photoreceptor
transmitters, (see Neal, 1976a for review) but
endogenous glutamate release from the rabbit (Neal et
al, 1979a) and chicken retina (Pasantes-Morales et al,
1974) were unaffected by light. However, in one study,
the release of endogenous aspartate was significantly
decreased by light flashes, a result consistent with
this amino acid being a photoreceptor transmitter, or
possibly a hyperpolarising bipolar cell transmitter
(Neal et al, 1979a).

Cholinergic Neurones in the Retina

There is strong evidence that ACh is a synaptic
transmitter substance in the vertebrate retina, but the
function of the cholinergic neurones is unknown (for
reviews, see Graham, 1974; Neal, 1976b; Masland, 1980).
In the rabbit retina, autoradiographical studies
revealed that ^{3}H choline was selectively accumulated
by a sub-population of amacrine cells and by photoreceptors. However, only the uptake into amacrine cells
was associated with ACh synthesis, indicating that these
amacrine cells are the only cholinergic neurones present
in the rabbit retina (Masland & Mills, 1979; Masland &

Mills, 1980). The cholinergic amacrine cells are
divided into two layers. One group of cell bodies
occurs in the inner part of the inner nuclear layer but
the other group are displaced amacrine cells and are
located in the ganglion cell layer (Haydon et al, 1980).
The cholinergic amacrine cells in the rabbit retina have
been tentatively identified on circumstantial evidence
as "star-burst" amacrines (Famiglietti, 1981).

     Little is known of the characteristics or the
detailed synaptic connections of the cholinergic
amacrine cells. Therefore, in the present study, we
have taken the release of ACh to be a measure of
cholinergic amacrine cell activity, and have attempted
to examine possible synaptic inputs to these cells by
measuring the effect on ACh release, of other transmitters (and their analogues) present in the retina.
The results of some of these experiments have been
published previously (Neal & Cunningham, 1981;
Cunningham & Neal, 1981a; 1981b; Dawson & Neal, 1981;
Neal et al, 1981).

METHODS

     The methods have been described in detail
previously (Massey & Neal, 1979; Neal & Massey, 1980;
Neal & Cunningham, 1981). Briefly, adult albino
rabbits were anaesthetized with urethane (1.5 g/kg I.P.)
and a stainless steel ring was sutured to the episclera
to prevent collapse of the eye-cup. The cornea and iris
were removed and this was followed by an intracapsular
lens extraction and vitrectomy. The resulting eye-cup
was filled for 30 min with Krebs Ringer bicarbonate
containing ^{3}H Ch and then the retina was continuously
irrigated for 60 min with medium containing eserine
sulphate (30 uM). A syringe mounted on a micromani-
pulator was used to place 0.5 ml of eserinized medium
in the eye-cup and this was replaced at 5 min intervals.
The total radioactivity in the resulting samples was
measured by liquid scintillation counting   In some
experiments, ^{3}H ACh and ^{3}H Ch were separated by high
voltage electrophoresis before counting. However,
previous experiments indicated that ^{3}H ACh represented
95 - 100% of the increase in total radioactivity evoked
by light flashes (Neal & Massey, 1980).

     The light source was a quartz halide bulb (100 watt)
and the initially dark-adapted retina was stimulated for
5 min periods by flashes of light at 3 Hz (25% duty

cycle, retinal illuminance = 1650 photopic lux).

The viability of the preparation was assessed by electroretinography (Neal & Cunningham, 1981).

RESULTS AND DISCUSSION

Effect of GABA Agonists

The effect of exposing the retina to medium containing muscimol (1 uM) is illustrated in Fig. 1. Muscimol was strikingly potent in the retina, and the light evoked release of ACh was almost abolished by this concentration of drug.

The results with GABA, muscimol and also 3-amino-propane sulphonic acid (3-APS) are summarized in Fig. 2, where the inhibitory effects of these compounds on the light evoked release of ACh are plotted against the log of the concentration. From these results, the concentrations of GABA, 3-APS and muscimol which reduced the

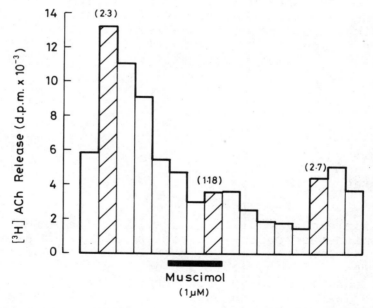

Fig. 1. Effect of muscimol on the release of ^{3}H ACh from the retina. In this and in all similar Figs., the number in parentheses indicate the ratio of light evoked release (hatched columns) to the spontaneous resting release.

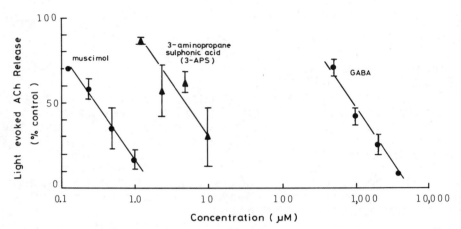

Fig. 2.   Effect of different concentrations of GABA, 3-aminopropanesulphonic acid and muscimol on the light-evoked release of ^{3}H ACh.   The light evoked release of ^{3}H ACh in the presence of the drug is expressed as a percentage of the evoked release in the absence of drug (controls).   Each point is the mean of 3 to 6 separate rabbit experiments.   The vertical bars indicate the S.E.M. and the lines were fitted by the least squares method.

light evoked release of GABA by 50% (EC_{50}) were found to be 900, 5 and 0.3 uM respectively.

GABA Antagonists

We have previously shown (Massey & Neal, 1979) that picrotoxin and bicuculline cause large increases in both the spontaneous resting release and the light evoked release of ACh from the retina.   Because of the effects on the resting release, it was difficult to demonstrate convincingly that these drugs antagonized the inhibitory effect of GABA agonists on the light evoked release of ACh from the retina.

For this reason, the effect of bicuculline on the resting release of ACh was examined in the presence of muscimol, which completely blocked the effect of bicuculline on the resting release of ACh (Fig. 3).

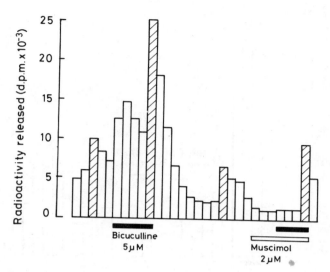

Fig. 3. Antagonism by muscimol of the effects of bicuc--
ulline on the spontaneous and light-evoked release of
^{3}H ACh. This experiment was repeated 3 times with
identical results.

        Bicuculline does not increase ACh release merely by
a non-specific effect on the neuronal membrane because
exposure of the retina to Ca-free, high-Mg medium, which
inhibits synaptic activity in the retina, reversibly
abolished the effect of bicuculline on the resting
release of ACh (Fig. 4).

Glycine, Taurine and Strychnine

        Glycine (Fig. 5) and taurine (Fig. 6) both reduced
the light-evoked release of ACh from the retina, without
affecting the spontaneous release. The EC_{50} values for
the inhibitory effect of glycine and taurine were
approximately 1.5 mM and 0.3 mM respectively. Strychnine
(20 uM), unlike the GABA antagonists, had no obvious
effect on either the spontaneous resting release or the
light-evoked release of ACh. However, strychnine at
this concentration completely blocked the inhibitory
effects of glycine and taurine on the light-evoked
release of ACh (Figs. 5 and 6). This action of
strychnine was specific and the drug did not
significantly antagonise the effect of muscimol on ACh
release (Fig. 5).

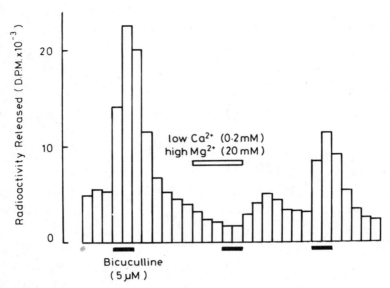

Fig. 4.   Exposure of the retina to low–Ca, high–Mg
medium reduced the spontaneous resting release of ^{3}H –
ACh and completely abolished the effects of bicuculline
on the resting release of ^{3}H ACh. This experiment was
repeated twice with the same result.

Peptides, Dopamine and 5HT

        Compounds which had no significant effect on the
spontaneous resting release or light evoked release of
ACh are shown in Table 2. Somatostatin (10^{-7}M) reduced
the amplitude of the b-wave of the ERG by approximately
60%, but no other electroretinographic changes were
observed.

        These results show unequivocally that the release
of ACh from the retina is unaffected by dopamine, 5HT,
morphine and all the peptides studied, indicating that
the activity of the cholinergic amacrine cells is
unlikely to be modulated by other retinal neurones
using these substances as transmitters.

        In contrast, the cholinergic amacrines were strongly
affected by GABAergic and glycinergic compounds,
suggesting that amacrine cells using these amino acids as

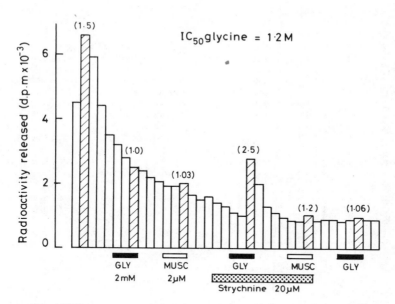

Fig. 5. Effects of glycine and muscimol on ^{3}H ACh
release from the retina. The light-evoked release of
^{3}H ACh was completely abolished by these drugs.
Strychnine blocked the action of glycine but not that
of muscimol. This experiment was repeated 3 times with
the same result.

transmitters may have an important influence on the
cholinergic amacrines. It is not clear whether the
GABA and glycine receptors involved are on the cholinergic amacrine cells themselves, or whether the effects
of the amino acids are indirect. In the case of GABA,
the ERG b-wave amplitude was not decreased, suggesting
that the amino acid had no significant effect on the
bipolar cells. In the mudpuppy retina, the amacrine
cells are amongst the most sensitive to GABA even in
the presence of Co^{++} to prevent synaptic transmission
(Miller et al, 1981). Thus, it is likely that in the
present experiments, GABA is acting directly on the
cholinergic amacrine cells. The possibility that GABA
might be inhibitory on an excitatory amacrine cell with
an input to the cholinergic amacrine neurones cannot be
excluded, but as far as I am aware, no such excitatory
amacrine cells have been reported in the rabbit retina.

Glycine and taurine clearly act at different
receptors to GABA as their effects were blocked by

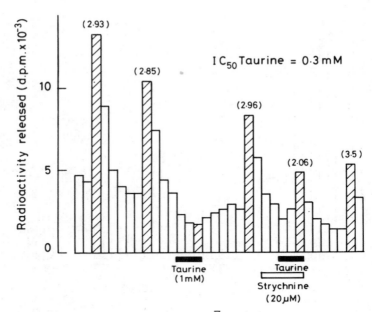

Fig. 6. Effect of taurine on ^{3}H ACh release from the
retina. Taurine (1 mM) abolished the light-evoked release
of ^{3}H ACh, an effect which was antagonised by strychnine
(20 uM). This experiment was repeated 3 times with the
same result.

Table 2.   Compounds Not Affecting the Release of ACh
           From the Rabbit Retina

Compound	Concentration (mM)
Substance P	10^{-6}
Somatostatin	10^{-7}
Cholecystokinin sulphate	10^{-6}
Thyroid Releasing Hormone (TRH)	10^{-6}
Leutinising Hormone Releasing Hormone (LHRH)	$10^{-8} - 10^{-6}$
Angiotensin	$10^{-8} - 10^{-6}$
Morphine	10^{-5}
Dopamine	$10^{-5} - 10^{-3}$
5HT	10^{-3}

Retinae were exposed for 15 min to medium containing the
above compounds at the concentrations indicated.   Each
compound was tested on at least two preparations.   No
attempt was made to prevent the inactivation of the peptides but ascorbic acid was present in the dopamine
solutions.

strychnine but not by bicuculline. However, as they
also reduced the amplitude of the ERG b-wave at
concentrations necessary to reduce the light-evoked
release of ACh, it is not clear whether the effects of
glycine and taurine on ACh release result from a direct
action on the cholinergic amacrine cells or by effects
on more distal neurones such as the bipolar cells. (For
a more extensive discussion, see Cunningham & Neal,
1981b).

Cholinergic Autoreceptors

      In other cholinergic systems, there is evidence
that the nerve terminals possess so called autoreceptors
(Szerb & Somogyi, 1973; Fosbraey & Johnson, 1980). The
presence of cholinergic autoreceptors in the retina was
studied by examining the effects of cholinergic agonists
and antagonists on ^{3}H ACh release in the presence and
absence of eserine.

Table 3.   Effect of Cholinergic Drugs on the Light-
           Evoked Release of ^{3}H ACh From the Rabbit
           Retina.   Each Result is the Mean $\pm$ S.E.
           Mean of 4 Experiments.

Drug	Light-evoked release / Resting release	P
Control Muscarine (10 uM)	1.56 ± 0.1 1.28 ± 0.1	< 0.02
Control Atropine (10 uM) + eserine (30 uM)	2.8 ± 0.5 4.4 ± 0.7	< 0.01
Control Atropine (10 uM)	2.1 ± 0.2 2.2 ± 0.3	N.S.

Muscarine (10 uM), in the absence of eserine reduced
the light-evoked release of ACh by 50%. In contrast,
atropine (10 uM), in the presence of eserine almost
doubled the light-evoked release of ACh (Table 3). In
the absence of eserine, atropine had no effect on ACh
release. The nicotinic antagonists hexamethonium and
pempidine had no effect on ACh release in the presence
or absence of eserine. These results suggest that as in

other areas of the CNS, and in the peripheral nervous
system, the cholinergic amacrine cells possess
inhibitory muscarinic autoreceptors.

Effect of 2,Amino-4-Phosphonobutyric Acid (APB). Evidence for On-Channel Input to Cholinergic Amacrine Cells

Recently, Slaughter & Miller (1981) reported that
in the mudpuppy retina, (±)-2-amino-4-phosphonobutyric
acid (APB) selectively blocked all responses in the ON-
channels but left intact the OFF-responses, probably by
mimicking the photoreceptor transmitter. In the present
study, we have used APB to investigate the relative
importance of ON-channels and OFF-channels as inputs to
the cholinergic amacrine cells.

It was necessary to demonstrate that APB also
selectively blocked ON-channels in the rabbit and the
effect of (±) APB (200 uM) on the ON and OFF responses
of a ganglion cell is shown in Fig. 7. The post-
stimulus histograms show clearly that APB reversibly
blocked the ON-response of the ganglion cells, whilst
the OFF-response was, if anything, increased in size.
At this concentration, the b-wave of the ERG was also
abolished. A lower concentration of (±) APB (100 uM)
reduced the ERG by 80% and the ON-response by 75% (data
not shown). Further ganglion cell recordings revealed
that (+)-L-APB was far more potent than (-)-D-APB in
blocking ON-responses (Fig. 8).

The effects of both (+) and (-) APB on the release
of ACh from the retina is illustrated in Fig. 9, where
it can be seen that both stereoisomers reduced the light-
evoked release of ACh but had no effect on the
spontaneous resting release. Consistent with the
ganglion cell recordings, the (+)-isomer was much more
potent, the concentrations of (+) and (-)-APB which
reduced the light-evoked release of ACh by 50% (EC_{50})
being 7.5 uM and 115 uM respectively (Table 4),with
an EC_{50} of 16 uM for the racemate.

2-Amino-5-phosphonovalerate (APV) also reduced
both the light-evoked release of ACh and the b-wave of
the ERG but was much less potent than APB. Again the
(+) isomer was the most effective stereoisomer; the
EC_{50} for the (+) and (-) compounds being 230 uM and
660 uM respectively. The efficacy of APB and APV in
reducing the amplitude of the b-wave closely paralleled

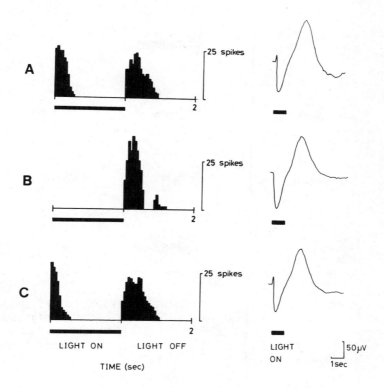

Fig. 7.   Post-stimulus histograms (LEFT) from a single
ON-OFF ganglion cell and E.R.G.s (RIGHT).   The horizontal bar indicates the duration of the light flash.
A control: B 3 min after exposure to DL-(±)-APB: C
5 min after removal of drug.   Note complete abolition
of the ON response and the ERG b-wave by APB.   This
experiment was repeated 4 times with the same result.

their effect on the light-evoked release of ACh
(Table 4).   In the case of both APB and APV, there
seemed to be a small proportion (about 10%) of the
light-evoked ACh release, which was not blocked at
concentrations up to 15 times the EC_{50}.   It is not
clear whether this residual release is due to a small
number of depolarising bipolars which are resistant to
the drugs or to a cholinergic amacrine cell input from
hyperpolarising bipolar cells.

The ω-phosphonic derivatives of 2-amino-proprionic,
-hexanoic and -heptanoic acid (APPr, APHex and APHep)
at concentrations up to 1 mM, had no obvious effect on

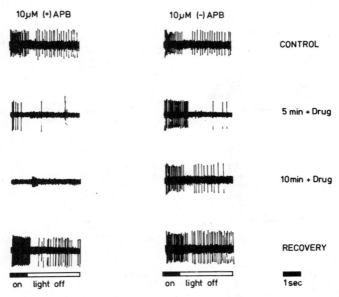

Fig. 8. Extracellular recording from an on-ganglion
cell. Note that (+) APB (10 uM) completely abolishes
the on-response but (-) APB (10 uM) has little effect.
When the concentration of (-) APB was increased to
100 uM the on-response was abolished (not illustrated).

either the light-evoked release of ACh or the ERG.

Collectively, these data indicate that the release
of ACh from amacrine cells is mediated mainly via the
ON-channels.

Previously, it has been shown that exposure of the
retina to chloride-free medium also selectively
abolished responses mediated via the ON-channels
(Miller & Dacheux, 1976). Thus, it is interesting to
note that chloride-free medium also abolished the light-
evoked release of ACh (Fig. 10) and produced changes in
the ERG similar to those produced by high concentrations
of APB. However, unlike APB, chloride-free medium
increased the spontaneous resting release of ACh approximately two-fold.

These experiments confirm that APB selectively
abolishes ON-channels in the rabbit retina (Massey et
al, 1981) and strongly suggests that the activity of
the cholinergic amacrine cells is determined mainly by

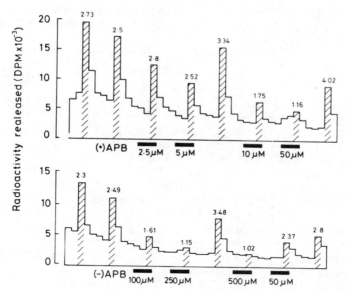

Fig. 9. Typical experiments showing the effects of L-(+)-APB (TOP) and D-(-)-APB (BOTTOM) ON ^{3}H -ACh release from the retina. Each column is a 5 min collection period and hatched columns indicate stimulation with light (3 Hz). Horizontal bars show exposure of the retina to APB and the numbers above the hatched columns give the peak release/resting release.

the depolarising bipolar cells. These ON-channels appear to require the presence of Cl⁻ ions (Miller & Dacheux, 1976).

     The mechanism by which APB blocks transmission of ON-channels in the rabbit retina is unknown, but in the mudpuppy it appears to mimic the endogenous photo-receptor transmitter (Slaughter & Miller, 1981), which is believed to be aspartate and/or glutamate (Neal, 1976a). Our experiments with APB and other ω-phosphono-2-aminocarboxylic acids are consistent with this suggestion. An alternative possibility, that APB and APV are acting as antagonists of aspartate or glutamate is very unlikely, because antagonistic activity is greater in the (-) isomers (Davies et al, 1981), rather than in the (+) forms which were most potent in our experiments. Furthermore, the order of potency in blocking N-methyl-D-aspartate receptors in the brain is APHep APV APB, (Perkins et al, 1981) again the reverse of the present results.

Table 4.   The Effect of ω-Phosphono-2-Aminocarboxylic
           Acids on the Light-Evoked Release of ACh and
           on the ERG b-Wave

| | EC$_{50}$ (uM) | |
Compound	ACh release	ERG b-wave
(±)2-Amino-3-phosphonoproprionic acid	N.E.	N.E.
L-(+)-2-Amino-4-phosphonobutyric acid	7.5	5.8
D-(-)-2-Amino-4-phosphonobutyric acid	115	140
DL-(±)-2-Amino-4-phosphonobutyric acid	16	11
L-(+)-2-Amino-5-phosphonovaleric acid	230	155
D-(-)-2-Amino-5-phosphonovaleric acid	660	680
(±)2-Amino-6-phosphonohexanoic acid	N.E.	N.E.
(±)2-Amino-7-phosphonoheptanoic acid	N.E.	N.E.

The results are expressed as the EC$_{50}$ (the concentration
which reduced the light-evoked release of ACh or the
amplitude of the b-wave by 50%). Each result was
obtained from graphs of log concentration against effect
using at least three drug concentrations. Each drug
concentration was the mean of at least 4 separate
experiments and S.E.M. of any point was not more than
10%. N.E.: no effect up to 1mM.

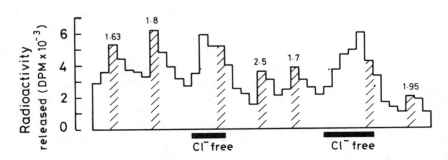

Fig. 10. Effect of Cl-free medium on ^{3}H ACh from the
rabbit retina. This experiment was repeated three
times with the same result.

CONCLUSIONS

In general, release studies of transmitters in the retina are lagging considerably behind anatomical and electrophysiological studies. Although the retina possesses certain advantages over other areas of the CNS in the study of transmitter release, it has proved unexpectedly difficult to measure, or even detect, light induced changes in the release of some important transmitters such as GABA. The reasons for the difficulties are not entirely clear. They may reflect the tonic nature of the retina, the use of inappropriate stimuli or other deficiences in experimental design. However, release studies are important, not only because they provide very strong evidence for the role of a substance as a transmitter, but also because they can provide information on specific types of retinal neurone which cannot easily be obtained by anatomical or electrophysiological methods. For example, the present studies on ^{3}H ACh release have shown that the cholinergic amacrine cells are transiently responding neurones whose activity is mainly stimulated by the depolarising bipolar cells. They also possess muscarinic autoreceptors and probably GABA and glycine receptors. On the other hand, the cholinergic amacrines apparently do not possess receptors for peptides, dopamine or 5HT.

ACKNOWLEDGEMENT

I am grateful to Mrs J. Cunningham, Miss C. Dawson, Mr T. James and Dr J. Collins for their collaboration in the present studies, to the S.R.C. and S.K.F. Foundation for grants, and to Mrs B.A. Klymkiw for typing the manuscript.

REFERENCES

Bauer, B., 1978, Photic release of radioactivity from rabbit retina preloaded with ^{3}H GABA, *Acta Ophthalmologica*, 56:270-283.
Bauer, B., and Ehinger, B., 1977, Light evoked release of radioactivity from rabbit retinas preloaded with ^{3}H GABA, *Experientia*, 33:470-471.
Bauer, B., and Ehinger, B., 1980, Action of α-MSH on the release of neurotransmitters from the retina, *Acta Physiol. Scand.*, 108:105-107.

Bauer, B., Ehinger, B., and Aberg, L., 1980, ^{3}H Dopamine release from the rabbit retina, Albrecht von Graefes Arch. Klin. Ophthalmol., 215:71-78.

Collins, J.F., Cunningham, J.R., James, T.A., and Neal, M.J., 1981, The effect of 2-amino-4-phosphonobutyrate (2-APB) on the release of ACh from the retina of the anaesthetised rabbit, J. Physiol., (in press).

Coull, B.M., and Cutler, R.W.P., 1978, Light-evoked release of endogenous glycine into the perfused vitreous of the intact rat eye, Invest. Ophthalmol, 17:682-684.

Cunningham, J.R., and Neal, M.J., 1981a, Effect of GABA agonists, glycine and neuropeptides on the release of acetylcholine (ACh) from the rabbit retina in vivo, Brit. J. Pharmac., (in press).

Cunningham, J.R., and Neal, M.J., 1981b, Effect of GABA agonists, glycine, taurine and neuropeptides on the release of ACh from the retina, J. Physiol., (in press).

Davies, J., Francis, A.A., Jones, A.W., and Watkins, J.C. 1981, 2-Amino-5-phosphonovalerate: a potent and selective antagonist of amino acid induced and synaptic excitation, Neurosci. Lett., 21:77-82.

Dawson, C., and Neal, M.J., 1981, Evidence for muscarinic autoreceptors on cholinergic neurones in the rabbit retina, Brit. J. Pharmac., (in press).

Djamgoz, M.B.A., Stell, W.K., Chin, C.A., and Lam, D.M.K., 1981, An opiate system in the goldfish retina, Nature, 292:620-623.

Ehinger, B., and Lindberg, B., 1974, Light-evoked release of glycine from the retina, Nature, 251: 727-728.

Ehinger, B., and Lindberg-Bauer, B., 1976, Light-evoked release of glycine from cat and rabbit retina, Brain Res., 113: 535-549.

Eskay, R.L., Long, R.T., and Iuvone, P.M., 1980, Evidence that TRH, somatostatin and substance P are present in neurosecretory elements of the vertebrate retina, Brain Res., 196:554-559.

Famiglietti, E.V., 1981, Starburst amacrines: 2 mirror-symmetric retinal networks, Invest. Ophthal. Suppl., 20:204.

Fosbraey, P., and Johnson, E.S., 1980, Modulation by acetylcholine of the electrically-evoked release of ^{3}H acetylcholine from the ileum of the guinea-pig, Brit. J. Pharmac., 69:145-150.

Graham, L.T., 1974, Comparative aspects of neurotrans-
        mitters in the retina, in: "The Eye", H. Davson
        and L.T. Graham, eds., 6: Comparative Physiology,
        pp. 283-342, Academic Press, New York.
Hayden, S.A., Mills, J.W., and Masland, R.M., 1980,
        Acetylcholine synthesis by displaced amacrine
        cells, Science, 210:435-437.
Lopez, B., Colomie, A.M., Salceda, R., and Pasantes-
        Morales, H., 1978, Potassium stimulated release
        of GABA, glycine and taurine from the chick
        retina, Neurochem. Res., 3:431-441.
Kennedy, A.J., and Neal, M.J., 1978, The effect of
        light and potassium depolarisation on the release
        of endogenous amino acids from isolated rat
        retina, Exp. Eye Res., 26:71-75.
Kramer, S.G., 1971, Dopamine: a retinal neurotransmitter,
        Invest. Ophthalmol., 100:438-452.
Marc, R.E., Stell, W.R., Bok, D., and Lam, D.M.K., 1978,
        GABAergic pathways in the goldfish retina,
        J. comp. Neurol., 182:221-246.
Masland, R.H., 1980, Acetylcholine in the retina,
        Neurochem. Int., 1:501-518.
Masland, R.H., and Livingstone, C.J., 1976, Effect of
        stimulation with light on synthesis and release
        of acetylcholine by an isolated mammalian
        retina, J. Neurophysiol., 39:1210-1219.
Masland, R.H., and Mills, J.W., 1979, Autoradiographic
        identification of acetylcholine in the rabbit
        retina, J. cell. Biol., 83:159-178.
Masland, R.H., and Mills, J.W., 1980, Choline
        accumulation by photoreceptor cells of the
        rabbit retina, Proc. Natl. Acad. Sci. U.S.A.,
        77:1671-1675.
Massey, S.C., Crawford, M.L.J., and Redburn, D.A., 1981,
        Many cholinergic amacrine cells in rabbit retina
        receive ON input, Invest. Ophthalmol. Suppl.,
        20:44.
Massey, S.C., and Neal, M.J., 1978, Light-evoked
        release of acetylcholine (ACh) from the rabbit
        retina in vivo, J. Physiol. (Lond.), 280:51-52P.
Massey, S.C., and Neal, M.J., 1979, The light-evoked
        release of acetylcholine from the rabbit retina
        in vivo and its inhibition by α-aminobutyric
        acid, J. Neurochem., 32:1327-1329.
Miller, R.F., and Dacheux, R.F., 1976, Synaptic organi-
        sation and ionic basis of ON and OFF channels in
        mudpuppy retina, J. gen. Physiol., 67:661-678.

Miller, R.F., Frumkes, T.E., Slaughter, M., and Dacheux,
      R.F., 1981, Physiological and pharmacological
      basis of GABA and glycine action on neurones of
      mudpuppy retina. II Amacrine and ganglion cells,
      J. Neurophys., 45:764-782.

Neal, M.J., 1976a, Mini review: Amino acid transmitter
      substances in the vertebrate retina, Gen.
      Pharmacol., 7:321-332.

Neal, M.J., 1976b, Acetylcholine as a retina transmitter
      substance, in: "Transmitters in the Visual
      Process", S.C. Bonting, ed., pp. 127-143,
      Pergamon, Oxford.

Neal, M.J., Collins, G.G., and Massey, S.C. 1979a,
      Inhibition of aspartate release from the retina
      of the anaesthetised rabbit by stimulation with
      light flashes, Neurosci. Lettr., 14:241-245.

Neal, M.J., and Cunningham, J.R., 1981, The vertebrate
      retina in vivo: A preparation for studying
      acetylcholine release from central cholinergic
      neurones, in: "Progress in Cholinergic Biology:
      Model Cholinergic Synapses", A.M. Goldberg and
      I. Hanin, eds., Raven Press, New York, (in press).

Neal, M.J., Cunningham, J.R., James, T.A., Joseph, M.,
      and Collins, J.F., 1981, The effect of 2-amino-
      4-phosphonobutyrate (APB) on acetylcholine
      release from the rabbit retina: evidence for
      on-channel input to cholinergic amacrine cells.
      Neurosci. Lettr., (in press).

Neal, M.J., Cunningham, J.R., and Marshall, J., 1979b,
      The uptake and radioautographical localisation
      in the frog retina of $^3H \pm$ 3-amino-cyclohexane
      carboxylic acid: A selective inhibitor of
      neuronal GABA transport, Brain Res., 176:285-296.

Neal, M.J., and Iversen, L., 1972, Autoradiographic
      localisation of ^3H GABA in rat retinae, Nature,
      New Biology, 235:217-218.

Neal, M.J., and Massey, S.C., 1980, The release of
      acetylcholine and amino acids from the rabbit
      retina in vivo, Neurochem. Int., 1:191-208.

Osborne, N.N., 1980, In vitro experiments on the
      metabolism, uptake and release of 5-hydroxy-
      tryptamine in bovine retina, Brain Res., 184:
      283-297.

Pasantes-Morales, H., Klethi, J., Urban, P.F., and
      Mandel, P., 1974, The effect of electrical stimu-
      lation, light and amino acids on the efflux of
      ^{35}S-taurine from the retina of the domestic fowl,
      Exp. Brain Res., 19:131-141.

Pasantes-Morales, H., Urban, P.F., Klethi, J., and
        Mandel, P., 1973, Light stimulated release of
        ^{35}S taurine from chicken retina, Brain Res.,
        51:375-378.
Perkins, M.N., Stones, T.W., Collins, J.F., and Curry, K.,
        1981, Phosphonate analogues of carboxylic acids
        as amino acid antagonists on rat cortical
        neurones, Neurosci. Lettr., (in press).
Salceda, R., and Pasantes-Morales, H., 1975, Calcium
        coupled release of ^{35}S taurine from retina,
        Brain Res., 96:206-211.
Schmidt, S.Y., 1978, Taurine fluxes in isolated cat and
        rat retinas. Effect of illumination, Exp. Eye
        Res., 26:529-535.
Slaughter, M.M., and Miller, R.F., 1981, 2-Amino-4-
        phosphonobutyric acid: A new pharmacological
        tool for retina research, Science, 211:182-184.
Szerb, J.C., and Somogyi, G.T., 1973, Depression of
        acetylcholine release from cerebral cortex by
        cholinesterase inhibition and by oxotremorine,
        Nature, New Biol., 241:121-122.
Thomas, T.N., and Redburn, D.A., 1979, 5-Hydroxytryp-
        tamine - A neurotransmitter of bovine retina,
        Exp. Eye Res., 28:55-61.

POSTNATAL DEVELOPMENT OF A MAMMALIAN RETINA:

NEUROTRANSMITTERS AS PHYSIOLOGICAL AND ANATOMICAL PROBES

Dominic Man-Kit Lam[*], Sek-Chung Fung and Yun-Cheung Kong

Kevin Hsu Research Foundation, Hong Kong
Department of Biochemistry
Chinese University of Hong Kong and
Cullen Eye Institute, Baylor College
of Medicine, Houston, Texas, U.S.A.

The emergence and maturation of specific neurotransmitter systems in different neurons is a characteristic feature of neural differentiation. In adult nervous systems, neurons which use γ-aminobutyric acid (GABA) and dopamine as neurotransmitters have been shown to contain high concentrations of these substances and their synthetic enzymes, to possess high-affinity transport mechanisms for the accumulation of these substances and to release them upon appropriate stimulations. In addition, putative glycinergic neurons also possess a specific high-affinity uptake mechanism for glycine and release it in response to depolarizing stimuli. We have recently used some of these transmitter-specific properties as physiological and anatomical probes to follow the emergence and maturation of identified neurons in *Xenopus* and rabbit retinas. (Hollyfield et al., 1979; Rayborn et al., 1981; Sarthy et al., 1981; Lam et al., 1980, 1981; Kong et al., 1980). This article summarises our studies to-date on the postnatal development of putative GABA-ergic, glycinergic and dopaminergic neurons in the rabbit retina.

*Please address all correspondence to Dominic Man-Kit Lam, Cullen Eye Institute, Baylor College of Medicine, Houston, Texas 77030.

GABA-ERGIC, GLYCINERGIC AND DOPAMINERGIC RETINAL NEURONS

There is considerable morphological and physiological evidence that GABA, glycine and dopamine may serve as transmitters for certain neurons in the adult rabbit retina. Autoradiographic, histofluorescence and immunocytochemical studies have localized putative GABA-ergic, glycinergic and dopaminergic neurons to a class of retinal interneurons with processes ramifying in the inner plexiform layer: the amacrine cells, which play an important role in information processing from bipolar to ganglion cells. Although direct evidence is still lacking, both morphological and physiological studies indicate that the putative GABA-ergic, glycinergic and dopaminergic amacrine cells probably belong to different distinct subpopulations of amacrine cells. (Figure 1b, d, f). Additionally, we have shown that the ^{3}H-labeled GABA, glycine and dopamine taken up by rabbit retinal neurons can be released in response to high K$^+$ concentrations in the medium, and that these releases are inhibited by 10mM Co^{++} in the medium (Lam et al., 1980, 1981; Kong et al., 1980).

GABA, GLYCINE AND DOPAMINE UPTAKE IN NEWBORN RETINAS

Since putative GABA-ergic, glycinergic and dopaminergic neurons in the adult rabbit retina possess high-affinity mechanisms for GABA, glycine and dopamine uptake respectively, we began our developmental studies by examining autoradiographically the time of appearance for this transmitter-specific neuronal uptake properties during postnatal retinal differentiation and maturation. As shown in Figure 1, we found that certain neurons in the newborn rabbit retina already selectively accumulate exogenous GABA, glycine and dopamine respectively (Figure 1a, c, e). The number, position and morphology of the GABA-, glycine- and dopamine-accumulating cells in the newborn retina are similar to those found in the adult retina (Lam et al., 1980, 1981, Kong et al., 1980). These results suggest that (1) the neuronal uptake mechanisms for GABA, glycine and dopamine are functional at, or prior to, birth, and (2) the commitments for certain neurons in the rabbit retina to be GABA-ergic, glycinergic or dopaminergic are all made prenatally. Indeed, preliminary studies of prenatal development indicate that these uptake systems are present in the rabbit retina 3 to 4 days prior to birth, although it is not yet certain whether mechanisms for GABA, glycine and dopamine emerge at different times during retinal differentiation (Fung, Kong and Lam, in preparation).

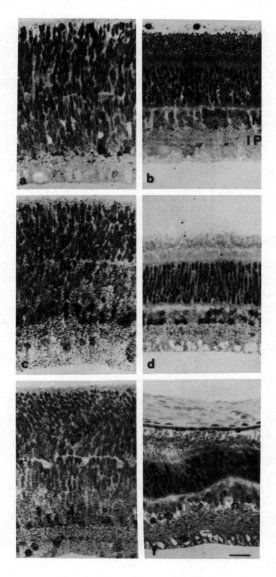

Fig. 1. Autoradiographs of adult (b,d,f) and newborn (a,c,e)
retinas following injections of ^{3}H-dopamine (a,b), ^{3}H-glycine
(c,d) and ^{3}H-GABA (e,f) respectively into rabbit eyes *in vivo*.
IN: inner nuclear layer; IP: inner plexiform layer. Scale 20μm.

TRANSMITTER RELEASE DURING RETINAL DEVELOPMENT

Unlike the uptake mechanisms for GABA, glycine and dopamine which are already functional in the newborn rabbit retina, the abilities for the neurons to release the accumulated GABA, glycine and dopamine by K^+ depolarization vary significantly among the different transmitter candidates. As shown in Figure 2, there is very little K^+-induced ^3H-glycine release at birth and only a small amount of ^3H-GABA release. On the contrary, the dopamine-accumulating neurons in the newborn retina are capable of releasing the accumulated dopamine at about half the rate of the adult retina. The rates of release reach 80% of the adult level at day 8 after birth for ^3H-GABA and ^3H-dopamine, and at day 12 for ^3H-glycine. These results indicate that the emergence and maturation of ^3H-GABA, ^3H-glycine and ^3H-dopamine follow different temporal patterns during development of the rabbit retina.

CONTENTS AND BIOSYNTHESES OF TRANSMITTERS DURING DEVELOPMENT

The endogenous levels of retinal GABA and dopamine as well as the specific activities of the GABA- and dopamine-synthesizing enzymes, L-glutamic acid decarboxylase (GAD) and tyrosine hydroxylase (TH) in the retina were measured throughout postnatal development. GABA contents in the retina generally follow closely the specific activity of GAD. Likewise, the increase in retinal dopamine levels follow the increase in the TH activities. The results suggest that during retinal differentiation and maturation, the endogenous contents of GABA and dopamine are regulated largely by their respective synthesizing enzymes.

GABA contents in the newborn retina are low at birth but increase steadily during the first 10 days of postnatal life, reaching 80% of the adult level at day 8 or 9. On the contrary, the increase in dopamine contents follow a biphasic pattern. Dopamine levels remain low for the first 6 days after birth, increasing 35% of the adult level by about day 13, at day 18, there is another abrupt increase in dopamine contents, reaching 50% of the adult level on day 21, 80% at day 23 and 100% by day 25 (Figure 2). Thus, similar to the patterns of GABA and dopamine release, the temporal pattern for the increase in retinal GABA contents during development is also vastly different from that for the increase in retinal dopamine contents.

LOGISTICS OF RETINAL DEVELOPMENT

Assuming that the GABA-accumulating neurons in developing rabbit retinas are also those that synthesize and release GABA, results presented in this study indicate that from about 9 days after birth, putative GABA-ergic neurons take up, synthesize, store, and release GABA at over 80% of the adult levels and may therefore be considered mature by these criteria. There is also

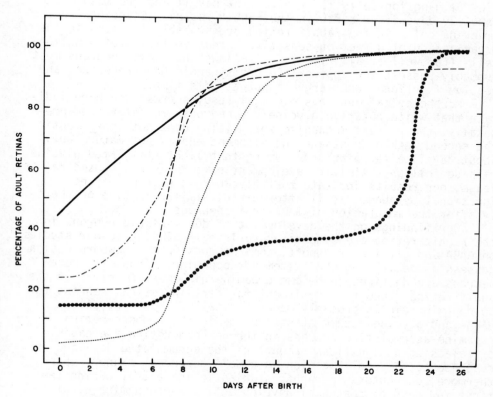

Fig. 2. A comparison of the development patterns of endogenous
dopamine concentrations (closed circles) and ^{3}H-dopamine release
(solid line) with those of endogenous GABA concentrations
(—.—.—.—), ^{3}H-GABA release (— — — —) and ^{3}H-glycine release
(-------) in the rabbit retina. The releases of ^{3}H-labeled
neurotransmitters candidates were measured by Ca^{++}-dependent
effluxes of preloaded ^{3}H-labeled transmitters into the medium in
response to 56 mM extracellular K$^+$.

electrophysiological evidence that GABA-ergic neurons may be
functional at this stage of development. For instance, Masland
(1977) has shown that during retinal development the number of
ganglion cells responsive to light increases from 0% on day 7
after birth to over 80% by day 10. Additionally, visual responsiveness, concentric field organizations and directional selectivi-
ties of ganglion cells first appear at day 11 and are mature by
about 20 days after birth in the rabbit retina. Since GABA-ergic
amacrine cells in the rabbit retina are probably involved in the
organization of direction-sensitive receptive fields of ganglion
cells (Caldwell et al., 1978), it follows that these neurons most
probably possess the appropriate postsynaptic GABA receptors and
receive functional GABA-ergic input at this time.

        Morphological and physiological results presented here indi-
cate that while putative glycinergic neurons are determined prenatally, the release mechanism for glycine does not appear until
the second week of postnatal development and is not mature until
about day 11 after birth. Assuming that light-stimulated glycine
release follows a similar development pattern as K^+-induced release, our results indicate that glycinergic neurons may be
functional by about day 11 after birth, similar in time or shortly after the maturation of GABA-ergic neurons.

        Our findings on the development of dopaminergic neurons in
the rabbit retina are somewhat surprising. Similar to our studies
on GABA and glycine transport, some neurons in the newborn retina
possess a specific uptake system for dopamine. Thus, if these
neurons are destined to become dopaminergic amacrine cells of the
adult retina, then the commitment for certain retinal neurons to
be dopaminergic is probably made prenatally. However, unlike
GABA- and glycine-accumulating neurons in the newborn retina,
dopamine-accumulating neurons in the newborn retina are capable
of releasing a significant amount of the accumulated dopamine in
response to K^+ depolarization in a Ca^{++}-dependent manner. Furthermore, our autoradiographic studies indicate that during the
first few days of postnatal development, these dopamine-accumulating cells already have long processes and extensive arborization in the inner plexiform layer (Lam et al., 1981). These
neurons are, however, functionally immature at this time because
they contain little endogenous dopamine and extremely low activities of tyrosine hydroxylase. The dopamine concentrations and
tyrosine hydroxylase activities increase in parallel and in a biphasic manner, reaching the adult level at about day 25. The
reason for this biphasic mode of maturation is unknown. By analogy to developmental studies in other nervous tissues, the
possibility that the second phase of dramatic increase in retinal
tyrosine hydroxylase activities which begins around day 18 may be
dependent on induction from other neurons deserves further studies.

        Our studies also raise a number of other questions regarding
the logistics in the development of retinal neurons and their
transmitter systems. For instance, it is puzzling why there is

a 2 to 3 week delay in the maturation of the dopamine-synthesizing mechanism and dopamine content compared to the dopamine uptake and release mechanisms. Additionally, our results that retinal GABA-ergic and glycinergic neurons are probably functionally mature shortly after the animals first open their eyes (about day 10) are consistent with the physiological maturation of ganglion cells (Masland, 1977) and morphological maturation synaptic connections (McArdle et al., 1977). It is therefore unclear why the dopaminergic neurons become mature many days after the functional maturation of GABA-ergic and glycinergic amacrine cells as well as most ganglion cells. In this regard, it would be of interest to compare the emergence and maturation of postsynaptic dopamine receptors with the differentiation of dopaminergic neurons. The rationale underlying the developmental pattern of dopaminergic neurons is, however, likely to remain unknown until the roles played by these neurons in the processing of visual information are elucidated.

Finally, in the *Xenopus* retina, our studies also indicate that the dopaminergic neurons become mature at a much later stage than putative GABA-ergic and glycinergic neurons (Hollyfield et al., 1979; Rayborn et al., 1981; Sarthy et al., 1981). In this retina, however, the last dopaminergic property to emerge is the dopamine release mechanism. Results presented in this paper therefore show that the emergence and maturation of dopamine uptake, synthesis and release mechanisms in different retinas may follow vastly different developmental patterns.

In summary, our studies have shown that certain neurotransmitter-specific properties in identified neurons of the rabbit retina emerge and mature in precise temporal patterns during retinal differentiation. Our results also indicate that the GABA-ergic, glycinergic and dopaminergic neurons, which constitute three separate subpopulations of amacrine cells in this retina, differentiate and mature not only in rather different manners but also at distinctly different times.

ACKNOWLEDGEMENTS

We thank Ms. Patricia Glazebrook, Dr. Jeanne Frederick and Ms. Patricia Cloud for valuable assistance. This work was supported by research grants from the National Institutes of Health (EY02608) and the Retina Research Foundation (Houston). D.M.K.L. was a visiting Research Professor of Biochemistry at the Chinese University of Hong Kong.

REFERENCES

Caldwell, J.H., Daw, N.W. and Wyatt, H.J., 1978. Effects of picrotoxin and strychnine on rabbit ganglion cells. Lateral reactions for cells with more complex receptive fields. J. Physiol. 276: 277-298.

Kong, Y.C., Fung, S.C. and Lam, D.M.K., 1980. Postnatal development of glycinergic neurons in the rabbit retina. J. Comp. Neurol. 193: 1127-2235.

Hollyfield, J.G., Sarthy, P.V., Rayborn, M.E. and Lam, D.M.K., 1979. The emergence, localization and maturation of neurotransmitter system during development of the retina in Xenopus laevis. I. γ-aminobutyric acid. J. Comp. Neurol. 188: 587-598.

Lam, D.M.K., Fung, S.C. and Kong, Y.C., 1980. Postnatal development of GABA-ergic neurons in the rabbit retina. J. Comp. Neurol. 193: 89-102.

Lam, D.M.K., Fung, S.C. and Kong, Y.C., 1981. Postnatal development of dopaminergic neurons in the rabbit retina. J. Neuroscience, in press.

Masland, R.H., 1977. Maturation of function in the developing rabbit retina. J. Comp. Neurol. 175: 275-286.

McArdle, C.B., Dowling, J.E. and Masland, R.H., 1977. Development of outer segments and synapses in the rabbit retina. J. Comp. Neurol. 175: 253-274.

Rayborn, M.E., Hollyfield, J.G., Sarthy, P.V. and Lam, D.M.K., 1981. The emergence, localization and maturation of neurotransmitter system during development of the retina in Xenopus laevis. II. Glycine. J. Comp. Neurol. 195: 585-594.

Sarthy, P.V., Rayborn, M.E., Hollyfield, J.G. and Lam, D.M.K., 1981. The emergence, localization and maturation of neurotransmitter system during development of the retina in Xenopus laevis. III. Dopamine. J. Comp. Neurol. 195: 595-603.

CYCLIC NUCLEOTIDES IN RETINA

James A. Ferrendelli

Division of Clinical Neuropharmacology and Departments
of Pharmacology, Neurology and Ophthalmology
Washington University School of Medicine, 660 South
Euclid Avenue, St. Louis, Missouri   USA   63110

Introduction

Although adenosine 3',5',-monophosphate (cyclic AMP) was
discovered only 25 years ago and the existence of other cyclic
nucleotides, particularly guanosine 3',5'-monophosphate (cyclic
GMP), has been known for a much shorter period of time, an immense
amount of information concerning these compounds has been
generated. It has been determined that both cyclic AMP and cyclic
GMP are present in almost all biologic systems examined, and it
appears that they are involved in several metabolic and functional
processes. The apparent multiple roles of cyclic AMP and cyclic
GMP have been suggested to reflect the presence of multiple
"cyclic nucleotide systems" within a single tissue or even in a
single cell type. Cyclic nucleotide system is an operational term
and consists of a synthesizing enzyme (cyclase); a catabolizing
enzyme (phosphodiesterase); and one or more cyclic nucleotide
dependent enzymes (kinases) that regulate phosphorylation of
proteins or lipids and their respective substrates and products.
Specificity and selectivity of a cyclic nucleotide system is
determined by the enzymatic properties of cyclases and
phosphodiesterases; by the individual substrates of cyclic
nucleotide dependent kinases; and by the cellular or sub-cellular
location of the various components.

The retina presents an especially intriguing problem with
regard to cyclic nucleotides. This structure has extraordinarily
high levels of cyclic GMP; its concentrations of both cyclic AMP
and cyclic GMP are regulated by light; and recent studies have
demonstrated that there are marked quantitative and qualitative
differences in cyclic nucleotide metabolism among different

795

regions of the retina. We carried out several studies of cyclic
nucleotides in mammalian retina in an effort to characterize and
localize individual cyclic nucleotide systems in this tissue.
Specifically, we measured guanylate and adenylate cyclase and
phosphodiesterase activities and the effects of various activators
and inhibitors on their activities in whole, biologically
fractionated and freeze-dried microdissected retinas. Tissues
from various animal species, including mouse, rabbit, and ground
squirrel, were examined and compared. In addition, the effects of
light and dark, cellular depolarization, and several
neurotransmitters on cyclic nucleotide levels in whole retina and
retinal layers were tested. The present report reviews and
discusses these studies with the purpose of demonstrating the
existence of multiple compartments of cyclic AMP and cyclic GMP in
retina.

Cyclic GMP

As in other tissues cyclic GMP in retina is formed by the
enzyme(s) guanylate cyclase which converts GTP to the cyclic
nucleotide and pyrophosphate. Cyclic GMP is degraded by
phosphodiesterases of which there are several in most tissues with
varying degrees of specificity for cyclic GMP and cyclic AMP.
Cyclic GMP is believed to influence tissue metabolism and function
by activating various kinases.

Guanylate Cyclases

Activity of guanylate cyclase in whole retina is
substantially higher than that in other parts of the CNS or in
other tissues. Early studies indicated that this is due to
extremely high enzyme activity in photoreceptor outer segments
(Goridis et al., 1973; Pannbacker, 1973; Bensinger et al., 1974;
Pannbacker, 1974). Enzyme activity in rod outer segments has been
reported by several laboratories to range from 1000-8000 pmoles
cyclic GMP formed/mg protein/min, while that in brain is only 10-
120 pmoles cyclic GMP formed/mg prot/min. In an attempt to
localize the enzyme, guanylate cyclase activity was measured in
various subcellular fractions of whole retina homogenates, and the
overwhelming majority of guanylate cyclase activity is associated
with the outer segment fractions (Virmaux et al., 1976; Zimmerman
et al., 1976). This distribution of enzyme activity was confirmed
in rabbit and ground squirrel retinas where guanylate cyclase
activity was measured in various layers throughout the retina
(Berger et al., 1980). Activity in the outer segment layer is
about 1200-1400 pmoles cyclic GMP formed/mg dry wt/min, which is
10-50 times that found in any other layer.

Both soluble and particulate guanylate cyclases have been found in a variety of tissues, including retina. Earlier studies of guanylate cyclase activities in retinal homogenates from normal and dystrophic mice suggested that at least two classes of enzymes might exist, one of which is preferentially associated with photoreceptor cells (Farber and Lolley, 1976). Later investigations indicated that there may be three guanylate cyclases in retina (Troyer et al., 1978). In their studies of mouse retina they found a soluble enzyme similar to that in mouse brain which has a Km-GTP of 70 μM, which is stimulated by Ca in the presence of low Mn, and which is not influenced by Triton X-100, NaN_3 or NH_2OH. In addition, two particulate enzymes were defined -- one which is similar to the particulate enzyme found in brain, and one that has a greater affinity for GTP, a very high Vmax and is inhibited by Ca. This latter enzyme seemed to be confined to photoreceptor cells, since it was not present in photoreceptorless retina from mice with retinal dystrophy. The other particulate enzyme and the soluble enzyme were present in both whole and dystrophic retinas, however. More recent studies in our laboratory (De Vries and Ferrendelli, in preparation) further support the idea of multiple guanylate cyclases in retina. Examination of microdissected freeze-dried retina demonstrated that guanylate cyclase activity in photoreceptor outer segments is regulated differently from that in the inner retina. The former is inhibited by high concentrations of divalent cations (Ca and Mn), whereas the latter is activated. Sodium nitroprusside stimulates enzyme activity in inner retina and has no effect in outer segments. Preliminary data suggest that enzyme activity in the inner segments and nuclear portions of the photoreceptor cells is a mixture of those activities found in the outer segment and in the inner retina. Thus, we suggest that not only are there two or three guanylate cyclases in retina, but that the photoreceptor cells may also have multiple forms of the enzyme.

Cyclic GMP Phosphodiesterase

A high level of cyclic nucleotide phosphodiesterase activity has been observed in whole retina and in rod outer segment preparations (2-6 times that reported for brain). The enzyme associated with rod outer segments hydrolyzes both cyclic GMP and cyclic AMP, but it has a greater affinity for cyclic GMP (Pannbacker et al., 1972; Goridis and Virmaux, 1974). It has been demonstrated that light activates this enzyme and that the light-activated PDE is probably the major regulator of cyclic GMP concentrations in photoreceptor outer segments (Miki et al., 1973; Chader et al., 1974a; Goridis and Virmaux, 1974; Manthorpe and McConnell, 1975). The cyclic nucleotide phosphodiesterase from frog rod outer segments was purified and shown to have an

approximate molecular weight of 240,000 and K_m values for cyclic
GMP and cyclic AMP of 70 μM and 3 mM, respectively (Miki et al.,
1975). In order to clarify the distribution of enzyme activity
throughout the retina, cyclic nucleotide phosphodiesterase was
measured in various subcellular fractions of bovine retinal
homogenates (Chader et al., 1974b). In whole retina homogenates,
cyclic GMP phosphodiesterase activity is three times that of
cyclic AMP phosphodiesterase. After fractionation, the specific
activity found in rod outer segments is significantly higher for
both enzyme activities, while that in the nuclear, mitochondrial
and microsomal fractions does not change. Cyclic GMP
phosphodiesterase activity was measured in various layers of
freeze-dried rabbit and ground squirrel retinas. Activity in the
outer segment layer ranges from 148-318 nmoles GMP formed/mg dry
wt/min, which is 15-300 times that found in any other layer.
Cyclic AMP phosphodiesterase was also measured in freeze-dried
retinal layers. This enzyme activity in outer segments is much
less than that of cyclic GMP-PDE (i.e., approx. 10 nmoles AMP
formed/mg dry wt/min) but still 5-10 times that of any other layer
(Carter et al., 1979).

Kinetic studies of cyclic GMP-PDE activity in mouse retinal
homogenates indicate the presence of two classes of enzyme
activity with apparent K_m-cyclic GMP values of 30 and 100 μM
(Farber and Lolley, 1976). In microdissected freeze-dried rat
retina, a cyclic GMP-PDE with a high K_m has been localized in the
photoreceptor cell layer, while an enzyme activity with a greater
affinity for cyclic GMP has been demonstrated in the bipolar-plus-
ganglion cell layer (Lolley and Farber, 1975).

Distribution and Regulation of Cyclic GMP Levels

The average concentration of cyclic GMP in whole mouse retina
is approximately 5 μM, 1-2 orders of magnitude higher than in
other regions of the CNS and substantially greater than the level
of cyclic AMP (Goridis et al., 1974; Ferrendelli and Cohen, 1976;
Goridis et al., 1977; De Vries et al., 1978). Examination of rod
outer segment preparations revealed very high levels of endogenous
cyclic GMP (Fletcher and Chader, 1976; Krishna et al., 1976),
implying that perhaps much of this cyclic nucleotide is in the
outer segment of photoreceptor cells. In support of this idea is
the finding that in retinas devoid of photoreceptor cells from
mice with an inherited retinal degeneration, levels of cyclic GMP
were only 1-2% of that found in normal mouse retina (De Vries et
al., 1978). Cyclic GMP levels also were measured in individual
layers of freeze-dried retinas from rabbit (Orr et al., 1976),
ground squirrel (De Vries et al., 1979), and frog (de Azeredo, et
al., 1979). In both rabbit and ground squirrel, the levels of
cyclic GMP are highest in retinal layers containing photoreceptor

cells, where they are at concentrations 10-25 times that found in the inner retinal layers. Furthermore, outer segments appear to have two to three times or more cyclic GMP than other portions of photoreceptor cells. Similar distributions of cyclic GMP occur in frog retina (de Azeredo et al., 1979). It is apparent, therefore, that in vertebrate photoreceptors cyclic GMP levels are very high and, unlike any other known cell, it is the predominant cyclic nucleotide. In contrast, in the inner retina the levels are similar to that in other regions of the CNS.

Some of the earliest studies of cyclic nucleotides in retina revealed that cyclic GMP levels are influenced by light and darkness. Initially it was reported that exposure of dark-adapted, isolated retinas to light produces a rapid fall in their cyclic GMP levels (Goridis et al., 1974). Subsequently, it was observed that the content of cyclic GMP in isolated rod outer segments could also be reduced by illumination (Fletcher and Chader, 1976; Woodruff et al., 1977). Measurements of cyclic nucleotides in individual layers of rabbit retina demonstrated that the changes in cyclic GMP levels after long (1 hour) light- or dark-adaptation occur in all regions of photoreceptor cells, including outer segment, but not in the inner retina (Orr et al., 1976). A most intriguing observation was reported by de Azeredo et al. (1979). These investigators found that exposure of dark-adapted frogs to 2 min of room light not only decreases photoreceptor cyclic GMP levels but also markedly increases its levels in the outer plexiform layer and in the outer portion of the inner nuclear layer. The levels of cyclic GMP in these areas then returned to normal after a longer (1 hour) exposure to light. Light and darkness was reported to influence cyclic GMP levels in rod-dominant retinas from mouse (De Vries et al., 1978), frog (Goridis et al., 1974), rabbit (Orr et al., 1976) and cow (Goridis et al., 1974). In contrast cyclic GMP levels seem to be unaffected by light and darkness in cone-dominant retinas from ground squirrel (Farber and Lolley, 1978; De Vries et al., 1979) and Anolis (De Vries, unpublished). At present it is unclear whether this difference is due to fundamental properties of cones and rods, species differences or some yet unresolved technical problems associated with examination of cone-dominant retinas.

As in other regions of the CNS, anoxia or ischemia has been reported to decrease cyclic GMP levels in mouse (Mitzel et al., 1978) and rabbit retina (Orr et al., 1976). Quantitative histochemical studies indicate that the effect of ischemia on cyclic GMP levels occurs only in layers of retina containing photoreceptor cells and the effect is much more pronounced in dark-adapted tissue.

The fact that isolated retina maintained, in vitro, possesses many of the characteristics of retina in situ has allowed study of

this tissue when its environment is modified in known ways. Using
mouse retina incubated in oxygenated physiologic buffers the
effect of Ca concentration on cyclic nucleotide regulation in this
tissue was studied (Cohen et al., 1978). Exposure of dark-adapted
retinas to Ca-free media in darkness causes a 5- to 6-fold
increase in cyclic GMP levels. This effect is not observed in
light-adapted retinas. Light still causes a rapid decrease of
cyclic GMP levels of retinas incubated in Ca-free media.
Suggestive that the increase in cyclic GMP levels induced by Ca-
lack occurs in photoreceptor cells is the finding that little or
no effect is seen in dystrophic, rodless retinas. These data
suggest that calcium has a strong regulatory influence on cyclic
GMP levels in dark-adapted photoreceptors but not in light-adapted
retina nor in the process responsible for the light-induced
decrease in cyclic GMP levels.

Cyclic AMP

    The enzyme responsible for the synthesis of cyclic AMP is
adenylate cyclase, which converts ATP to the cyclic nucleotide and
pyrophosphate. Cyclic AMP is degraded to AMP by
phosphodiesterase. Cyclic AMP appears to exert its action in
tissue via stimulation of specific kinases. There is much
evidence indicating that cyclic AMP is an intracellular second
messenger which mediates the action of several hormones and
neurotransmitters in various tissues.

Adenylate Cyclase

    In essentially all tissues adenylate cyclase is a membrane
bound enzyme under complex regulation. Although only ATP and Mg
are required to demonstrate its activity, multiple hormones,
neurotransmitters and other substances influence its activity.
Hormone or neurotransmitter-sensitive adenylate cyclase activity
has been well characterized in a number of tissues. It is
recognized that the hormone or neurotransmitter receptor is
separate from the catalytic portion of the enzyme (Maguire et al.,
1977) and that guanine nucleotides play an essential role in the
regulation of this enzyme (Rodbell et al., 1971). A series of
elegant reconstitution studies (Ross et al., Howlett et al.,
1979), in which separate components of hormone-sensitive adenylate
cyclase have been recombined to produce hormone- and guanyl
nucleotide-regulated activity in vitro, has resolved the enzyme
into at least three components: a hormone/neurotransmitter
receptor, a guanine nucleotide binding protein, and a catalytic
unit. The relationship between these components was examined in
liver (Salomon et al., 1975), erythrocytes (Schramm, 1975), fat

cells (Harwood et al., 1973) and other tissues. It is apparent
that the guanine nucleotide binding protein (N), in the presence
of GTP, complexes with the catalytic moiety (C), thereby
stimulating adenylate cyclase activity (Rodbell, 1980). Hormone
or neurotransmitter receptor, in the presence of its agonist,
facilitates the formation of the active N°C complex. The enzyme
requires the presence of divalent cations, moreover, with Mg.ATP
or Mn.ATP serving as the true substrate. Concentrations of Mg or
Mn in excess of ATP are required for optimal activity, which is
interpreted as demonstrating the presence of a second binding site
on the enzyme. Calcium has also been shown to modulate adenylate
cyclase activity and, in fact, in brain there are apparently both
Ca-dependent and Ca-independent forms of the enzyme (Brostrom et
al., 1978a). Low levels of Ca (0.02-0.1 µM) stimulate adenylate
cyclase activity, while higher levels (> 0.1 µM) inhibit the
enzyme (Piascik et al., 1980). That this actually represents two
forms of the enzyme is supported by the separation of brain
adenylate cyclase into two fractions (one insensitive to
calmodulin and only inhibited by Ca, and a second stimulated by
calmodulin and Ca) by calmodulin - Sepharose chromatography
(Westcott et al., 1979). The relationship between Ca and hormonal
regulation of adenylate cyclase activity, however, is not clear.

     Many laboratories have found adenylate cyclase activity in
retinal tissue from several animal species. In addition, a
dopamine-sensitive adenylate cyclase in retinal homogenates has
been reported (Brown and Makman, 1972; Bucher and Schorderet,
1975), with increases in enzyme activity ranging from 40-50% in
mouse and rabbit to 6- to 10-fold in monkey. In order to localize
enzyme activity, adenylate cyclase was measured in two strains of
dystrophic ("rodless") mice (Makman et al., 1975). The specific
activity of adenylate cyclase is higher in the mutant mice than in
controls. Furthermore, in rats in which neonatal glutamate
treatment selectively destroyed the inner retina, there is a
decrease in basal adenylate cyclase activity together with a
proportionate reduction in dopamine-stimulated activity. Similar
observations have been made in the RCS rat, where degeneration of
photoreceptor cells parallels an increase in adenylate cyclase
specific activity (Farber and Lolley, 1977). Direct measurement
of enzyme activity in microdissected mouse retina revealed much
higher adenylate cyclase activity in the bipolar-plus-ganglion
cell layer than in the photoreceptor layer. Recently we examined
adenylate cyclase activity in layers of retina from ground
squirrel and rabbit. The distribution of basal enzyme activity is
similar in both species, with the highest levels found in the
inner plexiform and photoreceptor cell inner segment layers. EGTA
inhibits adenylate cyclase in the inner retina of both species,
stimulates activity in rabbit outer and inner segment layers and
has no effect in these layers from ground squirrel. Enzyme
activity is stimulated in all regions by GPP(NH)P except in the

outer segments of the photoreceptors. Dopamine stimulates the
enzyme in the outer and inner plexiform and inner nuclear layers
in rabbit, but only in the inner plexiform layer in ground
squirrel.

The varying effect of EGTA on adenylate cyclase activity in
different retinal layers is the best evidence that there are two
or more forms of the enzyme present in the retina. It appears
that in the outer and inner segments of rabbit photoreceptors,
there is predominantly a Ca-independent form of the enzyme, whose
activity is enhanced in the presence of EGTA. Since EGTA did not
stimulate enzyme activity in ground squirrel photoreceptor cell
containing layers, the enzyme form (or forms) present in this
species may be different from those seen in rabbit. The proximal
third of the retina in both species appears to contain a
predominantly Ca-dependent form, since the addition of EGTA caused
a depression of activity in these layers. Stimulation by GPP(NH)P
indicates that adenylate cyclase is linked to a guanine nucleotide
binding protein throughout the retina, except for the outer
segments of the rod and cone photoreceptor cells. Adenylate
cyclase in the inner retina is probably associated with one or
more neurotransmitter and/or hormone receptors. We tried to
localize the effect of dopamine, which is known to stimulate the
enzyme in this tissue. In the ground squirrel, dopamine
stimulates adenylate cyclase activity only in the inner plexiform
layer. This is consistent with the distribution of dopaminergic
neurons in this species, where dopamine terminals are present in a
thin band at the border between the inner nuclear and inner
plexiform layers (B. Ehinger, personal communication). In the
rabbit, dopaminergic neurons are a small subclass of amacrine
cells whose terminals end in three bands within the inner
plexiform layer (Dowling and Ehinger, 1978). Dopamine stimulation
of adenylate cyclase activity in the inner nuclear and inner
plexiform layers is consistent with this distribution.
Stimulation of the enzyme in the outer plexiform layer points
either to the presence of dopamine receptors in an area normally
devoid of dopaminergic terminals, or to a stimulation of a non-
dopamine receptor in this layer. What other neurotransmitters or
hormones may be linked to adenylate cyclase in the retina is not
clear at present.

Cyclic AMP Phosphodiesterase

The existence of cyclic AMP phosphodiesterase in retina is
well known. Its activity in various regions of the retina was
briefly described in the study of Carter et al. (1979) (see
above). Since little else is known about this enzyme in retina it
will not be considered further here.

Distribution and Regulation of Cyclic AMP Levels

Cyclic AMP is much more evenly distributed than cyclic GMP in retina, and its concentration in whole mouse retina is approximately 1 µM. Examination of biologically fractionated mouse retinas and retinal layers from rabbit and ground squirrel indicates a slightly higher concentration in the inner retina than in photoreceptor cells.

Cyclic AMP levels in retina are also altered by light- and dark-adaptation. We observed that light depresses and dark elevates the levels of this nucleotide in intact mouse (Ferrendelli and Cohen, 1976; De Vries et al., 1978) and rabbit retina (Orr et al., 1976). In rabbit the change in cyclic AMP levels seems to occur primarily in the outer plexiform layer. We have found that, similar to cyclic GMP, cyclic AMP levels are unaffected by light and darkness in the cone-dominant retinas from ground squirrel (De Vries et al., 1979) and Anolis (De Vries, unpublished). However, Farber and colleagues (1981) reported that light depresses cyclic AMP levels in cone-dominant retina from ground squirrel. The reasons for these discrepant results are unclear at this time.

Ischemia or anoxia also affects retinal cyclic AMP. Associated with oxygen deprivation there is an increase in cyclic AMP levels, and this change occurs primarily in the inner retina.

Agents that are known to cause cellular depolarization alter levels of cyclic AMP in isolated incubated retinas. In intact bovine retina, both ouabain and high potassium have been shown to cause a two-fold elevation in cyclic AMP content (Brown and Makman, 1972). We examined the influence of depolarizing agents on cyclic nucleotide levels in incubated mouse retina. In intact normal retina, high concentrations of potassium increase cyclic AMP levels 2-fold in light-adapted retinas but have no effect on cyclic GMP levels; potassium depolarization has no effect on either cyclic nucleotide in dark-adapted retinas (Ferrendelli, unpublished).

The relationship between neurotransmitters and cyclic nucleotides is better understood and has been studied more extensively in brain than in retina. A dopamine-sensitive adenylate cyclase (see above) has been identified in retina. In addition, dopamine has been reported to cause an accumulation of cyclic AMP in retinal tissue (Makman et al., 1975; Schorderet, 1978; De Mello, 1978). Similar elevations have been reported in the presence of both epinephrine and norepinephrine (Makman et al., 1975; Schorderet, 1978). Preliminary studies in our labora-tory suggest that norepinephrine and adenosine can also elevate cyclic AMP levels in mouse retinas (Ferrendelli, unpublished).

Cyclic Nucleotide Dependent Kinases

The mechanism whereby cyclic nucleotides regulate cellular function and metabolism is believed to be mediated by cyclic nucleotide-dependent kinases acting to phosphorylate specific proteins, and perhaps lipids. This has been established in several tissues, but there is very little reported data in retina on this subject. Cyclic nucleotide dependent phosphorylation of endogenous proteins has been demonstrated in bovine (Farber et al., 1979) and frog (Polans et al., 1979) rod outer segments. In addition we have preliminary data suggesting the presence of a retinal protein which is phosphorylated by a cyclic nucleotide-dependent process. There is no information, however, concerning the localization of these proteins, the cyclic nucleotide-dependent kinases responsible for their phosphorylation or their biologic effect. The relationship, on a spatial or functional basis, of the kinases and their substrate proteins with specific cyclases and phosphodiesterase is also unknown.

Summary and Conclusion

There is much data presented in the preceding discussion which supports the idea that there are several cyclic nucleotide systems in retina and that these are compartmentalized. The best evidence for multiple cyclic GMP systems is the demonstration of three guanylate cyclases which can be distinguished by their enzymatic and/or physical properties. One of these cyclases is clearly localized to photoreceptor outer segments and may be functionally linked to a high activity cyclic GMP phosphodiesterase. This system seems to be regulated by light in rod photoreceptors, but perhaps not in cones, and by calcium. At present it is unknown if it is associated with the cyclic nucleotide-dependent protein kinase reported by Farber et al. (1979), or is related to other yet undefined kinases. The two other guanylate cyclases present in retina are not as well localized as the one in photoreceptor outer segments, but they certainly appear to be in the inner retina and may also be in the inner portions of the photoreceptor cells. These cyclases have not been associated with any specific phosphodiesterases. Light also seems to affect at least one of these cyclic GMP systems, but unlike the situation in outer segments, it causes transient accumulation of cyclic GMP. Calcium also influences this system, but it has the opposite effect from that in photoreceptors. The cyclic GMP systems in the inner retina have not been linked to kinases or other metabolic processes.

A similar argument can be made for the existence of multiple cyclic AMP systems in retina. Although there does not appear to be different forms of adenylate cyclase in retina, its activity is influenced differently by EGTA, guanine nucleotides and dopamine in various regions. The enzyme in outer segments is not influenced by calcium (or calmodulin) or any neurotransmitter tested so far. Guanine nucleotides also have little or no effect on its activity. Whether or not it is associated with a specific cyclic AMP phosphodiesterase has not been ascertained. This cyclic AMP system may be influenced by light in cones as suggested by the studies of Farber et al. 1981, but how it is regulated in rods is unknown at present. Cyclic AMP dependent kinases have not been identified in photoreceptor cells or associated with the adenylate cyclase in these structures. Clearly distinct from the enzyme in outer segments is adenylate cyclase in the inner retina. This latter enzyme is influenced by calcium (or calmodulin), guanine nucleotides and, in some regions, dopamine. Its location is poorly defined at present and it also has not been associated with specific cyclic AMP phosphodiesterases. What regulates cyclic AMP in the inner retina has not been ascertained, but it seems very likely that dopamine is one factor. Possibly other neurotransmitters have some effect on cyclic AMP regulation in inner retina, but probably not in the same regions as dopamine. Kinases that mediate the actions of cyclic AMP probably are present in the inner retina, but have not yet been identified.

The existence of three cyclic GMP systems and at least two cyclic AMP systems is suggested in the above discussion. It is possible that others may also exist. Obviously none is completely defined and additional research is necessary to characterize these systems, determine their cellular and sub-cellular localization and to explain their involvement in retinal function and metabolism. Certainly, these are necessary prerequisites for the eventual understanding of the roles of cyclic AMP and cyclic GMP in mechanisms underlying normal and abnormal visual function.

Acknowledgement

Supported in part, by USPHS grant EY 02294.

References

Bensinger, R.E., Fletcher, R.T. and Chader, G.T., 1974. Guanylate cyclase: Inhibition by light in retinal photoreceptor. Science 183: 86-87.

Berger, S.J., De Vries, G.W., Carter, J.G. Schultz, D.W.,
    Passonneau, P.N., Lowry, O.H. and Ferrendelli, J.A., 1980.
    The distribution of the components of the cyclic GMP cycle in
    retina. J. Biol. Chem. 255: 3128-3133.

Brown, J.H. and Makman, M.H., 1972. Stimulation by dopamine of
    adenylate cyclase in retinal homogenates and of adenosine -
    3';5' - cyclic monophosphate formation in intact retina.
    Proc. Nat. Acad. Sci. USA 69: 539-543.

Bucher, M.B. and Schorderet, M., 1975. Dopamine- and apomorphine-
    sensitive adenylate cyclase in homogenates of rabbit retina.
    Arch. Pharmacol. 288: 103-104.

Carter, J.G., Berger, S.J. and Lowry, O.H., 1979. The measurement
    of cyclic GMP and cyclic AMP phosphodiesterases. Anal.
    Biochem. 100: 244-253.

Chader, G.J., Herz, L.R. and Fletcher, R.T., 1974a. Light
    activation of phosphodiesterase activity in retinal rod outer
    segments. Biochim. Biophys. Acta. 347: 491-493.

Chader, G., Johnson, M., Fletcher, R. and Bensinger, R., 1974b.
    Cyclic nucleotide phosphodiesterase of the bovine retina:
    activity, subcellular distribution and kinetic parameters. J.
    Neurochem. 22: 93-99.

Cohen, A.I., Hall, I.A. and Ferrendelli, J.A., 1978. Calcium and
    cyclic nucleotide regulation in incubated mouse retinas. J.
    Gen. Physiol. 71: 595-612.

de Azeredo, F.A., Lust, W.D. and Passonneau, J.V., 1979. Guanine
    nucleotides in the frog retinal layers following light
    adaptation. Invest. Ophthalmol. Visual Sci., Suppl. ARVO 18,
    21: Abstr. 7.

De Mello, F.G., 1978. The ontogeny of dopamine-dependent increase
    of adenosine 3', 5'-cyclic monophosphate in the chick
    retina. J. Neurochem. 31: 1049-1053.

De Vries, G.W., Cohen, A.I., Hall, I.A. and Ferrendelli, J.A.,
    1978. Cyclic nucleotide levels in normal and biologically
    fractionated mouse retina: effects of light and dark
    adaptation. J. Neurochem. 31: 1345-1351.

De Vries, G.W., Cohen, A.I., Lowry, O.H. and Ferrendelli, J.A.,
    1979. Cyclic nucleotides in the cone-dominant ground squirrel
    retina. Exp. Eye Res. 29: 315-321.

Dowling, J.E. and Ehinger, B., 1978. Synaptic organization of the
   dopaminergic neurons in the rabbit retina. J. Comp. Neurol.
   180: 203-220.

Farber, D.B., Brown, B.M. and Lolley, R.N., 1979. Cyclic
   nucleotide dependent protein kinase and the phosphorylation of
   endogenous proteins of retinal rod outer segments.
   Biochemistry 18: 370-378.

Farber, D.B. and Lolley, R.N., 1976. Enzymic bases for cyclic GMP
   accumulation in degenerative photoreceptor cells of mouse
   retina. J. Cyclic Nucl. Res. 2: 139-148.

Farber, D.B. and Lolley, R.N., 1977. Influence of visual cell
   maturation or degeneration on cyclic AMP content of retinal
   neurons. J. Neurochem. 29: 167-170.

Farber, D.B. and Lolley, R.N., 1978. cAMP and cGMP content of
   cone-dominant retinas of ground squirrel. Invest. Ophthalmol.
   Visual Sci., Suppl. ARVO 17: 255 Abstr. 8.

Farber, D.B., Souza, D.W., Chase, D.G. and Lolley, R.N., 1981.
   Cyclic nucleotides in cone dominant retina. Invest.
   Ophthalmol. Vis. Sci. 20: 24-31.

Ferrendelli, J.A. and Cohen, A.I., 1976. The effects of light and
   dark adaptation on the levels of cyclic nucleotides in retinas
   of mice heterozygous for a gene for photoreceptor dystrophy.
   Biochem. Biophys. Res. Comm. 73: 421-427.

Fletcher, R.T. and Chader, G.J., 1976. Cyclic GMP: Control of
   concentration by light in retinal photoreceptors. Biochem.
   Biophys. Res. Comm. 70: 1297-1302.

Goridis, C., Urban, P.F. and Mandel, P., 1977. The effect of
   flash illumination on the endogenous cyclic GMP content of
   isolated frog retinae. Exp. Eye Res. 24: 171-177.

Goridis, C. and Virmaux, N., 1974. Light-regulated guanosine 3',
   5'-monophosphate phosphodiesterase of bovine retina. Nature
   248: 57-58.

Goridis, C., Virmaux, N., Cailla, H.L. and Delaage, M.A., 1974.
   Rapid, light-induced changes of retinal cyclic GMP levels.
   FEBS Letters 49: 167-169.

Goridis, C., Virmaux, N., Urban, P.F. and Mandel, P., 1973.
   Guanyl cyclase in a mammalian photoreceptor. FEBS Letters 30:
   163-166.

Harwood, J.P. Low, H. and Rodbell, M., 1973. Stimulatory and inhibitory effects of guanyl nucleotides on fat cell adenylate cyclase. J. Biol. Chem. 248: 6239-6245.

Howlett, A.C., Sternweis, P.C., Macik, B.A., Van Arsdale, P.M. and Gilman, A.G., 1979. Reconstitution of catecholamine-sensitive adenylate cyclase. J. Biol. Chem. 254: 2287-2295.

Krishna, G., Krishman, N., Fletcher, R.T. and Chader, G., 1976. Effects of light on cyclic GMP metabolism in retinal photoreceptors. J. Neurochem. 27: 717-722.

Lolley, R.N. and Farber, D.B., 1975. Cyclic nucleotide phosphodiesterases in dystrophic rat retinas: guanosine 3', 5' cyclic monophosphate anomalies during photoreceptor cell degeneration. Exp. Eye Res. 20: 585-597.

Maguire, M.E., Ross, E.M. and Gilman, A.G., 1977. β-adrenergic receptor: Ligand binding properties and the interaction with adenyl cyclase. Adv. Cyclic Nucl. Res. 8: 1-83.

Makman, M.H., Brown, J.H. and Mishra, R.K., 1975. Cyclic AMP in retina and caudate nucleus: influence of dopamine and other agents. Adv. Cyclic Nucl. Res. 5: 661-679.

Manthorpe, M. and McConnell, D.G., 1975. Cyclic nucleotide phosphodiesterases associated with bovine retinal outer-segment fragments. Biochim. Biophys. Acta. 403: 438-445.

Miki, N., Baraban, J.M., Keirns, J.J., Boyce, J.J. and Bitensky, M.W., 1975. Purification and properties of the light-activated cyclic nucleotide phosphodiesterase of rod outer segments. J. Biol. Chem. 250: 6320-6327.

Miki, N., Keirns, J.J., Marcus, F.R., Freeman, J. and Bitensky, M.W., 1973. Regulation of cyclic nucleotide concentrations in photoreceptors: an ATP-dependent stimulation of cyclic nucleotide phosphodiesterase by light. Proc. Nat. Acad. Sci. USA 70: 3820-3824.

Mitzel, D.L., Hall, I.A., De Vries, G.W., Cohen, A.I. and Ferrendelli, J.A., 1978. Comparison of cyclic nucleotide and energy metabolism of intact mouse retina in situ and in vitro. Exp. Eye Res. 27: 27-37.

Orr, H.T., Lowry, O.H., Cohen, A.I. and Ferrendelli, J.A., 1976. Distribution of 3'-5'-cyclic AMP and 3'-5'-cyclic GMP in rabbit retina in vivo: selective effects of dark and light adaptation and ischemia. Proc. Nat. Acad. Sci. USA 73: 4442-4445.

Pannbacker, R.G., 1973. Control of guanylate cyclase activity in the rod outer segment. Science 182: 1138-1140.

Pannbacker, R.G., 1974. Cyclic nucleotide metabolism in human photoreceptors. Invest. Ophthalmol. 13: 535-538.

Pannbacker, R.G., Fleischman, D.E. and Reed, D.W., 1972. Cyclic nucleotide phosphodiesterase: high activity in a mammalian photoreceptor. Science 175: 757-758.

Piascik, M.T., Wisler, P.L., Johnson, C.L. and Potter, J.D., 1980. Ca^{++}-dependent regulation of guinea pig brain adenylate cyclase. J. Biol. Chem. 255: 4176-4181.

Poulons, A.S., Hermolin, J. and Bounds, M.D., 1979. Light-induced dephosphorylation of two proteins in frog rod outer segments. J. Gen. Physiol. 74: 595-613.

Rodbell, M., 1980. The role of hormone receptors and GTP-regulatory proteins in membrane transduction. Nature 284: 17-22.

Rodbell, M., Birnbaumer, L., Pohl, S.L. and Krans, H.M., 1971. The glucagon-sensitive adenyl cyclase system in plasma membranes of rat liver. V. An obligatory role of guanyl nucleotides in glucagon action. J. Biol. Chem. 246: 1877-1882.

Ross, E.M., Haga, T., Howelett, A.C., Schwarzmeier, J., Schleifer, L.S. and Gilman, A.G., 1978. Hormone-sensitive adenylate cyclase: Resolution and reconstitution of some components necessary for regulation of the enzyme. Adv. Cyclic Nucleotide Res. 9: 53-68.

Salomon, Y., Lin, M.C., Londos, C., Rendell, M. and Rodbell, M., 1975. The hepatic adenylate cyclase system. I. Evidence for transition states and structural requirements for guanine nucleotide activation. J. Biol. Chem. 250: 4239-4245.

Schorderet, M., 1978. The interrelationship between dopamine receptors and cyclic AMP metabolism in rabbit retina and its importance for the mechanism of action of centrally active drugs. In: Molecular Biology and Pharmacology of Cyclic Nucleotides. Folco, G. and Paolette, R. (eds.), Elsevier-North-Holland Biomedical Press, Amsterdam, 259-263.

Schramm, M., 1975. The catecholamine-responsive adenylate cyclase system and its modification by 5' guanylylimido-diphosphate. Adv. Cyclic Nucleotide Res. 5: 105-115.

Troyer, E.W., Hall, I.A. and Ferrendelli, J.A., 1978. Guanylate
    cyclases in CNS: enzymatic characteristics of soluble and
    particulate enzymes from mouse cerebellum and retina. J.
    Neurochem. 31: 825-833.

Virmaux, N., Nullans, G. and Goridis, C., 1976. Guanylate cyclase
    in vertebrate retina: evidence for specific association with
    rod-outer segments. J. Neurochem. 26: 233-235.

Westcott, K.R., La Porte, D.C. and Storm, D.R., 1979. Resolution
    of adenylate cyclase sensitive and insensitive to Ca^{++} and
    calcium-dependent regulatory protein (CDR) by CDR-Sepharose
    affinity chromatography. Proc. Natl. Acad. Sci. USA 76: 204-
    208.

Woodruff, M.L., Bownds, D., Green, S.H., Morrisey, J.L. and
    Shedlovsky, A., 1977. Guanosine 3', 5'-cyclic monophosphate
    and the in vitro physiology of frog photoreceptor membranes.
    J. Gen. Physiol. 69: 667-679.

Zimmerman, W.F., Daemen, F.J. and Bonting, S.L., 1976.
    Distribution of enzyme activities in subcellular fractions of
    bovine retina. J. Biol. Chem. 251: 4700-4705.

NEUROTRANSMITTER-SENSITIVE ADENYLATE CYCLASE

IN THE TELEOST RETINA

K. J. Watling, R. G. Van Buskirk and J. E. Dowling

The Biological Laboratories
Harvard University
Cambridge, Massachusetts 02138
U.S.A.

There is now substantial evidence that several neurotransmitters activate the enzyme adenylate cyclase in the central nervous system (CNS). It has been proposed that the resulting increase in intracellular levels of cyclic AMP may mediate some of the postsynaptic effects of these neurotransmitters (Greengard, 1976, 1978; Daly, 1977). The best characterised neurotransmitter-sensitive adenylate cyclase is that activated by dopamine which has been identified in several regions of the CNS (Kebabian et al., 1972; Clement-Cormier et al., 1974; Iversen, 1975), including the retina (Brown and Makman, 1972; Schorderet, 1977). In addition, it has been reported that noradrenaline (Von Hungen and Roberts, 1973), histamine (Hegstrand et al., 1976) and the neuropeptide vasoactive intestinal peptide (Quik et al., 1978) also specifically stimulate cyclic AMP production in certain brain regions. However, despite the enormous amount of information which has been published concerning the biochemical characterisation, regional distribution and neuropharmacology of these neurotransmitter-sensitive adenylate cyclases, comparatively little information is available concerning their functional significance.

We have been investigating the presence of neurotransmitter-sensitive adenylate cyclases in the teleost retina, in the hope that the use of this simplified region of the CNS, with its well defined synaptic and functional organisation, may help to clarify and focus some of the current ideas concerning the role of these systems in neuronal function. This report summarizes our findings concerning the presence of a dopamine-sensitive adenylate cyclase in the teleost retina, together with recent investigations

regarding the cellular localisation of this response and the
observation that vasoactive intestinal peptide (VIP) also stimulates cyclic AMP accumulation in the fish retina.

DOPAMINE-SENSITIVE ADENYLATE CYCLASE

     In the retina of teleost fish, dopamine is confined to
interplexiform neurones that spread processes in both plexiform
layers of the retina. These cells receive their synaptic input
from amacrine cells in the inner plexiform layer and make synapses
on horizontal, bipolar and amacrine cells and their processes
(Dowling and Ehinger, 1978). In the fish, the majority of the
interplexiform cell synapses are made onto the perikarya of the
large, outermost (external) horizontal cells in the outer plexiform
layer (Dowling and Ehinger, 1978).

     In initial experiments (Watling and Dowling, 1981), retinae
were removed from mirror or common carp (Cyprinus carpio),
homogenised and assayed for adenylate cyclase activity using the
method of Kebabian et al. (1972). Twenty microlitre aliquots of
the homogenate (1 retina/500 µl homogenising buffer) were incubated
at 30°C for 5 min in the presence of 1mM ATP and various test
substances. Incubations were terminated by boiling for 3 min and
following microcentrifugation, supernatants were assayed for cyclic
AMP content using the method of Brown et al. (1972). These
experiments indicated the presence of a highly specific dopamine-
sensitive adenylate cyclase in homogenates of the carp retina.
Figure 1 shows the effects of increasing concentrations of
dopamine, noradrenaline and adrenaline on adenylate cyclase
activity. It can be seen that dopamine, with an EC50 value of
approximately 1µM (concentration producing 50% of the maximum
response), was ten times more potent than either adrenaline or
noradrenaline. Furthermore, the specific α- and β- adrenoreceptor
agonists, phenylephrine and isoprenaline, together with histamine
and 5-hydroxytryptamine were ineffective at stimulating adenylate
cyclase activity, demonstrating the dopaminergic specificity of the
response. In addition, various antagonists inhibited the dopamine
response (Watling and Dowling, 1981) with potencies which resembled
their ability to antagonise the dopamine sensitive-adenylate
cyclase in homogenates of rat striatum (Iversen, 1975).

     To examine the retina under more physiological conditions,
experiments investigating the factors affecting the accumulation of
cyclic AMP in intact pieces of retina were performed (Dowling and
Watling, 1981). Dissected retinae were removed onto small pieces
of Ringer's-soaked filter paper, receptor side up, and cut into
four or six pieces. Each retinal piece was placed in an oxygenated
vial and preincubated at 30°C for 2-5 min in 900 µl of oxygenated
carp Ringer's solution at pH 7.4 (Wu and Dowling, 1978) containing

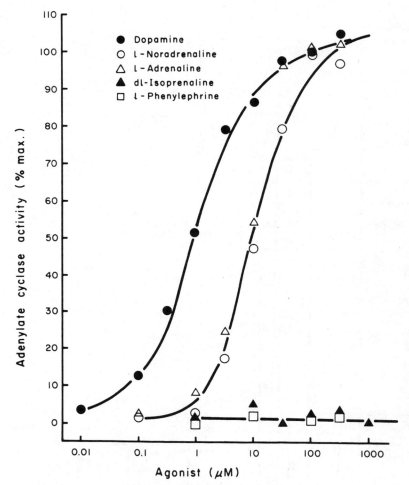

Fig. 1.   Effect of agonists on adenylate cyclase activity in
           homgenates of carp retina.   Each point is the mean of 2-6
           experiments involving quadruplicate determinations.
           S.E.M. values were less than 10% of the mean.   Results
           are expressed as percent maximum response elicited by
           100 μM dopamine.

2mM isobutylmethylxanthine (IBMX), a phosphodiesterase inhibitor.
Following the addition of 100 μl carp Ringer's containing test
substances, the tissue was incubated for a further 5-10 min.
Incubations were terminated by boiling, after which the Ringer's
was drawn off, microcentrifuged and assayed for cyclic AMP using
the method of Brown et al. (1972).   The protein contents of the
remaining retinal pieces were determined using the method of Lowry

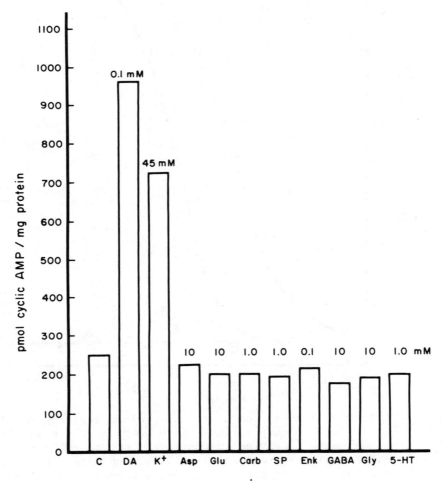

Fig. 2.   Effects of dopamine (DA), K$^+$ ions, aspartate (Asp),
glutamate (Glu), carbachol (Carb), substance P (SP),
enkephalin (Enk), γ-aminobutyric acid (GABA), glycine (Gly)
and 5-hydroxytryptamine (5-HT) on cyclic AMP accumulation in
pieces of intact carp retina.   All retinal pieces were
preincubated for 2 min in carp Ringer's containing 2mM IBMX
and for an additional 5 min in carp Ringer's containing 2mM
IBMX plus the indicated concentrations of test substance.
Results are expressed as pmol cyclic AMP/mg protein.   Each
histogram represents the mean of 2-4 experiments.

et al. (1951) and data were calculated as pmol cyclic AMP/mg
protein. Figure 2 illustrates the effects of a number of putative
retinal neurotransmitter agents on cyclic AMP accumulation in
pieces of intact carp retina. Whilst dopamine, at a concentration
of 100 µM, stimulated cyclic AMP levels approximately 6-fold as
compared to control levels, none of the other neurotransmitter
agents examined, including 5-hydroxytryptamine, carbachol,
aspartate, glutamate, GABA (γ-aminobutyric acid), glycine,
substance P and the metabolically stable enkephalin analogue, D-
Ala_2,-D-Leu_5-enkephalin had any significant effects on cyclic AMP
accumulation at concentrations ranging from 100µM to 10 mM. The
EC50 value for dopamine in pieces of intact retina was
approximately 10 µM.

Incubation of retinal pieces with 45 mM K^+ ions also
stimulated cyclic AMP accumulation (Fig.2). It is known that K^+
ions depolarise neurones and evoke the release of neurotransmitter
substances from presynaptic terminals. The ability of 100 µM
haloperidol, a dopaminergic antagonist, to inhibit almost
completely the stimulation of cyclic AMP production induced by
45 mM K^+ ions in pieces of intact retina strongly suggested that
this response was being mediated through the release of endogenous
stores of dopamine.

In summary, the results of these experiments, involving both
homogenates and intact pieces of tissue, confirmed the presence of
a dopamine-sensitive adenylate cyclase in the teleost retina.
Furthermore, the inability of any other known retinal
neurotransmitters to mimic this response led us to propose that the
dopamine-sensitive adenylate cyclase is the 'major or only'
neurotransmitter-activated adenylate cyclase in the teleost retina
(Dowling and Watling, 1981).

CELLULAR LOCALISATION OF DOPAMINE-SENSITIVE ADENYLATE CYCLASE

In an attempt to further our understanding of the possible
role of dopamine-sensitive adenylate cyclase in retinal function we
have recently undertaken experiments designed to determine the
cellular localisation of this response in the teleost retina. The
horizontal cells appear to represent one particularly likely locus
for dopamine-sensitive adenylate cyclase based on the anatomical
evidence of abundant dopaminergic synapses on these neurones and on
previous intracellular recordings which have shown that dopamine
can transiently depolarise carp horizontal cells and reduce the
amplitude of their light evoked responses (Hedden and Dowling,
1978). With the introduction in recent years of techniques for the
dissociation and isolation of retinal neurones (Sarthy and Lam,
1978; 1979), we have developed a procedure for isolating
populations of horizontal cells from the enzymatically dissociated

carp retina as follows: eight dissected retinae are placed in 20
ml of a solution containing 0.8% trypsin made up in a phosphate
Ringer's solution containing 80 mM NaCl, 22.7 mM NaHCO$_3$; 0.8 mM
Na$_2$HPO$_4$; 3.5 mM KCl; 0.1 mM KH$_2$PO$_4$; 2.4 mM MgSO$_4$; 10 mM dextrose
and 5mM ethyleneglycol-bis-(β-aminoethyl ether)-N, N'-tetraacetic
acid (EGTA), adjusted to pH 7.4 at room temperature following
thorough oxygenation with 100% O$_2$.   Retinae are gently bubbled with
95% O$_2$: 5% CO$_2$ for 1.5 hr at room temperature and transferred to 10
ml of oxygenated carp Ringer's solution (Wu and Dowling, 1978)
adjusted to pH 7.4.   Retinae are rinsed in two changes of this
Ringer's and dissociated at 9°C in a further 40 ml by repeated
withdrawal and ejection from a Pasteur pipette.   Having allowed any
undissociated material to settle, 2 ml aliquots from the upper cell
suspension are gently applied to the surface of each of 12
gradients, containing 50 ml of 0.8-4.0% Ficoll.   These gradients
are constructed at 9°C in 12 glass gradient vessels, each
possessing a diameter of 5 cm, a depth of 7 cm and a tap at its
base to permit the removal of various fractions.   Cells are left to
sediment in the Ficoll at unit gravity for 4 hr at 9°C.   Following
sedimentation, 9 X 5.5 ml fractions were initially run off in
series from each gradient and the cells in each fraction identified
under the light microscope.

      Figure 3 illustrates the distribution of various retinal cell
types throughout the nine 5.5 ml fractions of a typical small (50
ml) gradient.   Particularly striking is the presence of a wide band
of rod photoreceptors at the top of the gradient (Fractions 6-9).
These retinal neurones are easily recognisable by their
characteristic shape, and far outnumber the presence of any other
cell type.   In contrast, the other major class of photoreceptors,
the cones, migrate furthest through the gradient and are found in
fraction 1.   Also located in the lower half of the gradient
(fractions 3 and 4) are the horizontal cells.   These neurones may
be identified on the basis of their relatively large size with
respect to the other neurones present throughout the gradient, and
cells possessing processes spanning 100 μm are routinely
observed.   Furthermore, electron microscopy has confirmed the
identity of these large neurones as horizontal cells based on their
large size and the presence of a multi-lobed nucleus (Van Buskirk
and Dowling, 1981), features which are characteristic of horizontal
cells.   In addition, these studies indicate that the isolated
horizontal cells possess no associated axon terminals.

      Other retinal neurones, including bipolar, ganglion and
amacrine cells are more difficult to distinguish after
sedimentation although a mixture of these neurones may constitute
of the cells observed in fractions 5 and 6.   Finally, some non-
neuronal cells including red blood cells, pigment epithelial cells
and fibroblast-like cells are also observed in various fractions
throughout the gradient.

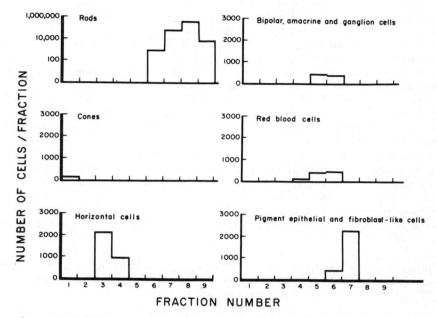

Fig. 3.   Distribution of various retinal cell types throughout
nine 5.5 ml fractions of a typical small (50 ml)
gradient. Results are expressed as the number of
cells/gradient fraction, as determined by placing each
5.5 ml fraction into a gridded culture dish, allowing the
cells to settle and then estimating the total number of
cells by counting the cells in a representative sample of
grids.   Cell number is on a linear scale except for the
rod photoreceptors where a logarithmic scale applies.
Fraction 1 represents the first 5.5 ml fraction removed
from the bottom of the gradient; fraction 9 represents
the uppermost fraction of the gradient.

The examination of retinal cell types in each gradient
indicated that a relatively pure population of horizontal cells
(fractions 3 and 4) and rod photoreceptors (Fractions 7,8 and 9)
could be obtained. These two regions of the gradient were
therefore individually pooled and the cells centrifuged and
subsequently examined for their ability to accumulate cyclic AMP.
The Ficoll solution remaining after centrifugation was gently
decanted and the isolated cells, present in approximately 100 μl of
residual Ficoll, were preincubated for 3-5 min at 30°C in 300 μl of

carp Ringer's, pH 7.4, containing 2mM IBMX. One hundred
microlitres of Ringer's containing various test substances were
added and the cells incubated for an additional 5-10 min.
Incubations were terminated by boiling for 3 min and following
microcentrifugation, triplicate 100 µl aliquots of the supernatant
were assayed for cyclic AMP content using an acetylated cyclic AMP
radioimmunoassay (Collaborative Research Inc., Waltham,
Massachusetts, USA) which increases the sensitivity of the assay to
approximately 0.0025 pmol cyclic AMP/100 µl sample. The increased
sensitivity of the acetylation method is due to the greater
affinity of the antibody for acetylated cyclic AMP as compared to
native (unacetylated) cyclic AMP (Harper and Brooker, 1975). The
small numbers of cells present in each incubation tube preclude a
reliable protein determination and as such it is impossible to
express data in terms of pmol cyclic AMP/mg protein. Results are
expressed therefore in terms of pmol cyclic AMP/pooled fraction or
pmol cyclic AMP/incubation tube (see individual Figure legends for
details).

Figure 4 illustrates the effects of increasing concentrations
of dopamine on pooled fractions of either isolated horizontal cells
or rod photoreceptors. In the horizontal cells it can be seen that
during a 5-7 min incubation in the presence of 2mM IBMX, dopamine
induced a dose-related increase in cyclic AMP accumulation.
Dopamine evoked a significant stimulation at a concentration of
1 µM, attaining a maximum response at concentrations of 300 µM or
greater. The EC50 value for dopamine in this system (concentration
producing 50% of maximum response) was approximately 30 µM. Based
on an estimate of approximately 3,000 horizontal cells in the
pooled horizontal cell fraction (see Fig. 3), the maximum response
to dopamine corresponds to an accumulation of approximately 0.18
fmol cyclic AMP per horizontal cell, assuming that all horizontal
cells are responding to dopamine. Of particular interest was the
absence of any detectable basal cyclic AMP levels following a 5 min
incubation in Ringer's containing only IBMX (i.e. cyclic AMP levels
were less than 0.0025 pmol/100 µl assay sample, or less than 0.0125
pmol/pooled fraction). Furthermore, if the basal level is just
below the detectable level of cyclic AMP in these fractions,
dopamine can induce at least a 30-40 fold increase in cyclic AMP
production in the isolated horizontal cell fraction. In contrast
to the isolated horizontal cells, the pooled rod photoreceptor
fraction demonstrated a substantial basal level of cyclic AMP.
However, the accumulation of cyclic AMP in the rod fraction was
unaffected by incubation with dopamine at concentrations up to
300 µM (Fig. 4). Further data presented in Fig. 4 indicates that
the response to dopamine in the isolated horizontal cell fraction
requires the presence of intact cells. If, prior to incubation,
the horizontal cells are homogenised using a glass rod, the
response to dopamine is abolished. Finally, isolated horizontal
cells incubated with 100 µM dopamine in the absence of 2mM IBMX

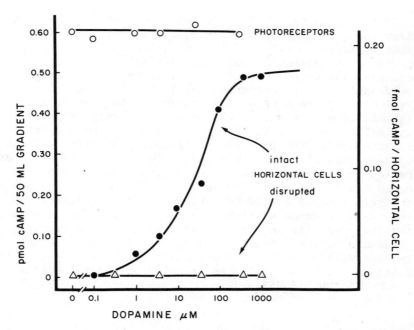

Fig. 4.   Effect of various concentrations of dopamine on cyclic
           AMP accumulation in fractions of isolated horizontal
           cells and rod photoreceptors. All fractions were
           preincubated in Ringer's containing 2mM IBMX for 3 min
           and for an additional 7 min in Ringer's containing 2mM
           IBMX plus dopamine. Results are expressed as pmol cyclic
           AMP/pooled fraction. Each point represents the mean of
           2-5 experiments involving triplicate determinations.

failed to accumulate cyclic AMP. This result emphasises the need
to include a phosphodiesterase inhibitor in the incubation Ringer's
when attempting to demonstrate dopamine-dependent cyclic AMP
accumulation in these cells.

     A number of other putative retinal neurotransmitters were
examined for their ability to induce the accumulation of cyclic AMP
in pooled horizontal cell fractions, including the amino acids
glutamate, glycine, aspartate and γ-aminobutyric acid (GABA). Each
was tested at concentrations of up to 1 mM, but all failed to
elevate cyclic AMP levels. Furthermore, phenylephrine, isoprenaline and 5-hydroxytryptamine, at concentrations up to 100 μM,
yielded similar negative results. In addition, no increase in
cyclic AMP levels was observed in isolated horizontal cells
incubated in the presence of 45 mM K^+ ions in contrast to results
obtained in pieces of intact retina (Fig. 2).

Several dopamine antagonists were examined for their ability to block the dopamine-dependent accumulation of cyclic AMP in isolated horizontal cell fractions as illustrated in Fig. 5. Haloperidol and (+)-butaclamol were particularly effective in this respect inducing a complete inhibition of the normal response to 100 µM dopamine at concentrations as low as 0.01 µM. Indeed, the IC50 value for these antagonists (concentration required to induce 50% inhibition of the normal 200 µM dopamine response) was approximately 1 nM. Fluphenazine was also able to completely abolish the normal 100 µM dopamine response, but with an IC50 value of approximately 0.03 µM, was somewhat less potent than either haloperidol or (+)-butaclamol. In contrast, domperidone was unable to induce a 50% inhibition of the normal 100 µM dopamine response at concentrations up to 100 µM. Likewise (-)-butaclamol was ineffective at a concentration of 1 µM. Whilst these data are qualitatively similar to results obtained in either carp retinal homogenates or intact pieces of retina (Watling and Dowling, 1981; Dowling and Watling, 1981) the effective antagonists appear to be substantially more potent in the isolated horizontal cell system (see COMMENTS AND DISCUSSION).

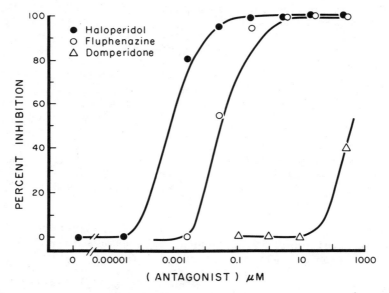

Fig. 5.   Inhibition of dopamine-stimulated cyclic AMP accumulation in isolated horizontal cell fractions by various dopaminergic antagonists. Results are expressed as the percentage inhibition of the normal response produced by 200 µM dopamine. Each point is the mean of 2-3 experiments involving triplicate determinations.

In conclusion, the results of these experiments involving the use of isolated retinal neurones, and reported in greater detail by Van Buskirk and Dowling (1981), demonstrate that the horizontal cells represent a major locus of dopamine-sensitive adenylate cyclase in the teleost retina.

VIP-STIMULATED CYCLIC AMP ACCUMULATION

During the past few years the recognition of several neuropeptides in the retina of many species (Karten and Brecha, 1980; Brecha et al., 1979; Krisch and Leonhardt, 1979) has raised the possibility that these agents may be acting as neurotransmitters in the retina. The current list of putative retinal neuropeptide transmitters includes leu-enkephalin, somatostatin, neurotensin, glucagon, substance P and VIP although to date there is very little evidence other than immunohistochemical data to support this contention. For example, little is known about what biochemical processes or physiological responses these peptides may be controlling in the retina (Glickman et al., 1981; Dick and Miller, 1981; Djamgoz et al., 1981). However, the recent observation that VIP, a twenty eight amino acid residue peptide, will stimulate cyclic AMP accumulation in both homogenates of bovine and rabbit retinae (Longshore and Makman, 1981) and intact pieces of rabbit retinae (Schorderet et al., 1981) prompted us to investigate its effect on cyclic AMP accumulation in the teleost retina.

Experiments were performed in pieces of intact retina according to previously described techniques except for the inclusion of a peptidase inhibitor, bacitracin (30 µg/ml), in the carp Ringer's in an attempt to inhibit the degradation of VIP by proteases possibly present in the retina. VIP induced a dose-related stimulation of cyclic AMP accumulation, as illustrated in Fig. 6, with a concentration of 10 µM VIP producing a 5-fold stimulation with respect to control levels. This dose-response curve closely paralleled that obtained for dopamine in this series of experiments (Fig. 6). However, whilst dopamine clearly induced a maximum response at concentrations of 100 µM or greater, the limited amount of VIP available did not permit a similar measurement to be made for VIP, although the results of two experiments did suggest that 30 µM VIP can stimulate cyclic AMP production to levels well in excess of 1000 pmol/mg protein. Thus, whilst the EC50 value for dopamine was approximately 3 µM, the concentration of VIP eliciting half maximal activation of cyclic AMP production could not be determined. Additional experiments indicated that various other neuropeptides including glucagon, α-melanocyte stimulating hormone, secretin and cholecystokinin octapeptide were ineffective at stimulating cyclic AMP production at concentrations up to 10 µM.

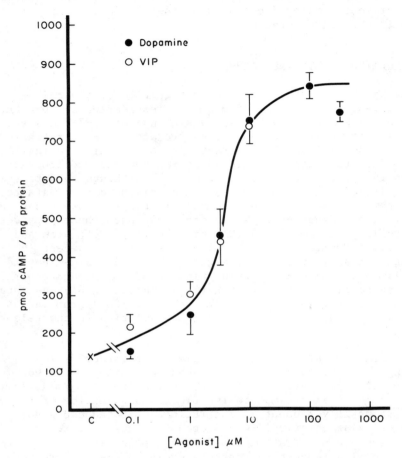

Fig. 6.   Effects of various concentrations of dopamine and VIP on
           cyclic AMP accumulation in pieces of intact carp
           retina.   In these, and subsequent experiments, retinal
           pieces received a 5 min preincubation in carp Ringer's
           containing 2mM IBMX followed by a 10 min incubation in
           carp Ringer's containing 2mM IBMX plus test substance.
           Results are expressed as pmol cyclic AMP/mg protein.
           Each point is the mean of at least 8 experiments
           involving triplicate determinations and is given with the
           S.E.M.

The effect of time on the accumulation of cyclic AMP induced by either 100 µM dopamine or 10 µM VIP was also investigated as shown in Fig. 7. Dopamine induced a comparatively rapid response with the majority of the cyclic AMP being formed during the initial 5 min of incubation. Furthermore, this maximal level of cyclic AMP accumulation remained constant throughout a 40 min incubation. In contrast, the response to 10 µM VIP was initially much slower with cyclic AMP accumulation after 5 min being approximately 50% of that observed with 100 µM dopamine. However, following a 40 min incubation, the VIP-induced accumulation of cyclic AMP appeared to surpass that induced by 10 µM dopamine. Although these data may reflect the presence of different dopamine- and VIP-stimulated adenylate cyclase mechanisms in the retina, possible access problems associated with the larger VIP molecule cannot be overlooked.

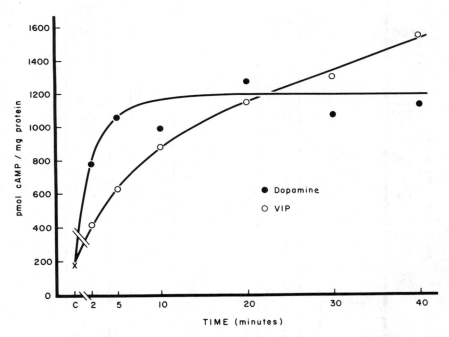

Fig. 7.   Effects of time on dopamine-stimulated (100 µM) and VIP-stimulated (10 µM) accumulation of cyclic AMP in pieces of intact retina. Each retinal piece received a 5 min preincubation in carp Ringer's containing 2mM IBMX followed by an incubation for a varying period of time in Ringer's containing 2mM IBMX plus test substance. The control value represents the accumulation of cyclic AMP following a 10 min incubation in the absence of test substance. Results are expressed as pmol cyclic AMP/mg protein. Each point is the mean of two experiments involving triplicate determinations.

These results clearly indicated that VIP is capable of
stimulating cyclic AMP accumulation in the teleost retina, but did
not discount the possibility that VIP was activating dopamine
receptors linked to adenylate cyclase or that the effects of VIP
may involve the release of endogenous stores of dopamine. These
hypotheses were investigated by examining the effects of the dopaminergic antagonist, haloperidol on the increase in cyclic AMP
production induced by either 100 μM dopamine or 10 μM VIP (Fig. 8).

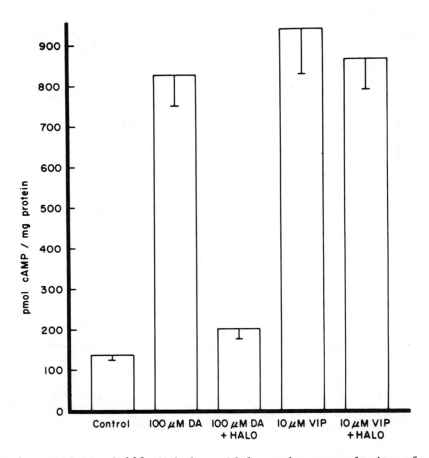

Fig. 8.   Effect of 100 μM haloperidol on the accumulation of
           cyclic AMP in pieces of intact retina induced by either
           100 μM dopamine or 10 μM VIP. Results are expressed as
           pmol cyclic AMP/mg protein. Each histogram represents
           the mean of 4-6 experiments involving triplicate
           determinations and is given with the S.E.M.

As in previous experiments, 100 µM haloperidol, added to the retina
during the 5 min preincubation period, almost completely abolished
the response to 100 µM dopamine. On the other hand, 100 µM haloperidol had no effect on the response to 10 µM VIP. These data indicate that the teleost retina possesses pharmacologically distinct
dopamine-sensitive and VIP-sensitive adenylate cyclase systems.

CELLULAR LOCALISATION OF VIP-STIMULATED CYCLIC AMP ACCUMULATION

        Having established the presence of separate dopamine-sensitive
and VIP-sensitive adenylate cylcases in the teleost retina, the
question arises as to whether these systems are also located in
separate populations of retinal neurones. Experiments performed
with pieces of intact retina suggested that this is not the case.
Figure 9 illustrates the results of experiments where both 10 µM
VIP and 100 µM dopamine were added to the retina simultaneously.

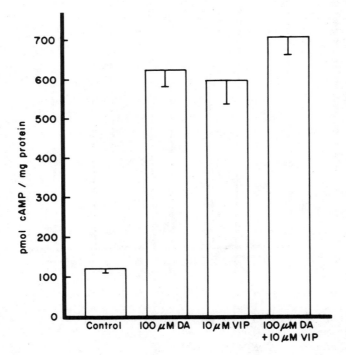

Fig. 9.   Effect of 100 µM dopamine and 10 µM VIP, alone or in
            combination, on cyclic AMP accumulation in pieces of
            intact carp retina. Results are expressed as pmol cyclic
            AMP/mg protein. Each histogram represents the mean of
            6-8 experiments involving triplicate determinations and
            is given with the S.E.M.

It can be seen that the resulting response is no greater than the
individual responses obtained with either 100 μM dopamine or 10 μM
VIP alone. If dopamine and VIP are stimulating separate populations of adenylate cyclase, an additive response would be expected
when these two agents are added together. As such, the lack of
additivity indicates that both VIP- and dopamine-stimulated adenylate cyclase activity may reside within the same population of
retinal neurones.

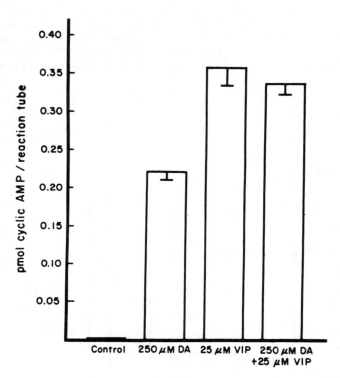

Fig. 10.   Effect of approximately 250 μM dopamine and 25 μM VIP,
           alone or in combination, on cyclic AMP accumulation in
           fractions of isolated carp horizontal cells.   Each
           fraction received a 5 min preincubation in carp Ringer's
           containing 2mM IBMX followed by a 10 min incubation in
           carp Ringer's containing 2mM IBMX plus test substance(s).
           Results are expressed as pmol cyclic AMP produced/
           reaction tube.   In the absence of added dopamine or VIP,
           cyclic AMP levels were below the level of detection.
           Each histogram is the mean of four experiments involving
           triplicate determinations and is given with the S.E.M.

We have been able to test this hypothesis more directly by examining the effects of VIP on cyclic AMP accumulation in fractions of isolated horizontal cells. The results illustrated in Fig. 10 indicate that VIP, like dopamine, can stimulate cyclic AMP production in preparations of horizontal cells. Furthermore, the effects of VIP and dopamine are not additive. These data argue strongly that not only are the VIP-sensitive and dopamine-sensitive adenylate cyclase systems present within the same population of retinal neurones in this species, but that they are also present on the same, rather than different, populations of horizontal cells.

COMMENTS AND DISCUSSION

We have identified an adenylate cyclase system, sensitive to dopamine, in both homogenates and intact pieces of the teleost retina (Watling et al., 1980; Watling and Dowling, 1981; Dowling and Watling, 1981). However, these data do not provide evidence as to the cellular localisation of this response, or whether it represents a pre- or postsynaptic event. Using techniques involving the enzymatic dissociation of the teleost retina and the subsequent separation and isolation of fractions of particular retinal cell types, we have been able to demonstrate the presence of a postsynaptic dopamine-dependent adenylate cyclase system in horizontal cells. As to whether such a system also resides in bipolar and amacrine cells and/or on the presynaptic dopaminergic terminals is for future work to determine.

The response to dopamine in the isolated horizontal cells displays similar characteristics to that observed in intact pieces of retina. For example, a similar range of dopamine concentrations (1-300 μM) is required to stimulate cyclic AMP accumulation in both isolated cells and intact pieces of retina. In contrast, we have previously shown that dopamine is effective over a lower range of concentrations (0.1-30 μM) in broken cell preparations (Watling and Dowling, 1981). In addition, the accumulation of cyclic AMP observed in either pieces of intact retina or intact horizontal cells requires the presence of a phosphodiesterase inhibitor, namely 2mM IBMX. This result is important as it suggests that in the intact functioning retina, dopamine probably induces only a very transient increase in cyclic AMP levels within the horizontal cells. The loss of the dopamine response when the isolated horizontal cells are homogenised almost certainly relates to the dilution of endogenous ATP levels. It should be remembered that 1mM ATP is routinely added to the incubation mixture when investigating dopamine-sensitive adenylate cyclase activity in homogenates (Watling and Dowling, 1981).

In contrast to the results obtained in intact pieces of retina, 45 mM K^+ ions failed to raise cyclic AMP levels in

preparations of isolated horizontal cells. Having previously
attributed the K^+ ion response to its ability to release endogenous
presynaptic dopamine stores, the lack of an effect in the isolated
cells may be explained by the absence of presynaptic terminals
associated with these cells. Histological examination confirmed
that there are no presynaptic terminals impinging on these
neurones.

The increased potency of several dopamine antagonists at
inhibiting dopamine-induced cyclic AMP production in the isolated
horizontal cells represents a major anomaly as compared to data
previously obtained in the intact or homogenized retina. For
example, whereas in retinal homogenates micromolar concentrations
of the butyrophenone derivative haloperidol are required to inhibit
the dopamine response; in the isolated horizontal cells a
concentration of 1nM haloperidol produces an approximate 50%
inhibition of dopamine-stimulated cyclic AMP accumulation.
Although the possibility exists that the trypsin treatment of the
retina may be modifying the dopamine receptors associated with
adenylate cyclase, we have encountered no such increased
sensitivity to antagonists in retinal homogenates treated with
trypsin. The increased potency of antagonists in the intact cells
is particularly interesting in view of recent attempts to classify
dopamine receptors into various sub-types (Seeman, 1981). It is
generally believed that dopamine receptors possessing a nanomolar
affinity for various butyrophenone dopaminergic antagonists, as
identified by radioligand binding studies (Burt et al., 1975;
Fields et al., 1977) constitute a subclass of dopamine receptors
which are not associated with adenylate cyclase. These receptors
have been designated D2 receptors, as opposed to dopamine receptors
which are associated with adenylate cyclase and are referred to as
Dl receptors (Kebabian and Calne, 1979). As such the isolated
horizontal cells may prove to be an interesting system in which to
pursue the concept of multiple dopamine receptors, in addition to
furthering our understanding of how dopamine-induced increases in
intracellular levels of cyclic AMP contribute to the physiological
response to dopamine.

The observation that VIP will also stimulate cyclic AMP
accumulation in the teleost retina raises the question as to
whether this neuropeptide may be acting as a neurotransmitter in
this tissue. Unfortunately, this contention is not supported by
any published reports indicating the presence of VIP in the teleost
retina, although VIP-immunoreactive neurones have been localised to
a population of amacrine cells in the rat retina (Lorén et al.,
1980), and are believed to be present in the retinae of the rat,
cat, rabbit and mudpuppy (Brecha - personal communication). VIP-
immunoreactive neurones have been identified in the teleost
peripheral nervous system where they have been observed in some
nerve fibres of the principle pancreatic islet and surrounding
tissues, the vagus and splanchnic nerves, the coeliac ganglion and

the walls of the intestine (Van Noorden and Patent, 1980) and an investigation of their presence in the teleost retina is currently in progress.

In an attempt to test for the possible presence of VIP in the teleost retina, we have reexamined the accumulation of cyclic AMP induced by 45mM K^+ ions in pieces of intact carp retina, and have investigated the presence of a non-haloperidol blockable component. We previously found that 100 µM haloperidol 'almost completely' inhibited the accumulation of cyclic AMP induced by 45 mM K^+ ions (Dowling and Watling, 1981). That is, cyclic AMP levels in the presence of 45 mM K^+ ions and 100 µM haloperidol were essentially similar to those observed in the absence of any added test agent. However, the results of recent experiments detailed in Table 1 indicate that 100 µM haloperidol alone causes a significant reduction in cyclic AMP accumulation with respect to control levels (P = ≤0.001 - one tailed, two sample t-test).

Table 1. Effects of haloperidol on control, dopamine-stimulated and K^+ ion-stimulated accumulation of cyclic AMP in pieces of intact carp retina. Retinal pieces were preincubated for 5 min in the presence of carp Ringer's containing 2 mM IBMX, with or without 100 µM haloperidol, followed by an additional 10 min in Ringer's containing 2mM IBMX plus either 3 µM dopamine, 45 mM K^+ ions or no test substance. Results are expressed as pmol cyclic AMP /mg protein and are given as the mean ± S.E.M. Numbers in parenthesis represent the number of experiments.

Additions	pmol cyclic AMP/mg protein	
None	151.6 ± 6.1	(20)
Haloperidol (100 µM)	116.4 ± 5.0	(16)
Dopamine (3 µM)	668.0 ± 92.7	(8)
Dopamine (3 µM) + Haloperidol (100 µM)	100.4 ± 7.8	(8)
K^+ ions (45 mM)	674.7 ± 58.4	(8)
K^+ ions (45 mM) + Haloperidol (100 µM)	166.2 ± 11.0	(20)

See text for further details and statistical analysis.

This result presumably reflects an antagonism of cyclic AMP
accumulation induced by endogenous dopamine present in the
retina. In addition, the response to exogenously applied 3 μM
dopamine is totally blocked by preincubation of the retina with
100 μM haloperidol, and as might be predicted, cyclic AMP levels
are reduced to those observed in the presence of 100 μM haloperidol
alone. However, the recent experiments indicate that 100 μM
haloperidol fails to completely antagonise the cyclic AMP
accumulation induced by 45 mM K^+ ions, and as such cyclic AMP
levels observed in the presence of 45 mM K^+ ions and 100 μM
haloperidol are significantly different from those seen with 100 μM
haloperidol alone (p = <0.001 – one tailed, two sample t-test).
The data suggest about 10% of the K^+ response can not be accounted
for by the release of endogenous dopamine. Whilst we have no way
of proving the hypothesis, it is tempting to speculate that the
small non-haloperidol blockable component of the response to 45 mM
K^+ ions may be due to the release of endogenous stores of VIP.

The ability of VIP to stimulate cyclic AMP accumulation in
isolated horizontal cells suggests two possible locations for VIP
in the teleost retina based on the cell types known to make
synaptic connections with the horizontal cells. Both the
photoreceptors and the dopamine-containing interplexiform cells
thus emerge as possible candidates for the localisation of VIP in
the teleost retina. Furthermore, the latter alternative also
raises the possibility of the co-existence of neurotransmitters in
the same retinal neurone, a phenomenum so far not reported in the
retina of any species. Finally, the presence of both VIP-sensitive
and dopamine-sensitive adenylate cyclase systems on the horizontal
cells raises the question as to how different physiological
responses to these neurotransmitters might be mediated since both
systems appear to reside on the same postsynaptic cell.

ACKNOWLEDGEMENT

K.J. Watling gratefully acknowledges the receipt of a
Travelling Fellowship from the Medical Research Council, England.
The authors also acknowledge the excellent technical assistance of
B. Saxon. This work was supported by grants from the National
Institutes of Health (EY-00811 and EY-00824).

REFERENCES

Brecha, N., Karten, H.J. and Laverack, C., 1979, Enkephalin-
    containing amacrine cells in the avian retina:
    Immunohistochemical localisation, Proc. Natl. Acad. Sci. USA.,
    76: 3010-3014.

Brown, B.L., Ekins, R.P. and Albano, J.M.D., 1972, Saturation assay
    for cyclic AMP using endogenous binding protein, in: 'Advances
    in Cyclic Nucleotide Research'. pp. 25-40, P. Greengard and
    G.A. Robison, eds., Raven Press, New York.

Brown, B.L. and Makman, M.H., 1972, Stimulation by dopamine of
    adenylate cyclase in retinal homogenates and of adenosine
    3',5'-cyclic monophosphate formation in intact retina, Proc.
    Natl. Acad. Sci. USA., 69: 539-543.

Burt, D.R., Creese, I. and Snyder, S.H., 1976, Properties of [^{3}H]
    haloperidol and [^{3}H] dopamine binding associated with dopamine
    receptors in calf brain membranes, Mol. Pharmacol., 12: 800-
    812.

Clement-Cormier, Y., Kebabian, J.W., Petzold, G.L. and Greengard,
    P., 1974, Dopamine-sensitive adenylate cyclase in mammalian
    brain. A possible site of action of antipsychotic drugs,
    Proc. Natl. Acad. Sci. USA., 71: 1113-1117.

Daly, J.W., 1977, 'Cyclic Nucleotides in the Nervous System',
    Plenum Press, New York.

Dick, E. and Miller, R.F., 1981, Peptides influence retinal
    ganglion cell, Neurosci. Letts., (In press).

Djamgoz, M.B.A., Stell, W.K., Chin, C.-A. and Lam, D.M.K., 1981, An
    opiate system in the goldfish retina, Nature, 292: 620-623.

Dowling, J.E. and Ehinger, B., 1978, The interplexiform cell
    system. I. Synapses of the dopaminergic neurons of the
    goldfish retina, Proc. R. Soc. Lond. B., 201: 7-26.

Dowling, J.E. and Watling, K.J., 1981, Dopaminergic mechanisms in
    the teleost retina. II. Factors affecting the accumulation of
    cyclic AMP in pieces of intact carp retina, J. Neurochem., 36:
    569-579.

Fields, J.Z., Reisine, T.D. and Yamamura, H.I., 1977, Biochemical
    demonstration of dopaminergic receptors in rat and human brain
    using ^{3}H-spiroperidol, Brain Res., 136: 578-584.

Glickman, R.D., Adolph, A.R. and Dowling, J.E., 1981, Inner
    plexiform circuits in the carp retina: Effects of cholinergic
    agonists, GABA and substance P on the ganglion cells, Brain
    Res., (In press).

Greengard, P., 1976, Possible role for cyclic nucleotides and
    phosphorylated membrane proteins in postsynaptic actions of
    neurotransmitters, Nature, 160: 101-107.

Greengard, P., 1978, 'Cyclic Nucleotides, Phosphyorylated Proteins and Neuronal Function,' Raven Press, New York.

Harper, J.F. and Brooker, G., 1965, Femtomole sensitive radioimmunoassay for cyclic AMP and cyclic GMP after 2'0 acetylation by acetic anhydride in aqueous solution, J. Cyclic Nucleotide Res., 1: 207-218.

Hedden, W.L. and Dowling, J.E., 1978, The interplexiform cell system. II. Effects of dopamine on goldfish retinal neurones, Proc. R. Soc. Lond. B., 201: 27-55.

Hegstrand, L.R., Kanof, P.D. and Greengard, P., 1976, Histamine-sensitive adenylate cyclase in mammalian brain, Nature, 260: 163-165.

Iversen, L.L., 1975, Dopamine receptors in the brain, Science, 188: 1084-1089.

Karten, H.J. and Brecha, N., 1980, Localisation of substance P immunoreactivity in amacrine cells of the retina, Nature, 283: 87-88.

Kebabian, J.W. and Calne, D.B., 1979, Multiple receptors for dopamine, Nature, 277: 93-96.

Kebabian, J.W. Petzold, G.L. and Greengard, P., 1972, Dopamine-sensitive adenylate cyclase in the caudate nucleus of the rat brain and its similarity to the 'dopamine receptor', Proc. Natl. Acad. Sci. USA., 69: 2145-2149.

Krisch, B. and Leonhardt, H., 1979, Demonstration of somatostatin-like activity in cells of the retina, Cell Tissue Res., 204: 127-140.

Longshore, M.A. and Makman, M.H., 1981, Stimulation of retinal adenylate cyclase by vasoactive intestinal peptide (VIP), Eur. J. Pharmacol., 70: 237-240.

Lorén, Il, Tornqvist, K. and Alumets, J., 1980, VIP (vasoactive intestinal polypeptide)-immunoreactive neurons in the retina of the rat, Cell Tissue Res., 210: 167-170.

Lowry, O.H., Rosenbrough, N.J., Farr, A.L. and Randall, R.J., 1951, Protein measurement with the Folin phenol reagent, J. Biol. Chem., 193: 265-275.

Quik, M., Iversen, L.L. and Bloom, S.R., 1978, Effect of vasoactive intestinal peptide (VIP) and other peptides on cAMP accumulation in rat brain, Biochem. Pharmacol., 27: 2209-2213.

Sarthy, P.J. and Lam, D.M.K., 1978, Biochemical studies of isolated glial (müller) cells from the turtle retina, J. Cell Biology, 78: 675-684.

Sarthy, P.J. and Lam, D.M.K., 1979, Endogenous levels of neurotransmitter candidates in photoreceptor cells of the turtle retina, J. Neurochem., 32: 455-461.

Schorderet, M., 1977, Pharmacological characterisation of the dopamine mediated accumulation of cyclic AMP in intact retina of rabbit, Life Sci., 20: 1741-1748.

Schorderet, M., Sovilla, J.-Y. and Magistretti, P.J., 1981, VIP- and glucagon induced formation of cyclic AMP in intact retinae in vitro, Eur. J. Pharmacol., 71: 131-133.

Seeman, P., 1981, Brain dopamine receptors, Pharmacol. Rev., 32: 229-313.

Van Buskirk, R.G. and Dowling, J.E., 1981, Isolated horizontal cells from the carp retina demonstrate dopamine-dependent cyclic AMP accumulation, Proc. Natl. Acad. Sci. USA., (In press).

Van Noorden, S. and Patent, G.J., 1980, Vasoactive intestinal polypeptide-like immunoreactivity in nerves of the pancreatic islet of the teleost fish, Gillichthys mirabilis, Cell Tissue Res., 212: 139-146.

Von Hungen, K., and Roberts, S., 1973, Adenylate cyclase receptors for adrenergic neurotransmitters in rat cerebral cortex, Eur. J. Biochem., 36: 391-401.

Watling, K.J. and Dowling, J.E., 1981, Dopaminergic mechanisms in the teleost retina. I. Dopamine-sensitive adenylate cyclase in homogenates of carp retina; effects of agonists, antagonists and ergots, J. Neurochem., 36: 559-568.

Watling, K.J., Dowling, J.E. and Iversen, L.L., 1980, Dopaminergic mechanisms in the carp retina: Effects of dopamine, K^+ and light on cyclic AMP synthesis, in: 'Neurochemistry of the Retina', pp. 519-537, N. Bazan and R. Lolley, eds., Pergamon Press, Oxford.

Wu, S. and Dowling, J.E., 1978, L-Aspartate: Evidence for a role in cone photoreceptor synaptic transmission in the carp retina, Proc. Natl. Acad. Sci. USA., 75: 5205-5209.